ANIMAL SANITATION AND DISEASE CONTROL

by

R. R. DYKSTRA
Dean Emeritus, School of Veterinary Medicine,
Kansas State University

THE INTERSTATE
Printers & Publishers, Inc.
Danville, Illinois

PREFACE

In the preparation of the subject matter for this book two thoughts have animated the writer:

First, to impress the young mind with the importance of adequate veterinary service, and the role that the veterinarian has played in conserving America's immense livestock industry, as well as the favorable influence this has had upon human health and welfare. During many years of experience the writer has found it impossible to greatly influence the mature mind in its preconceived erroneous notions of the veterinarian and veterinary service. It is hoped, therefore, that young people with open minds will study this book.

Second, to lay a genuine foundation for the prevention of animal ailments. It is the writer's impression that many of these are at least controllable if care, based on established principles, is followed.

The thought farthest from the writer's mind has been to provide a text for the treatment of animal ailments by those lacking formal professional veterinary training. The disease problem is far too complex for anything of this nature to be attempted and, therefore, the matter of treatment has been purposely avoided; the employment of the skilled veterinarian has been emphasized.

This book is for the teacher, the student, the sanitarian, and for all those interested in conserving livestock health.

R. R. DYKSTRA.

TABLE OF CONTENTS

PART ONE

Some Animal Health Factors

CHAPTER I

Ill-health a serious drain on the livestock industry. Disease more easily spread. Prevention and control of disease more important than cure. Some diseases may be controlled only by sanitation. Losses. Human welfare involved. Many sick animals point to a common cause. Horses relieved of some diseases because of the automobile.

CHAPTER II

The organs of digestion. The lips and their action. The teeth in the horse. Why the teeth need care. "Wolf" teeth. The teeth in cattle, sheep and goats. The dog and cat and their teeth. The tongue and cheeks and their function. The palates. The saliva and its uses. The pharynx as a cross-road. The oesophagus in domesticated animals. The stomach of the horse. Vomiting in animals. Ruminants or animals that "chew the cud." Ruminants (cattle, sheep, goats, etc.) not developed at birth. Origin of rumen organisms. Function of rumen organisms. Some effects of disturbed bacterial content in the rumen. Calf feeding on roughages. "Chew-the-cud." "Loss of cud." Hair balls and their nature. The gizzard in poultry. The intestines and their uses. The liver and pancreas.

CHAPTER III

Normal temperature range. Fever. Pulse rate. Breathing rate.

CHAPTER IV

Feeding practices. Animal "conditioners" and "tonics." Composition of foods. Sanitary feeding.

Greedy feeding and its prevention. Methods of feeding. Clean storage of feeds. The effect of sudden changes in the feed. Not enough food. Too much food. Protein and its value. Indigestible foods. The "essential" amino acids. An unknown growth factor. The role of APF. Protein for dairy cattle. Poor quality hay and alfalfa pellets. Diarrhoea and lack of protein in pigs. Properly heated garbage a safe feed. Temperature required and methods. Mechanical removal of harmful things. State law requirements. Other method of handling. So-called protein poisoning. Production feeding of swine. Flushing ewes. Feed for weanling colts. Feed and care of brood mares. Steers in dry lots. Replacements save milk for sale purposes. Method of feeding the "replacement." "Starters" in calf feeding. Milk substitutes for pigs? Sow furnishes heat and care. Must have water. Pigs weaned earlier. Sanitation essential in feeding pigs on substitutes. A unique system of swine sanitation. Operation is technical. Feed for the piglets. Natural selection of foods. Urea is a urine constituent. Digestive upsets due to urea. Increased carbohydrate is helpful. Indigestible feed made digestible. Urea is poisonous in the larger doses. Urea not a protein. Urea and bacteria. Value of antibiotics in weight gain of pigs. Method and results questioned. Do antibiotics cause more fat? Helps runty pigs. Effect on beef cattle.

CHAPTER V

Vitamins, Minerals and Hormones as
Health Requirements _____ 63

The vitamins. Vitamins stable and unstable. Vitamin A and sore eyes. Relative value of vitamin A and carotene. Night blindness in swine. Vitamin A deficiency in cattle. Vitamin B not stored in the body. Sore feet in chicks. Vitamin C and scurvy. Vitamin D and rickets. Vitamin E and fertility. Vitamin K not important in animals. Lack of vitamins. Vitamins and cottonseed meal "poisoning." The minerals. Salt aids in the functions of the body. Salt needed for gains. Adequate lime, phosphorus and sodium are essential. Deficiency of lime and wheat-plant "poisoning." Egg layers need lime. Phosphorus sources. Phosphorus needs. Fluorine danger. Phosphorus and egg laying. Prevention of rickets. Trace elements or minerals essential. Lack of iodine causes abnormal conditions. Iron and copper are essential. Manganese essential for reproduction in rats, mice, poultry and rabbits. Magnesia and spasms. Cobalt a part of vitamin B_{12} molecule. Coal slack—is it harmful? No superhealth possible. Urinary calculi (stones). Deficiency of some minerals a rare condition. Hormones and their nature. Effects of removal. The adrenals and activities. The thyroid and its action. Is thyroprotein harmful? Pineal function. The thymus a mystery gland. The hormone of the testicle. The ovary has two functions. There are three gonadotropins. Controlled breeding of swine. Hogs must be vigorous. Insulin and its function. Other hormone or hormone-like substances.

CHAPTER VI

The purpose of water in the body. Water from various sources. Intake must equal outflow. Pure water—what is it? Transmission of germs by means of water. Flowing waters. Classes of waters. Alkali or "hard" water. Salt water and the limit of tolerance for it. Warming water before it is consumed. No heated water for poultry. How to have water analyzed. Sterilizing water. Disinfecting water. Chlorination of water. Iodine as a water purifier. Water requirement. Higher production with enough watering.

CHAPTER VII

Why is housing necessary? Losses from lightning. Bad effects of housing. Location of buildings for animal occupancy. Some desirable features in buildings. Good lighting desirable. Size of living quarters. Larger stalls and more space for cattle. Chain-tie stanchions. Comfort stalls. Newly born calves die if too cold. Pens with raised floors. A "loose housing barn." Adequate space essential in loose housing. Bedding removal. Poultry houses need special features. Moisture from hens. Space for feeding and drinking equipment. Special features for animal houses. Gutters for cattle. Running water in the dairy barn. A special room as a milk house. Code requirements for the milk house. Dropping boards for poultry. Dropping pits a new feature. Electricity to stimulate egg production. Homemade electric brooders popular. Space and warmth for pigs. Temperature drops in new-born pigs. Space for hogs. Portable farrowing stalls. Feeding and watering space. Tying horses. Control of cattle. Ringing bulls. A guard rail to protect pigs.

CHAPTER VIII

The need for ventilation. The composition of air. Not enough oxygen. Impure air. Moisture in air and its effect. Moisture from the animal. Harmful gases in the air. Amount of air space needed. Heat and ventilation. Methods of ventilation. Average barn permits outside air to infiltrate.

PART TWO

Some Animal Disease Factors

cattle diseases. Preventable injuries to animals in transit result in large losses. Some causes of losses in transit. Means of preventing transit losses. The "carrier" of animal diseases.

PART THREE

Some Methods of Disease Control

CHAPTER XIII

PART FOUR

Infections and Their Handling

CHAPTER XIV

CHAPTER XV

sick animals. Disinfect clothing. Drinking water a source of danger. Contaminated feeds to be treated. Desirable qualities in disinfectants. How disinfectants exert their action. Carbolic acid not effective against viruses. Manure limits the action of disinfectants.

CHAPTER XVI

Dampen material before removal. Some germs are removed mechanically. Windowglass stops the germicidal action of sunlight passing through it. Heat, in a sufficient degree, is destructive to germs. Burning substances on germ-contaminated ground of some value. Cold slows germs. Filtered water is better. All life destroyed in time. Blood and gastric juice germicidal. Germs destructive to each other. Recent antibiotics.

CHAPTER XVII

Use only disinfectants of established value. The significance of the "phenol coefficient." Soap and its limitations. Lye effective against viruses. Lye valueless against tuberculosis. How to use lye as a disinfectant. Lime and its uses as a disinfectant. Whitewash for foot-and-mouth disease infection. Whitewash seals up cracks in wood and thus imprisons germs. A calcium salt or compound. A sodium salt or compound. Chlorinated lime a good source of the gas chlorine. Chlorinated lime without value against tuberculosis. A good household disinfectant. A method of disinfecting milking machines. How to make a wound disinfectant. A water of limited disinfectant value. An excellent deodorizer. Another chlorine preparation. Carbolic acid has many advantages. Some disadvantages of carbolic acid. Crude carbolic acid of uncertain strength, and therefore not reliable. Compound solution of cresol is one of the best all-round disinfectants. Cresol effective against viruses and tuberculosis. Cresol must be diluted with soft water. Formalin, which is a water solution of formaldehyde gas, has many valuable properties. Formalin is the best gaseous disinfectant by means of fumigation. A method of disinfecting a room. One method of disinfecting a hatchery house. How to disinfect poultry incubators. Some disadvantages of formaldehyde. Permanganate of potash not so effective clinically. It has one decided advantage in being non-irritating. It should not be used as a routine disinfectant of poultry drinking water. It stains. "Peroxide" rapidly loses strength. Peroxide is effective against fowl-pox virus. A very powerful disinfectant though having decided disadvantages. How to deal with accidental bichloride poisoning. The origin of iodine. Iodine is highly effective in the handling of many diseases. Iodoform is a valuable iodine-containing compound. Sulphuric acid is too dangerous for general use. Boric acid is very mild, but its presence controls germ growth. Vinegar is a good household disinfectant. A comparatively new disinfectant. Not equally effective against all bacteria. Sulfonamides are bacteriostatic. Questions bearing on the use of "sulfas." The invading germs destroyed by the blood. Chemotherapy and infections.

PART FIVE

Some Insecticides, Larvicides and Their Use on Premises and on Hosts

An infestant defined. The nature of repellents. Prevention of poultry lice. Pasture rotation to control ticks. Mechanical agencies to control insects. Building disinfestation. Insects controlled by D.D.T. D.D.T. not effective. Resistance to insecticides. D.D.T. not a repellent. A valuable characteristic. Surface effect on D.D.T. D.D.T. and whitewash. D.D.T. as a poison. D.D.T in an oil solvent dangerous. Use of D.D.T. in buildings. Not for dairy cattle. Ticks on sheep controlled by spraying. Dusting with D.D.T. for lice control. Commercial D.D.T. preparations. Precautions in the use of D.D.T. Physical properties of chlordane. Compared with D.D.T. Effective against animal parasites. Strong preparations kill sheep and goats. No offensive odor. Poisonous nature of chlordane. Not as poisonous as D.D.T. Musty odor objectionable. Highly effective against ticks, mites and lice. B.H.C. has a musty odor, but it's a good disinfectant. Sheep tick dipping. A purified B.H.C. A new "smear" for screw-worm control. Greater diffusion along wool fibers. Some more precautions. Carbon bisulphide a good disinfectant, though it must be kept away from heat and flame. A method of disinfecting grain. Hydrocyanic gas a deadly poison. Burning sulphur is an established method of disinfecting. Kerosene emulsion sprayed on roosts controls mites. Persian insect powder an excellent delouser. Methods of using Persian insect powder. Pyrethrum against stable flies on dairy cattle. Derris root a highly lauded new disinfectant. Derris for ticks on dogs and warbles on cattle. Louse powder. Dipping for sheep ticks. Best time to dip sheep. Fluoride of soda a favorite remedy to rid poultry of biting lice. Use in drinking water for humans. Highly chemical poisons no longer used. Spinose ear ticks in cattle controlled by means of pine tar. Benzene, not benzine, is destructive to screw-worm maggots. A screw-worm specific. Applying No. 62 to wounds. Coal-tar dips are useful against lice on cattle and horses. "Lime and sulphur" dip is a standard against mange mites. A dog wash to combat fleas and lice. Oily repellents on horses result in a loss of hair. A good fly repellent. A method of preventing "grubs in the head" in sheep.

PART SIX

Non-Infectious, Sporadic Ailments

tions are prolific sources of trouble in young animals. The prevention of navel infections. Loosening of the wool in sheep may be due to excessive moisture. Animals likely to consume hardware with their food; it frequently results in a serious heart ailment. Prevention. Mine-detector use for diagnosis. X-ray diagnosis. A magnet in the rumen or paunch to attract metals. Bloat is a frequent cause of death in several species of animals. Surface tension and bloat. The cause of a sudden cessation in the secretion of milk. It is important to know how to stop the milk secretion. Drying the ewe. How to guard against teat eversion. Other "vacuum" injuries. Small stalls and "spider" teat. Milk from the side of the teat. Green feed and off flavors. Upsets in digestion cause off flavors. Testing for rancidity. Why cream fails to rise. Some sweet curdling bacteria in the udder. A test for udder infection. Paralysis of the facial nerve is of frequent occurrence as a sequence of injury. Anatomy of sheath in boars and barrows. Feather plucking is a common vice in poultry. Cannibalism of poultry is quite easily prevented. For cannibalism and associated vices. Male turkeys injure the females. Protecting the hen with a canvas "saddle." Vent cleaning during mating. Bumble-foot in fowl is due to an infection and is preventable. Sows that eat their offspring need protein. Snake bites are common though in the larger animals the termination is seldom fatal. Electricity a danger to animals. A source of danger. A human disease.

CHAPTER XXII

Restraining cattle. Special methods of restraint. Casting cattle. Casting individuals. Disadvantages of the "half-hitch." An improved cattle-casting hitch. Death as a result of back or side recumbency. Lashing cattle against a board fence. Twitching the horse's nose. Casting a horse a major step. Boars snubbed to a post. How to prevent biting of wounds and "self sucking." A simple device. The ringing of bulls is necessary to control them as they are usually very vicious. The correct method of inserting a ring in a bull. Restricting free bulls. How to ring a hog. A good protein ration obviates the necessity of ringing hogs. How to prevent horn growth. The removal of new horn growth is described. The relation between the horn core and the frontal sinus. Instruments and dehorning. Sinus infection following dehorning. Method of weighting. The method of docking and castrating lambs. A new instrument for castrating and docking lambs. Still another method of castrating and docking. Tetanus may be a sequel of filthy methods of operating on lambs. Amputation of the wattles necessary to prevent infection. Claw and spur trimming prevents injury to the back of the female. Place needed brands only on the jaw, neck or shoulder. A sheep branding formula. Scouring fluids used. Location of the male process. When a male and when a female. Clipping wing feathers. The use of a brail. Division of a tendon. The wing-tip removal. Surgical caponizing. Feminizing by means of a hormone. Correction by the use of bad tasting drugs. By means of a jockey stick or cradle. By mechanical means. A dangerous device. Surgical steps. Not hereditary but a decided tendency in this direction.

Dental troubles rare in cattle. The effect of fluorine on the teeth of cattle. Dogs have dental ailments comparable to those in the human. Why bunches form following the castration of pigs, and their prevention. Actinomycosis occurs in various locations. A disease resembling actinomycosis in the soft tissues. Fistula of the withers, and poll-evil are serious infections. Hernia in pigs inherited and its control. Bleeding warts of cattle are contagious; they spoil many otherwise good hides. Blue bag of ewes is a contagious condition; its prevention is of the most importance. Eye-lid pigmentation and cancer. Extra teats may discharge milk. Why do cows leak from the teats? Cause of hard milking. When no milk can be drawn from the teat. How to remove warts from teats. Teat tampering dangerous.

Many poisonous plants. The control of many poisonous plants is one of general weed eradication. Cattle and sheep most susceptible, and horses and swine are almost entirely free from this form of poisoning. Sudan grass less than two feet high is dangerous. Stunted plants are dangerous. There are many tests for prussic acid content. Symptoms of prussic acid poisoning. Emergency treatment of prussic acid poisoning. What use to make of prussic acid containing plants. A method of crop management and growth to control prussic acid content in plants. Cockle-bur poisoning common in pigs. Prevention of cockle-bur poisoning. Oakleaf poisoning most frequently observed when other forms of vegetation are scarce. "Acorn calves." Seleniferous plants cause losses at times. "Alkali disease" a form of selenium poisoning. Preventing selenium poisoning. Loco-weed disease was formerly quite common in certain sections of the western U.S. Symptoms. Eating loco an acquired habit. Prevention of loco growth. An ailment due to poisonous plants. Seeds poisonous. Crotalaria may result in quick death. A very deadly plant. Animals do not like its odor. Occurs in wheat fields in the middle west. Animals with simple stomachs more susceptible. A test for this poison. Description of the bracken fern. The effect on cattle. A year-around poisonous plant. A water plant causes trouble. The plant does not thrive under competition. Oxalic acid the poison. The white snakeroot is responsible for "trembles" in cattle. Poisoning from cottonseed meal may be due to a poisonous principle or it may be caused by lack of vitamins. Sweet clover disease is due to a chemical poison; it causes easy bleeding. A test to determine whether sweet clover is harmful. Cornstalk disease of cattle has not been entirely solved. "Big-head" in sheep due to sensitization by a plant and sunshine. Moldy foods are unwholesome, not desirable. "Forage poisoning" is a general classification, and means that the animal is receiving something harmful with its food. Horses succumb to prolonged consumption of moldy corn. Prevention of moldy corn poisoning. A food poisoning caused by a germ. Loin disease of cattle a germ disease. Prevention of loin disease. A smut of rye and other grasses causes serious trouble at times. Vermin infested foods are not wholesome. The over-feeding of lambs on grain may result in a form of food poisoning. Laboratory diagnostic aid. Acute salt poisoning is not of common occurrence. Cattle dead from eating oat hay. Saltpeter the real cause. Marsh lands frequently have nitrates causing cattle abortion. Harmful substances to be removed. Symptoms in cattle. Chemical poisonings occur more frequently during recent years. A wood preservative and lubricating oil ingredient the cause. A disease of economic importance. Symptoms of X-disease. Source of the lead that causes poisoning of livestock. Chronic lead poisoning rare in animals. Orchard grass and grasshopper poisons cause losses. Sources of arsenic. Symptoms of arsenic poisoning not characteristic. An effective antidote for humans. Sheep poisoned by copper. Fluorine poisoning rare in animals. A chemical used to kill weeds. Known for a hundred years in England. The disease in America.

Chapter XXV

Soil conditions and deficiencies. Other factors in deficiency conditions. An ailment due to lack of soil contact, with subsequent iron and other mineral impoverished blood. Prevention by giving access to soil. A practical method of getting iron and copper to pigs and sows. Shivering of newly born pigs. Diseases due to a lack of iodine. This ailment is an avitaminosis. The handling of nutritional blindness. Pregnancy disease of ewes caused by a deficiency of carbohydrates in the ration. The prevention of pregnancy disease. Blood changes in wheat "poisoning." Similar symptoms produced experimentally. Paralysis in pigs due to a lime deficiency and an avitaminosis. Rickets in cattle a phosphorus deficiency. Irradiated yeast in calf meal as a preventive of rickets. An ailment due to a low intake of carbohydrate.

A test for "false milk fever." A new test for the detection of ketosis. Prevention of "false milk fever." Milk fever is a disease closely associated with calving. Prevention of milk fever. The early air treatment productive of unfavorable results. Modern treatment and nursing. "Crazy chick" disease prevented by the use of vitamin E. Curled toes due to riboflavin deficiency.

CHAPTER XXVI

An ailment observed in horses, accustomed to regular work after a day of rest on full feed. Prevention of azoturia. An ailment of lambs characterized by stiffness and thought to be the result of improper feeding of the ewe. Severe exercise a predisposing factor. Is there an incompatibility in the blood of the sire and dam? Blood reactions occur. Don't let colt have mare's milk for 48 hours after its birth. Jaundice and anemia when the bloods of parents are not compatible. A mysterious periodic eye ailment frequently erroneously associated with the phase of the moon. High temperatures, humidity, hard work, loss of salt and low water intake are contributing factors in causing this condition. An accumulation of chemical substances in the urinary organs. A change of feed recommended as a method of prevention. Swollen eyelids an important symptom. Fluid in many tissues.

PART SEVEN

Infectious and Communicable Ailments of Farm Animals

CHAPTER XXVII

A germ gains entrance to the soft tissues of the mouth and nose. Prevention is by sanitary methods. An ailment associated with insanitary corrals. Success in treatment depends upon clean surroundings. A serious dysentery of swine believed to be one of a so-called group of filth borne ailments; a lack of vitamins is said to be a predisposing cause. When hog cholera and "necro" appear simultaneously the situation is grave. A method of prevention. An ailment of calves resembling human diphtheria though it is not related. Sanitation a preventive. A brain disease; sheep circle. Recovered animals are carriers for many weeks. Urine of infected animals may contaminate human foods, etc. An infection gains entrance through the navel of foals; it results in a general poisoning. A method of disinfecting the navel. A highly infectious diarrhoea in calves occurring within a few days

after birth. Prevention after the most rigid sanitary
steps have been adopted. A method of feeding is
helpful in affected animals. Link's colostrum formula.
Other preventive steps. A new sanitary device for
the control of calf scours. One of the grave commonly
observed ailments of man and animals due to a wound
infection. The termination of the disease is frequently
a fatal one. Prevention consists in thorough disinfection of all wounds as shortly as possible after their
occurrence. A disease that is more and more becoming
a serious menace to human and animal welfare. No
workable method of prevention. Vaccination is the
best protection for the dog but it is not perfect. A
person bitten by a supposedly rabid animal should
have the attention of a physician. In cattle the disease
occurs when associated with swine. A frequently diagnosed disease of animals. The causative germ a
normal inhabitant of the respiratory tract. The
symptoms vary depending on the localization of the
ailment. Prevention is difficult and necessitates special precautions. An ailment affecting isolated groups
of cattle and believed to be due to a virus. Infection
persists. A widespread cattle ailment preventable by
vaccination. A complicating disease. An ailment that
will require additional research to clarify all phases
of it. The application of sanitary steps is a sound
preventive measure. Sleeping sickness assumed epizootic proportions during recent years. Annual vaccination a preventive. A later method of vaccination.
Other preventive steps. Bleeding and swelling the outstanding symptoms. Safe in high places, and during
daylight hours. A disease of mature sheep. Vaccines
not effective. Control the disease early. Dangerous
to man. Symptoms in man. A danger to humans.
Cattle and sheep are reservoirs of the infection.

CHAPTER XXVIII

Devitalizing factors make animals susceptible to this
infection. Preventive steps are of a sanitary nature.
A contagious ailment due to a fungus. A very serious
udder disease spread in various manners. Early
diagnosis of great importance. Methods of diagnosis.
Methods of control. How to clean an udder before
milking. Injuries to be avoided. An old disease that
still is a source of trouble; it is related to human
smallpox. Characterized by sores on the teats. Care
must be taken to prevent its spread. Spread by means
of the hog louse. A disease of young sheep. One of
the most serious of animal infections; humans also
susceptible. A blood test to diagnose the disease.
A new milk test for Brucella infection. The nature
of the ring test. Value of the ring test. Another
accurate test. Method of control. Calfhood vaccination
in the control of the ailment. Diseases and conditions
other than Bang's disease in which abortions are
observed. Undesirable to attempt to stop an impend-

ing birth. An ailment of swine usually manifesting itself by premature births. The swine ailment may be transmitted to cattle. Preventive measures. Man susceptible to what is primarily an animal ailment. Complicates the abortion problem in Bang's disease-free herds. Common in Europe now also in U. S. A deadly infection of warm blooded animals. Its spore lives permanently in contaminated soil. Symptoms in man. How to prepare tissues for shipment to a diagnostic laboratory. Vaccination of some value. An anthrax cure. A contagious disease of man and animals. Modes of contracting the ailment. Symptoms differ depending upon the center of localization of the infection. Methods of diagnosis. The tuberculin tests. The control of tuberculosis rests upon the destruction of the tuberculous animals. Vaccination not successful. The use of meat derived from tuberculous animals for human consumption. A false tuberculosis of cattle. Symptoms of Johne's disease. A test for Johne's disease. The control of Johne's disease has not been entirely encouraging. A common eye ailment of cattle. Most prevalent in animals subjected to bright summer light. A plague of cloven-footed animals that has repeatedly made its appearance in the United States, and that has as frequently been stamped out. Humans also susceptible. Must be distinguished from foot-and-mouth disease. Clinical symptoms of vesicular exanthema. Shipping regulations. A disease most common in young horses and mules. An ailment of horses that usually makes its appearance wherever large numbers of these animals are brought together. A strange form of disease-spread and development. The disease usually of short duration. A highly contagious disease of swine only. Means of spread. A method of diagnosis when in doubt. Death rate very high. The disease is preventable by a highly efficient form of vaccination. A lately developed effective vaccine. Sanitary steps to hold the disease in check. A disease of swine—man also is susceptible—that is assuming greater importance. A laboratory test may be necessary to establish the diagnosis. A method of protection by immunization. Penicillin in swine erysipelas. Due to an unknown infection. One of the animal "national defense" diseases. A "Defense Against Animal Diseases" entity.

PART EIGHT

Some Infectious and Communicable Ailments of Barnyard Fowl

Chapter XXIX

A thorough understanding of basic sanitary principles essential to the control of poultry ailments. The right soil important. Limited shade desirable. Small portable brooder houses are recommended. Poultry netting to keep birds away from droppings boards. Wet foods should be kept cleaned up. Danger in the promiscuous use of feed bags. Sanitary drinking arrangements. A frequent change of range desirable. Remove old disease-carriers before young susceptible stock is added to old flocks. Keep newly acquired birds in quarantine. A wide spread disease of poultry. Poultry tuberculosis transmissible to swine. May occasion a reaction in contaminated cattle. The disease in poultry not transmitted through the egg. Symptoms uncertain. The best means of diagnosis is by an autopsy. A tuberculin test for flock diagnosis. Control not entirely satisfactory. The best approved clean-up plan. A highly contagious disease of the preliminary respiratory organs affecting chickens of all ages. Recovered birds are carriers. Symptoms are those of difficult breathing. Sanitary steps are not entirely satisfactory. Vaccination is successful, though dangerous in the hands of those that are technically untrained. A respiratory disease in chicks less than three weeks of age. Difficult to distinguish between respiratory ailments. No form of immunizing in areas that are free from this disease. An ailment of chickens characterized by inability to control the action of the legs and wings. Sometimes the ailment settles in the eyes. Occasionally there are large tumor-like masses involving various organs. Until more information is available sanitary measures offer the best means of control. A highly contagious disease of poultry—not communicable to mammals. Recovered birds are immune to future attacks. Vaccinate before the third and fourth months. Methods of vaccination. Danger in improper vaccination. A very virulent disease of barnyard fowl. The ailment appears very suddenly. Sanitation offers most for the control of the ailment. All barnyard fowl with the exception of water-fowl are susceptible. Sanitary measures most successful in the attempts at control. A form of food poisoning in poultry. Early symptoms of paralysis observed. Prevention by withholding contaminated foods. A highly fatal diarrhoea of young chicks. Mature birds are the source of the ailment, and the blood test should be used for its detection. Control rests in sanitation. A serious threat to the fowl industry in the U.S. A new safe vaccine. Handle as if contagious. A differential diagnosis important. Destroy ailing fowl. Symptoms of "vent gleet." Vigilance by sanitary authorities has kept this disease out of the United States. One of the "Animal Defense" ailments. A spreading disease.

PART NINE

Parasites and Disease

A livestock disease caused by a leaf-shaped parasite; it is found in swampy places. The parasite destroys the liver tissue, and unthriftiness ensues. Prevention. Prevention of tapeworm infestation in meat eaters is on a rational basis. Intermediate hosts necessary for tapeworm development. Prevention of tapeworm infestation. A diagnosis based on the passage of segments. Poultry acquire tapeworms by eating intermediate hosts such as flies, beetles, snails and others. This parasite is present wherever swine are raised. When the parasite finally lodges in the intestines it has already inflicted much damage. The McLean County system of prevention also controls other filth borne diseases of swine. Effective medication not always satisfactory. Life cycle of the thorn-headed worm. Damage of the larvae of the kidney worm. Kidney worm symptoms. Prevention of kidney worms. Lungworms of hogs are acquired following the eating of infested earthworms. Prevention not entirely satisfactory; in general, it consists in keeping hogs from areas where earthworms abound. The trichina worm is of importance because of the possibility of its transmission to man through the eating of insufficiently cooked pork. Man must be certain that pork products are well cooked before eating. A very serious worm disease of sheep. A very common parasite of sheep. The effects of stomach-worm infestation. Horses and swine may graze on sheep pastures. Separate pastures for young and old sheep. A parasitecide for several sheep worms. Phenothiazine and its properties. Round worms of poultry are commonest in the younger members of a flock. A method of prevention. Gapeworms of fowl lodge in the windpipe. A home treatment. The cecal worm is important because it transmits the cause of black-head in turkeys. A worm under the gizzard lining.

The battle for supremacy between man and insects. The housefly is a filthy transmitter of disease. A biting blood sucker. Stable fly a blood sucker. Methods of control. Another blood sucker. A large biting fly. Horse-fly control. Losses due to biting flies. The Tsetse fly not an American problem. Blow-flies usually deposit their eggs on dead animal tissue. True screwworms eat deeply into the tissues of the host, and may cause his death. A unique though biological method of control. The stomach bot of horses is responsible for large annual losses because it is responsible for loss of vigor in the host. When to medicate horses for the control of stomach bots. Grubs in the backs of cattle constitute a serious condition. The life history of the parasite. Economic loss is great. Prevention. Systemic insecticides. It is absorbed into the animal's tissue so as to kill the larva. Spraying with a systemic insecticide. Prevent screwworms in sheep. Grubs in the heads of sheep are a source of great annoyance. A practical method of prevention. Ticks are a menace to the livestock industry. A method of eradicating Southern Fever ticks by a system of pasture rotation. Importance of discovery of the role of the Southern Fever tick. A common infestant in the ears of animals. Practically impossible to control. Lice are very common on all domesticated animals. The life history of the mosquito. Mosquitoes bearers of many diseases. The distinguishing feature of fleas is that they do not remain continuously on the host. Mites are responsible for many animal ailments. A new skin mite of sheep.

CHAPTER XXXII

A bloody diarrhoea of cattle due to a small parasite. The parasite is readily spread. Prevention consists largely in sanitation. A micro-parasitic disease of poultry. The milk-flush to control coccidiosis in fowl. The feeding of sulphur may be harmful. Exposure and immunity as methods of prevention. A vaccine to protect chickens against coccidiosis. Handling in smaller flocks. Sanitary steps are effective. Blackhead of turkeys was formerly the major hazard in the raising of these birds. Keeping turkeys away from chickens is the best means of control. A unique surgical operation. Phenothiazine helpful though not a specific. A serious micro-parasitic disease of cattle. Detection of carriers a needed step. A simple test. Prevention only partly understood. Southern cattle fever for many years prevented the development of the cattle industry in the southern American states. Dipping and pasture rotation have practically stamped out the disease. A disease of the organs of reproduction of cattle. A final positive diagnosis depends on demonstrating the protozoa. Prevention and control. No known cure. A serious disease of poults. Sanitation as a preventive. A disease stamped out by sanitation. Is it a cause of disease?

PART TEN

Miscellaneous Information

CHAPTER XXXIII

The diagnosis of animal diseases is a complex problem. Laboratory aids are sometimes needed. During recent years blood tests are extensively employed in the diagnosis of animal diseases. The allergic tests are accurate, and much used. These are usually tests of last resort. Feeding tests may be applied by any intelligent person. An examination of abnormal tissues. Chemical tests are of great value in the diagnosis of animal ailments. Pregnancy tests have a limited value in animals. An examination made of the organs of a dead animal is a source of valuable information. A limited or partial post mortem examination is frequently all that is needed to establish a diagnosis. Skin parasites. Stool or fecal examinations. Rabies or dog madness. Poultry examinations. Help the laboratorian. Blood specimens. A photograph of very small objects.

CHAPTER XXXIV

Newly born orphaned animals need artificial feeding. Danger in over-feeding. Cleanliness is very important. The mother's first milk is believed to protect against infections. Substitutes for colostrum. Colts need their milk with sugar and lime water added. Cow's milk which is the natural food for calves is abundantly available, though it must be fed in limited amounts and in a clean manner. A foster mother should be provided. Lambs need milk rich in fat. Sweet whole cow's milk is satisfactory for pigs. Artificial foods for puppies should be rich in fat content.

CHAPTER XXXV

Care required in administering medicine. Channels for administering medicine. Giving medicine to a horse. Coughing on the part of the animal when medicine is given by way of the mouth is an indicator of trouble. Do not rub an animal's throat. Giving medicine to cattle. More than usual care must be taken in administering medicine to sheep. As individuals, hogs are difficult to medicate; medicine, in the hands of the amateur, is best given mixed with the food. Dogs must usually be forcibly restrained when being medicated. Cats because of having a small mouth are difficult to medicate. Medicating fowl is as a general rule not to be encouraged.

mon. Breeding unsoundness is serious. Hereditary
unsoundness is most serious. A blemish does not
interfere with usefulness of the animal. Bad habits
and vices reduce the animal's usefulness.

CHAPTER XXXIX

Financial investments in horse racing. Identification
by tattooing. Photographing the chestnuts. Some
drugs used. Tests to detect "dope." A federal offense.

CHAPTER XL

Actinomycosis or Actinobacillosis. Anthrax. Botulism.
Brucellosis. Bubonic plague. Asiatic cholera. Gas
gangrene. Glanders. Equine encephalomyelitis,
Equine encephalitis. Leptospirosis. Salmonellosis;
food infection. Swine erysipelas, diamond-skin disease.
Tetanus. Tuberculosis. Tularemia. Foot-and-mouth
disease. Psittacosis. Pox. Rabies.

PART ELEVEN

Livestock Sanitary Bureaus, Boards and Commissions, and the Veterinarian

CHAPTER XLI

A federal bureau that has demonstrated its usefulness. State veterinarians render an important
service.

CHAPTER XLII

The veterinarian is the keystone of the arch supporting livestock well-being in America. Veterinary vocations. The veterinarian an asset to a community.

PART ONE

Some Animal Health Factors

⚓⚓⚓⚓

CHAPTER I

INTRODUCTORY STATEMENT

Without question the most serious menace threatening the interests of the livestock, dairy and poultry producer is animal ill-health. This has been broadly

Ill-health a serious drain on the livestock industry
defined as any condition in which there is a deviation from health or normal functioning of any or all of the tissues and organs of the body. There are degrees of ill-health varying from a mild deviation of function in a comparatively unimportant part of the body to impairment of function of a vital organ of such a severe character as to result in quick and certain death of the affected animal. Furthermore, by far the greatest loss from ill-health is the result of those diseases that are due to a common, animal-to-animal transmissible cause. These are the infectious, contagious, and parasitic diseases—all theoretically controllable.

The constant problem of maintaining the health of livestock is causing federal and state agencies to expend enormous sums of money yearly in an effort to increase the knowledge of the causes of, and the methods of controlling and handling animal diseases. In the earlier days of this work the problem was a comparatively simple one, and many notable discoveries of far reaching importance were made. This was especially true in the decades immediately following Pasteur's contributions demonstrating bacteria as causes of disease, but as the simpler problems were solved, more complex and elusive ones presented themselves. The numbers of livestock increased enormously; the areas for rearing them were frequently diminished and thus became disease-contaminated in a concentrated

Disease more easily spread

form; there was much more traffic in livestock, animals frequently being shipped to extreme points, so that a single diseased animal served as a focus for starting disease in new areas. Also, methods of human transportation added to the problem because the bacterial cause of a disease making its appearance in one section of America might easily be carried through the agency of the airplane to a far distant point in twenty-four hours or less.

The result today is that though well in hand there must not be one moment of relaxation in the steps to conserve America's livestock from loss due to controllable diseases. Public agencies daily receive and answer many inquiries from teachers and students in vocational agricultural high schools, and from animal owners, about the deaths of animals and the control of disease. Those receiving these communications can not help being impressed by the general lack of knowledge about the fundamental principles of disease control.

Prevention and control of disease more important than cure

Though an animal owner is usually much more concerned in regard to the immediate pressing problem of saving the life of an already ailing animal, sanitarians everywhere are convinced that the far more important problem is the prevention, control and eradication of communicable diseases. During recent years there has been a good deal of changed thought and action in one important phase of animal disease prevention, the process of artificial immunization such as the vaccination of swine against hog-cholera—the use of virus is now prohibited in many states

—and cattle against blackleg. Many diseases, however, do not lend themselves to this form **Some diseases may be controlled only by sanitation** of protection, and this leaves sanitary methods as the only reasonably reliable safeguard against these enormous potential losses from actual death, as well as from those conditions where the animal recovers incompletely, or remains in a state of chronic illness, so that the economical production of meats, milk, wool, and eggs becomes impossible.

In order to have statistical information about animals, the following figures for the United States are presented:

Livestock on U. S. Farms
(in 000 head)

	Jan. 1, 1960	Jan. 1, 1955	Jan. 1, 1960	Jan. 1, 1960
			Total Value	Per Head
Horses and Mules.............	3,089	4,309	$ 347,689	$113.00
Cattle and Calves...........	96,236	96,592	13,149,813	210.00
(All cattle)				
Milk Cows............................	19,527	23,462	—	—
(Kept for milk)				
Sheep and Lambs................	33,170	31,582	545,684	16.50
Hogs......................................	59,026	50,474	1,091,896	18.50
Chickens	389,464	390,708	390,733	1.06
Turkeys.................................	5,633	4,917	27,547	4.89

All figures from U.S.D.A. Statistical Bul. No. 278.

The average per capita consumption of meat in the United States in 1960 was 89.5 lbs. of beef; 6.7 lbs. of veal; mutton and lamb, 4.3 lbs.; pork, excluding lard, 64.6 lbs.; turkey and chicken, 35.2 lbs.

Losses of livestock are impossible to determine accurately because there are no formal agencies engaged in collecting and compiling data. However, based on inventory numbers, births, sales, animals slaughtered, **Losses** and in shipments the final balance sheet tends to give a good estimate of losses from disease, predators, accident and other causes. Based on such an estimate the figures for 1959 include: Death losses of more than 1,452,000 cattle;

2,315,000 calves; 2,476,000 sheep; and 11,136,000 hogs and pigs. During the same period about 250,000,000 chickens and 72,000,000 turkeys died from disease and other causes. A rough financial estimate is a loss of more than one billion dollars from all causes, and death losses from parasites exceeded ½ million dollars.

The statistics cited give only a small estimate as compared to total losses from all sources, including inability of an ailing farm animal to work, to secrete milk, to lay eggs; failure to produce maximum amounts of wool, and mohair; and the production of reasonably good calf, pig, and lamb crops—all conditions that may be ascribed to malnutrition and ill-health. Only those actively engaged in the growing and raising of live-stock and the production of livestock products are thoroughly familiar with the bitter disappointments, financial reverses, and losses brought to them by their unthrifty, unhealthy animals. The hidden losses such as condemnations of meats, injured hides, edible offal, etc. when included in the total for the period 1942-51 represent six per cent of the potential agricultural production and about 15 per cent of the average annual value of farm marketings and home consumption of livestock and products. (1956 Yearbook, U.S.D.A.)

Also because many animal diseases are transmissible to humans (page 823) it is highly important to have an animal population free from diseases that
Human   may affect human well-being. One of the
welfare   more populous American states, through
involved   its department of health, indicates that
out of 65 reported diseases 23 were found to be intercommunicable between man and animals, or that have an animal reservoir. The diseases listed are actinomycosis, ankylostomiasis, anthrax, blastomycosis, botulim, cholera,* diphtheria,* amebic dysentery, bacillary dysentery,* equine encephalitis—horses are not reservoirs but birds are so that mosquitoes transmit the

---

*Frequently milk-borne.

infection from birds to horses and in horses the ailment is designated a "dead-end" condition, erysipelas, favus, glanders, infectious jaundice, paratyphoid B, psittacosis, rabies, ringworm, Rocky Mountain spotted fever, salmonella infections, scabies, scarlet fever,* streptococcic sore throat,* trichinosis, tuberculosis, tularemia, typhoid and undulant fever. Since foot-and-mouth disease is sometimes prevalent in America it is well to list it as a disease occasionally affecting man. Poliomyelitis (infantile paralysis) could possibly be conveyed through milk if its causative virus (this has been recovered from stools of infected persons and from sewage) should contaminate milk intended for human consumption. The foregoing facts indicate the significance of the close relationship existing between animal and human diseases.

Whenever several animals on the same farm become ill at about the same time, it is reasonably con-

Many sick animals point to a common cause clusive evidence that a common disease-producing factor has gained admission. This may be due to spoiled, contaminated, and improper food, or still more likely to a disease-producing agency in the form of parasites and bacteria. Care in using foods of a known wholesome character and the rigid exclusion of parasites and bacteria in so far as possible and practicable, or their destruction if they have gained admission, are logical steps in the control of animal ailments. Although not necessarily harmful, unwholesome foods are always to be viewed with suspicion.

On some of America's livestock farms, and notably on its most profitable fox and mink ranches, because these animals are very susceptible to disease due to extremely artificial conditions of living, there is practiced the most rigid form of food sanitation and exclusion of infection by the "no visitors allowed" rule. Another good illustration of the value of segregation and sanita-

---

*Frequently milk-borne.

tion as a step in disease prevention is afforded by the
enforced isolation of farm horses. Former-
Horses relieved of some diseases because of the automobile
ly these animals were frequently driven to
town, there to rub noses on the common
hitching post and thus contracting a variety of infectious and contagious diseases.
With the advent of the automobile, however, the horse remained at home, and
many of these diseases have almost disappeared. A
more general application of these practices would conserve the health and lives of many farm animals.

CHAPTER II

THE ANATOMY AND PHYSIOLOGY OF THE ORGANS OF DIGESTION IN ANIMALS

The utilization of foods by the animal, and the elimination of many of the waste products of digestion take place in a series of organs collectively known as the alimentary tract. Named in sequential order these organs are the mouth, pharynx, oesophagus, stomach, intestines, and anus.

The mouth includes the lips, teeth, tongue, and cheeks, and the closely related salivary glands. The pharynx is a vestibule succeeding the mouth from which it is separated by an incomplete curtain, the soft **The** palate, and continued by the oesophagus. **organs of** The pharynx may be called a vestibule be- **digestion** cause it is a cross-road, as it were, serving for the passage of both food and air, as well as maintaining intimate relations by means of the eustachian tube with the ear. The oesophagus is the tubular passageway leading from the pharynx to the stomach. The term gullet is often applied to it alone or in combination with the pharynx. The stomach serves for storage purposes and for partial preparation of aliment to be passed into the intestines. In the latter additional changes, mostly chemical, take place, as well as absorption of the separated digestible portion of the food and the onward passage of indigestible waste to be discharged through the anus.

The organs named in the preceding paragraphs differ somewhat in the various species of domesticated animals not only anatomically, but physiologically as well.

The lips, especially the upper one in the horse, serve the purpose of directing food between the teeth;

The lips and their action in cattle the tongue largely acts in this manner, and sheep perform this function by means of the tongue and incisor teeth, thus enabling them to graze very closely. The sheep, as distinguished from other domesticated animals, has a cleft upper lip, each segment being independently motile, though not prehensile. Goats, lacking only the cleft lip, otherwise guide the food into the mouth in a manner similar to sheep. Hogs in a state of nature first root up the ground with the snout and then get the food with the pointed lower lip which acts very much like a shovel. When not rooting, the tongue, incisor teeth and an upward movement of the head direct food into the mouth. All domesticated mammals, with the exception of the dog and cat, suck liquids with the mouth through the combined action of the lips and tongue. Dogs and cats lap liquids, using the tongue as a spoon for this purpose.

The teeth differ markedly in the various species of domesticated animals, especially in their mode of action due to anatomical peculiarities, and owing to the nature of the aliment.

The horse has six upper and six lower incisor teeth, and twelve upper and twelve lower (six in each arcade) molar or grinding teeth. All of the incisor **The teeth in the horse** teeth are said to be deciduous, which means that the permanent ones are preceded by temporary or milk teeth. In a state of health or normal conformation, the table surfaces of the corresponding upper and lower incisors should meet each other, the angle gradually increasing as the animal ages. Malformed mouths consist in too much forward extension, or backward regression of the lower jaw creating the so-called "undershot," and "overshot" jaws. Certainly horses with this conformation are at a decided disadvantage in the prehension and grazing of foods, and they are usually unthrifty, or they are known as "hard keepers." Though the abnormality cannot be obviated, its evil effects may

fect is that the outer borders of the table surfaces of each upper arcade project laterally beyond the corresponding borders of the lower arcades, and the inner borders of the table surfaces of each lower arcade extend medially beyond the corresponding borders of the uppers. The result is that the projecting borders are not subjected to grinding wear so that the outer edges of the uppers and the inner edges of the lowers soon become elongated and very sharp thus inflicting lacerations on the cheeks and tongue so that the proper mastication of food is seriously interfered with. In order to avoid these consequences, the teeth of horses must frequently be rasped so as to remove the sharp edges, but in doing this care must be taken not to smooth the normal and highly essential rough grinding surface of the teeth—the edges only being rasped.

Why the teeth need care

The male horse, rarely the female, has four additional teeth appearing one on each side of both upper and lower jaws about midway between the corner incisors and the first molars. These are the canine teeth. If they appear in the female they are comparatively small and rudimentary.

Furthermore, all horses have four more teeth that only occasionally come to the surface. The ancestors of the horse of today had seven molars in each arcade—all coming to the surface or erupting. As time progressed the anterior one of the seven in each arcade retrogressed or atrophied probably because of disuse, and finally seldom erupted, a condition that persists in the modern horse. There are then still seven molars in each arcade, though normally only six of these are erupted, the other remaining embedded under the gums. Only occasionally do these remnant teeth erupt. When they do appear it is just in front of and very closely related to the first molar in one or all of the four arcades. When erupted these remnant teeth constitute the so-called "wolf-teeth." They are generally, though erroneously, said

"Wolf" teeth

to be related to diseased eyes. If there is a diseased condition of the eyes, and if at a corresponding period there are "wolf-teeth" it is a coincidence and not because of any biological relationship between the two conditions. It is usually recommended, and rightfully so, that wolf-teeth be extracted because like all rudimentary organs they are weak and therefore more than ordinarily susceptible of becoming diseased so as to result in impaired mastication, and to an extent they interfere with the bit when the animal is bridled.

Cattle, sheep, and goats of the domesticated animals differ in several respects in their dentition from that of the horse. These animals have only eight incisors and all are placed in the lower jaw. The upper jaw has no incisors though there is a very firm dental pad. Cattle differ from sheep and goats in that the incisors are loosely or movably implanted in their sockets. This must not be mistaken for a diseased condition. There are no important practical differences in the molar teeth of these animals and those in the horse. Age may be determined up to somewhat over three years of age. The first pair of permanent incisors frequently erupt at 18 to 21 months of age; the next pair at 27 to 30 months; the third pair at about 36 months, with the fourth pair appearing shortly thereafter. At three years of age, or possibly a little older, there is a full mouth of incisors. This seems to hold true, generally for well-nourished beef and dairy breeds, though the incisor teeth of Brown-Swiss cattle appear at a somewhat older age.

The teeth in cattle, sheep, and goats

The dog has a total of forty-two teeth—twelve incisors, four canines, and twenty-six molars. Of the latter, twelve are fixed in the upper and fourteen in the lower arcades.

The cat has thirty teeth—twelve incisors, four canines, and fourteen molars,

The dog and cat and their teeth

eight of the latter being implanted in the upper jaw and six in the lower.

The tongue and cheeks assist in various ways in the masticatory process. Both of these organs are largely muscular and therefore an important function is to keep the food between the teeth and to aid in its backward movement.

The tongue and cheeks, and their function

The tongue consists of a fixed portion and a free portion. Its outer covering is a mucous membrane. On the upper surface of the tongue the mucous membrane is covered with numerous projections or papillae. Certain groups of these have specialized functions to retain sapid foods on the tongue, and to act both as tactile and gustatory organs. The tongue of cattle is distinguished by its great muscular development and extreme motility, so that its tip may readily be made to enter the nostrils, and the papillae on the mucous membrane which are directed backward and have a horny sheath so as to impart a very rough reaction when grasped.

The inner lining of the cheeks is also a mucous membrane. In cattle and sheep there are on the mucous membrane some very prominent, backward directed papillae extending from the corners of the mouth to the first molar tooth, and continued backward by a single row of papillae corresponding in direction to the border of the teeth. In sheep, black patches are common on the mucous membrane. These should not be mistaken for evidences of disease.

The tongue and cheeks are frequently the seat of conditions interfering with mastication. Awns of grasses become embedded here, and may even fester. Sharp teeth in horses lacerate the tongue and cheeks. In cattle the tongue is not uncommonly invaded by a germ, the so-called "ray fungus," which in the region of the jaws causes "lumpy jaw" (page 422), and in the tongue by a somewhat similar organism causing "wooden tongue."

The *hard and soft palates* form the roof of the mouth and the latter marks the anatomical dividing line between the mouth and the pharynx.

The palates The former has numerous transverse ridges which sometimes in the region immediately back of the upper incisor teeth in the horse become engorged with blood and so prominent as to project beyond the table surface of the teeth. This condition is colloquially designated "lampas." It is the result of repeated bruising incidental to the eating of hard grains and especially corn on the cob. Withholding the offending grains and substituting soft material usually correct the trouble. The crude practice of incising or even burning of these engorged tissues is cruel and because of the resulting bleeding may be decidedly harmful. The soft palate is in the nature of a flexible curtain that varies in length in the different domesticated animals. In the horse, for example, it is so long that when food and water have passed it, and then are regurgitated, it is done through the nose and not by way of the mouth, though in cattle the soft palate permits food from the paunch to be passed back into the mouth in the physiological process of "chewing the cud."

The salivary glands are important organs anatomically closely related to the mouth. All of them are paired. The parotid salivary gland is located back of the jaw beneath the ear, the mandibular in the space between the branches of the lower jaw, and the sublingual beneath the tongue. Those named are the largest and most important ones. They discharge the saliva into the mouth through excretory ducts with openings either in the cheek opposite the third molar tooth, or under the tongue. The amount of saliva secreted varies not only in different species but in individuals, depending on their size, and also as the nature of the food changes, dry aliment stimulating its flow. In horses during an hour of dry hay consumption, the amount varied from

The saliva and its uses

5000 to 8800 grams, and grass consumption stimulated only fifty per cent as much salivary secretion.

It has been determined that a horse in health on dry aliment may secrete as much as ten gallons of saliva in twenty-four hours, and cattle fourteen gallons under comparable conditions. The chemical composition of the saliva of the various named glands is not identical in all animals, and necessarily the reaction with the food varies. In general it may be said that the chief functions of the saliva are to lubricate the preliminary digestive tract, to ease the passage of food, to soften food and mechanically assist in its reduction to a less solid and more soluble form, and to convert the starches of the food into sugar.

The pharynx is the anatomical structure succeeding the mouth and separated from it by the soft palate.

The pharynx as a cross-road The degree of separation depends upon the development of the soft palate from an extreme length in the horse to no soft palate at all in poultry. It has been aptly stated that the pharynx is the cross-road in the animal's body. There are seven distinct openings into the pharynx, as follows: The opening from the mouth, two openings from the nasal cavities, two openings from the eustachian tubes, the opening from the larynx, and the opening from the oesophagus. This necessarily means that both food and air are almost continuously meeting each other and passing each other in the pharynx. Nature has placed there many safeguards to prevent misdirection of any of these substances. For example, when the opening into the oesophagus is open for the reception of food, the opening into the larynx automatically closes. If perchance a particle of food succeeds in passing the laryngeal safeguards, nature has made the interior of the larynx so very highly sensitive that violent expulsive efforts connected with coughing at once expel the invading substance. The same sort of protection is not present at the opening of the oesophagus, because an animal can inhale a good deal of air into its stomach, sometimes with the production of considerable bloating in the digestive tract. Whenever the pharynx becomes diseased because of mechanical influences, or inflammatory process as a sequence of colds especially, there is at once the gravest disturbance not only in the breathing, but in the swallowing of food as well.

The oesophagus is the tubular passageway extending from the mouth to the stomach. Measured outwardly in the horse it may be said to extend from the region of the throat to a point corresponding to the upper third of the sixteenth rib. At its origin the opening of the oesophagus is just above the opening in the larynx. It continues backward in this position for a short distance and then deviates to the left side of the trachea. It continues in the latter position until it is well within the chest, and there it again assumes a position above the trachea to enter the stomach after passing through the diaphragm. The oesophagus is lined by the usual mucous membrane, and to the outside of this, for all practical purposes, we may consider that there is a muscular coat.

The oesophagus in domesticated animals

In the horse, the half of the oesophagus succeeding its origin has voluntary muscle fibers, the lower half of the oesophagus consisting of involuntary muscle fibers. In cattle, sheep, swine, and other domesticated animals the entire muscular coat of the oesophagus is of a voluntary character. This means, then, that in the horse, once food has progressed beyond the first half of the oesophagus, it is beyond the animal's control, though in other animals it may almost be forced back into the mouth at will. Though the oesophagus is a tubular passageway, it differs considerably anatomically in regard to its caliber. In the horse, for example, and in a measure because of its relationship to other organs, the oesophagus is constricted at its origin, again at the point where it enters the chest, and finally just before its passage through the diaphragm. In cattle, swine, and dogs, the oesophagus is dilated at its origin, that is, somewhat funnel-shaped, and again at its entrance into the stomach. In poultry, the oesophagus is capable of enormous dilatation throughout its entire extent.

These anatomical peculiarities in the caliber of the oesophagus are in a measure responsible at times for difficulties in deglutition. The horse, for example, is occasionally greedy and attempts to swallow too rapidly, so that aliment is not properly moistened and the lumen of the oesophagus is not lubricated, with the result that the food becomes impacted, especially at those points where the lumen is constricted. This gives rise to the so-called pharyngeal, thoracic and diaphragmatic "choke" (page 36). Though this choke or impaction may take place at any point throughout the course of the oesophagus, it certainly occurs most frequently at the constrictions. Cattle, swine, and dogs having a funnel-shaped opening at each end of the oesophagus, sometimes become too ambitious and attempt to swallow very large bodies, with the result that they choke on these. On the other hand, with the exception of the horse, domesticated animals can quite easily force food from the stomach back into the mouth through the oesophagus. In poultry there is another anatomical peculiarity consisting in a distinct diverticulum attached to the oesophagus and in communication with it, located at about the entrance to the chest. In ducks and geese, instead of a distinct diverticulum, there is a decided spindle-shaped dilatation of the oesophagus at the entrance to the chest. In pigeons there are two diverticuli side by side. These diverticuli or dilatations constitute the so-called crop of birds. Their function in most instances is to serve as a storage place for hastily swallowed food, though in both male and female pigeons at the time of the hatching of the eggs, the crop secretes a fatty fluid which serves the purpose of nourishment for the young when first hatched.

The stomach is the organ succeeding the oesophagus. So great are the anatomical differences in this

organ in species of animals that two general groups
are recognized, i.e., ruminants and non-ruminants. The
former grouping includes cattle, sheep and goats, and
the latter most other animals such as the horse, swine,
dog, and cat.

In the horse the stomach has a capacity of about
three and one-half gallons. The oesophagus enters it
through a narrow opening with the mu-
The
stomach
of the
horse
cous membrane arranged around it in
many folds. This arrangement has been
asserted to offer a partial explanation attending the extremely difficult vomiting
in the horse, but other factors are probably involved.
The mucous membrane of the oesophagus is continued
apparently unchanged in the first half of the stomach,
then changes to the true gastric-juice-secreting mucous
membrane. This transition from one type of mucous
membrane to another is sudden, the line of demarcation
being very abrupt and immediately noticeable when the
stomach is opened. To laymen it frequently seems
that a diseased condition is present, because of the
marked difference in the appearance of the mucous
membrane in the left and right halves of the stomach.
The darker colored mucous membrane in the right half
secretes the digestive or gastric juice. This juice consists of various enzymes and hydrochloric acid, and
serves to break down by chemical means the complex
substances consumed by the animal as food. So abundant is the hydrochloric acid that it gives the horse a
large measure of protection against the highly poisonous prussic acid (page 437) formed under certain conditions of growth in many plants, especially the sorg-
hums, kafir, sudan grass, Johnson grass and others.
Food arranges itself in the stomach in layers which do
not seem to be much disturbed by water ingested at a
later period. The old precaution, therefore, not to
water a horse after the animal has eaten its solid food
is not well founded. Other non-ruminants such as the

Vomiting in animals

hog, dog and cat, have stomachs quite comparable to the horse, though the oesophageal opening in these animals is funnel-shaped, so that they vomit easily and almost at will. There are other important and not fully explained factors in the act of vomiting, but certainly an absence of mechanical obstruction to retrograde outflow of ingesta is helpful to the process.

The group of animals classed as ruminants include cattle, sheep and goats. These animals are said to have

Ruminants or animals that "chew the cud"

four stomach compartments, known technically as the rumen (paunch), reticulum, (honeycomb), omasum (manyleaves, manyplies, etc.), and the abomasum or true stomach. At birth the rumen, reticulum and omasum are undeveloped. Formerly regarded in their development as oesophageal (gullet) dilatations

Ruminants (cattle, sheep, goats, etc.) not developed at birth

it is now known from research on the embryo that they develop from the embryonic stomach—during this process the forestomachs lose their gastric glands and under the stimulus of coarse feeds they grow rapidly. At 10 to 12 weeks of age the change is distinctly noticeable and at the age of a year and a half the four compartments have reached their permanent comparative or relative sizes.

In cattle the rumen (paunch) is a voluminous hollow organ capable of holding forty to fifty gallons of liquid. It is located largely in the left side of the abdomen and is in direct contact with the left upper flank. It is entered by the funnel-shaped end of the oesophagus and is succeeded through a large opening by the reticulum. The mucous membrane lining the rumen is but feebly adherent in places so that on autopsy patches of it may be quite easily rubbed off. This is not to be considered an evidence of disease.

The reticulum or second stomach is in direct communication with the rumen by means of a large opening, and is continued by the third stomach. The reticulum has its lining mucous membrane arranged in the form of a honeycomb, which accounts for its common name. The reticulum is closely related to the heart sac in front, being separated from it by the diaphragm. Under certain conditions the actual space separating the two organs is less than one-fourth of an inch, which explains the ease with which swallowed sharp pointed foreign bodies that have lodged in the reticulum pass to the heart, with a fatal termination (pages 23 and 356).

The omasum or third stomach is peculiar as an anatomical organ in the arrangement of its mucous membrane in prominent longitudinal leaves covered with hard elevations the size of grains of sand. This arrangement of the mucous membrane is responsible for the names "manyleaves," and "manyplies" applied to this organ. The omasum has two openings at its extremities placing its cavity in communication with the reticulum and the true, or fourth stomach, the abomasum. The latter has all the characteristics found in the glandular portion of the stomach in non-ruminants. It is continuous through a muscular ring-like opening with the intestines.

The functions of the various compartments of the stomach in ruminants are quite well understood. The rumen has correctly been compared to a vast fermentation vat where bacteria play an important role in food digestion. This bacterial action may be seriously impeded by the drinking of very cold water; the removal of ice in cold weather, especially for housed animals, is recommended.

Since it is well known that the rumen and reticulum secrete no enzyme or leavening agent that is capable of digesting the cellulose or woody portion of the ration nature takes care of this by germs and protozoa which do produce enzymes. Under normal conditions shortly after birth the newly born creature by association with older cattle acquires these germs and protozoa—the latter small single-celled, microscopic animals that pro-

Origin of rumen organisms

duce four generations a day—that are present in the rumen of older animals and therefore in the "cud." These organisms by their rapid multiplication—they originate mostly in crevices of the reticulum which serves as a "starter" tank for these ana-
Function of rumen organisms erobic organisms—soon constitute a considerable portion of the contents of the paunch—they collectively constitute about 10 percent of the dry matter present in the rumen. Not only do they digest cellulose to a considerable extent, but by their very presence they produce food because the rumen organisms synthesize many—reported to be ten—amino acids that are necessary for animal growth. Furthermore these organisms are capable of artificially building up all the known vitamins except A, D and E. Since the organisms must have food for their own growth, and as they cannot satisfy their needs from poor quality roughages, therefore it is a sound practice to fortify such feeds with a limited amount of some carbohydrate such as molasses but not to an excess as the bacteria become indolent when there is more carbohydrate than enough to satisfy their needs. The bacteria must also have nitrogen which is utilized in the form of ammonia broken off from the amino acids, or added as urea (page 58), and minerals especially phosphorus and cobalt both usually present in the ration. It is informative to note that unless the bacteria get very small amounts of cobalt (page 91) administered *by way of the mouth* either as a constituent of the food or otherwise they cannot synthesize vitamins. Under some conditions the bacterial content is upset by
Some effects of disturbed bacterial content in the rumen improper or poisonous feeds, by sudden changes to an unaccustomed ration, by the administration of some drugs, by inadequate amounts of food, by extreme chilling, by toxic infections or almost any factor inimical to health. Many of the conditions are manifested by loss of appetite, rumen impaction, acute

and chronic bloat, and other digestive dysfunctions. Relief from some of these conditions may in some instances be afforded by the artificial inoculation of the rumen contents. This is the so-called "rumen seeding." In a crude way the "cud" from healthy cattle has been used, but there is danger in this messy practice as harmful infections of the donor animal may thus be inadvertently given to the recipient. Refined products are available commercially through the veterinarian.

Calf feeding on roughages   Taken as a whole it is asserted that improved health in some herds where calf pneumonia, calf scours, and coccidiosis were rampant, has been observed from the feeding of limited amounts of milk to which has been added some feeding of soft green alfalfa from birth, plus weekly rumen inoculations—about 25 grams of dried rumen culture daily is the usual dosage. Undoubtedly the voluminous rumen and the reticulum also

"Chew-the-cud"   serve for the storage of food. Ruminants must ingest enormous quantities of comparatively non-nutritious material in order to obtain enough nourishment to sustain the body. They consume this food hastily and with incomplete mastication. Then when the animal is at rest, it has the physiological ability to force food from the rumen back into the mouth for more thorough chewing, when it is again swallowed to find its way to the third and fourth stomach compartments, there to be subjected to more thorough and complete digestion. This regurgitation of food with its more thorough mastication is called rumination, or "chewing the cud." Necessarily when an animal becomes ill, this function is discontinued, and the beast is said to have "lost its cud" (page 348). This must not be interpreted too literally, as it is sometimes

"Loss of cud"   done, people actually hunting for "the lost cud," and sometimes substituting for it by forcing into the animal's mouth a greasy rag or a piece of pork in the hopes that the "chewing of the cud" may be resumed. It is almost needless to state that such practices are to be discouraged as harmful, and at any rate, when the animal's general health returns the physiological regurgitation of food will again be resumed, and "chewing the cud" reestablished. In a state of health the rumen also undergoes certain peristaltic or churning motions for the purpose of mechanically aiding in the mixing of the ingesta. These movements are at the rate of two or three each minute. They may be quite readily felt by placing the hand in the left upper flank. When absent, it is an indication of a lack of function most frequently associated with some form of impaction of the rumen.

Hair balls and their nature It is very common to find hair balls in the rumen varying in size up to that of a man's head. When a ruminant licks itself, a good deal of the hair is swallowed, to be gathered in the rumen in the form of balls (page 349). They are usually harmless, apparently causing no inconvenience. The physiological functions of the reticulum do not differ materially from those of the rumen other than the starting area for the micro-organisms needed by the rumen. It is very common on a post mortem examination to find in this compartment such foreign bodies as nails, pieces of bailing wire, cinders, and the like. Occasionally these foreign bodies penetrate the wall of the reticulum, pass into neighboring organs, and because of its proximity, into the heart (page 20), usually with a fatal termination. In the omasum very little if any digestion takes place, though there is a marked reduction in the fluid contents of the food to one-half that in the rumen. Finding these contents, then, in a comparatively dry condition is not to be considered as evidence of disease. In the abomasum or true glandular stomach the digestive processes are very similar to those taking place in the simpler stomachs of non-ruminants. The contents of the abomasum in contradistinction to the omasum are in a state of health quite fluid.

In domesticated poultry the stomachs also vary from the simple non-ruminant type. The oesophagus and crop have already been described. Food enters an oval sac known as the glandular stomach which secretes an acid juice. Ingested material quickly passes through it and goes into a second compartment known as the gizzard, characterized by the muscular development of its walls, and by a thick horny mucous membrane for lining. The gizzard always contains grinding material in the form of sand and pebbles, and when these are activated by the powerful muscular and the hard mucous coats, disintegration of the food particles takes place.

The gizzard in poultry

The intestines succeed the stomach. Because of a difference in volume the intestines are classified as small intestine and large intestine. The small intestine is arbitrarily divided into duodenum (twelve fingers' breadth), jejunum ("empty"), and ileum ("to twist"). The large intestine is in turn subdivided into the caecum, large or double colon, and small or floating colon. The rectum, about twelve inches long in the larger animals, succeeds the floating colon, and it communicates with the exterior through the anus. In fowls at the point of union of the small and large intestines two blind sacs enter the intestines. These are from four to six inches in length. The pouches are known as "ceca." (Page 24.) Any material entering the ceca must pass out at the same place it enters—in a retrograde manner.

The intestines and their uses

Also in poultry there is the "cloaca." This is a short passage-way terminating the large intestine, and the outer opening of the cloaca is the anus or vent. In addition to being a terminus for the large intestine the cloaca also is the urinary reservoir because poultry have no urinary bladder—the urine is in the form of semi-solid whitish urates mixed with feces at the time of defecation. Finally the cloaca also receives the oviduct—usually on its left side. Therefore the cloaca is a final passage way or reservoir for feces, urine and organs of generation in both male and female.

All of the intestines have the usual mucous membrane as a lining, and to the outside of this, a coat of involuntary muscle fibers arranged longitudinally and circularly. In and beneath the mucous membrane of the entire intestinal tract there are glands singly or in groups, and either microscopic or macroscopic in size. The size and function of the intestines vary in different species. Those with functionally well developed stomachs such as carnivorous animals, the dog and cat, have comparatively small intestines because most of the digestive processes are completed in the stomach, and their food is in a concentrated form. Cattle have more voluminous intestines than the carnivora because their food is very bulky and it does not have the same degree of concentration. Horses use about the same kind of food as cattle, but horses have a simple stomach in which the digestive processes are limited, while cattle complete more of the digestion in the stomach, with the result that the intestines in the horse are much more voluminous.

Other than the glands in the intestines proper, there are two additional ones, i.e., the liver and the pancreas that pour their secretion into the lumen of **The liver and pancreas** the intestines, there to aid the various intestinal digestive juices to reduce aliment largely by chemical and mechanical means to such a state that it may effectively and beneficially be absorbed from the intestines to be taken up by the blood and lymph streams to be carried to distant parts of the body. Neither must bacterial action in relation to carbohydrate fermentation and non-putrefactive protein decomposition be ignored in the digestive process.

After the extraction of the nutritive material from the ingested food, the residue gathers in the small colon and rectum to be expelled through the anus. The frequency of defecation varies depending upon the species involved and the nature of the aliment. On dry feed it is less frequent than on highly succulent material, and in debilitating non-feverish diseases it is increased. Foods that are very woody or fibrous such as second and third cuttings of alfalfa, sweet clover, oats-straw and similar materials have a definite retarding action on the number of defecations. The horse usually defecates from five to ten times daily, cattle from ten to twenty times, and dairy cattle have as many as twenty-four evacuations in twenty-four hours. Dogs perform the act two or three times daily. When passages are suppressed, peristalsis, that is the normal contractions of the intestines that can so easily be heard by placing the ear against the animal's side, is also suppressed, or greatly increased under contrary conditions. Frequent listening to the peristalsis soon educates a person to be able to distinguish between the normal, subnormal and abnormal sounds. Valuable diagnostic evidence may thus be obtained.

Chapter III

PULSE, RESPIRATION AND TEMPERATURE

In humans any deviation from a temperature of 98.6° F. is looked upon as evidence of an abnormal con-

Normal temperature range

dition in the body. In some animals there is more range or it may be stated that there exists a minimum normal and a maximum normal temperature as the following table indicates:

	Normal Temperature	Range
Horse _____	100.5° F.	
Cattle _____	101.5 "	100–102.4
Sheep _____	103.0 "	102–104
Goat _____	103.0 "	
Pig _____	102.6 "	102–103
Dog and Cat_____	101.5 "	101–102.5
Fowl _____	106.0 "	105–107

Temperature recordings in animals as in man are taken by means of a clinical thermometer. Animal thermometers are of heavier or more rugged construction than those intended for use in humans. This prevents breakage. For animal use the end having the mercury-bulb is blunt pointed—either pear-shaped or spherical —to prevent injury when inserted, after lubrication, into the rectum. Human clinical thermometers, except for their comparatively frail construction, are also satisfactory for animal use.

All clinical thermometers are so constructed that the mercury in the recording column rises under the influence of warmth and remains stationary. This means that before the instrument may again be used the mercury column must be mechanically lowered by downward hand swinging, or by lightly jarring it downward while holding the thermometer in one hand and striking this hand against the other.

Whenever the temperature of an individual is elevated above the normal there is said to be fever or

27

Fever
the individual is feverish. Always regard such an elevation as a possible evidence of disturbed health. However, many things other than ill health can influence the temperature; excitement, exercise, digestion, rest, high surrounding temperatures, etc. Usually an animal's temperature is lower in the morning than later in the day. A temperature below normal in a sick animal is a very serious symptom.

Pulse rate
The pulse rate indicating the rapidity of heart action is subject to an even wider range than is the temperature. Below is given the normal range or number of pulse beats per minute for various animals:

	Range and rate per minute
Horse	32–44
Cattle	60–70
Sheep	70–80
Goat	70–80
Pig	60–80
Dog	70–120
Cat	110–130
Fowl	200–400

In general the pulse rate varies with the size of the animal in that small animals have a more rapid pulse than large ones—a small dog has a faster pulse than a large dog, and a dog of any size has a faster heart rate than a horse or cow. Very small animals such as the mouse will have a pulse rate of 600 per minute while an elephant's rate is from 30 to 45. Also the heart action is more rapid in young animals than in the older. Other factors that tend to cause acceleration of heart action are excitement, exercise, digestion and high temperature.

Veterinarians attach a good deal of importance to the character of the pulse such as the force and fullness of the beat, and form of the pressure wave. Thus, the beat may be quick and abrupt, hard, or long, slow and soft; at other times it may be fast, thin, thready and arythmic. In health the rhythm in horses and cattle is steady, though in the dog there is frequently irregularity. If these abnormal characters are maintained over more than a comparatively short period of time they should be considered as evidence of a disturbed bodily function.

The sites for taking the pulse vary in domesticated animals. In the horse the favorite and preferred site is the external maxillary artery located at the lower border of the jaw at a point where it is superficial and rests against the underlying jaw bone. If the foregoing artery is not available—this sometimes occurs when the area is diseased and swollen—the median artery at the inner surface and upper extremity of foreleg is quite accessible. In cattle correspondingly located arteries may be used, or the saphenous artery on the plantar surface of the hind limb just above the hock joint. In dairy and thin cattle this artery is quite available. In still other cases the coccygeal artery high up on the under surface of the tail is the preferred site. In sheep the femoral artery high up on the inner surface of the thigh at a point where it emerges from the groin muscles is the preferred site. This artery is also used for pulse palpation in pigs, dogs, and cats.

Breathing rate Respiration rate or the breathing rate is subject to some normal variation as it is perceptably influenced by excitement, exertion, plethora, size of the animal, as well as some extraneous factors, Abnormally it is increased by fever, pain, weakness, infections, and notably by lung ailments. The range and rate per minute in domesticated animals is approximately as follows: Horse 8 to 16; cattle 10 to 30; sheep and goat 12 to 20; pig 8 to 18; dog 10 to 30; cat 20 to 30; and fowl 15 to 30.

In order to know and appreciate the difference between health and disease as evidenced by the temperature, pulse, and respiration, constant and frequent practice is necessary. Only after repeated observations of these health functions can the deviations in them as caused by disease be determined. Practice makes perfect. (Consult Chapter VI, regarding influence of water, outside temperature, etc.)

CHAPTER IV

FOODS AND HEALTH

To live, an animal must eat and this necessitates the use of foreign materials to become a part of the body. The method of obtaining these **Feeding practices** foods, the nature of the food, and its proper amount constitute *feeding practices*. Domestication of animals, the demands upon them in the form of work, and in the production of milk, meat, eggs and wool, are all beyond the original physiological intents and purposes of nature. Furthermore, the character of the soil and its influence upon growing crops, as well as the growing of feeds for economical reasons in certain sections of the world not their habitat, and the use of these strange plants as livestock foods, affect animals in various ways; however, certain fundamental principles in feeding are not materially altered. Sound production of animals that receive most of their nutrients from home grown feeds should start with the soil since there is always the cycle of soil, plants and animals. Also, the chemical composition of the soil is reflected in the chemical composition of the plants grown on it. Therefore, under apparently normal feeding there may be ill-health from mineral deficiency if the soil is not adequate in essential minerals.

The first essential in handling a lack of well-being in animals is a correct diagnosis of the cause. It may be malnutrition because of improper balance of nutrients; it can be parasitism; **Animal "conditioners" and "tonics"** physical conditions surrounding the animals; chronic ailments and a host of others. Certainly the graduate veterinarian is the person best qualified by training and experience to investigate and advise in these situations. To place one's trust in "tonics" and "conditioners" of unknown formulation for ill-health the nature of which has not been determined is entirely out of line with the modern animal-husbandman's ideals and training. Fortunately Federal and State Agencies have stepped in to curtail the sale of live-stock remedies of questionable merit, as well as the activities of unscrupulous manufacturers and venders. Unless a livestock remedy offered for general sale has real merit to warrant registration by official agencies, or unless it has the endorsement of the veterinarian its use is inadvisable.

Certainly the food or combination of foods must have the essential ingredients of carbohydrates (sugars, starches, gums, etc.), fats (neutral **Composition of foods** fat, fatty acids, vegetable wax, resins, lecithin), protein (albumens), and ash (phosphate of lime, magnesia, chlorides, salt, etc.).

The first point of importance is that the food shall be offered in a reasonably clean manner (Fig. 2). The **Sanitary feeding** very general practice of throwing food, especially the grains, on the ground so that it is impossible for the animal to get these without at the same time getting a liberal amount of foreign matter, is to be condemned. Unfortunately the space of feeding is usually one where animals generally congregate, with the result that the ground is soon very badly contaminated with worm eggs and all the dangerous forms of infection to which the species is heir.

In an effort to overcome this, and it has met with a reasonable degree of success, various so-called self-feeders (Figs. 1 and 3) have been developed. These self-feeders should have certain features such as inability of the animal to get into it, or to deposit intestinal evacuations in it, ease of cleaning with no sharp corners or angles (Fig. 4) to harbor decomposing old

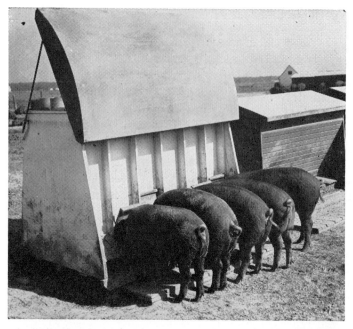

(Photo supplied by Douglas Fir Plywood Assn., Tacoma 2, Washington)

FIG. 1. A plywood hog-feeding crate as developed at Purdue University, Lafayette, Indiana.

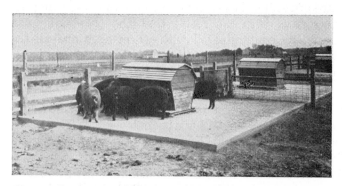

FIG. 2. Concrete feeding floors are sanitary and practical.

food, and a readily accessible trough with safeguards to prevent greedy feeding or gulping. They are usually constructed of wood, because this material lends itself readily to the necessary construction work by the average individual; it is everywhere available, and racks and self-feeders made out of wood can easily be moved to some other part of the farm. The chief disadvantage of wood is that it absorbs disease-producing agencies, and is disinfected with difficulty. Whenever feasible and when it may profitably be done, and in their proper place, cement, galvanized iron, tin-covered iron, and comparable materials should be used for the

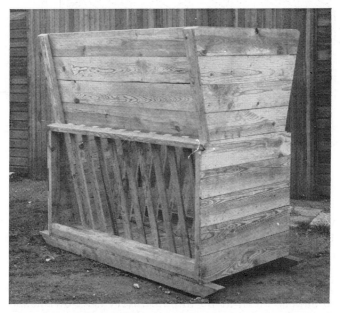

(Courtesy Dept. of Agricultural Engineering, Kansas State University)

Fig. 3. A movable substantial feed rack.

building of all utensils, feed racks and troughs, self-feeders, feed platforms and similar devices. Agricultural colleges through their Experiment Stations have done valuable work in the matter of the most efficient and sanitary method of feeding and watering livestock and poultry. Their publications are available to all those requesting them. For poultry, an additional safeguard against infections in the drinking water consists of preparing a saturated solution of permanganate of potash and, because of their habit of picking up food particles from soiled surroundings, an elevated platform with a wire screen floor on which the

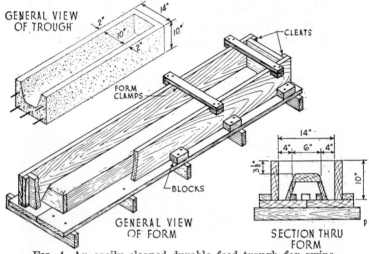

FIG. 4. An easily cleaned durable feed trough for swine.

water container is placed is to be recommended (Fig. 160). An automatic poultry feeder (Figs. 5 and 6) developed at the Penn. Agr. Exp. Sta., has much to commend it. It is energized by an electric motor. Its operation is controlled by a timer and a time-clock so as to supply mash at 30 minute intervals. Fowl hearing the hum of the feeder are attracted to it.*

In offering foods that are highly relished, such as grain, horses should not be permitted to gulp it hastily

---

*Also consult "Penn State Mechanical Dairy Feeder," Progress Report No. 110, Pennsylvania State University, University Park, Penn.

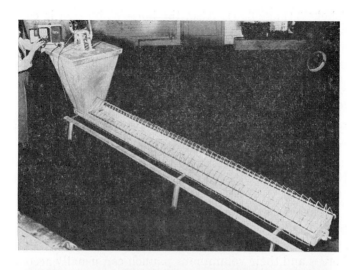

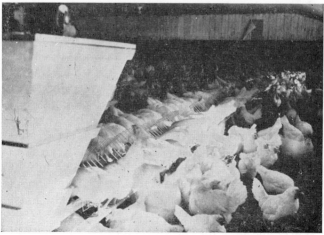

(Courtesy Pennsylvania Agricultural Experiment Station)

FIGS. 5 and 6. An automatic, clock-controlled poultry feeder.
(Lower picture) The feeder in action; it is sanitary.

Greedy
feeding
and its
prevention

as they are so likely to do. Greedy feeders
do not mix the food thoroughly with saliva,
and therefore the necessary lubricating
quality of this substance is lacking, and
the food gathers in the gullet, there to constitute a

"choke" (page 350). Also, the horse's stomach is comparatively small and when hastily filled with dry grain or easily swelling and fermenting food, trouble ensues in the form of stomach bloat or colic, and not infrequently with death as a sequence. Let **Methods of feeding** horses have both their grain and roughage at the same time, and place the grain in a shallow box so that big mouthfuls cannot be taken. In the case of excessively greedy eaters it is sometimes a practice to place a few stones in the feed box so that the animal is compelled to pick the grain from between the stones.

Though cattle do suffer from "choke" because of attempting to swallow large pieces of beets, potato, corncobs, and similar feed, they can eat more rapidly than horses and their voluminous paunch can usually accommodate it, though there are many recorded instances where free access to a forbidden grain bin has caused the cow to overestimate the capacity of her stomach, with distressing and not infrequent fatal outcome. Sheep prefer fresh, fine food, with grain and roughage fed separately. Swine masticate food very imperfectly and they swallow it hastily. For these reasons foods offered them in the trough should be neither coarse nor woody, and not in large pieces. Dogs and cats are capable of digesting pieces of soft food as large as they can swallow, though bones are chewed so as to reduce them to at least a coarse state of division, and the highly acid reaction of the stomach quickly finishes their complete dissolution.

Lofts and bins for the storage of foods should keep these foods dry. If repeatedly moistened and with no compensatory exposure to the sun's action, **Clean storage of feeds** the growth and development of germs, molds, and fungi are unhampered, and decomposition soon takes place (page 474). Bins for the storage of grains should be vermin and rodent proof; otherwise contamination of the food with the ejecta of these parasites soon renders it undesirable for feeding purposes. Though it has not been positively demonstrated that decomposed, moldy, and germ-infected, and parasite excreta-contaminated foods are harmful, they certainly cannot be classed as wholesome feeds, and the extent of their contamination is a good criterion of their undesirability as food for animals.

No single factor in feeding practice causes trouble as frequently in animals as a sudden change from a food to which they are accustomed to a new and unaccustomed food. Usually the new food is highly relished by the animal, and not only is the body suddenly called upon, without gradual preliminary preparation to handle this, but gorging with its attendant evils also takes place. In ruminants, germs and food are in close relationship with each other—no single germ species is responsible for the complete digestion of a particular food. Therefore if the proper balance is upset by inadequate food intake, by gorging, and a sudden change of feed, the function of the rumen is impaired. If animals are to be changed to a new ration, and especially if the change is one from that to which they have become accustomed over a more or less long period of time, the change should be made gradually. A good practice is during the first day of the new feeding to let the animal have its usual accustomed ration, and then offer it some of the new food in addition. Gradually from day to day the old ration may be reduced in amount and the new ration correspondingly increased. The abrupt change in diet is most likely to be harmful when a dry ration has been fed and then changed to a green succulent one. The change from old prairie hay to new prairie hay or alfalfa, and from old seasoned corn to new or green corn is frequently a cause of trouble. Sometimes animals are on a large grain ration because heavy work is demanded of them, and under these circumstances they are able to utilize this food. Sudden discontinuance of labor

The effect of sudden changes in the feed

for a day as over Sunday or a holiday without a corresponding decrease in the grain ration is likely to cause horses to contract the serious so-called "Monday disease" or "holiday disease." Veterinarians speak of it as azoturia (page 513) or "hemoglobinuria" because of the presence of the red coloring matter of the blood in the urine. Horse owners do not find it practical to withhold or materially reduce the grain ration on Sundays or holidays because then the animal is not in the best of condition for the work to be done when it is resumed after the day of idleness. A better plan is to continue these animals on their full ration during days of freedom from work but to compel them to take some exercise on these days.

Another example of the evils attending a sudden change to a new diet as well as the gorging is the development of inflammation in the feet known as "founder" or laminitis. There seems to be a sympathetic relationship between inflammatory processes in many of the bodily organs, and the deeper sensitive portion of the feet so that the latter frequently become secondarily inflamed to produce "founder." This reaction in the feet is most likely to occur as a sequence to inflammatory processes in the digestive tract as induced by sudden changes and gorging, though other accessory causes and conditions are also frequently simultaneously operative. Such meat eating animals as the dog and cat and the omnivorous hog are not susceptible to these conditions as nature has endowed them with ability to unload their stomachs by the act of vomiting.

Underfeeding is not nearly so likely to result in an acute disturbance as gorging. Probably its opposite **Not enough food** is manifested as obesity but even this in animals is not as likely to have such grave consequences as chronic starvation or underfeeding, or the more opposite acute condition of gorging. Underfeeding may be the result of deficient amounts of a well balanced ration, or apparently there are sufficient amounts though there is a lack of some essential constituent in the ration fed. If carbohydrates, fats, protein and minerals as well as essential supplementary items such as vitamins are not supplied the animal in regular and sufficient amounts, slow starvation is the result. It is not possible to outline any one food or combination of foods that will adequately supply all species of animals under various conditions of bodily metabolism such as engendered by idleness, heavy work, heavy milk production, or repeated and almost continuous rearing of young.

A condition almost equally serious for most animals is too heavy feeding on concentrates and a deficiency in bulk. For normal intestinal function, a reasonable degree of bulk is essential.

Too much food

Empty or partially filled intestines lose their tone or power of contracting simply because they lack a resistance which can only be supplied by bulk. Again, an opposite evil is excessive bulk as is frequently the case when exclusive rations of corn stover, oats straw and comparable materials are used. In this event the intestines lose tone because of a ceaseless effort to dislodge the bulk. The animal ultimately becomes "pot-bellied," and in some instances the inhibitions placed upon the digestive tract result in complete stasis and death.

All of the foregoing factors constitute underfeeding or slow starvation, in itself a serious condition especially when recuperative powers are slow as in the aged, and even the young may be permanently stunted as a result. Furthermore, starved or undernourished animals are much more subject to attacks by germs, the higher parasites, and other specific disease-producing agencies made possible because the bodily tissues and juices are so undernourished as to have lost their maximum powers of resistance.

On many farms there are evidences of slow starvation, though it may not be the result of actual underfeeding. "Pregnancy disease" in ewes (page 499) is due to a lack of carbohydrate; "wheat poisoning" (page 501) or grass tetany is due to a deficiency in lime and magnesium; posterior paralysis in pigs (page 503) is caused by a lack of lime possibly aided by deficient amounts of vitamin D (page 71) ; sore eyes in poultry, and other animals as well, may be Xerophthalmia (page 63), a vitamin A deficiency; slow breeding or delayed settling to service during early spring months may be due to a reduced supply of the sex vitamin E (page 123), ordinarily obtained from green feeds; and so on. The list of slow-starvation or deficiency diseases could be lengthened almost indefinitely. In general, a good ration must consist of correct amounts of wholesome feeds with the necessary supplemental factors.

Protein (page 44) is the nutrient most likely to be deficient in home grown feeds. And since protein con-

Protein and its value

centrates are more expensive than grains and roughages, it is not always an easy matter to convince farmers that it pays to balance animal rations. The statements which follow are based upon the results of carefully controlled experiments and thus are convincing proof that protein supplements merely "look" high priced.* (Fig. 7).

One pound of tankage, a rich protein substance, will replace 7 pounds of corn when fed to pigs in dry lot or 4 pounds of corn when fed to pigs on pasture. The protein supplement may be self-fed to hogs. From $\frac{1}{4}$ to $\frac{1}{3}$ pound of tankage or $\frac{1}{4}$ to $\frac{1}{2}$ gallon of skim milk per pig daily usually balances hand-fed grain rations.

One acre yielding 30 bushels of grain sorghum, if fed alone to hogs, will produce only about 120 pounds

---

*A 1959 U. of Ill. report in regard to soybean meal as the exclusive source of protein indicates that when pigs weighing less than 100 pounds received soybean meal only as protein they gained more than a pound a day while those receiving either fish meal, or meat and bone scraps gained only about ¾ pound daily. The difference in weight gains tends to disappear when the pigs weigh more than 100 pounds. The belief that pigs must have animal protein does not seem to be well founded. Soybean meal is cheaper than animal protein.

of pork; but one acre yielding 30 bushels of grain sorghum plus 150 pounds of protein supplement will produce about 360 pounds of pork.

For fattening calves, one ton of cottonseed meal equals 100 bushels of corn when fed at the rate of 1½ pounds per head daily in conjunction with grain,

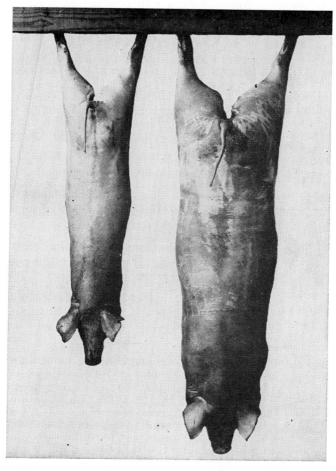

(Courtesy Dr. C. E. Aubel, Kansas State University)

FIG. 7. Litter mates. The smaller pig had corn alone; the larger one corn and protein. At the time of slaughter the smaller animal weighed 120 pounds, the larger 300 pounds. Both remained in good health during the test.

ground limestone, and a low-protein roughage like silage, ground fodder, or prairie hay. However, cottonseed meal fed in excess of 1½ pounds per head daily in this ration is worth no more per ton than corn.

One ton of prairie hay will produce only about 50 pounds of beef; but one ton of prairie hay plus 100 pounds of cottonseed cake will produce at least 150 pounds of beef.

Each ton of cottonseed cake or equivalent high-protein supplement fed at the rate of one pound per head daily in conjunction with silage for wintering stock calves will increase the gain approximately 1100 pounds. However, since cottonseed meal contains less lysine—an essential amino acid—than needed by growing swine and poultry, it should be combined with either soybean meal, fish meal, meat scraps, or milk, or be fortified with lysine itself.

A protein supplement sharpens an animal's appetite, improves thrift, increases gain, makes better finish on full-fed animals, and results in greater profit.

There are some foods that are relatively indigestible because of the large amount of fiber or woody material they contain. Outstanding among

Indigestible foods

these are the dried corn plant,* straw, and to a less degree the woody cuttings of alfalfa, sweet clover and other plants. It is not uncommon for animals fed largely on these foods to become badly constipated and in the more serious cases the indigestible fiber lodges as a tangled mass in the intestines, and all efforts to dislodge it prove to be unavailing. When foods of this nature must be fed, the animal should be induced to take large quantities of water by salting them regularly and by making water readily available. If this diet can be supplemented by occasional feedings of succulent foods, or

---

*Without attached grain it is "stover"; with attached grain it is "fodder."

such laxatives as linseed meal or linseed oil cake, decided benefit results.

In feeding animals for the best results the following points may well be kept in mind:

1. In general roughages are high in fiber and comparatively low in digestible nutrients. Concentrates are high in total digestible nutrients. High fiber feeds are relatively low in net energy content. A good roughage should be palatable; it should contain ample protein (most animals refuse to consume freely over a prolonged period if the protein is low) ; it must be rich in calcium to make up for the deficiency of this element in the concentrates; it should have high total digestible nutrient or net energy; and it should contain a liberal amount of carotene or pro-vitamin A as the latter is low or entirely lacking in most concentrates. Roughages are usually better sources of minerals and vitamins.

If the foregoing factors are lacking there results retarded growth and, in the case of dairy cattle, lowered milk production. A 1000 lb. dairy cow for example should receive at least eight pounds of good roughage daily for maintenance, plus 0.32 pound for each pound of 4% milk produced by her. It is rightfully contended that an inadequate supply of good roughage is probably the most frequent of all dairy cattle deficiencies. In the feed lot roughages of good quality may be fed in any quantity without serious effects. If the concentrates are corn, barley, milo, or kafir they should be ground. For fattening purposes* in the Corn Belt area, and to increase the palatability of the ration, not to exceed three pounds of molasses per head per day, providing its cost does not exceed that of corn, is fre-

*Farmers Bulletin No. 1549 U.S.D.A. "Feeding Cattle for Beef" for sale at 10 cents a copy by the Superintendent of Documents, Washington 25, D.C., is recommended.

quently added in diluted form to roughages. Over-ripe grass hays, cottonseed hulls, straws, and dried pasture grass contain no carotene.

2. Protein (page 40) for herbiverous animals is sometimes a problem when legume roughages are not available. Earlier, protein of animal origin, was said to be superior to that of vegetable origin—the former mostly meat scrap, tankage, fish meal and dried milk, and the latter soybean meal, cottonseed meal and linseed meal. However, with more knowledge when vegetable proteins are fortified by the addition of such non-protein substances as calcium and phosphorus, and the water soluble vitamins such as ribo-flavin, niacin and choline the seeming difference between the two proteins vanished. Therefore when vegetable proteins are the exclusive source of protein there should be added calcium and phosphorus, and water-soluble vitamins, or in place of these a small amount of animal protein. Proteins are made up of at least 22 different amino acids listed as "essential" and "non-essential" the former being those the body cannot synthesize and therefore the "essentials" must be supplied from extraneous sources.

The essential amino acids are lysine, tryptophane, histidine, phenylalanine, leucine, isoleucine, threanine,

The "essential" amino acids

valine, arginine and methionine. Late literature records that there appears to be in protein of animal origin a non-isolated unidentified "animal protein factor" (page 69) that is not an amino acid. Since it is not an amino acid it seems that the designation "unidentified growth factor" would be better. It in-

An unknown growth factor

fluences metabolism. It is found in fish-meal, liver-meal, meat scraps, tankage, milk by-products and dried cattle manure. It is carried through the egg, or when added to vegetable protein in amounts of 1¼ ounces per ton influences growth materially. It has been claimed to be identical to vitamin B_{12} which in a pure form is a red crystalline substance containing cobalt and phosphorus. The cobalt may be an explanation of the role APF has in the nutrition of animals. APF is produced commercially as a by-product in the

The role of APF

production of such antibiotics as penicillin, aureomycin and streptomycin. It is not improbable that the antibiotics mentioned may be contained in the commercial APF, and this is offered as an explanation of the beneficial results obtained by the feeding of APF supplements. Experiments have demonstrated that good rations having only plant sources of protein plus approximately 3.3 to 6.6 pounds of APF supplements per ton of feed meet a pig's nutritional requirement. Expressed in terms of B_{12} this means between 5 and 10 micrograms per pound of total feed. However, the conservative opinion is that tankage and meat scrap, minerals, amino acids, etc., are still necessary for a balanced ration.

The minimum amounts of the "essential" amino acids for normal growth in white rats vary from 0.2% to 1.0% in the food, provided the "non-essentials" are included in the ration. The minimum total for white rats of the "essential" amino acids is 5.8%. Amino acids provide material for antibody production in bacterial infections, they maintain nitrogen equilibrium, they help to overcome gastric hyperacidity, they supply needed protein for blood regeneration in anemia, and they speed recovery following operations.

In dairy cattle, especially when the rations are of the non-legume kind, protein deficiency, as exemplified

Protein for dairy cattle

by retarded growth and decreased milk production, is a problem. Where legumes constitute the bulk of the roughage protein shortage is unlikely especially if the grain concentrate has from 12 to 14% protein; if the roughage is non-legume the grain concentrate should have at least 16 to 18% protein.

When only poor quality hay is available for dairy cows, dehydrated alfalfa pellets may be used for re-

Poor quality hay and alfalfa pellets
inforcement. Cows having a reduction of 27.2 per cent in milk production when poor hay was fed increased so that the drop was only 15.2 per cent when 0.5 pound of alfalfa pellets were added for each 100 pounds of body weight. When one pound of pellets for each 100 pounds of weight were fed, the decrease in milk production was 3.6 per cent, and when the pellets were increased to 1.5 pounds for each 100 pounds of weight the milk reduction was only 0.7 per cent.

Protein intake for bulls can be kept relatively low. The highest level of fertility is obtained when bulls are on a relatively low protein intake. Grain and quality hay fed at the rate of 0.4 to 0.5 and one pound per 100 pounds of body weight, respectively, provide about the right amount of feed for active bulls. On this basis, grain containing 12 per cent protein when fed to a 2,000-pound bull will provide 0.96 to 1.20 pounds of protein. Hay with a protein content of 12 to 15 per cent fed to a bull of the same weight at the rate of one pound for every 100 pounds body weight will supply 2.4 to 3.0 pounds of protein. When fed as recommended, large bulls will receive a total of 3.36 to 4.20 pounds of protein daily (consult pages 40 and 44).

Pigs fed either on a low or very high (19.2%) protein corn ration developed a severe diarrhea during

Diarrhea and lack of protein in pigs
the fourth week though when this ration was supplemented with either the amino acid tryptophane, or the vitamin nicotinic acid no diarrhea appeared. When oats was the grain fed the pigs remained normal. These results are of course inconclusive but they are significant. In pigs there may be many other factors responsible for the appearance of the diarrhea.

Heat-Treatment of Garbage.* If garbage contains raw or improperly heated, or otherwise insufficiently processed pork products, it may be a reservoir of parasites and germ life capable of transmis-
sion of these to swine consuming the gar-
bage. The trichina spiralis (page 681) parasite, and the viruses of vesicular ex-
anthema, foot-and-mouth disease, and hog cholera may be so spread. Tuberculosis, erysipelas and other germ ailments have also been spread by contaminated garbage.

Properly heated garbage a safe feed

When garbage is sufficiently heated the transmis-
sion of swine diseases and parasites can be controlled. Certainly there are other methods of spread such as direct contact between diseased and susceptible animals, and indirect contact through contaminated premises, but the heat-treatment of garbage intended for swine consumption will control one of the most important avenues of disease spread.

The trichina spiralis can be destroyed by tempera-
tures ranging from 121° to 131° F. (see page 682) held there for 30 minutes. The virus of vesicular exanthema (page 611) is destroyed by a temperature of 140° F. for a 30 minute period. However, the tem-
peratures mentioned may be insufficient to penetrate to the necessary degree to the center of thick pieces of pork or large masses of other material in the garbage. To insure thorough penetration at the temperatures named, the garbage must first be ground or, in the absence of grinding, the temperature must be maintained at 212° F. for a period of not less than 30 minutes. At this latter temperature the living material

Temperature required and methods

---

*The U.S.D.A. has issued the publication, "Equipment and Methods for Heat-treating Garbage for Hog Feed," also desig-
nated "Program Aid No. 370," Nov., 1958. No price is indicated.

in the garbage is destroyed, and the value of the garbage for feed purposes is not affected. Held for more than 30 minutes at the 212° temperature the feed value is somewhat lowered. Animals relish cooked garbage and clean it up much better than when it is in the raw state.

Mechanical removal of harmful things
Garbage may contain used razor blades, broken glass, pieces of cloth or leather and other foreign matter. These must be removed. Also, the grease should be skimmed from the top of cooked garbage since its consumption by swine frequently results in digestion upsets.

Garbage may be heated to the required degree by:

1. "Wet-steaming, or boiling in an open vat."

2. "Dry-steaming, or boiling in a jacketed kettle or cylinder."

3. "Steaming in a pressure cylinder."

4. "Direct heating over an open fire."

State law requirements
Since the extensive occurrence of vesicular exanthema (page 611) during the early fifties, several states now have laws requiring the heating of publicly collected garbage when intended for use as swine feed.

Other method of handling
When not intended for swine feed garbage may be buried in trenches, treated with an odorous disinfectant, and soil covered. Rats must be controlled (page 325) when burial of garbage is the method used.

So-called protein poisoning
Frequently the assertion is made that a group of animals is affected with "protein poisoning." However, a ration high in protein, when properly balanced, does not result in poisoning. Nutrition authorities do not recognize "protein poisoning" as a phenomenon of

animal nutrition, but consider any harmful effects accompanying high protein rations as due to a deficiency of some vital nutrient. So-called "cottonseed meal poisoning" (pages 74 and 460) is a good example.

For maintenance and production it is indicated that a 50-pound pig will eat about 2.7 pounds of a balanced ration daily, a 100-pound pig 5.0 pounds, **Production** a 200-pounder 7.5 pounds of feed. Preg- **feeding of** nant gilts will need 1.6 to 1.8 pounds of **swine** feed daily for 100 pounds of live weight, while bred sows in the dry-lot will need 1.4 to 1.6 pounds daily per 100 pounds of live weight. If the animals are on good pasture somewhat less concentrates are needed. Sows with six or more pigs may be self-fed after the pigs are two weeks of age. Sows that are nursing pigs will consume 10 to 15 pounds more of feed daily depending on the size of the litter and the weight of the sow.

In ewes there is a system of feeding colloquially spoken of as "flushing." After the lambs are weaned the ewes are put on drier pasture, and **Flushing** then two or three weeks before the begin- **ewes** ning of the fall breeding season they are to be changed to better pasture supplemented by legume hay and some grain. Equal parts of oats and corn constitute a satisfactory grain ration for this purpose. "Flushing" is claimed to be beneficial in the production of a larger and a more uniform lamb crop.

Colts should be weaned when they reach the age of six months. During the first winter they should receive from one-half pound to one pound **Feed for** of grain per day for each 100 pounds of **weanling** live weight in addition to hay. This is **colts** enough grain up to two years of age. In addition there should be liberal roughage such as good pasture, or well cured hay. Increase the grain allowance as the colt goes over two years. Excellent grain mixtures are as follows:

Parts by weight

Corn	2
Oats	5
Wheat bran	1
Linseed meal	1
or	
Oats	4
Corn	1
Wheat bran	1

(Both formulas are from U.S.D.A. Bul. No. 2052)

Brood mares should be kept at light work, or turned out to pasture for ten days preceding foaling. Alfalfa hay not excessively stemmy is recom-

Feed and care of brood mares

mended for roughage. A good laxative grain ration, not to exceed five pounds daily, consists of two parts by weight of wheat bran, one part linseed meal, and six parts crushed oats. A week after foaling the mare may be permitted to take exercise in a pasture, and at two weeks after foaling she may be put to light work on full feed.

Care must be exercised not to overfeed as it will result in digestive upsets. Start the animals on all the roughage they will take, and gradually

Steers in dry lots

increase the ration of concentrates so that at the end of a month they will be on full feed. Fattening rations vary in a geographical area as large as the United States. In general the Agricultural Experiment Stations of the various states are the best sources of information about local feed requirements, and the feeder must operate at a chance for a reasonable profit from his venture. A two-year-old steer of about 1000 pound weight can handle each day twenty pounds of ground corn and eight to ten pounds of a legume hay such as alfalfa or clover. If hogs follow the cattle grinding the corn is not so important.

Milk Replacements: Dairy calves, if during the first four days of their lives, they are given the milk from their dam (colostrum or "Kafmalak") (page 540) can be raised to be entirely normal in every

Replacements save milk for sale purposes

respect on formulae containing a minimum amount of milk, thus saving several hundred pounds of saleable milk. A formula developed at Pennsylvania State University has the following composition:

	Pounds
Dried whey	50
Distillers dried solubles	10
Oat flour	5
Soluble blood flour	10
Dextrose	7
Dicalcium phosphate	2.0
Vitamin A and D feed (500 U.S.P. units D_2 and 4000 I.U. A per gram)	0.5
Mineral mix (Calcium 32%, magnesium 2.6%, manganese 1%, iron 0.175%, cobalt .002%, and copper 0.125%)	0.5

How Is It Fed? The replacement should be mixed in warm water and fed at 100 degrees Fahrenheit. It can be fed in open pails placed at 14 to 18 inches from the floor at the following rates:

Feeding Schedule—Twice Daily

Days of age	Lbs. Milk		Lbs. Water		Lbs. Replacement	
	HB*	LB*	HB	LB	HB	LB
1—4	4	3			.0	.0
5—7	2	2	2	1	.2	.2
8—10	1	1	3	3	.4	.3
11—28	0	0	5	4	.5	.4
29—42	0	0	6	5	.6	.5
43—49	0	0	7	6	.7	.6
50—56	0	0	7	6	.7†	.6

*LB means light breed, HB means heavy breed.
†Feed once daily.

In addition to the "replacement" the calves at weaning time should receive up to five pounds of good quality "starter" per day and all the high quality grass-legume hay they will consume. The time varies from 30 to 50 days, depending on the stage of development of the organs of digestion (see page 19).

Method of feeding the "replacement"

Where there is a heavy demand for market, milk "starters" are in general use. In this system the calf is started on whole milk, and is taught to eat a dry calf starter and hay at an early age. Milk is withheld from the ration at seven to ten weeks of age and thereafter the calf is fed "starter," hay and water. At about four months of age a cheaper concentrate mixture is substituted for the "starter."

"Starters" in calf feeding

A simple "starter" mixture—demonstrated to be as effective as the more complex mixtures, has the following formula for one ton:

	Pounds
Cracked corn	956
Wheat bran	200
Ground oats	500
Soybean oil meal	300
Mineral mixture, containing calcium phosphorous, and trace minerals	20
Salt	20
Vitamin A and D supplement containing 4000 U.S.P. units of vitamin A, and 500 U.S.P. units of vitamin D in each	4
Total	2000

The above outlined mixture is estimated to have a 15.7 per cent total protein value. "Starters" having granular texture are preferred to those of a finely ground consistency, and laxative substances in milk substitutes should be avoided.

Milk substitutes or replacements in the raising of pigs are successful in the controlled laboratory, but field experiences are usually not so successful. The starting point of attempts for more economical pork production is to wean the pigs at an early age—at birth or two days of age—so that the sow may be rebred. Normally the sow does not come in "heat" so long as she is being nursed. Almost all come in "heat" at two to three days after the pigs are removed, but this is in most instances a non-ovulating heat so that conception does not follow the insemination. Furthermore, when

Milk substitutes for pigs?

Sow furnishes
heat and
care

pigs are left with the sow she furnishes warmth, and care, as well as regular feeding from a sanitary source of production.

It seems also that the pig does not synthesize its own vitamin C until it is about one week of age—it receives this vitamin from the abundant supply in its mother's milk. Research workers in this field are optimistic that in time artificial rearing of pigs will result in economy, and a steadier supply of pork.

In one project the pigs were removed from the sows when two to three days of age. A milk substitute or replacement having the following formula was used:

```
Dried  skimmed  _____ 76%
Lard _____  5
Rapeseed oil _____  5
Lecithin _____  1
Dried  sulphite  yeast_____  3
Glucose  _____  5
Cane sugar _____  5
                                              ───
                                              100
```

To the above a mineral mixture having the following formula was added to the extent of 0.2%:

```
FeSO₄ _____ 60 parts
MnSO₄ _____ 50   "
CoSO₄ _____ 15   "
CuSO₄ _____ 10   "
KI _____  1   "
```

$FeSO_4$ 60 parts, $MnSO_4$ 50, $CoSO_4$ 15, $CuSO_4$ 10, KI 1.

Furthermore the mixture was fortified with the following:

```
Vitamin  A_____22,000 I.U./kg
Vitamin  D₂_____ 3,000 I.U./kg
Thiamine  _____    10  mg/kg
Riboflavin  _____    10  mg/kg
Niacin  _____    50  mg/kg
Calcium  pantothenate  _____    80  mg/kg
Pyridoxine  _____    15  mg/kg
Ascorbic  acid  _____   250  mg/kg
Vitamin  B₁₂ _____    40  mg/kg
Terramycin  _____    50  mg/kg
```

This synthetic formula should be mixed with six parts of water so as to give it a milk-like consistency and appearance. At first, feed six times daily and at the end of a week four to five times a day. The pigs

Must have water   must have free access to fresh drinking water, in addition to the milk replacement.
At three weeks the pigs may be removed from the brooder, and at four to five weeks artificial heat is dispensed with. The replacement milk is discontinued at 20 pounds.

At another Experiment Station pigs were weaned at three weeks of age because at this time the sow's milk flow is much reduced. At the 3 weeks age—or by some at 5 weeks—they were given replacement milk and *dry feed* along with it. A pig starter used has the following formula:

Pigs weaned earlier   Table sugar, 300 pounds; coarse ground yellow corn, 350 pounds; rolled oats, 800 pounds; 60 per cent fish meal, 50 pounds; dried whey, 50 pounds; soybean oil meal, 400 pounds; ground limestone, 20 pounds; steamed bone meal, 30 pounds; salt, 10 pounds; trace mineral mix, 4 pounds. Vitamin and aureomycin are added according to manufacturer's recommendations. In addition the pigs are offered shelled corn in a creep, and an abundance of drinking water must be available at all times. With this formula pigs required from 1.5 to 1.8 pounds of feed for each pound of gain, while in old style feeding they consumed 2 to 2.5 pounds of feed for each pound of gain.

Sanitation essential in feeding pigs on substitutes   It has been ascertained in attempts to raise pigs on substitutes that it is necessary during the early days of life they be kept in heated draught-free brooders; that strict sanitation be practiced such as daily cleaning of feed vessels and brooders, and that at two or three weeks of age they have access to a palatable pig *starter* rich in protein.

Aseptic Delivery and Rearing for disease control in pigs is the object of research (Young of Minnesota and Nebraska). This system has potentialities for the con-

A unique system of swine sanitation

trol of infections of pigs on the farm, especially for those interested in rebuilding their herds from nuclei of disease-free stock. Many pig infections are contracted not only during birth through the vaginal and vulvar passage-ways, but later from surroundings. Basically the method consists of removing piglets aseptically from their dam at the termination of pregnancy, or a day or two before this, by Caesarean section (birth through a surgically made opening through the wall of the abdomen either into the uterus or removing the uterus entirely with its contained piglets.) If the uterus is removed the sow is salvaged immediately after the operation for pork—since she was anesthetized with dry ice the meat is edible. If the uterus is not removed she may later be used for rebreeding.

This operation is highly technical. Many veterinarians have established fully equipped laboratories, usually known as "Pathogen-free Swine Laboratories" or "Swine Disease-free Laboratories."

Operation is technical

A fairly effective method is to have the pigs born naturally and as aseptically as possible to meet the most rigid requirements—though by this method infection of the piglets in their passage through the birth canal cannot be avoided; to prevent some of this, tincture of iodine is at once applied to the navel.

The pigs delivered surgically are kept for a time in special equipment so that all infection is kept from them. Those delivered naturally must be placed in disinfected quarters, fed on clean food, and have separate attendants. The dam of these pigs may be rebred at the second or third heat period.

Cow's milk, homogenized and pasteurized, to which one whole egg is added to the quart, is fed every two hours between four A.M. and midnight during the first

Feed for the piglets

month after delivery, and gradually reduced to three daily feedings. By the surgical method of pig delivery and raising, it has been possible to bring pigs to maturity free from host-specific obligate parasites, swine dysentery, transmissible gastro-enteritis, atrophic rhinitis and mange. This method has also been suggested for the control of infectious rhinitis and virus pneumonia, both usually contracted from the sow.

Dr. George A. Young, of the University of Nebraska who originated this plan to have pathogen-free swine said the following:

"These techniques may be effectively used to control and eradicate swine diseases in a practical manner. The approach we plan to use is as follows:

"1. OBTAIN ASEPTIC PIGS. These would be obtained from good breeding stocks by hysterectomy* and handled as reported previously.

"2. REAR PIGS IN ISOLATION. Pigs would be housed in individual isolation units from birth by hysterectomy until one week old. During this period they would be fed cow's milk modified by addition of egg, vitamins, and mineral. From one week until four weeks of age they would be housed in groups of 8-12 in isolation brooders. They would be adapted to eating solid feed during this period.

"3. MATURE   ON   FARMS. Pigs   previously adapted to eating solid feed and water would be placed in groups of 10-20 on farms from which all other swine had been removed. Ordinary rearing methods would be employed except that no new so-called "normal" stock would be introduced and contact with other swine would be avoided by the farmer. Stock would be raised to maturity.

"4. RESUME NORMAL BIRTH. The stock which was reared to maturity on farms would be kept there and used as brood stock. Normal farrowing would be resumed, with precautions to avoid introduction of disease. When additional blood lines need to be added,

---

*Hysterectomy: Excising the uterus through an abdominal incision.

boars from other farms on the same program could be introduced.

"5. RESTOCK OTHER FARMS. The clean stock obtained on primary farms by steps 1-4 would be used to repopulate other farms. These considerations for disease control should be observed: (a) complete depopulation of swine from the premises; (b) mechanical cleansing and disinfection of premises; (c) introduction of stocks only from farms which are on the same program or from the central agency providing primary stocks; (d) avoidance of direct contact with other swine by the farmer and indirect contact in so far as possible.

"From what we have already learned about disease-free swine, the program just outlined has good likelihood of being immediately applicable to disease problems of swine. A five-year pilot study was initiated at the University of Nebraska Agricultural Experiment Station in the spring of 1956. It is hoped that such a study will make it possible for us to develop specific recommendations for the swine industry to aid in disease control."

Can Animals Exercise Instincts in the Selection of a Diet? It is debatable. In favor of this theory the following instances are cited: A group of pigs on a balanced ration acted contented, though those fed a ration low in calcium spent much time licking whitewash and attempting to root up cement and mortar from brick work. The pigs on a vitamin A deficient ration searched all the time for any chance sprig of grass or other green vegetation growing in the cracks of the floor; cattle fed on grass growing on soil deficient in phosphorus develop osteophagia or craving for bones. Young cattle on a continuous low phosphorous diet in an area cleared of bone debris satisfied their craving the moment bone in some form was made available to them.

Natural selection of foods

If they have a choice, cattle prefer hays of high

nutritive value—grown on fertilized soil. Laboratory rats will invariably select a balanced ration though it may be low in calories. Chicks allowed a free choice of foodstuffs consume less protein, less fat, somewhat more carbohydrate, and 10% less calories than those on a mixed diet of similar ingredients; however, growth and egg laying were the same in both groups.

In spite of the foregoing fragmentary evidence some researchers have reported contrary findings. If there is such a thing as the selection of correct foods by animals then they do this to satisfy a craving for something different from their regular ration. At times this leads the animal into grievous dietary errors— they will eat paint, poisonous plants, poisonous insecticides, indigestible substances such as hardware, glass, and osage orange and many other materials.

Urea in cattle feeds. Research at the time of this writing in regard to the role of urea, in dairy cattle rations was not sufficiently advanced to justify final conclusions. It has gained wide acceptance in beef cattle rations. Under natural conditions urea is the chief nitrogenous constituent of the urine, and it is the form in which the nitrogen of the body is eliminated. Therapeutically, urea is a uric acid solvent and it has diuretic properties. It does not produce off-flavor in milk except under the most unusual conditions. Neither does its use as a feed additive predispose to mastitis and other infections. Also it is poisonous in higher than therapeutic doses. Since in cattle feeds urea is often mixed with oil meals and other concentrates so as to furnish nitrogen for the building of proteins by microorganisms in the rumen (paunch) of cattle and sheep it may result in digestive upsets manifested by inappetance, bloating and even death if the urea is not thoroughly mixed in the protein feed. Urea has a tendency to become lumpy on standing and if these white lumps of urea, vary-

Urea is a urine constituent

Digestive upsets due to urea

ing in size from one-fourth inch in diameter to two or
three inches, it should not be fed, because in this form
of localized concentration it can be harm-
Increased ful. It has been shown that larger a-
carbohydrate mounts of urea may be fed in the presence
is helpful of carbohydrate. In animals dead as a result of improper or overconsumption of urea there is
usually a strong odor of ammonia in the rumen
contents.

It is of historic interest that in 1828 Wöhler synthesized urea by heating ammonium cyanate—this being the first recorded instance of an organic substance
from an inorganic compound. As an addition to the
protein ration—soybeans, linseed, alfalfa, etc. of
cattle and other ruminants—it is valueless for non-
ruminants such as horses, swine, etc., it has been
demonstrated that urea increases the activity of the
microorganisms normally present in the rumen
(paunch) so that much of the cellulose portion of it
that under ordinary conditions is not di-
Indigestible gestible becomes so. Under normal feeding
feed made practices, it appears to take 250 pounds of
digestible soybean meal to get 100 pounds of protein, but when urea is added a much larger amount of
protein is the result.

The excessive use of urea is harmful. In England
Urea is it was shown that when more than three
poisonous ounces of urea was fed per day there was
in the a depressant effect on milk production in
larger doses high producing cows.

"Most all the experimental data show quite definitely that urea is not effective when added to high-
protein grain rations for milk production purposes.
Thus, urea should not be added to grain rations already
containing 14 to 18 per cent of protein. It is most effective when added to grain rations containing 10 per
cent or less of protein, such as home-grown grains. It
appears that when urea is added to a mixture contain-

ing 10 to 11 per cent of protein, it may be utilized to the extent of 60 to 80 per cent; but if it is added to a mixture already containing 16 to 18 per cent of protein it will be utilized to the extent of 40 per cent or less." (Bur. Dairy Ind.)

"Urea can be used for wintering dry dairy cows and growing heifers. With dry cows and heifers it is possible to utilize some of the poorer quality forages along with urea and a source of readily available carbohydrate such as cereal grains and molasses. Of course, if good quality legume hay is made available to growing dairy heifers they will make normal gains without a grain supplement, according to recent work by the Bureau of Dairy Industry." (U. S. Bur. of Dairy Industry.)

Since urea has no energy value, carbohydrate must constitute a larger than usual portion of the ration.

Commercial urea is known to the chemist as carbamide. It is produced from ammonia and carbon dioxide under high pressure and temperature.

Actually urea is not a protein. However, it can be used as a substitute for protein by ruminants such as **Urea not a protein** cattle, sheep and goats. Ruminants which all have four-compartment stomachs are able to utilize the urea because the bacteria in the rumen (paunch) can convert it into amino acids and protein. The protein is stored in the bacteria **Urea and bacteria** and becomes available to the host animal as the bacteria are digested during their passage from the rumen into the true stomach and intestines.

A new concept in ruminant nutrition has been stated as follows:

"We do not actually feed cattle and sheep in a strict sense. We feed the bacteria, protozoa, and yeast in the rumen, and these billions of micro-organisms feed the animal. We are, therefore, performing a job of plant nutrition within the body of an animal."

Antibiotics: (page 248) Such antibiotics as aureomycin, procaine penicillin, terramycin and bacitracin

Value of antibiotics in weight gains of pigs
when added at the rate of 5 mg. per pound of ration, provided the pig is otherwise fed an adequate ration, either in drylot or pasture feeding, and apparently not related to the protein in the feed, will result in a 15 per cent to 30 per cent increase in the rate of gain of pigs from weaning time to 125 pounds liveweight. After the 125 weight is reached the effectiveness of these agents is very much reduced, though the value of antibiotics supplementation during the feeding period is recognized. Bred sows or gilts are not helped by the addition of these supplements, but the response in the creep-feed of nursing pigs is valuable. Runt pigs are usually helped by these agents.

In regard to bacitracin it is claimed that a single 1000-unit pellet subcutaneously placed at the base of

Method and results questioned
the ear of two day old pigs resulted in continued substantial growth-increase in pigs at least to weaning age. This growth stimulation in pigs and lambs by this method has not been substantiated in an Exp. Sta. research project.

Pigs fed 5 milligrams of aureomycin or terramycin per pound of ration, and the antibiotics

Do antibiotics cause more fat?
otics discontinued at 75 pound weight did not result in the production of an excess of fat—in fact the University of Wisconsin reported improved carcasses.

In runty pigs the growth rate has been improved as much as 100 per cent. Research indicates that the

Helps runty pigs
antibiotics are more than ordinarily valuable in creep rations for nursing pigs. There is no indication that the use of antibiotics added to sow rations during the gestation period increases litter size, pig weight, or pig health.

If pigs are handled in an approved sanitary manner (McLean County system of swine sanitation, page 672), then the addition of antibiotics to the ration seems to exert a favorable influence in the prevention of bloody diarrhoea of a vibrionic nature. Their value as curative agents has not been established.

In general it has been asserted that antibiotics influence the rate of gain in pigs (1) by reducing the numbers of harmful organisms in the intestines, and (2) by decreasing the incidence of disease.

Diethylstilbestrol (Stilbestrol) in Beef Cattle Feeding:

Diethylstilbestrol is an artificial chemical having estrogenic action (page 104) similar to natural "heat" (estrus) producing hormones, and as a feed additive for more economical gains.

It must not be included in the *feed of breeding cattle*. It may be included in the feed of beef cattle intended for slaughter and that have attained a weight of 600 pounds. Its feeding must be discontinued 48 or more hours before slaughter. Ten milligrams a day for each animal is the approved dosage, but because of the danger of excessive dosage only approved mixes may be used, i.e., 1000 milligrams of stilbestrol per pound of premix and this in turn is to be incorporated by authorized feed manufacturers at the rate of ten pounds of premix per ton of mixed feed, or this makes a level of five milligrams per pound. Unless thus thoroughly mixed the feeding is *not* approved by the Federal Food and Drug Administration. All other precautions as outlined in this paragraph are required safeguards, and under these conditions there is no data indicating a carry-over in the meat intended for human consumption.

Effect on beef cattle

When fed with an otherwise balanced ration of good feeds, it does not make good feed out of bad or poor quality feed, it resulted in increased gains of 19 per cent in steers—somewhat less in heifers—over controls not receiving it, or a saving of an estimated 10 per cent in feed costs. (Consult page 104.)

In poultry stilbestrol is used as a feed additive, and in chemical caponizing (see page 415).

CHAPTER V

VITAMINS, MINERALS, AND HORMONES AS HEALTH REQUIREMENTS

It is well known that fats, carbohydrates, proteins and minerals are not sufficient as foods to maintain life, and that there are needed other ac-

The vitamins cessory substances to sustain it. These substances are known as vitamins. For some time after their discovery their composition was unknown, though now some of them are synthetically prepared, so that they are no longer known, as formerly, by their action only. Vitamins are given an alphabetical designation.

Under ordinary storage conditions vitamins E and K are quite stable in farm roughages and grains.

The instability of vitamin A is in marked

Vitamins stable and unstable contrast to E and K. Thirty minutes of exposure of milk to direct sunlight will eliminate all of vitamin C and about 20 per cent of vitamin B_2 (riboflavin) in the milk. An overcast sky does not prevent this serious problem. Fat soluble vitamins, especially vitamin E, are quickly and almost completely destroyed by contact with rancid fats and oils in general. Avoid long storage of mixed feeds.

Vitamin A (Carotene). Occurs in butter, fish-liver oils, spinach, carrots, egg-yolk, milk, green leaves and

Vitamin A and sore eyes in the embryo of many seeds. It is fat soluble. It is absent from grains—including white corn though present in yellow corn—straws, millet, soy beans, and most peas. It promotes growth and maintains health when it is present in food stuffs, while its absence from the ration causes the sore-eye disease known as xerophthalmia (Fig. 11), (page 40) as well as emaciation and a rough coat; it is believed to increase resistance to infections. It is stored in the body as a reserve supply, but with its prolonged absence from the diet, as when animals are fed on grains other than yellow corn and if at the same time on such roughage as straw or improperly cured hays, it does not take long for the deficiency to

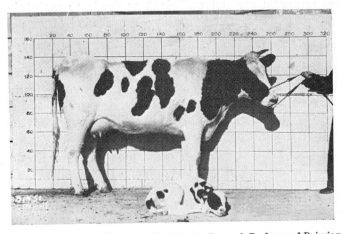

(Courtesy C. F. Huffman, Research Professor of Dairying, Michigan State University)

FIG. 8. A weak blind calf that failed to survive because the cow was fed a ration too low in vitamin A.

manifest itself by general unthriftiness. This is also shown by the appearance of sore eyes because of involvement of the cornea and also by night blindness (page 497), as it is needed for the making of visual purple of the eye, and in some cases because of constriction of the optic nerve (Fig. 9). Young calves are very likely to be deficient in this vitamin especially if the dam has been on a ration of low vitamin A potency. Since calves must obtain most of their initial vitamin from the colostrum it is important that they be permitted to have this. Whenever calves are weak and rough coated at birth, and when the blood plasma level

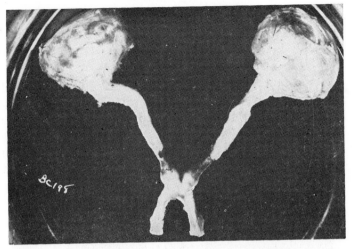

(Courtesy C. F. Huffman, Research Professor of Dairying,
Michigan State University)

FIG. 9. Constriction of optic nerves in calf as a result of low
vitamin A (carotene) supply.

of vitamin A is less than ten micrograms* per 100 cc.,
it is advised to administer 15,000 units of pure vitamin
daily. Carotene is much less effective for calves. Also
continue to give the calf the dam's milk for at least a
week of extra-uterine life, and the calf should be encouraged to eat soft, green, high-carotene hay after the
second week.

Pregnant cows—especially those calving in late
winter and early spring—may develop a vitamin A deficiency as indicated in giving birth to weak or dead
young—and when brucella negative—and blindness
(Fig. 8) or even total lack of eyes occurs in the newborn. Such cows should receive a high carotene roughage during the dry period or a high-carotene dehydrated leaf meal. A ration rich in carotene increases
the vitamin A potency of milk, but under farm conditions supplementation of concentrates for milking

*Micrograms, International or U. S. P. units are identical,
and in general are equal to 0.000,001 gram or 1/1,000,000 of a
gram.

cows is not warranted. The bull's vitamin A needs are the same as those of the pregnant cow. One-half pound of sun cured hay per day carries enough carotene to supply the needs of cattle for vitamin A.

Vitamin A deficiency in chicks, three weeks old and older, is characterized by general weakness, emaciation, staggering gait and ruffled plumage. The mucous glands of the intestines, the salivary and tear glands fail in their functions. On a post-mortem examination an outstanding lesion consists in the presence of

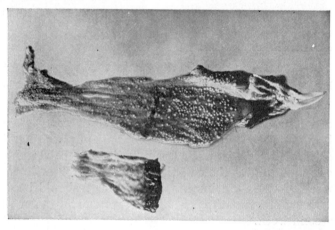

(Courtesy Department of Bacteriology, Kansas State University)

Fig. 10. Vitamin A deficiency lesions in the gullet (oesophagus) of chicken.

creamy white pustules in the roof of the mouth and extending along the lining of the gullet (oesophagus) (Fig. 10). The kidneys are enlarged and creamy white in color because of an accumulation of urates. Eye lesions (Fig. 11) are common. Egg production and hatchability are markedly reduced. Turkeys are similarly affected though usually more acutely.

Vitamin A for Swine: The National Research Council's daily vitamin A allowances for pregnant sows and gilts were 13,000 I.U. vitamin A or 20 mgs.

Relative value of vitamin A and carotene

carotene. This is based on the factor of 1.6 as the approximate conversion of crystalline carotene to vitamin A. The limited data do not give consideration to the needs of swine during pregnancy and beginning lactation. Research has shown that unit for unit carotene is less effective than preformed vitamin

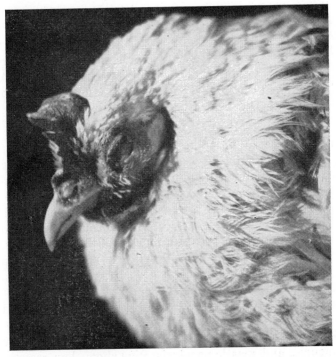

(Courtesy Department of Bacteriology, Kansas State University)

Fig. 11. Nutritional disease due to lack of vitamin A. Note the swollen condition of the eyes.

A for swine during gestation and early lactation. However, the evidence did not show that carotene supplemented sows or gilts suffer from vitamin A deficiency. In swine, partial posterior paralysis occurs, when there is deficient vitamin A before night-vision

Night blindness in swine impairment. Pigs become easily excited, fall over on one side in a spasm, squeal, and there is usually labored breathing. In the later stages, after the early symptoms of staggering gait, there is nerve degeneration and loss of use of the hind legs. Premature births are common in advanced pregnancy.

Vitamin A deficiency is probably the commonest vitamin deficiency disease of cattle. Forage, fresh or cured, is the chief source of carotene for **Vitamin A deficiency in cattle** livestock. Green pastures and properly cured green grass or legume, or silage in winter will prevent or cure vitamin A deficiency in cattle, sheep and swine. (Consult page 71 for vitamin D deficiency.)

Vitamin B (Thiamin). This is a water soluble vitamin. It occurs in milk, yolk of eggs, the husks of **Vitamin B not stored in the body** grain, leaves, roots and fruits of growing plants, and in yeast. It is also essential for growth, and it is not stored in the body, therefore a continuous supply is essential. When not supplied, it causes an abnormal reaction to take place in the nerves and muscles in fowls and rats, and shrinking of the muscles with nerve pains in man (beriberi), and a skin disease with mental disorders. There are several subdivisions of it. Ruminants appear to synthesize thiamin in the digestive tract and are not subject to a deficiency of it. Dogs show a deficiency by lack of appetite, loss of weight, convulsive seizures, and spastic paralysis. Pigs show slow growth, lack of appetite and leg weakness. Poultry are unthrifty with head retraction, and unless the deficiency is corrected death ensues. Chicks and laying hens should receive 180 International Units per pound of total ration; dogs 12 micrograms daily per pound of body weight. For pigs the required amount has not been determined. Ruminants do not need it in the ration as it is synthesized by rumen flora though within recent months the theory has been advanced that the synthesis of this vitamin is due to an interaction between the mineral cobalt and infusoria of the rumen (page 91). Also, that so-called "cobalt deficiency" is in fact a vitamin B deficiency because the cobalt is not present to stimulate the infusoria in the production of this vitamin. Under ordinary conditions there will be no thiamin deficiency in animals that receive a high proportion of whole grains in the ration, but if whole grains—"whole grains" means those grains that retain all their natural constituents—are absent from the ration, or present in small amounts, a deficiency may occur.

Vitamin B_2 complex: This complex includes many components as follows: thiamine hydrochloride, riboflavin, (page 511) niacin (nicotinic acid), vitamin B_6 or pyrodoxine hydrochloride, pantothenic acid, choline, biotin, inositol, para-amino-benzoic acid, folic acid which consists of two factors B_{10} and B_{11} which influence growth and feather production of chicks, B_{12} isolated from liver found to be of value in treating pernicious anemia. There also has been announced factor X or animal protein factor (page 44) which now seems to appear as B_{12}; isolated in 1949, B_{14} is said to have high activity on cell proliferation. All of these are water soluble vitamins. They are contained in soybean meal, grains, alfalfa and other green feeds. For optimum performance in dry lot feeding of pigs certain "unidentified factors" (vitamin B_{12}) (page 44) contained in plant, animal, and fish by-products (dried corn distillers' solubles, condensed fish solubles—usually combined with alfalfa meal, AB liver extract, fortified dried whey products, and meat scraps) are to be added. Taken as a whole swine raised on green succulent forage obtain all the water-soluble vitamins they need. When changed to the dry lot they carry enough of these substances in their tissues to last them for some time. This is known as "residual effect."

When the residual effect wears off supplements containing the water-soluble vitamins need to be supplied. Now that vitamin B_{12} is available synthetically to add as a feed supplement it is more economical than when it had to be supplied in poultry and pig feed as high priced fish and meat meals and dried skim milk. In dogs "black-tongue" (pellagra) is a niacin (nicotinic acid) deficiency (page 511).

A biotin deficiency in chicks (Fig. 12) characterized by foot changes is quite common. First the bottoms of the feet become rough and calloused, and finally the entire bottom of the foot becomes encrusted

Sore feet in chicks   with the appearance of bleeding cracks; the toes may even become necrotic and slough off. Later changes occur in the angles of the mouth, and the eyes are swollen and the lids adhere to each other. In mature fowl biotin deficiency results in lower egg hatchability.

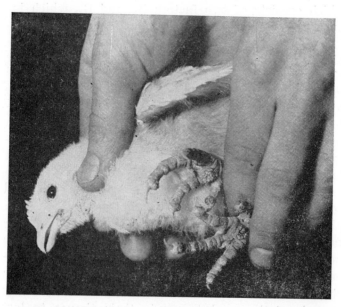

(Courtesy National Research Council)

FIG. 12. Biotin deficiency. Note the lesions on the bottom of the feet and in the corner of the beak.

Vitamin C, also known as ascorbic acid, cevitamic acid and avitamic acid. This is a water soluble vitamin of vegetables and of juices of such fruits as tomatoes, oranges, lemons and grapes. It is not stored in the body. The effect of its prolonged absence in the diet manifests itself in laboratory animals and man in the well known disease scurvy in which there are sore joints, bleeding and sore gums, loosening of the teeth, and fragile bones. This disease was formerly very common in sailors compelled to subsist during long trips on sailing vessels on a diet devoid of fresh vegetables and fruit juices.

Vitamin C and scurvy

Vitamin D (Calciferol). A fat-soluble vitamin contained in butterfat and fish-liver oils, irradiated dry yeast, sun-cured legume hay, alfalfa meal made from sun-cured alfalfa, but poor in artificially cured hay. It is only fairly present in whole milk. Vegetable oils do not ordinarily contain it. There are several forms of this vitamin such as D_2 or ergosterol which is in irradiated yeast, and D_3 or 7-dehydrocholesterol which predominates in fish liver oils. The action of this vitamin appears to be identical to that of direct sunlight or certain electric lights known as ultra-violet radiation. This radiation is not effective if the sunlight is filtered through window glass. Vitamin D is concerned with a proper deposition of lime (page 80) ; its absence in the body—phosphorus is a factor—is followed by the appearance of the disease rickets (Fig. 13) (page 504) in young animals, and in older animals by a harmful change in the existing lime or calcium balance in the body. It has the power to control the development of a satisfactory skeleton even when the calcium-phosphorus ratio is unfavorable, provided the supply of neither of these two minerals is below the mineral requirement (page 80). In housed animals during winter months when solar radiation is at a minimum, and if such animals are not consumers of large

Vitamin D and rickets

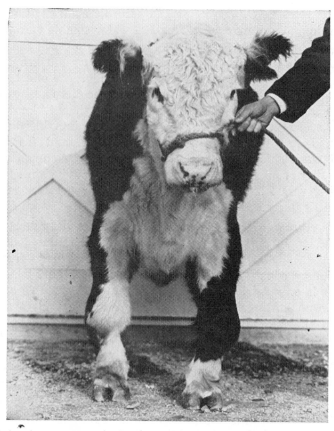

(Courtesy Animal Husbandry Division, Bureau of Animal Industry, U.S.D.A.)

FIG. 13. Experimentally produced rickets because the animal from early in life was maintained on a ration deficient in vitamin D, and no exposure to direct sunlight.

amounts of sun-cured roughages—especially pigs, young calves and poultry (page 162)—they are likely to show evidence of vitamin D inadequacy such as rickets (page 504).

Vitamin E (Alpha Tocopherol). This is the reproductive vitamin contained in lettuce leaves, vegetable

Vitamin E and fertility oils, whole oats and wheat, egg-yolk, beef liver, and in unusual potency in the embryos of wheat. It is not present in milk.

Alpha tocopherol occurs as a viscous, nearly colorless oil. It is stable to heat, but is destroyed by association with rancid fats. In sheep, swine and rats a deficiency results in reproductive failure, though goats are not similarly affected. In suckling pigs defective muscular nutrition resulted when the vitamin was withheld from the sows. In female rats a deficiency of it results in embryonic mortality and in males degeneration of the testes. In cattle the effect of an inadequate supply of this vitamin has not yet been sufficiently clarified to warrant an authoritative statement. Because of the general tendency to use the vitamin E, rich germ of cereals in human foods, animals get the left overs, livestock feeders should not overlook supplying their charges adequately. Absence of vitamin E, which is stored only to a slight extent in the body, is especially noticed in animals during the late winter months when the previously stored vitamin E is exhausted, and the animal has not yet had an opportunity to replenish its supply by the consumption of green growing feed. Adequate amounts of it prevent and even correct "white muscle disease" in calves and lambs. (Page 514.)

Vitamin K. In order that coagulation of blood will take place whenever bleeding is an outstanding symptom, certain substances normally present in the blood of individuals must interact. These substances are an enzyme, thrombin, prothrombin and fibrinogen. Prothrombin for its synthesis in the liver requires some form of vitamin K. Therefore in the absence of vitamin K—this vitamin is in alfalfa, though low in solvent extracted soybean meal—the chain of events in normal clotting is not complete, and the resulting bleeding may go on to a fatal termination. The substance used for the destruction of rats and other rodents known as "Warfarin" produces internal bleeding; in this instance dicoumarin which is at times present in sweet-

Vitamin K not important in animals

clover is the agent in "warfarin" (page 335). Vitamin K has therefore been suggested in the handling of "sweetclover disease," and in accidental "warfarin" poisoning.

Vitamin deficiency disease or conditions are relatively uncommon in animals when they are kept under reasonably natural conditions, because **Lack of vitamins** their diet is then so varied that it is almost impossible to miss receiving all the required vitamins. Under artificial feeding practices and housing, the situation changes, however, and unthriftiness, eye diseases, bone diseases, forms of barrenness and others are observed with surprising frequency. As soon as these deficiencies are observed, the ration should be balanced, and if intense structural or pathological changes have not taken place, recovery may follow the adoption of the improved feeding regime.

The latest available information seems to indicate that the condition formerly spoken of as cottonseed **Vitamins and cotton-seed meal "poisoning"** meal poisoning may be very largely a vitamin deficiency disease. (Page 49.) Cottonseed meal is one of the economical and very valuable sources of vegetable protein in the animal diet, but unfortunately its continuous feeding in amounts not exceeding from one to one and one-half pounds daily to a steer on feed is followed by an abnormal condition in the eyes, urinary and digestive disturbances, and incoordination of movement. These symptoms were originally entirely ascribed to an active principal in the cottonseed meal known as gossypol which was assumed to produce a gradual poisoning of some highly susceptible animals, and though gossypol has not been entirely eliminated as a source of trouble, it has been established that animals fed on roughage having a high vitamin A content such as good leafy pea-green alfalfa in addition to the cottonseed meal allowance do not develop the symptoms previously ascribed to the over-consumption of cottonseed meal.

The fact that the symptoms do not appear when all the other conditions are identical, though with the addition of vitamin A containing roughage, to the ration, is reasonably conclusive evidence that most of the so-called cottonseed meal "poisoning" is in fact a vitamin A deficiency disease. To avoid cottonseed meal "poisoning," give the animals leafy alfalfa in moderate amounts daily. For swine the treatment of cottonseed meal with iron, or autoclaving it, seems to make it better tolerated.

Minerals must also be included in the ration to maintain the nutritional requirements, and to permit

The minerals many physiological processes to take place. Minerals include such substances as salt (chloride of soda), lime, (calcium), phosphorus, iron, copper, iodine, potash, magnesium, manganese, zinc, cobalt, and possibly others. These substances are needed by the animal body for its actual growth as well as for the performance of physiological and physical functions. Most of the minerals, with the possible exception of salt, are contained in sufficient amounts in the grains and roughages of the average well balanced ration. Grains and straw are poor in phosphorus, though this element is usually abundant in well cured hays, and it is unusually plentiful in the tips of the growing wheat plant, as well as in bran. Lime is present in hay, and it is low in grains. Iodine, iron, copper, cobalt, and other minerals are needed only in infinitesimally small amounts.

As an example of these mineral needs of the body, it is well to consider salt and its uses. In the digestive processes hydrochloric acid, a substance rich in chlorine, is very essential and it obtains its chlorine from salt, salt being a chemical combination of soda and chlo-

Salt aids in the functions of the body rine. It is furthermore necessary in the body that some liquids shall pass through some of the animal membranes. This takes place only when the amount of salt in solution in the liquids on one side of the membrane exceeds the amount of salt in solution on the opposite side. Under the foregoing conditions, the liquids will pass from one side of the membrane to the opposite side until there is an exact balance between the salt content of the liquids on both sides of the membrane. This process is known as osmosis. Also, salt is a constituent of many of the tissues of the body such as the blood, tears and other secretions. Salt must always be supplied to animals in addition to the amounts contained in the usual well balanced ration. Swine especially because of their rapid growth, and frequently they are not pastured, need a good supply of salt. They can be made to mature earlier and on less feed if their ration includes 2½ pounds of salt in every 100 pounds of meal. Dairy cows should have one pound of fine salt with each 100 pounds of grain and in addition an available supply where they can help themselves.

Good livestock management calls for free access to salt at all times for cattle. Whether on dry-lot roughage rations, or on grass, salt may mean the **Salt needed for gains** difference between a profit or a loss. In winter feeding tests steer calves on a roughage ration, with free access to salt, gained an average of 40 pounds more per head in 138 days than similar steers which got no salt. Larger amounts of feed were consumed by the "salted" calves . . . and they made more efficient gains.

Two trials were conducted in dry lot. The calves which had free access to salt produced 100 pounds of gain at a feed cost of $12.21 for one lot and $16.04 for another. With two similar lots, which got no salt, the feed costs were $19.99 and $19.62 respectively. (1953).

Steers on a full feed of grain with salt free-choice for 210 days averaged 2.21 pounds of gain per head daily. Steers on the same ration without salt gained 2.15 pounds per head per day. This test showed little difference in feed consumption or economy of gain

TABLE NO. 1—Mineral Requirements of Swine*

(Data Taken From National Research Council Bulletin Recommended Nutrient Allowances For Swine)

Live Weight of Animal (lbs.)	Pounds of Total Feed Dry Basis (Per Animal Per Day)	Calcium		Phosphorus		Potassium		Sodium	
		Grams Per Day	Per Cent in Ration	Grams Per Day	Per Cent in Ration	Grams Per Day	Per Cent in Ration	Grams Per Day	Per Cent in Ration
50................	2.7	7.4	.60	4.9	.40	1.3	.11	2.7	.22
100...............	5.	13.7	.60	9.1	.40	2.5	.11	5.0	.22
150...............	6.6	15.8	.53	10.5	.35	3.8	.12	6.6	.22
200...............	7.5	17.9	.52	11.9	.35	5.0	.14	7.5	.22
250...............	8.3	17.9	.47	11.9	.31	6.0	.16	8.3	.22
Pregnant Gilts and Sows, Young Boars......	6.	16.4	.60	10.9	.40	6.0	.22	6.0	.22
Lactating Sows, Breeding Boars............	10 to 15	27 to 41	.60	18 to 27	.40	12.5	.22	12.5	.22

*"Trace elements" (page 85) not included.

TABLE NO. 2—Average Mineral Content of Some Hog Feeds

	Per Cent Calcium	Per Cent Phosphorus	Per Cent Sodium	Per Cent Potassium	Per Cent Magnesium	ppm Manganese	ppm Cobalt	ppm Copper
Corn	.02	.27	.02	.27	.08	5.	.1	3.
Barley	.05	.38	.07	.5	.17	8.	.01	4.
Oats	.09	.33	.16	.43	.16	40.	.05	5.
Wheat	.03	.43	.05	.55	.16	110.	.1	10.
Kafir-Milo	.04	.30	.04	.34		13.	.05	10.
Soybean Oil Meal	.28	.65	.45	1.8	.26	25.	.10	22.
Peanuts (shelled)	.06	.38	.56	.54	.18			
Peanut Oil Meal	.17	.55	.07	1.5	.36			
Linseed Meal	.35	.75	.14	1.1	.42	40.	.1	25.
Cottonseed Meal	.24	1.10	.25	1.5	.64	16.	.1	8.
Fish Meal (60 per cent)	5.	3.3	.55	.33	.15	20.	.16	8.
Tankage (60 per cent)	6.2	4.3	1.0	.46	.75	20.	.20	40.
Meat Scrap (55 per cent)	8.5	4.3	1.5	.55		9.	.15	11.
Alfalfa Hay, Sun Cured	1.5	.20		1.7	.30	15.	.05	5.
Alfalfa Hay, Dehydrated	1.81	.31	.04	2.1	.33	14.	.09	5.
Alfalfa Pasture	.35	.07	.54	.56	.05	12.		2.
Skim Milk, dry basis	1.24	1.0		1.46	.12	2.5	.15	11.
Bone Meal	25.0	11.				2.	.06	18.
Limestone	38.0					40.		

when steers were on full feed of grain. It was also observed that steers wintered on dry grass consumed as much or more salt than those on summer pasture.

At the Kansas Agricultural Experiment Station steers consumed 1½ pounds of salt per month when on pasture; three pounds per month on alfalfa hay, and nine pounds per month when on corn ensilage. It is generally advised to provide at least 20 pounds of salt per head per year. Sheep and lambs have a very high salt requirement; tests prove that for the fastest gains lambs should receive ½ pound of salt per month, and ewes one pound. Sheep fed on a ration containing 0.5, 4.8, 9.1, and 13.1 per cent of salt were not harmfully affected during a growing, fattening, breeding, gestation and lactation period extending over 253 days —the ewes on the high percentage suffered the greatest weight loss during the lactation period. Horses lose 30 grains of salt in every pound of perspiration and therefore when worked on hot days salt should be added to their drinking water. (Page 521.)

Since milk is rich in both sodium and chlorine calves that are either nursing or handfed do not as a rule need additional salt. However, since many calves are weaned at an early age the addition of one per cent of salt to the calf starter is advisable.

The data in the two tables reveal several facts of great importance in swine feeding:

1. Rations composed entirely of cereal grains are always deficient in calcium, phosphorus and sodium. However there is no deficiency of potassium.

2. Rations of cereal grains supplemented with oil meals such as soybean, cottonseed, linseed and peanut are deficient in calcium and border line deficient in phosphorus and sodium. While these meals are much better sources of phosphorus and sodium than cereal grains, they are not usually

consumed in sufficient amounts to overcome the deficiencies of the grains.

3. Animal by-products such as tankage, meat and bone scrap, fish meal, steamed bone meal, and skim milk are excellent sources of calcium and phosphorus. Swine allowed free access to these products will usually consume enough to satisfy their calcium and phosphorus needs. Defluorinated rock phosphate is a fairly satisfactory substitute for steamed bone meal.

4. Legume hays and pastures are good sources of calcium but are deficient in phosphorus and sodium.

In swine feeding, therefore, calcium (lime), phosphorus, and sodium are a necessity to prevent weak bones as shown by rickets (Figs. 13, 14 and 15), lameness, easily broken bones, impaired growth; also in sows poor lactation, and "down in the back" or hind limbs at the time of nursing the young. In the way of feed requirement for swine there should be free access to such animal products as fish meal, tankage, meat and bone scrap, bone meal or skim milk and salt—the latter iodized in some areas where iodine is deficient in the soil as evidenced by hairlessness and "big-neck" in newly born pigs. If a mineral mixture is used in dry-lot feeding it should contain steamed bone meal or a defluorinated calcium compound, with an added twenty-five per cent level of sodium chloride (salt) in the mineral mixture either plain or iodized as the requirement may be.

Adequate lime, phosphorus and sodium are essential

It is not enough to simply supply the animals with the required amount of lime and phosphorus, because for lime utilization by the body the additional action of ultraviolet radiation is necessary (vitamin D, page 71). This may be obtained by direct exposure to the sun's rays daily, or the simultaneous administration of a fish-liver oil. Regarding the utilization of lime by the

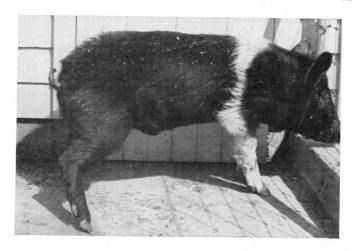

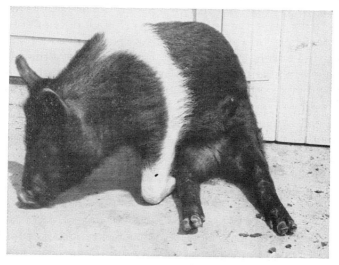

(Courtesy of Dr. C. E. Aubel, Kansas State University)

FIGS. 14 and 15. These conditions developed after 12 weeks on a ration deficient in calcium.

cooperative action of the sun or a fish-liver oil, the theory is that cod, halibut and other fishes exist largely on very minute forms of marine life. These minute forms live mostly on the surface of the water where they are continuously exposed to the ultra-violet sun radiation; their bodies thus become heavily impregnated with the vitamin which is in turn imparted to their devourer the large cod, halibut or shark, and stored in the livers of these fish, to be later expressed in combination with the oil. In other words, the fish-liver oils with their high vitamin content are essentially bottled sunshine, and either exposure to sunshine or ingesting a fish liver oil is needed in order that the body will utilize the lime offered it.

So called wheat plant "poisoning" or grass tetany (page 501) in cattle frequently develops in those animals grazed on winter wheat pasture **Deficiency** without a supplementary lime-containing **of lime and** ration. It is reasonably well established **wheat-plant** as being a lime or calcium and magnesium **"poisoning"** deficiency disease. Affected animals have spasms of the muscles of the extremities which may develop into convulsions of the entire body. That the symptoms are the result of a deficient calcium intake—though magnesium sulphate is also required—is demonstrated by prompt recovery following the intravenous administration of a calcium salt. In the light of this knowledge, it is reasonable to recommend that animals offered no other ration than wheat pasture should have before them at all times a mineral mixture from which they may partake at will. Either finely ground limestone, or a mixture of equal parts of finely ground limestone, hard wood ashes and salt is satisfactory for preventive purposes.

Usually the roughages are good sources of calcium —especially the legumes, and therefore when an animal receives good alfalfa or clover it gets much more calcium than it can utilize. There is usually no justification for feeding dairy cattle a calcium supplement with rations of grain and timothy hay; or with rations of grain, timothy hay and silage; or with rations of grain, timothy hay and pasture. Only when grasses, corn ensilage and the straws of the cereal grains are grown on acid soils is there likely to be a deficiency of calcium.

Chickens also are usually urgently in need of lime or calcium, especially when they are not permitted free range. They need it for physiological bone building and for egg shell production. The most acceptable form of lime for poultry is found in crushed oyster shell, and fowl under confinement should be given free access to this, especially if there is some evidence of leg weakness.

Egg layers need lime

Phosphorus is found abundantly in wheat bran, linseed meal, cottonseed meal, soybean oil meal, and wheat middlings. Other cereal grains are only medium in their phosphorus content, while root crops, sugar beet pulp, molasses, and corn gluten are very low in this element. Corn seems to be the cereal grain that is lowest in phosphorus. Milk, either whole or skimmed, is rich in phosphorus. Bonemeal is an excellent source of supplementary phosphorus.

Phosphorus sources

Numerous experiments have demonstrated that during drought conditions the phosphorus content of plants is low (page 499). Phosphorus fertilization seems to influence favorably the amount of phosphorus in a plant but here again the pH of the soil has a significant bearing.

In dairy cattle fed on alfalfa hay containing at least 0.18 per cent of phosphorus—even when the concentrate ration was the low-phosphorus-containing corn—the supply was adequate. If a deficiency exists—less than four milligrams per 100 cc. of blood plasma—then the addition of equal parts of odorless steamed bone meal and salt offered free-will, or added to the extent of two per cent to the grain will supply all requirements. Raw rock phosphate and the phosphorus containing limestones are not usually to be recommended owing to their frequently comparatively high fluorine content—

Phosphorus needs

Fluorine danger over 3½ to 4 per cent—as the fluorine has an unfavorable effect on the teeth (pages 419 and 490). Only defluorinated phosphates containing less than 0.2 fluorine should be fed to supply a phosphorus deficiency. However, fluorosis is not nearly as serious in animals as in man.

The usual evidences of phosphorus deficiency are loss of appetite and a depraved appetite—though in a severe phosphorus deficiency this latter symptom is frequently absent in milking cows. A decrease in milk production—when other factors are adequate—is a most suggestive symptom. "Bone-chewing" by cattle is of little—if any—significance as a symptom of phosphorus deficiency. Farm animals—with the possible exception of poultry—are seldom sufferers from a phosphorus deficiency.

As to poultry the phosphorus situation still needs some clarification. Phosphorus in the feedstuffs of vegetable origin is in the form of phytin (according to Dorland phytin is the proprietary name of a calcium-magnesium salt of inositol hexaphosphoric acid), and this seems to be usable by poultry to only a limited extent—in fact it requires 16 times as much vitamin D to promote phytin absorption as to cause phosphorus utilization when in the form of inorganic salts. Latest figures indicate that growing chicks for proper bone development require a minimum of 0.4 of phosphorus in readily available form in the ration.

Phosphorus and egg laying Laying hens must have at least 0.75 per cent of phosphorus—balanced with 2.25 per cent of calcium—in the ration to meet the requirements of the bones and eggs—lecithin and vitellin in the latter. This comparatively high phosphorus need is because of the rapid turnover of this element in laying hens.

The lowest calcium and phosphorus requirements of growing turkeys, because of their rapid growth, have been set at 2.0 per cent and 1.0 per cent respectively of the ration. The calcium phosphorus ratio for breeding turkeys has been set at 2.25 and 0.75 per cent, respectively in the ration. In order to assist in the utilization of both calcium and phosphorus—both for bone formation and the avoidance of rickets, and for egg production—extra vitamin D should be supplied either as 1.0 per cent of cod-liver oil (page 71) in the ration, or ultraviolet energy from direct sunlight, or from artificial sources.

Prevention of rickets

Then there are the group of minerals referred to as "trace elements" because the animal economy needs these only in very minute quantities—but for well being they are nevertheless absolutely essential.

Trace elements or minerals essential

The "trace elements" or "trace minerals" are iodine, iron, copper, zinc, manganese, magnesia, potassium and cobalt.

The *iodine* requirements of the animal body—in comparatively infinitesimal amounts are very specific. In most parts of the United States with possibly the exception of those in the great lakes region and in the far northwest, there is enough iodine in the soil to supply in adequate amounts by means of vegetation, the needs of man and animal. In those sections of the country where the soil is deficient in iodine so that people and animals do not receive the necessary maintenance amounts, it is a legal requirement that a small amount of iodine shall regularly be incorporated in table salt, and this is marketed as iodized salt. This same iodized salt is usually offered for sale in states in which there is no need of extra iodine, but the amount is so small that its consumption is free from known harm, and the addition of iodine has not increased to the consumer the cost of the salt. Deficiency of iodine is manifested in people in a form of enlargement of the thyroid gland of the neck called goiter. In little pigs a comparable condition, frequently present at birth and due to the same cause, is designated "big-neck" (page 497), and a deficiency of iodine also is responsi-

Lack of iodine causes abnormal conditions

ble for the naked or hairless condition of the body at birth (Fig. 129). In the case of animals the addition of as little as two grains of iodide of potash daily, this chemical being very rich in iodine, to the ration of the sow during the last three or four weeks of pregnancy, or, giving the animal its usual salt allowance in the form of iodized salt will prevent the "big-neck" and the hairlessness of new born pigs.

Iron and copper are equally as important in small amounts as iodine, because the blood soon becomes impoverished without a regular supply of
Iron and copper are essential these substances. Little pigs especially contract the so-called little-pig anemia (page 494) if they do not receive iron and copper. The disease is essentially a very low number of red blood cells and decreased hemoglobin so that all the visible mucous membranes assume a pale color; at the same time the pig gradually weakens and frequently dies during the nursing period of its existence. The disease is almost certain to make its appearance when the little pigs receive as nourishment only their mother's milk *without having access to soil, cinders, or comparable material.* All soil and cinders contain the small amounts of iron and copper so necessary for the pig's health, and the pig usually gets these minerals even during the nursing period of its existence by rooting or licking the dirt.

The disease is far more prevalent in early spring litters, because the weather is too cold for an out-of-door life with access to soil, and then if kept indoors and on permanent flooring, such as cement or planks, they are denied the soil containing the necessary iron and copper. It is claimed that much of this trouble may be prevented by throwing into the pig pen each day a piece of sod which the little pigs may lick. A better form of prevention is to daily paint the mammary gland and nipples of the sow with a solution consisting of one-tenth of one per cent of commercial copperas (iron sulphate, which has copper as an impurity) in water and corn syrup. During nursing, the little pig will get enough of the iron and copper to prevent the development of pig anemia. Iron dextran (commercially "Imferon") for quick results, administered intramuscularly, has received favorable reception by physicians and veterinarians.

In South Australia there is a condition in sheep known as "coast disease" in which an observed symptom is a loss of crimp in the wool. It has been demonstrated that the trouble is due to a copper deficiency—cobalt has nothing to do with it—because it can be prevented by the daily administration of five milligrams of copper sulphate. Fifty milligrams of copper daily produced symptoms of copper poisoning. In the Gulf Coast region of Texas "creeps" of cattle is a phosphorus deficiency.

From a reliable source in Scotland comes information that in addition to hemoglobin formation the addition of one per cent of copper sulphate in the ration of animals, that were pastured on copper deficient grasses, and that were affected with incoordinated gait, abnormal wool production, sway-back, degenerative changes in the central nervous system, "falling disease," and sudden death, was beneficial. This diagnosis was confirmed by an abnormally low concentration of copper in the liver, blood and milk of affected animals.

Zinc is believed to be necessary to the animal body for the operation of certain enzyme actions. It influences the rate of absorption of carbohydrates and proteins from the gastro-intestinal tract. A deficiency of zinc results in impaired growth, and the depression of certain enzyme actions. In swine a lack of it is the cause of a skin condition known as *parakeratosis*.

A review of research on the nutritional significance of zinc (Nutr. Rev., Oct., 1955: 303) indicates how its association with *parakeratosis* in swine was discovered. A severe dermatitis in swine, resembling parakeratosis, developed when a processed peanut meal was the source of protein in the ration. However, pigs with access to clover or alfalfa were not affected. This dermatitis was then produced in ten weeks by adding 2.0 per cent bone meal or 1.5 per cent calcium carbonate to certain rations, but it could be prevented by the further addition of 0.02 per cent zinc carbonate. The therapeutic effect of this zinc was prompt, the appetite and weight gain being resumed within one week.

Which ion aggravates the zinc deficiency is not known, but it might be presumed that calcium phosphate blocks the absorption of the zinc ion rather than competing with zinc in the body. Factors which may combine to produce parakeratosis are: a relatively low zinc content in the feed, increased quantities of calcium or phosphate, and relatively higher requirements of the pig for zinc. In regard to zinc, federal research workers (reported in the November 1956, issue of the Journal of Animal Science) state as follows: "When the diets of growing pigs contain up to 1.0% of calcium, the minimum zinc content for the prevention of parakeratosis is between 44 p.p.m. and 80 p.p.m." When there were only 32 p.p.m. of zinc in the diet parakeratosis appeared in three of six animals—when this was changed to 80

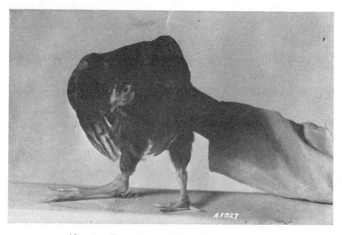

(Courtesy Department of Bacteriology, Kansas State University)

FIG. 16. Perosis or slipped tendon in a chicken due to lack of mineral—probably manganese.

p.p.m. the pigs in 28 days were as good as normal, though the scabs were not all shed.

Manganese is found in wheat bran, wheat middlings and hays grown on acid soils. A ration low in manganese interferes with reproduction in swine, and this element is also necessary for their normal growth. However, the quantity required is low even for sows and on the basis of present knowledge it seems evident that nature will take care of the needs of the body in this respect. In poultry, however, it is an element of major importance. In growing birds a deficiency of it is manifested by slow growth, shortening of the wing and leg bones—in the latter it is followed by so-called "slipped tendon" or perosis (Fig. 16) (page 511), and decreased enzyme—phosphatase to split the phosphoric acid esters of carbohydrates—in the blood and bones.

In producing hens loss of weight, lower egg and shell strength, decreased hatchability with nutritional disturbance in cartilage formation are characteristics; spasms of the head and neck in chicks have also been observed. The amount of manganese needed by growing chicks seems to be subject to some variation depending in a measure on the size of the breed. From 35 parts of manganese to one million parts of the diet for the lighter breeds and up to 50 parts per million for the heavier breeds prevented perosis. However, this latter statement carries with it the implication that the diet is balanced and adequate in other minerals and in biotin, choline and folic acid (page 69).

It has been established that a dietary deficiency in this element results in testicular degeneration in males, and depressed lactation and maternal instinct in females, as well as depressed growth in both sexes. The element has a tendency to accumulate in the gonads.

Manganese essential for reproduction in rats, mice, poultry and rabbits

Pigs have been reported to grow normally and reproduce successfully on rations containing less than ten parts of manganese per million. However, recent work at the University of Wisconsin indicates that significantly faster growth in pigs can be secured on rations containing higher levels. In these tests the basal ration of corn, soybean oil meal, gluten meal, alfalfa meal, limestone and salt which assayed 12 ppm of manganese was improved by adding enough manganese sulfate to bring the total manganese content of the ration up to 55 ppm. No advantage was obtained at higher levels and toxicity symptoms began to appear at a level of 500 ppm. This work indicates that swine growing rations consisting principally of cereal grains, all of which are low in manganese, may not always supply enough of the element to support optimum growth. It would seem to be wise to supplement swine rations with enough manganese sulfate to bring the total manganese content of the ration up to around 50 ppm. It seems probable that traces of manganese are also nutritionally essential for cattle, sheep and horses but this has not as yet been demonstrated.

Magnesia deficiency in most farm animals is not a problem under ordinary conditions. Many still hold that the muscular spasms—tetany—observed in so-called "wheat-poisoning" are in a measure the results of a hypomagnesemia or lowered magnesia level in the bodily tissues. Others contend that these spasms are due to a faulty calcium-potassium ration in the plasma and serum of the blood. It has been demonstrated that rats and dogs on diets low in magnesia develop symptoms almost paralleling those observed in grass tetany. Magnesium deficiency symptoms have been induced in rats, rabbits and chickens by placing them on a highly purified diet and in calves by keeping them a long time on a straight milk diet, however, such symptoms have not been reported to occur in swine. Since the feeds commonly fed to swine supply several times the amounts of magnesium required by these other animals

Magnesia and spasms

the danger of a magnesium deficiency on any type of practical ration is remote.

Potassium, another trace element, is widely distributed in feed stuffs of both vegetable and animal sources. In fowl at least there is three times as much potassium as sodium in the soft tissues—in the bones they are about equal in amount. On the heart's activity potassium favors relaxation or the opposite of calcium, and its ions are believed to enhance tissue permeability or osmosis. Chicks should have from 0.20 to 0.24 per cent in the diet; usually these amounts are present in vegetation and animal proteins.

Cobalt (pages 21 and 69) has received a good deal of attention as a required trace element and there is still some confusion about it. As an example of the incomplete knowledge it has been determined that cobalt administered by way of the mouth is very much more effective than when injected into the blood and this has given rise to the belief that the cobalt is essential in the animal's rumen or paunch—only cattle and sheep are known to suffer from so-called cobalt deficiency—in order that the synthesis of vitamin B—especially nicotinic acid and riboflavin—by rumen infusoria may take place. It is known that cobalt is an essential part of the vitamin B_{12} molecule (page 69). This vitamin is needed for the normal formation of and metabolism of the red constituent (hemoglobin) of the blood. In animals with a single stomach such as the horse, hog, dog, cat, etc. there does not appear to be a direct relationship between cobalt and hemoglobin formation, though in animals having a multiple stomach as in cattle, sheep, goats, etc. one of the symptoms of cobalt deficiency that has existed for some time is a profound paleness of the visible mucous membranes indicating an anemia.

Cobalt a part of vitamin B_{12} molecule

It has been pointed out that many of the symptoms observed in avitaminoses B such as loss of appetite and

general starvation are also noticeable in so-called
cobalt deficiency (page 69) ; in fact, it is at times not
clinically possible to distinguish between phosphorus
and cobalt deficiencies, and in this connection veterinarians usually adopt the attitude that if the symptoms
are observed in calves only, or in both cows and calves,
suspect cobalt deficiency, but if the symptoms are
noticed in cows only suspect phosphorus deficiency.
When cobalt is needed either cobalt chloride, cobalt
acetate, or cobalt sulphate may be used for calves at
the rate of a teaspoonful daily of a solution made by
dissolving one ounce of the cobalt salt in one gallon of
water; for mature cows one half ounce of the cobalt is
added to 100 pounds of salt and this mixture is then
fed at the usual rate. If cobalt deficiency is the trouble
then recovery is almost dramatic after three days to a
week of cobalt treatment. Some of the diseases of cattle
that have disappeared following cobalt administration
are "Grand Traverse or Lake Shore Disease" in Michigan; "Salt Sickness" in Florida; "Bush Sickness" in
New Zealand; "Pine Disease" in Scotland; Enzootic
Marasmus; Nutritional Anemia, and others.

Slack Coal for Hogs. Since minerals have been the
subject for discussion it seems appropriate to bring in
here the matter of allowing hogs free-
choice coal-slack, especially as they seem
to relish it—some swine producers furnish
it regularly to their hogs as a part of the
animals' diet.

Coal slack— is it harmful?

Chemically a sample of soft coal contained 19.05
per cent water, 19.19 per cent ash, most of which was
iron oxide, 66.6 per cent carbon, 3.25 hydrogen, 0.49
per cent sulphur, and 1.42 per cent nitrogen. In other
words more than two-thirds is carbon, with a minute
amount of iron—the latter also abundant in the soil.

Cornell University bulletin No. 836 reports on a
carefully controlled research project in which one to
three per cent of carbon was added to the swine ration.
It had no observable effect, except as one authority re-

marks rather facetiously it may have made them happier. Coal-slack will certainly not take the place of calcium, phosphorus, iodine and others.

Many hog raisers commonly have before their hogs as free-choice a mineral mixture made of two parts of steamed bone-meal, two parts of powdered limestone and one part of salt. In regions where iodine deficiency is common use iodized salt in the mixture. It is estimated that such a mixture need not constitute more than two per cent of the total ration of swine.

In concluding the minerals discussion there is good reason to emphasize their importance. Not a single muscle fiber can contract if mineral activated enzymes are not present. In other words they have a vital role in life's processes, but with animals, as well as man, it is not necessary to give minerals in excess of their normal requirements; in fact, a great excess, even in the case of ordinary salt (page 75) may produce results as harmful as a deficiency in minerals. Ordinarily, with the exception of salt, the animal receives more than enough minerals in the ration. If it receives moderately in excess of its needs, nature will simply get rid of the extra amount through the normal excretory processes, though if its needs for minerals are not met, the animal will soon show evidences of it in well marked and easily recognizable ill health. The foregoing thought is stressed because of so much misinformation brought about largely through the efforts of some people who seek to create the impression that the health of healthy animals may be improved—creating

No super-health possible a state of superhealth—by feeding minerals in excess of the normal requirements. A good rule to bear in mind is not to feed minerals until an animal in a herd shows evidence of needing these substances. If one or more animals in a herd are unquestionably suffering from a lack of minerals, then those other members of the same herd not yet giving outward evidence of ill health also are doubtless in need of these substances.

The 1952 Report of the Chief of the U.S.D.A. Bureau
of Animal Industry in discussing the
Urinary rather common formation of "stones" or
calculi calculi in the urinary tract of steers and
(stones) wethers (Figs. 135, 136 and 137) states:
"Observations on the occurrence of calculi in steers
and in wethers and experiments with rats have indicated that the amounts of silica (this is usually either
silicon dioxide, SO_2, or silicic anhydride a very abundant non-metallic natural substance, sand is an impure
silica, R.R.D.) and of vitamin D in the feed influence
calculi formation."

In concluding the statement about minerals it may
be summarized by the fact that other than
Deficiency calcium, phosphorus, sodium, iodine, iron
of some and copper, and the occasional deficiency
minerals a of magnesia, manganese and cobalt the
rare needs of animals are met by a well bal-
condition anced ration and good feeding practices.
Vegetation in the ration must be from soils containing
adequate minerals.

The Hormones. These chemical substances secreted
by the endocrine organs—usually classed under the
general heading of "ductless glands"—are
Hormones under certain circumstances poured into
and their the blood and lymph stream so as to be
nature transported to various parts of the body
so as to produce, excite, or depress a specific activity
in metabolism. Some of the hormones have been synthesized. If the secretion is a depressant or inhibitor
of metabolism it is designated a colyone or chalone.

Some of the endocrine organs have no other known
function than the elaboration of their specific product,
while others have at least a dual activity. In the former
group there are included the pituitary, adrenal, thyroid, parathyroid, pineal and possibly the thymus;
in the latter group there are the testicles, ovaries,

pancreas, and others. A summary of these organs and their activities follows:

The *pituitary* is located at the base of the brain. It may be divided into two or three physiological entities known as the anterior, posterior and intermediate lobes. In a measure because of the general action of its activities in relation to other endocrines it is frequently considered to be the master gland of the body.

The *anterior lobe* secretes six identified hormones that (1) stimulate the outer portion of the adrenals; (2) that stimulate growth; (3) that influence thyroid secretion; (4) and three hormones influencing ovary activity. The surgical removal of the anterior pituitary lobe results among other things in stoppage of growth and of ovarian activity. On the other hand unusual activity of this lobe results in giants and bone deformities.

The *posterior pituitary lobe* has at least two hormones—one that influences constriction of involuntary muscle fibres and is thus related to a rise in blood pressure, and stimulation of the uterus, intestines and urinary bladder, and possibly the mammary gland so as to result in what appears to be increased milk flow. This however has not proven to be of permanent value in an increased milk production. The *intermediate* lobe and its function are not well understood; it is said to influence color change in those animals—chameleons and others—that measurably harmonize with their surroundings in time of danger. In spite of the great influence of the pituitary organ in many processes of the body its complete surgical removal does

Effects of removal not necessarily result in the death of the individual though such removal does produce a definitely lower plane of existence and well-being.

The *adrenals (suprarenals)* are located below the vertebral region—one in front of each kidney—in humans above the kidneys. Each of these glands is physiologically divided into an outer cortical portion and an inner medullary part. The cortical portion is

The adrenals and activities responsible for several hormones that maintain (1) muscular activity; (2) that control water metabolism; and (3) assist in reducing the harmful effects of such things as poisons, injuries, low temperatures and others. In man a disturbed function of this cortical portion is responsible for excessive skin pigmentation observed in so-called Addison's disease which was a fatal condition until it was discovered that the administration of cortin—an active principle of the cortical portion of the adrenal—holds it in check. There is an interaction between the pituitary and the adrenal cortex but while removal of the former does not have death of the individual as a sequence, the removal of the latter is fatal.

The *medullary* portion of the adrenals may be removed without a resulting fatality. It is responsible for the hormone adrenalin—this has been synthesized —which is poured out continuously in minute quantities, though under excitation as a consequence of excitement, danger and emergencies its secretion is stimulated so as to increase the blood supply of various organs—it is sometimes called the emergency hormone. In a measure its action, depending on various factors, may be antagonistic. Thus it may be either a dilator or a constrictor of the vascular system; it may increase or retard the heart's activity; it definitely dilates the bronchi thus affording almost instantaneous relief in allergic asthma in humans; it may cause contraction of both the gravid and nongravid uterus though producing relaxation in the nongravid organ; it bulges the eyeball and dilates the pupil; it ruffles the feathers and erects the hairs. It is a valuable chemo-therapeutic agent that finds extensive use in human and animal medicine.

The *thyroid*. This one gland consists of two lobes usually connected by an intervening isthmus. It is

The thyroid and its action
located in the upper part of the neck region just below the wind-pipe and almost at the junction of the latter with the voice box. The hormone secreted by the thyroid is thyroxine which gains access to the tissue of the body by means of the very rich blood supply with which this gland is endowed. The gland serves in a sense as a repository for iodine, and when this element is low or absent in the gland hypothyroidism sets in characterized by goiter, or in human "juveniles" by arrested physical and mental development, and faulty nutrition of the bones and soft tissues, or all of these manifestations.

The effect is known as cretinism in the young or in the mature it is myxedema. In certain parts of the United States the so-called "big-neck" of pigs (page 497) is of this nature. When cretinism is due to an inability of the thyroid to build the hormone thyroxine, relief can be obtained only from the daily administration of the hormone. In the unborn young iodine administrations to the mother, however, are a preventive. Sometimes the thyroid gland is in a state of excessive functioning or hyperthyroidism. There is an inter-relationship between the pituitary and the thyroid and the most generally accepted theory regarding the cause of hyperthyroidism is that it is due to excessive stimulation of the thyroid by an anterior pituitary hormone. Hyperthyroidism in animals is characterized by a very rapid tissue change and restlessness. In addition in humans those affected are frequently "pop-eyed" (exophthalmic goiter). Malignant tumors of the thyroid may develop during hyperthyroidism.

The interrelations of the thyroid with other endocrines are quite numerous and complicated in the present state of knowledge. For example the thyroid and adrenals seem to assist each other; the thyroid and pituitary in health have a balancing action in regard to some of their secretions as between the stimulating action of an anterior pituitary hormone and the activity of the thyroid. The thyroid gland and the sex glands are apparently physiologically closely related because the thyroid enlarges as sex development begins, and if the sex glands are removed the thyroid slowly undergoes retrograde changes. The thyroid seems to be larger at the time of milk secretion, and the administration of thyroxine raises the level of milk secretion, while removal of the thyroid reduces milk yield.

Whenever there is clear evidence of thyroid insufficiency as indicated by lowered metabolism it may be corrected either by feeding thyroid substance or by the use of thyroxine. If the gland is too active inhibitory drugs such as thiourea—urea in which the oxygen has been replaced by sulphur—, and thiouracil —structurally 2-mercapto-4-pyrimidone—have been used. In fact thiouracil—0.2 per cent added to the ration of pigs has reduced the metabolic rate by its depressive action on the thyroid; more rapid weight gains are recorded for Chester White and Poland China crossbreeds, but other researchers using 0.25 per cent thiouracil in the ration of Durocs and Hampshires observed a depressed growth rate—greater in the Hampshires than in the Durocs. More research work is needed to determine the effects of feeding different levels of thiouracil to the several breeds.

Research literature issued in 1942 by the Missouri Agricultural Station concerns itself in a discussion of the chemical combination of iodized proteins containing the hormone thyroxine which when fed to dairy cows increased metabolism and with this the milk yield by as much as 20 per cent. The 1949 Report of the Chief of the U.S.D.A. Bureau of Dairy Industry conservatively states the synthetic material "thyroprotein" administered to cows to induce an increased milk flow may have unknown harmful effects on the

Is thyro-
protein
harmful?

health of the cows, and the economy of milk production over long periods. Initially there is increased milk production when thyroprotein is fed but this was not maintained. In B.D.I., Inf., Sept. 1953 it is indicated that "The feeding of extra nutrients to a level of 125 per cent of Morrison's maximum total digestible nutrient requirement was found to help sustain these increases." A final conclusion is that "The results seem to indicate that under a favorable milk-feed price relationship, the feeding of thyroprotein for 60 day periods may prove to be a profitable procedure." The service-per-conception rate in Jersey cows was not affected by thyroprotein feeding. The mortality rate from birth to 90 days of age in 22 calves from thyroprotein fed cows was 41 per cent compared with 24 per cent of 25 calves from cows in the same herd that received no thyroprotein.

There is voluminous research literature concerning the value and effect of thyroprotein but at this time it lacks conclusiveness. The U. S. Bureau of Dairy Industry indicates that thyroprotein sold under the name of "Protamone" when mixed with a concentrate mixture so that three pounds of this hormone product is in the mixture per cow per day, the correct amount of hormone will be consumed.

The *parathyroids*. There are two pairs of these glands in most species—in fact small accessory parathyroids are observed along the course of the cervical carotid. The main glands are anatomically closely related to the thyroid—one pair above and one pair below. The hormone is a protein known as parathormone. Usually in determining the function of an endocrine the gland under investigation is surgically removed and the resulting reactions noted. Because of the difficulty or impossibility in removing all of the thinly spread out accessory parathyroid tissue conclusions regarding the effects are not accurately measurable. In general in all species parathyroid hypofunction results in a greater or less extent in producing muscular twitching, convulsions and cramps—all included under the general name of tetany. This is due to an abnormal calcium metabolism.

Whenever the parathyroids do not function as they should the blood calcium is greatly reduced, and at the same time excretion of phosphorus is reduced so that the normal ratio between the calcium and phosphorus in the tissues is disturbed. In dogs death usually results, though less severe sequelae are observed in other species and in the mature. All of the symptoms resulting from parathyroid hypofunction in the living animal may be overcome by the administration of the active principle parathyrone; however, here again overdosing with this powerful hormone may have dire results, possibly death. There is basis for the belief that vitamin D (page 71), which improves calcium metabolism, in a measure overcomes the harmful effects of parathyroid disturbance especially as it is manifested in some forms of rickets (Figs. 13 and 130) (pages 72 and 504).

The *pineal.* This organ is lodged in the brain so that it is attached by a short stalk to the roof of the third ventricle. It is so named because in shape it resembles a pine cone. It is generally regarded as rudimentary glandular structure said to produce an internal secretion or hormone the function of which is unknown. It has been hinted that it plays a part in the changes observed in the body at the time of puberty. Surgical removal of this structure does not have a

Pineal function

fatal sequence. Rather, the results of such interference are either entirely negative or inconclusive. This also applies to feeding or injection experiments involving the pineal. For the time being it is shrouded in mystery.

The *thymus.* This is a ductless gland-like body situated at the entrance to the chest close to the heart and extending into the neck on the sides of the windpipe. A curious phenomenon in regard to this gland is that it reaches its greatest size and development in the young up to the time of puberty, and then it re-

The thymus a mystery gland

gresses though frequently vestiges of it may be observed in the aged. There seem to be interrelations between this and other glands though apparently not of great significance. For example castration in early life retards thymus development, but on the other hand removal of the thymus does not in any manner result in testicular or ovarian dysfunction or development. The removal of the adrenals results in a measure of retrograde changes in the thymus; here again the thyroid is involved.

The *testicle*. Located in most species outside of the abdominal cavity in the scrotum, though in some others—the elephant and birds—their situation is always intra-abdominal. In some species such as rodents and insectivores, the testicles leave the abdominal cavity only during the breeding season. When the testicles fail to descend into the scrotum in species in which they should do so it is known as cryptorchidism, or the animal is a ridgling—sometimes colloquially termed an "original." The castrate is known as a eunuch (man), steer (bovine bull), barrow (porcine boar), capon (avian rooster), and wether (ovine ram).

The glandular elements of the testicle consist of the seminiferous tubules which secrete the external secretion or seminal fluid containing the spermatozoa. The real internal secretion or hormone comes from the interstitial cells of Leydig. The hormone, known as testosterone, is a crystalline steroid usually obtained

The hormone of the testicle

for commercial or medicinal purposes from the testicles of the bull, and it is also prepared synthetically. All changes observed in the male animal body as the result of castration, or to overcome changes resulting from deficiencies in the natural secretion of the testicular hormone, may be overcome by the use of testosterone. The seminal fluid (semen) or external secretion is not essential to health although it has a bearing on virility. The internal secretion, testosterone, controls the development of the male sex characteristics and promotes sexual activity. It increases the size of the capon's comb, and the prostate gland and penis in castrated mammals. The castrate—when testosterone is administered—except for the fact that he is sterile or unable to beget his kind, retains all other male characteristics. These results are largely due to nitrogen retention.

The *ovary*. These female organs like the testicles of the male have a dual purpose, i.e., the production of the egg or ovum, and an endocrine or hormonal function. Since this treatise is concerned with a discussion of hormones the egg producing function will not be touched upon except to state that following the extrusion of the egg from the ovary there is left behind on the surface of the ovary a temporary endocrine body known as the "yellow body"; technically it is the corpus luteum. It remains fully developed so long as pregnancy persists—except in the mare where it regresses during late pregnancy. In pathological conditions it persists in the nonpregnant female thus inhibiting heat and conception. In some species it persists so long as the mother is nursing the young thus preventing "heat" (estrous cycle) during this period.

The ovary has two functions

Lutein which is in the nature of a yellow pigment is prepared from the dried corpus luteum of the sow. It is also in fat cells, and in egg yolks. Lutein is the hormone which causes ovulation or egg laying after an inter-action from the anterior lobe of the pituitary or master gland. The corpus luteum secretes the hormone progesterone which is concerned with the development of the maternal placenta in the uterus so that the membranes of the unborn young may have a place of attachment. The final act of parturition is probably the result of a complicated interaction between the pituitary, corpus luteum hormones, and other forces not yet fully understood. (For those interested in detailed information of the sexual cycle in the female a perusal of texts dealing primarily with endocrinology and physiology is recommended.)

Gonadotropins: These are substances that have an affinity for or a stimulating effect on the gonads (ovaries or testicles). There are three varieties; i.e., (1) chorionic gonadotropin from the urine of pregnant women. It is predominantly luteinizing in its action and is known as LH or luteinizing hormone; (2) equine gonadotropin (PMS) is a pregnant mare serum (serum is the clear portion of the blood as it separates in the clotting process). It contains both

There are three gonad-otropins

follicle stimulating (FSH) hormone, and luteinizing hormone (LH); (3) anterior pituitary gonadotropin obtained from pituitary glands of slaughtered animals; this gonadotropin has not been standardized but it is generally conceded to be both follicle stimulating (FSH) and luteinizing hormone (LH).

The equine gonadotropin (PMS) is used by some swine breeders to make sows come in heat at a definite

Controlled breeding of swine

period and thus have all pigs at approximately identical ages and sizes. Five hundred rat units of PMS will when injected subcutaneously or intramuscularly cause a sow to show heat and ovulate within three to five days. This effect is observed even when the sow is still nursing her young. The highest conception rate seems to take place if the PMS is used on the 38th to 40th day following farrowing. Several sows would thus show heat on about the same day, and there it is advisable, though not absolutely necessary, to give the boar 750 rat units about two weeks before he will be used and again at the same time that the sows are injected.

Guard against anaphylactic shock from foreign serum
or protein. The hogs must be vigorous.
Hogs must be vigorous Those that are in a poor state of nutrition,
or are unthrifty because of parasitic infestation are not good subjects for this type of stimulated breeding.

During recent years there have appeared on the medicinal market certain synthetic compounds—testosterone may be so prepared—that are not related to the natural hormones but that have an activity closely related to the natural products. One of these is diethylstilbestrol—also erroneously known as stilbestrol—that has equal ability in the causation of "heat" or estrus than the natural products estriol (theelol) and estrone (theelin) obtained from pregnancy urine. Also it is the agent of choice as compared with posterior pituitrin in aiding in the expulsion of retained "afterbirth" (foetal membranes or secundines). Recently it has received favor in the chemical caponizing of young roosters (page 415). Broodiness in chickens and turkeys may be overcome by injecting subcutaneously with diethylstilbestrol—for chickens 30 mg. in 3 cc. of sesame oil, for turkeys 200 mg. in 6 to 8 cc. of oil are required. Until the diethylstilbestrol has spent its action, laying will be resumed. Pellets are not to be used; because of their slow absorption egg laying is delayed too much.

The *pancreas*. Again this is an organ having a dual function or it might be said to consist of two glands in one. It is located in close anatomical relationship to the stomach, spleen, and at the beginning of the intestines. Its strictly glandular portion secretes the pancreatic juice which is concerned in digestion by means of its four ferments, i.e., amylopsin, trypsin, steapsin and rennin. It also has other tissue lying in the framework of the gland known as the "Islands of Langerhans" that elaborate the internal secretion known as insulin which is a hormone of a protein nature that effects sugar

Insulin and its function metabolism. In the treatment of diabetes in humans—a comparatively unrecognized condition in animals—it raises the body's power to metabolize sugars so as to reduce the blood and urinary sugars to a normal basis thus relieving the symptoms of this otherwise highly fatal human disease.

There are many other hormones and hormone-like substances obtained from both natural and synthetic sources. The placental membrane of pregnancy is rich in these substances. Enough has been indicated in this highly elementary treatise to indicate the complexity of the entire endocrine system and its interrelationships, as well as the high degree of physiological power exerted by its products. Outside, not exceedingly well versed, interference with endocrine action, well intentioned as this may be, is likely to set up a chain of reactions in the pre-existing delicate balance that may well be catastrophic. The medicinal use and the administration of hormones to animals is best left to the trained veterinarian.

Other hormone or hormone-like substances

CHAPTER VI

WATER AND ITS INFLUENCE

As a causative factor in the production of diseased conditions, water assumes a very important part in various ways. It is almost unnecessary to state that life is impossible without the required amount of water. More than 90 per cent of the weight of the newly born creature is water, though when the animal is three months of age or older, the water content is reduced to slightly above two-thirds of its weight. Whenever there is a loss of ten per cent of the total water content,

The purpose of water in the body the animal is seriously distressed, and a loss of twenty per cent causes death. In a broad sense it may be said that water is essential to dissolve all food before it may be utilized by the body. The blood, lymph, gastric juice, joint-water, and spinal fluid are largely water. The very essential part of the microscopic cells of which all living matter is composed, known as protoplasm, is largely water. The waste product of the body is mostly removed in solution in water such as in the urine, perspiration, and tears. The refuse of the digestive tract cannot be removed until it has been softened with water. The normal temperature of the body will not be maintained without an adequate supply of water.

Some animals apparently get along without water for prolonged periods without suffering, but though it may be true that they do not actually drink water, they do obtain it from the food they consume. Most foods

Water from various sources contain a high percentage of water, and this is frequently augmented by moisture in the form of dew on vegetation consumed by the animal. Physiologists have

106

also established that animals may manufacture a good deal of fluid in their own bodies out of such substances as fat, starch, glucose and others. The camel is said to go without an intake of water longer than other animals because it makes water in its body rather than because it has an unusual storage capacity. Shepherds are entirely familiar with the ability of sheep to thrive without an intake of water, and this is because they make it in their bodies and they obtain it in their food.

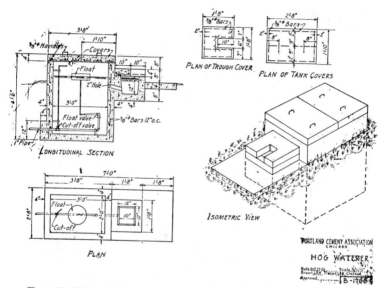

Fig. 17. This hog waterer will provide clean, fresh water. The dangers of extraneous contamination are largely prevented.

Whenever there is a large outflow of water from the body because of excessively high outside temperatures or for other reasons, fluid must be **Intake must equal outflow** taken in above the amount that the animal may make in its body or that taken in with the food. In fact, the entire matter of the need of the animal body for water is largely one of balancing the intake with the outflow. If this principle is disregarded as is so often the case with working animals during days of hard work and high temperature, disaster in the form of heat stroke (page 521) sets in, or if there is insufficient intake to moisten fibrous foods such as straw, cornstalks and similar materials in the digestive tract, constipation and its attendant evils follow.

Such an item as water, so important to animal well-being, should be pure (Fig. 17), but this statement needs qualifying. The word "pure" as ap-

Pure water— what is it? plied to water in this dissertation signifies an absence in it of harmful qualities in the the form of extraneous substances. Pure water is water that has been converted into steam, and the steam condensed back to water. It is known as distilled water. It is neither desirable nor practical to furnish it for animal or human use. It is necessary only when water is used for certain scientific purposes as in a laboratory in chemistry. Neither is it practical, nor has it been demonstrated to be essential that animals shall receive water of the same degree of pureness as that desirable for people. Furthermore, it is

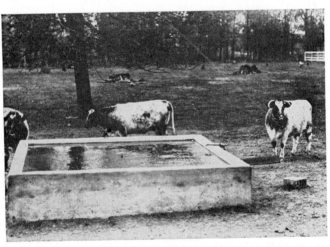

(Courtesy Dept. of Agricultural Engineering, Kansas State University)

Fig. 18. A concrete water tank; substantial and sanitary.

useless to supply animals with a relatively pure water (Fig. 18) if at the same time they may satisfy their craving for water from known polluted sources such as water standing on the surface near drinking tanks, or that in low places in barnyards or hog wallows.

It is well known that the germs of some animal diseases will live in water for a short time, and water **Transmission** may under these conditions be the carrier **of germs by** of the causes of such diseases as hog chol- **means of** era (page 616), foot-and-mouth disease **water** (page 605), strangles (page 614), chicken cholera (page 647), anthrax (page 591), and others, but unless there is frequent and repeated pollution of the water by these germs, the water will in the course of time be cleansed by natural processes. No sensible person denies that there is a real danger in the transmission of germs by water with the possibility of spreading diseases, but it does not follow that waters once polluted will remain permanently harmful if the source of germ pollution is removed.

There is doubtless greater danger to animals from the drinking of water that has been contaminated with intestinal discharges (Fig. 19), because the latter usually has a rich intermingling of worm eggs and these live for a comparatively long period in water. It is not implied that water is the natural habitat for many varieties of worm eggs, and prolonged soaking in water with attendant changes in temperature will vitiate the eggs, nevertheless the drinking by animals of water obtained from sources where it is subject to contamination by intestinal discharges is responsible in a large measure for the almost universal infestation with intestinal parasites.

The influence of flowing streams may not be disregarded in the spread of animal diseases. Most flowing streams are badly polluted with human and animal fecal material. The virus of hog cholera (page 616) may be carried for some distance by the flowing stream, as witnessed when an up-river outbreak of it is followed by successive outbreaks of the disease on bordering down-stream farms. The spores of anthrax (page 591) and blackleg germs (page 551) will live for some time in the slime of flowing streams, finally con-

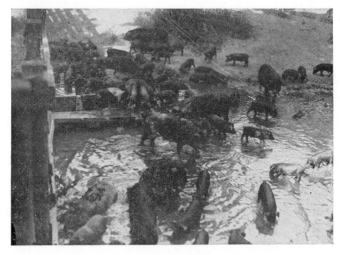

(Courtesy Associated Serum Producers, Inc.)

FIG. 19. Insanitary surroundings make favorable breeding places for parasites and infectious diseases. This is really a wallow though animals drink the water.

centrating at some point where, because of overflow and subsequent drying with the appearance of vegetation and the grazing of the same by livestock, the disease in question becomes rampant, as in the deltas of great rivers. There are sections in the southwest where the raising of calves to maturity without protective vaccination against blackleg is practically impossible because flowing streams have generally deposited on contiguous soil the highly resistant spores of the blackleg germ. The eggs of many animal parasites may be similarly transported.

Contaminated flowing water undergoes a certain degree of self-purification because of the exposure to

Flowing waters
action of the sun's rays and also by virtue of the consuming and destroying action of harmless bacteria and by other forms of vegetable life, as well as by fishes and other forms of aquatic life. Furthermore, some of the harmful germs settle to the bottom of the stream, thus reducing their numbers, and pure water flowing into the main stream from springs and the smaller streams has a still further diluting action. The time required for limited self-purification to take place depends upon several factors, such as the rapidity of flow of the water in the polluted stream, the numbers of brooks and springs flowing into it below the point of pollution, the forms of aquatic life it contains, the temperature of the water, and the nature of the pollution. (The latter is well exemplified by the resistance to destruction of anthrax spores). (Consult page 591). There is a limit to the waste loads waters can carry without exhausting their supply of dissolved oxygen. Most American states have agencies regulating the amount of sewage or other wastes that may be discharged into streams.

Taken as a whole, river water does not become fit for human use through self-purification. Its use for animals is also to be condemned, and especially so when it flows through extensive livestock producing territory. It is best to fence it off. So long as the water flows only through wooded and sparsely animal-populated territory, it is reasonably safe for animal consumption.

Waters are commonly classified as rain water, surface water, artesian water and spring water. Rain **Classes of waters** water is reasonably free from germ impurities, though it always has mixed with it materials floating in the air such as dust, some germ life, and gases, especially carbon dioxide. Residents of the so-called "dust bowl"—a section of the southwest where high winds frequently raise clouds of dust—are well aware of the large amount of the dust held in suspension by falling rain. Furthermore, rain water becomes badly contaminated when it flows down from the roofs of buildings in the collection of "cistern water." Also, the moment rain water comes to rest on the surface of the ground it at once becomes the abode of much of the surface organic material resulting from manure deposits, decaying animal flesh and inorganic chemicals from rocks and otherwise. During this period the rain water becomes surface water and it remains so classified even after it passes into the ground for a varying distance. It is only after it has passed through enough layers (page 246) of the soil that it becomes reasonably free from surface impurities, which is usually quite true of the water derived from deeply driven wells, artesian wells and some spring wells.

Flowing surface water exposed for some time to full sunlight and air is frequently freer from contamination than some waters that are presumably from deep sources, though a carefully conducted investigation of the latter may disclose that they are surface waters rather deeply deposited in the soil. A decided disadvantage of many deep waters is that in their subterranean travels they dissolve much material from rocks, chemicals and iron in the soil. It is these substances that make these waters "hard" or "alkali."

Alkali or "hard" water

The degrees of hardness in some sections of the United States may vary from 36,000 to 200,000 parts of minerals to one million parts of water. In other words, 3.6 per cent to 20 per cent of the weight of the water consists of these dissolved solids. One of the solids frequently present is common salt, and when it is present to the extent of 3.6 per cent, there is approximately between four and five ounces of it in each gallon of water. The disposal of "salt" water is one of the serious problems in "oil country" where it occurs in large quantities from some deep oil wells. If pumped onto the

Salt water and the limit of tolerance for it

surface it destroys vegetation, or put into streams it may make the latter unpalatable for consumption by livestock. Annually there are many claims for damages against oil producers by livestock owners for alleged damage to, or death of animals (pages 75 and 521) because of consuming these waters.

The U. S. Public Health Service has set up the following mineral tolerances for human drinking water.

	Mandatory Upper Limits ppm	Non Mandatory Upper Limits ppm
Lead	.1	
Fluoride	1.5	
Arsenic	.05	
Selenium	.05	
Chromium hexavalent	.05	
Copper		3.0
Iron and Manganese		.3
Magnesium		1.25
Zinc		.15
Chloride		250.
Sulfate		250.
Total Solids Desirable		500.
Total Solids Permitted		1000.

Carefully conducted research projects have established that in general when water contains more than 15,000 parts of total solids (total solids may be salt alone or a mixture of various inorganic chemicals) in a million parts of water, and if animals have no other source of supply, it becomes dangerous to their well being. Sheep seem to tolerate these waters better than other animals, though this may be explained on the basis of lower water consumption by these animals. They have been known to get along fairly well even though the water consumed by them contained as much as 2.5 per cent or 25,000 parts of solids per million. Cattle not producing milk and during the cooler months of the year when a minimum of water is consumed, have apparently suffered no harmful effects from the daily consumption of water containing 2 per cent of total solids.

It seems astonishing that animals can adjust themselves to these high levels. Of the animal functions lactation and reproduction are generally the first to be disturbed by a continuous intake of highly saline water. Milk and egg production may be much reduced or even terminated.

Water may become harmful to animals when the inclemencies of the weather have altered it physically. The harmful effects of sudden chilling of the animal following the unaccustomed consumption of quantities of ice water are well known. In part at least very cold water will inhibit the very important bacterial action in the rumen (page 20) which is so essential in the preliminary digestion processes. Thus, a decrease or even complete stoppage of the milk flow, (page 365) and also the premature birth of young are ascribed apparently on a sound basis to this factor. Strange as it may seem, animals accustomed to the regular daily consumption of very cold water are seldom or never harmed by it. Taken

Warming water before it is consumed as a whole, for domesticated stabled animals it is best not to permit of the free consumption of highly chilled water, and it is well to remove the chill by raising its temperature by means of one of the approved heating devices to about 45 degrees to 60 degrees Fahrenheit. This is particularly the point when stabled animals consume large amounts of water in out-of-doors tanks no oftener than once or twice daily. Stabled cattle having continuous free access to water from automatic fountains can consume it whenever it is not frozen and without harm. Even water at 45° F. may be harmful to heated work animals, and if there is any doubt about the matter, a good plan is to permit the animal to first quench its thirst only in part, then give it some food, and after it has cooled off, give it access to more water. Poultry, even baby chicks, gain nothing from warmed

No heated water for poultry water. When water containing ice particles was consumed by chicks they gained as rapidly as those receiving water at 75° F.; nor could any difference be detected in speed of yolk absorption. So long as an animal has ready access to unfrozen water so that it can drink anytime it wants to, there is no advantage in warming water. If the water is frozen part of the time and not readily available it is best to warm it.

How to have water analyzed There may be situations when it is desirable to know exactly what materials are in water obtained from a definite source, or an analysis becomes necessary. Generally such analyses may be classified as bacteriological and chemical, the former being to determine the absence or presence of harmful germs, and the latter the amount of chemicals and other inorganic and organic substances in the water. Occasionally the examination is to determine whether pollution exists with the higher types of life such as the animal parasites and their eggs. When such analyses are wanted, the water should be submitted to the proper public analyst, together with a general statement concerning the purpose for which it is to be examined. A good method of collecting and shipping the specimen of water is to gather at least one-half gallon in a glass container that has previously been sterilized in boiling water. The specimen should be an average sample—that is, it is to be collected from wells after a few bucketfuls have been discarded so that contamination from the pump itself may be largely eliminated. In very warm weather the water and its container should be surrounded with ice, and in cold weather it is to be protected from freezing during shipment to the laboratory. It should reach the laboratory within twenty-four hours of the time of its collection. It is sometimes necessary to submit for analysis several samples collected at different times, before definite conclusions may be drawn from the results.

The sterilization of water or its disinfection is not usually practical nor is it an entirely desirable procedure for potable water. Sterilization may **Sterilizing water** be accomplished by boiling the water, which destroys all forms of living matter, but it does not remove this material from the water and therefore when this water is consumed, the dead material is taken with it. For animal consumption, the boiling of large quantities of water is entirely out of the question.

Water of questionable purity, intended for use by poultry, is occasionally treated with a disinfectant in **Disinfecting water** the form of permanganate of potash (pages 34 and 271) to render it more safe. Water in wells may be so treated if necessary. A tablespoonful of the permanganate of potash crystals is dissolved in a quart of water and this is stored in a fruit jar to serve as a "stock" solution. Enough of this "stock" solution is added to the drinking water to impart a pink color to it. Whenever the pink color disappears during the course of the day, it is an indication that all of the permanganate of potash previously added has become neutralized and more of the "stock" solution should be added, or better still, fresh, newly treated water should be supplied. There is satisfactory evidence that many harmful forms of germ life are destroyed by the permanganate of potash, though the fowls consuming it are not harmed if it is not continued for too prolonged periods, that is, no longer than the duration of a disease outbreak.

Water intended for human consumption whenever there is reason to suspect pollution is usually treated with chlorine to the extent of one-half part of free chlorine in one million parts of water. In a more practical manner, calcium hypochlorite or bleaching powder that is fresh and that has a chlorine content of 24 to 35 **Chlorination of water** per cent is mixed with a little water and then this mixture is quickly added to the water to be treated at the rate of one and one-half pounds of the hypochlorite to each one hundred thousand gallons of water. After the elapse of one hour, when settling is complete, then water may be used. See additional statement about chlorine (bleach), (page 257).

The use of copper sulphate in water for the control of the growth of algae ("green scum" and others) is well known. (Consult page 275.)

Iodine (page 276) has also been recommended in the purification of water, but it is objected to because of its **Iodine** expense, and as large amounts of water are **as a water** used for purposes other than human or **purifier** animal consumption, the objection seems to be well founded. For emergency purposes, as when campers question a source of water supply, or for the disinfection of water intended for poultry, the addition of one drop of the tincture of iodine to one quart of clear water, or up to five drops when the water is turbid, may be recommended for occasional human use or more frequent animal use. The brown color produced by the addition of the iodine to the water which some people object to may be removed by adding a very small amount of sodium thiosulphate (this is the "hypo" of photographers). In the handling of coryza in fowl—when due to the organism known as the Hemophilus gallinarum (see page 659)—the addition of one teaspoonful of Lugol's solution of iodine to every gallon of drinking water, and vaporizing ten grams of resublimed iodine crystals for each 200 cubic feet of air space in the poultry house—to be inhaled by the fowl—are said to exert a favorable reaction in the control of the condition. At least there seemed to be a higher degree of recoveries.

Within recent years comparatively new bactericidal agents—the quaternary ammonium compounds (page 279)—have received favorable comment.

This agent has no favorable effect when these diseases are well established as when there are destructive cellular changes in the liver, intestines and other organs. However in chronic and sub-acute coccidiosis in chicks it may be helpful. In protozoa-contaminated drinking water this quaternary ammonium compound quickly inhibited all motility of the organisms usually indicating approaching death.

The exact water requirement of an animal cannot be definitely stated since it varies so widely with the amount and nature of the ration, with the stage in life cycle and with environmental conditions. To say that an animal needs a definite amount of water is meaningless unless all the conditions are specified. For example it is a matter of common observation that cows and horses on alfalfa hay drink more water and urinate more freely than on timothy or other non-legume roughage. This is due in part to the larger amount of waste matter excreted through the kidneys. Swine on corn and cob meal are reported to drink a third more water than on corn meal due perhaps to the greater amount of undigested material excreted through the feces. Well known to the poultry man is the fact that certain types of rations induce a higher water intake, produce wetter droppings and require more frequent removal of litter than other rations.

Water requirement

Of interest also is the observation that size of feed particles affects the water intake of broilers and that soybean oil meal increases water intake over meat scrap by 25%. (Poultry Sci., Vol. 27, 660; Vol. 28, 465; Vol. 29, 496). Laying hens in heavy egg production need to double their water intake to supply the extra amounts needed for the metabolism of extra food, the extra amount vaporized in the regulation of body temperature and the water put out in eggs. Similarly a cow in heavy milk production may drink up to four or five times as much water as when dry. Particularly striking is the extra water needed for regulation of body temperature in hot weather. Experiments at the Missouri and California Stations show that high producing cows cannot vaporize water fast enough in hot weather to maintain normal body temperature. The critical continuous surrounding temperature for a high producing Holstein is around 70 to 75° F. Above this temperature she reacts to eat less feed and thus to produce less body heat to be removed. At 90° F. milk production may cease entirely. The critical continuous temperature of Jerseys is around 85° F. and for Indian Cattle around 90° or higher. The difference in ability of the breeds to dissipate heat is not clearly understood but is perhaps related to differences in hair coat and skin texture.

Frequency of watering is an important factor in assuring an adequate water intake. For animals like poultry and swine which drink small amounts at a time and which subsist largely on rations naturally low in moisture it is advisable to provide a constant water supply in close proximity to the feed with the proper allowance of drinking space per animal. The minimum drinking space allowances for several ages and sizes of poultry and swine consistent with good feeding results are given below:

Nutrition Council

American Feed Manufacturers Association

Standardized Drinking Space Recommendations

1. *Chicks and Broilers:* Drinking space per 100 birds—

Day Old through 2 Weeks—*20 linear inches or two 1 gallon fountains.

7 Weeks through 12 Weeks—40 linear inches or two 3 gallon fountains.

Additional space should be provided in warm weather. (For feeding space see page 134.)

2. *Laying Flocks:* A minimum of one eight gallon waterer or equivalent should be provided for each 100 layers. When automatic float waterers or continuous

---

*For example, a 4-foot water trough open to birds from both sides provides 96 linear inches of drinking space.

jet waterers are used, one should be sufficient for each 300 layers. (Fig. 159).

3. *Dairy Calves:* Automatic drinking cups are preferred for calf waterers. When pails are used for watering, they should be kept clean and well filled with fresh water. Where watering tanks are used for calves in outside runs, the water should be fresh and the tanks should be kept in sanitary condition. Automatic drinking cups are preferred for calves housed in pen groups.

4. *Swine:* (Tentative Recommendations) One automatic watering cup should be provided for each twenty pigs (an automatic waterer with two openings should be considered two cups).

The minimum capacity waterer required for ten pigs should be 25 gallons per day in summer and 15 gallons per day in winter.

These recommendations are based on carefully controlled tests. Failure to allow proper drinking space is not uncommon in crowded poultry and hog houses and is a common cause of failure to obtain optimum feeding results. The cost of providing a constant water supply with ample drinking space may be thought to be too high for swine but tests show that it pays to do so. For example a test survey on Indiana farms showed that an average of twenty per cent of the labor of hog raising was in the watering and that the cost of a constant supply near the feed troughs where the hogs could drink at will was good economy (Indiana Agr. Experiment Station, Bulletin No. 506).

Less frequent watering is required by ruminants on green pasture since they drink large amounts at a time and since the grass is naturally high in moisture. If the grass is lush they may get enough from this source alone to supply their needs, four or more pounds of water for each pound of dry matter in the grass. On such pasture one watering per day is ample. On dry pasture more frequent watering is advisable.

Individual drinking bowls in close proximity to the feed trough have been recommended for dairy cows in barns or dry lots on winter rations naturally low in moisture. At Iowa State University cows so watered were observed to drink many times during the day and sometimes at night when in the dry lot and not confined outside the barn and 9% more than cows watered from inside tubs (Maine Agr. Exp. Station Bull. No. 408-409). At the Beltsville Station cows with a constant water supply yielded nearly 3% more milk and 2% more fat than cows watered twice per day (U.S.D.A. Technical Bull. No. 268).

Higher production with enough watering

In conclusion it must be emphasized that from the sanitary standpoint, harm to animals incidental to the consumption of water may to a considerable extent be minimized if watering troughs and other containers are kept clean by frequent scrubbing, if the water is placed in containers where it will not be subject to contamination by animal droppings, and if animals are kept away from sources of water supply other than that supplied for them in a reasonably sanitary manner.

CHAPTER VII

ANIMAL HOUSING AND CONTROL

Animals must frequently be housed in order to comply with the demands of domestication, for the safety of their keepers, during illness, and as protection against the elements and predatory foes.

Why is housing necessary? Newly born young creatures must be given protection from chilling. Hail storms have resulted in havoc to young poultry. Even the larger animals at times succumb to the terrific assaults of nature by cold winds, rain, snow and ice. Sheep with heavy fleece exposed for days at a time to soaking rains frequently become affected with so-called rain-rot in which patches of wool loosen from macerated skin. (Page 356.) Insufficiently drained and filthy feed lots are always a most prolific cause of foot-rot in cattle.

Probably not in the same category, though incidental to confinement and occasioning large yearly losses is the death of animals from electrical (page 383) currents induced by lightning discharges into wire fences that are not grounded, though the use of metal fence posts serving also as grounders for electricity has reduced these losses (page 383). Natural protection from heat, cold and hail is in a measure furnished by shade trees, and artificially by open sheds; these should be provided if at all possible.

Losses from lightning

Though housing and close confinement are frequently indispensable to either combat inclement weather or to facilitate the handling of animals, they do deprive them of the highly essential solar action and at the same time expose them by close contact to diseased members of

Bad effects of housing

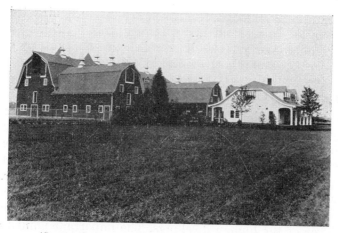

(Courtesy Dept. of Agricultural Engineering, Kansas State University)

Fig. 20. An attractive grouping of house and farm buildings, though they are rather closely placed.

the group. Solar exposure either direct or through light-pervious material other than ordinary glass (the latter does not permit ultra violet radiation) is necessary so that the animal may biologically absorb the calcium it gets in its food which is impossible without direct sun action, or as a substitute, indirect solar action through the ingestion of fish-liver oils. To indicate the danger in contact of closely grouped animals the rapid spread of tuberculosis (page 595) from one center of infection in a diseased animal to its healthy companions may be cited. Furthermore, though not of equal importance, is the fact that stabled animals are usually to a greater or less extent denied participation in green pastures. In winter months this latter factor frequently reduces the reserve in the body of the sex vitamin E to such a low limit that the normal reproductive function is impaired in some species (see page 72). The use of solar-radiated green sprouted oats, well prepared wheat-germ-oil, or the lush grasses of early spring pastures is helpful in correcting the sexual functional disturbance in those species that are affected by it such as sheep—not goats—swine and some laboratory animals. Nature seems to recognize this situation in most of her wild creatures in which the breeding seasons closely parallel the appearance of green foodstuffs in the spring of the year.

The correct site of farm buildings is a matter of importance as a factor in maintaining the health of those animals compelled to live in them (Fig. 20). Animal buildings should be placed low enough and far enough away from human dwellings to avoid the flow of barnyard effluvia in the general direction of the latter. Each of the two groups of buildings should preferably be on high, well-drained ground, with the advantage in favor of the human dwellings. The important point to bear in mind in the erection of all buildings is that they shall occupy sites higher than their immediate surroundings. If the natural lay of the land does not provide for this sort of a location, then it should be man made.

Location of buildings for animal occupancy

Good drainage away from buildings is so generally recognized as an essential that it is seldom overlooked. Buildings should not be near to bodies of stagnant water or swamps. Usually such locations are breeding or living places for molds, fungi, and bacterial, parasitic, and insect life; any one or all of which may make the preservation of nearby animal health an extremely difficult matter. Also, there is a well founded general belief that buildings with their long axis in a northern-southern direction, which means an easterly exposure, are the best placed. A northern exposure is usually avoided as it is cold, and because of a lack of direct sunlight it is frequently damp, though it does offer the advantage of coolness during the hot months of the year. A southern exposure is hot and more likely to subject animals housed in such buildings to the annoyance of insect pests. An eastern exposure in a measure at least obviates many of the disadvantages of either a northern or southern exposure.

Some of the general desirable features in buildings intended to house animals, and provided they are eco-

Some desirable features in buildings

nomically feasible and practical, include a good, reasonably high foundation. Double walled buildings, or walls of porous material afford better protection against cold than those otherwise constructed. Floors of broom finished cement, though difficult to keep clean, do give the animals a good footing. The coldness of cement floors with their harmfulness in relation to rheumatic conditions may be largely prevented by insulation with a thick layer of cinders, or of either hollow tile or hollow brick under the concrete. Cement floors without this insulation may be made quite satisfactory by placing loose, properly fitted wooden platforms on top of the cement floor. Floors to be as sanitary as possible for animal habitation should be provided with drains to carry away and sanitarily dispose of liquid waste. This does not necessarily involve the construction of an extensive system, as it may be quite satisfactorily attained by shallow gutters, except for cattle, directed towards a common conduit (page 139).

The ceiling of the quarters occupied by the animals, which in many instances is the floor of the loft, must be so closely constructed as to prevent any materials, including dust, from sifting down on the occupants. Dust from hay lofts is rich in disease-producing factors, and should not be permitted to excessively infiltrate the atmosphere that animals are compelled to inhale.

Windows are of importance both from the standpoint of ventilation and sanitation (Fig. 37). Their

Good lighting desirable

chief importance otherwise is because of the sun-light and air they admit and light exposes dirt so that it may be removed. Sun-light that passes through *ordinary* window glass is not destructive to germs. Furthermore, well lighted places are more conducive to essential physiological changes in the animal. This latter fact is sometimes taken advantage of by keeping fattening animals in darkened enclosures to delay tissue change and loss. In general, it is best to have windows at the rear of animals (Fig. 37), and if they must be placed in front, they should be high enough to throw the light over the animals rather than directly into their eyes. The glare may also be controlled by the use of frosted glass, and awnings. Animal houses should have approximately one-half as much light as human habitations.

In a succeeding chapter (Chapter VIII) general mention will be made of the approximate amount of air **Size of** space that should be made available to **living** housed animals, but this is not the entire **quarters** story because the extent of the air space permitted an animal must be closely related to the dimensions of height, width and length of their quarters. A good general height of living quarters for the usual numbers of housed large farm animals is ten feet, with an increase to as much as twenty feet for very large barns.

For cattle occupancy, stalls should be long enough so the animal will not be compelled to stand with the hind feet in the gutter, and short enough so that the droppings will fall in the gutter. As cattle vary in length, this necessitates placing the gutter slightly diagonally to the general direction of the stalls, rather than at right angles, so that the shorter animals may be placed in those stalls where stanchion and gutter are relatively close together, and the longer cattle at the end of the series of stalls where stanchion and gutter are most widely separated. (See additional statement about stanchions on page 152.) For the larger dairy breeds—Holstein, Brown Swiss, Shorthorn and Ayrshire, weighing 875 to 1,575 pounds—the length of the stall should be from 4 ft. 6 in. to 5 ft. 8 in., with width of stall from 3 ft. 6 in. to 4 ft. The smaller breeds—Guernsey and Jersey, weighing from 775 to

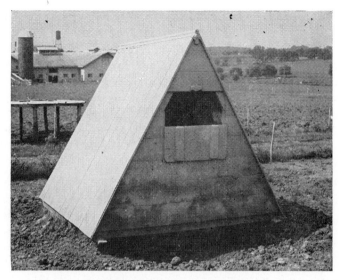

(Courtesy Dept. of Agricultural Engineering, Kansas State University)

Fig. 21. A-shaped individual hog house.

1,275 pounds—the length of the space for each cow may vary from 4 ft. 6 in. to 5 ft. 2 in., and the width from 3 ft. 4 in. to 3 ft. 8 in. In order to reduce the danger of udder injury by having curbs between stalls the width dimensions may be increased by six inches.

Some dairymen want even longer stalls. It is a known fact that a stall of 62 inch length is frequently **Larger stalls** not long enough for Holstein cows; dur- **and more** ing recumbency udders are often injured **space for** by hanging over the edge of the gutter **cattle** (Fig. 22).

The situation in connection with length of stall, may be further improved with a chain-tie stanchion substituted for the conventional type, **Chain-tie** since the former permits greater freedom **stanchions** of movement both fore and aft in lying down, and in moving about in the stall. However, stalls unnecessarily long usually have wet and dirty litter and this results in insanitary conditions. Therefore,

Comfort
stalls

on some dairy farms there is in use the so-called "comfort stall." It is 48 by 75 inches and each stall has a transversely placed, movable, four inch rear retainer curb to hold the bedding in place. By moving this curb forward or backward, as necessity demands for varying lengths of cows, the stall is adjusted. The stanchions are chain-tie for additional freedom. Then the cow can move for-

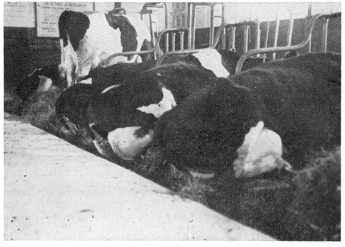

(Courtesy Dr. A. H. Groth of Missouri University)

FIG. 22. Udders injured by hanging over gutter.

ward in lying down and thus be completely on the curbed portion of the platform. Swollen hocks and knees are reduced to a minimum in these stalls. In a still later "comfort stall" developed at Penn State University the retained curb is adjustable fore and aft, and pipe partitions extend back within 16 inches of the gutter between each cow. It has a chain-tie. The grain and hay mangers are suspended on rods projecting from the stall partitions making them also adjustable fore and aft.

Bull pens may be 10 ft. by 12 ft. to 12 ft. by 12 ft. for the Jersey and Guernsey, and 12 ft. by 12 ft. to

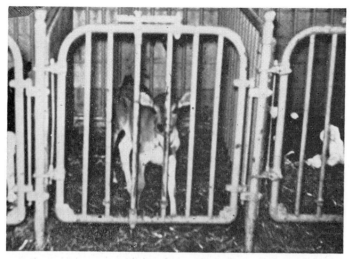

(Courtesy Dr. A. H. Groth of Missouri University)
FIG. 23. Individual calf pens.

12 ft. by 14 ft. for the larger breeds; partition heights
are recommended to be 5 ft. 3 in. If cows are kept in
pens the size of the pens may vary from 10 ft. by
10 ft. to 12 ft. by 12 ft., with partitions 4 ft. 6 inches
high.

Individual calf pens (Fig. 23) vary in size from
4 ft. by 6 ft. to 6 ft. by 6 ft. with height of partition 3
ft. 9 in. If there are to be a number of calves in a pen
allow 20 square feet per calf, and 20 inches to 25 inches
per calf for stanchion and manger space. Since young
creatures are susceptible to cold it is sometimes advisable for purposes of warmth to have them in the same
barn compartment with older cattle. In this case the
calf pens should be in that part of the
Newly born barn reached by direct sunlight and free
calves die from drafts. Calf groups should be about
if too cold the same age so that there are pens for
those from one to three weeks of age, three to six
weeks, and six to nine weeks. After nine weeks there
is not the same danger of spreading infection so a somewhat greater variation in ages is permissible. Floors

should be of the insulate-type—others are cold and wet. Slatted wood or welded wire with one inch mesh on a **Pens with raised floors** substantial frame elevated 18 to 24 inches above the permanent floor makes a very satisfactory device for a calf pen. It is readily cleaned and disinfected.

Some farms are supplied with a "loose-housing barn" (for details consult Bulletin 470—Sept., 1946— **A "loose housing barn"** Wisconsin Agricultural Experiment Station, or Agricultural Information Bulletin No. 98 of the U. S. Dept. of Agr. entitled "Loose Housing for Dairy Cattle"), as distinguished from the stanchion barn. In the "loose-housing barn" the animals can move about at will. If there is ample daily thick bedding above a firm layer of straw and manure, heat is generated and the bed is warm. Also the animal can get out of draughts. There should be concrete flooring along the mangers and the outside entrance (Fig. 24).

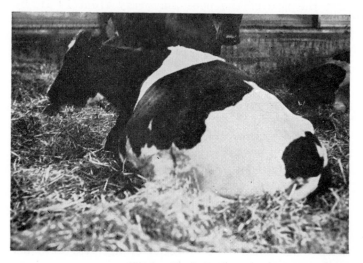

(Courtesy Dr. A. H. Groth of Missouri University)

FIG. 24. Cow in loose-housing type of shelter is free from udder, knee or hock injuries; also the animal is warm from the bedding, and is relaxed.

These hard surfaced areas must be cleaned daily, though in other areas the manure accumulates in a firm thick layer which may be removed when convenient to arable portions of the farm. High producing cows may be housed in the coldest weather without losing in production, though food consumption is somewhat higher. High quality milk can be produced if the cows are kept clean by frequent grooming, and if the bedding is two or three times as liberal as in a stanchion type. There must of course be a milking room (Figs. 30 and 31) into which the dairy animals may be placed at milking time. Animals with horns do not fit into this type of housing. Taken as a whole in this style of housing udder injuries are reduced, sore and swollen knees and hocks are lessened and the animals are more comfortable. These latter advantages in the opinion of many, at least, balance the insanitary features as compared with the stanchion type. The secret lies in ample dry bedding, and keeping the cows clean. If the litter becomes wet or soggy, mix in it 10 pounds of powdered limestone for each 100 square feet of floor space. Repeat the limestone every four weeks.

The Utah State University found that for each Holstein cow at least 75 square feet of space was necessary **Adequate** in the loose-housing type of shelter. When **space** only 40 square feet were available per cow **essential** it required three per cent more bedding **in loose-** and the cows were not as clean as in a **housing** larger space allotment. Also there was some mastitis in the 40 foot areas.

When animals are housed in closed buildings, as distinguished from a "loose housing-barn," different factors are imposed. There must still be ample satisfactory bedding. Included are either wheat straw, **Bedding** (oat straw is more edible and therefore **removal** more expensive) pine needles, leaves, sawdust, shavings, peat moss, or sand. All of these except sand absorb moisture such as urine,

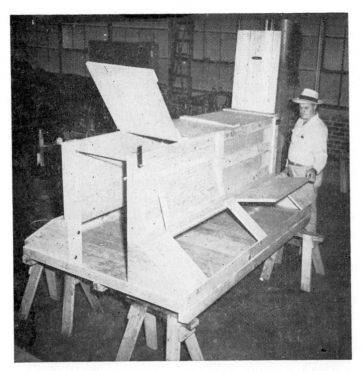

(Photo supplied by Douglas Fir Plywood Assn., Tacoma 2, Washington)

FIG. 25. A hog farrowing crate made out of plywood. Design developed at Colorado State University, Fort Collins, Colorado. Crate is 8 ft. long, 3 ft. high, with vertical box 1' 10" wide which can be increased 2" to 4" for larger sows. Bottom of crate is 5 ft. wide. Flooring is 1" x 8" t & g flooring.

which is desirable. The shorter materials are best suited when an animal is sick as well as for the very young as their feet do not become entangled in it. It is also easier to remove manure from it. Soiled bedding should be removed frequently from this type of housing and not less often than daily in case of the larger animals; somewhat less often is permissible for the smaller ones though at no time should this be delayed so long that the gases resulting from decomposition such as ammonia and others render the surrounding air insanitary.

Insufficient bedding on cold hard cement or other

hard surfaced floors is a cause of bone and muscle ailments in young animals, udder troubles in dairy animals, and lamenesses in those intended for work purposes. Wood platforms on cement floors are in a measure helpful.

Sheep should be allowed about twelve square feet of space per head, including feeding cribs. Sows with pigs need fifty square feet, and if several pigs are in one pen, they should be allowed on an average of ten square feet for each animal until they pass one year of age; they then need more room. During recent years the so-called colony house (Figs. 21 and 26) for swine has become very popular because it is comparatively small and may easily be moved from place to place in order to be in a more sanitary location. For a sow and her litter as soon as the pigs are large enough to be cold-resistant or when the weather warms, and to protect the young from worm infestation and filth-borne diseases, these houses are almost ideal. They afford protection from the weather, ventilation and light are adequate, and because of their small size a sanitary condition is easily maintained.

Poultry houses require somewhat different consideration than that accorded the houses intended for **Poultry houses need special features** other farm animals. Poultry have an internal temperature several degrees higher than other farm animals—an average of 106° F. for poultry as compared with about 101° F. for other farm animals— and therefore their abodes need not be kept as warm during winter months. Poultry exhale a comparatively large amount of moisture during breathing and therefore, ventilation must be better. They breathe much more rapidly than the larger farm animals and they utilize about three times as much air per live weight as a cow, so that they need more air space and a more frequent change of air. An estimate is that one hundred birds in high production produce from five to

five and one-half gallons of moisture each day. Stated
another way, this means that during the
Moisture from hens four months extending from Nov. 1 to
March 1—the months that high producers
are more or less continuously housed—they produce
over two and one-half tons of moisture. (See water
requirement page 119.) One-third of this moisture is
in the exhaled air and two-thirds in the droppings and
eggs. Poultry have no urinary bladder so that the
urates are discharged or voided with the feces. If the
"deep litter" system of housing is followed it must be
kept dry. (Page 170.)

The American Feed Manufacturers Association
recommends the following feeding space
Space for feeding and drinking equipment for chicks. (Consult page 119 as to drinking space.)

Allow chicks the following feeder space:

Per 100 chicks
Day old through 2 weeks_____100 linear inches*
3 weeks through 6 weeks_____175 linear inches*
7 weeks through 12 weeks_____300 linear inches*

Additional space should be provided in warm weather.

(Consult page 119.) (Consult Circular 406 en-
titled "Early Care of Chicks," issued by Agricultural
Extension Service, Pennsylvania State University,
University Park, Penn.)

Lower poultry house temperatures, and better ventilation is secured by the construction of approved-
type poultry houses. These usually are built with the
back and ends of closely boarded lumber, and a southern exposure is left from one-third to one-fourth open.
The opening is only covered by wire netting during the
warm days, and by muslin or burlap during cold or
blustery days (page 162). There are no drafts in a
building open on one side only, provided there are no
knot holes or cracks in the other three sides. Further-

---

*For example, a 4-ft. hopper open to birds from both sides
provides 96 linear inches of feeding space.

more, end-to-end whirling air currents will take place so as to set up drafts if the room is too long and, therefore, cross partitions built of impervious material must be placed in position every twenty or thirty feet. (Consult Kans. State University, Manhattan, Kansas, Extension Circular L 22, entitled "The Kansas Pole Type Laying House.")

The general rule followed in estimating the amount of space for each bird is four square feet of floor space when there are one hundred birds housed in one flock, and probably slightly less for the lighter breeds. A house 16 x 16 feet is ample for fifty of the heavy breeds, or sixty of the lighter breeds, and 20 x 80 feet will accommodate 450 to 500 birds. Both square and rectangular houses have advantages and disadvantages. The former permits the birds to roost farther back so that the front of the building need be closed only during the colder days, but the latter permits more of the floor space to be sun exposed, and therefore avoids damp floor spaces. Windows may be placed in the rear and end walls. If there are closed windows to

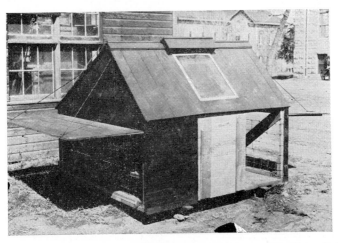

(Courtesy Dept. of Agricultural Engineering, Kansas State University)

FIG. 26. A movable hog house that is easily cleaned and disinfected.

the south, material permeable for the ultra-violet rays of the sun should be used. Tests indicate that ten per cent of the ultra-violet rays penetrate glass-cloth, twenty-five per cent goes through cel-o-glass, and thirty-three per cent goes through medium weight muslin. Adequate ventilation is highly important when the deep litter system is followed (pages 134 and 170).

Valuable and special features in animal buildings include smooth, impervious inside walls to avoid harboring places for germs and parasites, and to facilitate cleansing and disinfection. All angles and corners should be concaved or rounded, window sills sloped downward, and door handles and locks recessed to avoid places for accumulations of dirt or to prevent mechanical injuries to passing animals. High or overhead hay mangers for horses are not recommended, as they favor injuries to the eyes.

Special features for animal houses

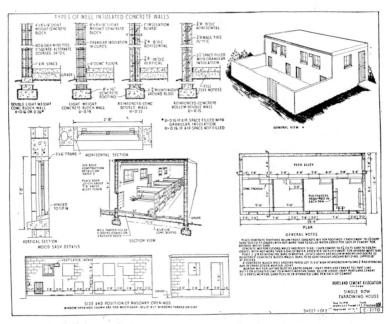

FIG. 27. A well planned and arranged farrowing house.

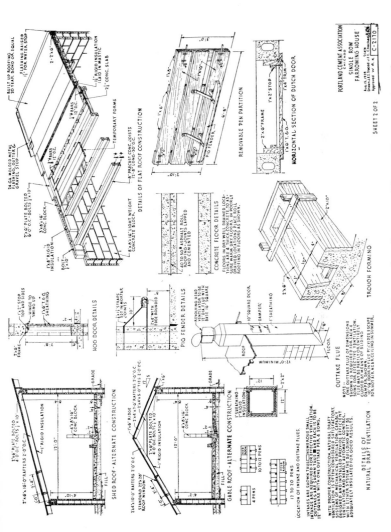

Fig. 28. An excellently arranged farrowing house, with sanitary construction.

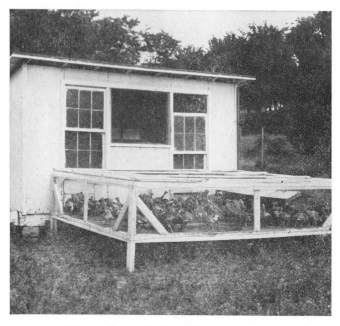

(Courtesy Dept. of Poultry Husbandry, Kansas State University)
FIG. 29. A sanitary runway for young poults.

Cattle barns need a gutter (page 138) six inches deep and wide enough to accommodate a scoop shovel, or large enough to hold the accumulated droppings of twenty-four hours, and supplied with drainage facilities to collect liquid waste. A special feature that discourages cattle from standing in the gutter with the hind feet is to make the anterior wall of the gutter a rather sharply inclined plane, rather than an abrupt vertical one. Cattle that are disposed to stand back in the type of gutter described, set their feet on the sloping surface so that they slip suddenly backward, and this reaction causes them to promptly step forward out of the gutter.

Gutters for cattle

It is well to know that electrically operated manure removers (Figs. 49 and 50) are on the market. They are so constructed that they discharge the manure directly into the spreader. The apparatus consists of a traveling chain with paddles the width of the gutter. It cleans the gutters in a few minutes. It is said to be economical for any dairy farm that has ten stalls or more. A three-fourths of one horse power motor supplies the necessary energy. The "cleaners" or manure removers are claimed to be almost trouble-free.

Also in the dairy barn there should be ample provision to supply the cows with drinking water at will, and for use in milk houses, at fire **Running** hydrants, and at tanks in pastures and **water in** corrals. Water under pressure with auto**the dairy** matic water cups, or float controlled, will **barn** not only, in the cold months, provide the housed, dairy and high producing animal with water free from ice or unduly cold, and the hazards incidental thereto for these pampered beasts. In these systems there is waste water which is usually tiled to a gravel bed, settling or septic tank, or disposed of in an isolated ravine. The danger in the latter (page 139) lies in the fact that disease producing germs—the brucella and tuberculosis organisms for example—may thus be transported and then become a source of contamination for other cattle having access to the ravine. Therefore, this method of disposal, unless rigid safeguards are practiced, is to be avoided.

A dairy barn, in order to comply with sanitary regulations, must have a separate room for the straining, cooling, storing and other handling of **A special** the milk (Figs. 30, 31 and 55). Otherwise **room as a** undesirable barn odors, and air infections **milk house** which are always present in suspension because of animal movements, will contaminate the milk. (Oklahoma Farm Structure Service of the Oklahoma Agricultural Station, Oklahoma State University, Stillwater, Oklahoma, has issued plans for "Grade A Dairy Barns for Plant Producer Dairies.")

According to more commonly used code requirements the following specifications are presented: "The

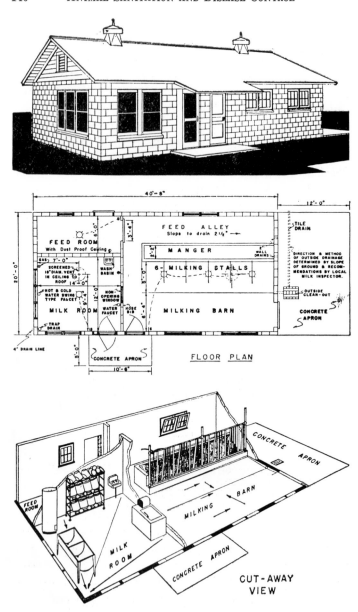

(Courtesy Hoard's Dairyman)

FIG. 30. Milking barn plans as planned by Oklahoma State University.

Code requirements for the milk house milk house should have a smooth concrete floor with a 4 inch drain. The walls and ceilings must be smooth, waterproof, suitable for painting and easy to clean. The room should be well lighted and ventilated. All windows should be open when desired, and the ventilator and the windows should be screened. Doors should be open outward to keep out flies and not lead directly into the barn, (the milk house should be separated from the barn by an open or ventilated passage and by two self-closing doors) or into any room used for living purposes. There should be a cooling tank, and hot and cold water. Arrangements for the loading of the milk are desirable. The milk house should be 25 to 50 feet from the barn yard.

In poultry houses, dropping boards are recommended built under the roosts to collect the night droppings. **Dropping boards for poultry** Level dropping boards are preferred to inclined ones, as the former do not so extensively prevent light from reaching the recesses under the boards.

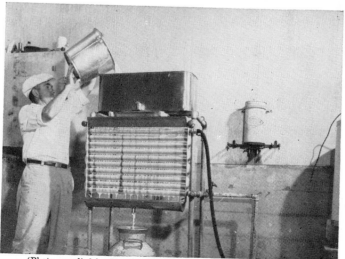

(Photo supplied by Douglas Fir Plywood Assn., Tacoma 2, Washington)

FIG. 31. Douglas Fir plywood paneling in milk room. Easily cleaned, and simplifies sanitation.

These boards permit removal of the droppings frequently with a minimum utilization of energy, and they promote sanitary surroundings. The droppings may be scattered on fields to which poultry do not have access. Roosts should be of two by two inch material with the upper edges rounded so as to reduce foot injuries, especially infections including bumble foot (page 381) to a minimum. They may be hinged to permit them to be raised during cleaning. Depending on the size of the bird, each should be given not less than six to eight inches of space on the roost. Nests fourteen inches square and twelve inches deep attached to the walls are satisfactory if they are kept clean, not only for the general health of the hen but in helping to keep her free from parasites, and it is also conducive to clean egg production.

A somewhat later feature for poultry houses is the

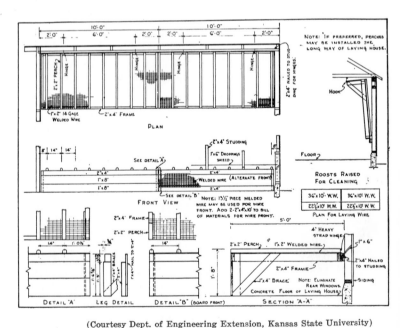

(Courtesy Dept. of Engineering Extension, Kansas State University)

FIG. 32. Plans for a "droppings pit" to supplant the "droppings board."

"droppings pit" (Fig. 32) to supplant the droppings board. This is a low frame about 20 inches high,
Dropping pits a new feature hinged to the rear wall of the laying house, supporting the perches, and enclosed so that the fowl do not have access to them. Immediately beneath the perches some one by two inch welded 14-gauge wire is placed so as to prevent eggs laid while the hen is roosting from falling into the pit. Frequently the fowl are encouraged to drink and eat by placing waterers and feeders directly on the perches. The droppings are gathered at the convenience of the owner. Ten pounds of hydrated lime on the droppings for each 100 square feet of space in the pit every two to four weeks will control undesirable odors. (Consult page 171 for the "deep or built-up litter" system.) ("Mechanical Cleaners for Droppings Pits" is the title of an illustrated circular issued by Pennsylvania State University Agricultural Experiment Station, University Park, Pennsylvania.)

Probably outside the realm of this treatise, but important for egg production is the use of electric lighting to stimulate laying in the pullet flock. One 40 to 60 watt light bulb for each 200 square feet of floor space for morning and evening lighting, or 15 to 25 watt bulbs for the corresponding space for all night lighting is recommended. Lighting is started as the
Electricity to stimulate egg production days shorten—usually about the middle of August to the middle of September, and continued to the spring. Gradual use of lights starting two weeks before heavy production is underway is satisfactory. Following this procedure hens will be brought out of the moulting season faster, and it results in higher fall and winter egg production. However, careful research indicates that this system does not increase the annual yield of eggs since this is controlled by heredity and environmental factors other than light; it simply changes the seasonal production of eggs.

An additional feature outside of, but attached to

and continuous with poultry houses and stationary brooder houses, is the wire platform. It is more correctly named "the sanitary runway" (Fig. 29), the floor of which is several inches above the ground; construction is of hardware cloth or wire netting having a mesh just large enough so that the droppings may pass through. By this means, chicks are kept off the ground and thus such conditions as worm infestation and coccidiosis (page 735) are largely controlled. As soon as the chicks are old enough to do without artificial heat, and if the outside temperature and other conditions are favorable, "summer range shelters" are desirable. These are made with sides of poultry netting and roofs of burlap or light lumber.

Possibly a word should be said here about brooder houses. For average farm use, a well built, movable brooder house 10 x 12 feet in size is very practical, and it will accommodate 350 chicks. Poultrymen do not advise crowding more than this number in the house. The brooder stove should be placed well back and towards one end so that there will be a good deal of space from the heated area where the chicks may find cooler, more comfortable atmosphere, and which also promotes feather growth. Rounding the corners with suitable material such as wire netting or roofing paper will prevent the chicks from smothering each other by crowding into corners; the latter is best if there are drafts. Homemade electric brooders (Figs. 33, 34, 35 and 36) have during recent years come into extensive use because of unavailability of those that may usually be purchased commercially. In the construction of brooders from the standpoint of sanitation the following points are of importance: 1. The hover should be well insulated in order that it may be operated economically and maintain the proper temperature; 2. At least 8 to 10 square inches of floor space is to be provided for each chick, and there should be from 10 to 13 inches of head room under the hover;

Homemade electric brooders popular

PLAN NO I

HOVER FOR COMMERCIAL HEATING UNITS

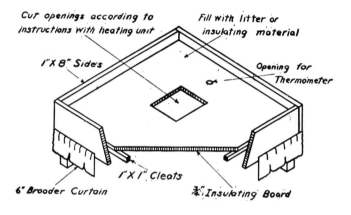

Cut openings according to instructions with heating unit

Fill with litter or insulating material

1"X 8" Sides

Opening for Thermometer

Cut openings according to instructions with heating unit

1"X 1" Cleats

6" Brooder Curtain

¾" Insulating Board

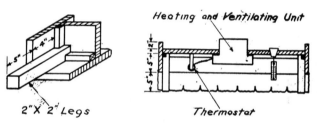

Heating and Ventilating Unit

2"X 2" Legs

Thermostat

BILL OF MATERIAL

No.	BROODER SIZE 4'x4' CAPACITY 225-275 CHICKS	BROODER SIZE 4'x6' CAPACITY 300-400 CHICKS	USE
1	¾" INSULATING BOARD 4'x4'	¾" INSULATING BOARD 4'x6'	TOP
2	1"x8"x48"	1"x8"x48"	SIDES
2	1"x8"x48"	1"x8"x72"	SIDES
4	2"x2"x10"	2"x2"x10"	LEGS
2	1"x1"x44"	1"x1"x44"	CLEATS
2	1"x1"x42"	1"x1"x66"	CLEATS
	17'6" CANVAS	21'6" CANVAS	BROODER CURTAIN
1	BROODER THERMOMETER	BROODER THERMOMETER	SET THERMOSTAT
1	ELECTRIC HEATING UNIT	ELECTRIC HEATING UNIT	PROVIDE HEAT
	SCREWS AND NAILS	SCREWS AND NAILS	ASSEMBLING BROODER

(Courtesy Extension Engineering, Kansas State University)

Fig. 33. Plans for hover and brooder.

PLAN NO 2

BROODER WITH ORDINARY LAMP BULBS

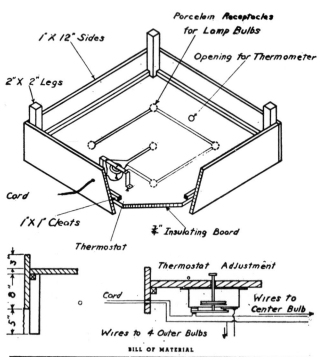

BILL OF MATERIAL

No.	BROODER SIZE 3'x3' CAPACITY 100-150 CHICKS	BROODER SIZE 4'x4' CAPACITY 200-250 CHICKS	USE
1	¾" INSULATING BOARD 3'x3'	¾" INSULATING BOARD 4'x4'	TOP
4	1"x12"x36"	1"x12"x48"	SIDES
4	2"x2"x13"	2"x2"x13"	LEGS
2	1"x1"x22"	1"x1"x44"	CLEATS
2	1"x1"x30"	1"x1"x42"	CLEATS
	13-6" CANVAS	17'-6" CANVAS	BROODER CURTAIN
1	BROODER THERMOMETER	BROODER THERMOMETER	ADJUST THERMOSTAT
5	75 W. LAMP BULBS	100 W. LAMP BULBS	PROVIDE HEAT
5	PORCELAIN RECEPTACLES	PORCELAIN RECEPTACLES	SOCKETS FOR BULBS
1	BROODER THERMOSTAT	BROODER THERMOSTAT	ADJUST TEMPERATURE
20'	RUBBER COVERED CORD	RUBBER COVERED CORD	WIRING
	SCREWS AND NAILS	SCREWS AND NAILS	ASSEMBLING BROODER

(Courtesy Extension Engineering, Kansas State University)

FIG. 34. Hover plans.

PLAN NO 3

RECTANGULAR HOVER USING ORDINARY LAMP BULBS

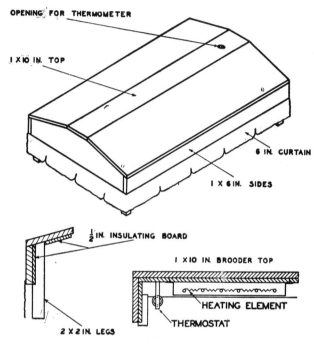

BILL OF MATERIAL

No.	BROODER SIZE 3'x4' CAPACITY 150-200 CHICKS	BROODER SIZE 3'x5' CAPACITY 200-225 CHICKS	USE
4	1"x8"x48"	1"x8"x60"	TOP
1	1"x10"x48"	1"x10"x60"	TOP
2	1"x6"x48"	1"x6"x60"	SIDES
2	1"x10"x36"	1"x10"x36"	ENDS
4	2"x2"x12"	2"x2"x12"	LEGS
	1—4'x8' SHEET ½" INSULATING BOARD	2—3'x5' SHEETS ½" INSULATING BOARD	INSULATION
1	THERMOSTAT	THERMOSTAT	ADJUST TEMPERATURE
1	BROODER HEATING ELEMENT	BROODER HEATING ELEMENT	PROVIDE HEAT
10'	RUBBER COVERED CORD	RUBBER COVERED CORD	WIRING
	15'-6" BROODER CANVAS	17'-6" BROODER CANVAS	CURTAIN
	NAILS AND SCREWS	NAILS AND SCREWS	ASSEMBLING
1	THERMOMETER	THERMOMETER	READ TEMPERATURE

(Courtesy Extension Engineering, Kansas State University)

FIG. 35. Hover plans.

PLAN NO 4

BROODER WITH REFLECTOR LAMP BULBS

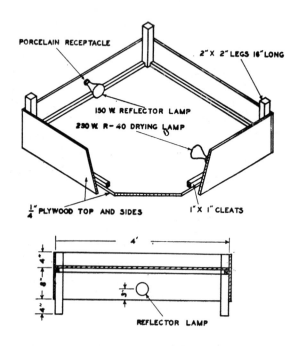

BILL OF MATERIAL

No.	BROODER SIZE 4'x4' —150-200 CHICKS	USE
1	4'x8'x¼" PLYWOOD	TOP AND SIDES
4	1"x1"x4' CLEATS	SUPPORT FOR TOP
4	2"x2"x16"	LEGS
2	PORCELAIN LAMP RECEPTACLES	SOCKETS FOR BULBS
1	150 W. PROJECTOR OR REFLECTOR LAMP	PROVIDE HEAT
1	250 W. R-40 DRYING LAMP	PROVIDE HEAT
20'	RUBBER COVERED APPLIANCE CORD	WIRING
	SCREWS AND NAILS	ASSEMBLING BROODER

(Courtesy Extension Engineering, Kansas State University)

FIG. 36. Plans for hover and brooder.

3. Ventilation is very important as well as the maintenance of the proper temperature. There may be provision for natural ventilation by raising the hover or by a fan-forced air heating and ventilating unit—the latter also controls relative humidity. Other methods used to solve the litter moisture problem are to use wire floors with either rough paper, cloth, or burlap placed under the brooder. The heating element is usually set at approximately the equivalent of that obtained from 35 watts for each square foot of floor space. (Plans for homemade brooders may usually be obtained from the Extension Service of the State College or University.)

Chilling of pigs causes an extensive annual death rate. Little pigs at birth have very low resistance to chilling because temperatures under ordinary barn conditions drop from 3 to 9 degrees below normal during the first hour after birth. The greatest drop is during the first 20 minutes of extra-uterine life. At the end of the hour the pigs' temperature starts to rise so that by the second day it is up to an approximate normal of 102.5° F. Hover type brooders, using electric heat lamps, have become very popular with advent of electricity on most of the nation's farms. ("Electric Pig-brooders" is the title of Leaflet 153 issued by the Agricultural Extension Service of Pennsylvania State University, University Park, Penn.)

Space and warmth for pigs

Temperature drops in new-born pigs

In order to prevent piling up with resulting overheating and later chilling out-of-doors so that respiratory diseases are more common, the hog should have ample space. If the barn is reasonably well constructed the square feet of recommended floor space for a hog is as follows:

Space for hogs

Size of Hog	Sq. ft. of floor space
50-100 lbs.	5- 6
100-200 lbs.	8-10
200-300 lbs.	10-14
300 and up	14-16

Portable farrowing stalls are favored by many small scale producers. Such stalls are easily constructed in such buildings as a garage, machine shed, etc. The building used must have hard surfaced floors to facilitate adequate cleaning, some auxiliary heat, such as a heat lamp for the piglets, and in some seasons a type of heating for the attendant.

Portable farrowing stalls
For the stalls use 2″ x 4″ uprights, and have slotted cleats to receive the partitions. In order that the stalls may be of the proper length for various sized sows, a board is placed cross-wise in slots at the entrance to this stall so as to be about 18 inches at the rear of the sow, to prevent her from backing. At the side of each stall, easily accessible to the piglets, though not to the sow, have a low boarded area to prevent their crushing. The sow must be let out of the stall twice daily for feed and water, and exercise. Usually she must be driven back to her stall. The sow is best placed in the stall a day or two before farrowing, to accustom her to the new surroundings. Also, it is an excellent plan to wash her with a mild antiseptic solution before she goes into the disinfected stall. (Consult page 672.) A week after the farrowing the sow and her pigs may be moved to permanent quarters. Then the farrowing stall is to be again disinfected for the next occupant.

The important point about portable stalls is that they may easily be taken down at the end of the farrowing season so that the building is again available for other purposes.

Feeding and watering space
The Nutrition Council of the American Feed Mfgs. Association after a survey of Agricultural Experiment Stations and the U. S. Dept. of Agriculture submits the following for swine feeding and watering space:

The number of pigs per linear foot of self-feeder space or pigs per self-feeder hole should be:

	On Dry Lot	On Pasture
Weaning to 75 lbs.	4	4-5
76 lbs. to market	3	3-4

(A ten-foot self-feeder open to pigs on both sides provides 20 linear feet of feeding space.)

The percentage of self-feeder space given to protein supplement should be:

	On Dry Lot	On Pasture
Weaning to 75 lbs.	25%	20-25%
76 to 125 lbs.	20%	15-20%
126 lbs. to market	15%	10-15%

Three self-feeder holes, or three linear feet of mineral box space, should be allotted for 100 pigs when salt or a mineral mixture is fed free-choice.

For hand feeding in troughs, or for hand watering, the length of the trough per pig should be:

Weaning to 75 lbs.	.75 ft.
76 lbs. to 125 lbs.	1.00 ft.
126 lbs. to market	1.25 ft.

(A ten-foot trough is considered to provide ten feet of feeder space whether pigs eat from one or both sides.)

When pigs are confined from weaning to market, 15 sq. ft. of feeding floor space should be provided per pig if the pigs are fed from troughs and 10 sq. ft. of feeding floor space if fed from self-feeders. This is in addition to sleeping space.

One automatic watering cup should be provided each 20 pigs. (An automatic waterer with 2 openings should be considered 2 cups.)

The minimum capacity waterer for 10 pigs per day should be 25 gallons in the summer time and 15 gallons in the winter time.

The drinking water should not fall below a temperature of 35 to 40 degrees Fahrenheit during the winter.

The use of sanitary hog wallows during hot weather is recommended. Up to 50 pigs can be accommodated per 100 sq. ft. of wallow providing shade or shelter is near-by.

On good legume or legume-grass pasture allow 20 growing-fattening pigs per acre on a full feeding program and 10 to 15 per acre on a limited-feeding program.

Pigs of widely varying weights should not be run together. It is recommended that the range in weight should not exceed 20% above or below the average.

Tying horses

Tying horses when this is necessary should approach the ideal of permitting sufficient slack in the tie-rope or strap so that the animal may rest and feed comfortably, but not so much slack as to endanger casting in the stall by becoming entangled in the tie-rope. The proper length for a head halter rope, or any other similar means of fastening, is the distance from the lower ring of the backstrap of the head collar to the ground when the horse is standing upright. A device occasionally used is to pass the free end of the rope, which has a snap hook attached, through a ring or through a ring-like aperture in the edge of the manger, and suspending a light weight from the snap-hook. If the weight is not too heavy it will not cause discomfort to the animal though it should be heavy enough that it will maintain the tie-rope at the proper degree of tautness. Some horses acquire the habit of "halter-pulling." There are many methods of trying to cure this. A simple one is to pass the free end of the halter rope through a ring in the edge of the manger and finally tie it around one fore pastern so that the pull is equal on the head and foot. This method is simple, safe and reasonably efficient.

Control of cattle

Cattle are controlled in barns, and when not in box-stalls or in a "loose-housing barn" (page 130) by placing them side by side with the neck in a stanchion (page 127) suspended by means of a chain from a rigid frame and attached below in a similar manner. This arrangement permits so much movement on the animal's part that it can lick itself as well as easily reaching all food intended for it, though inhibiting free movement of the body as a whole (Fig. 38). However, some more improved barns have discarded this type of stanchion and have substituted for it "chain-tie" stanchions in the so-called "comfort stalls." (See page 128.)

Bulls are controlled by the placement of a ring in the nose (page 394). The best procedure is to punch a circular disk of tissue out of the nose partition or septum just back of the muzzle. Punching **Ringing** a hole without removing a disk may be **bulls** productive of harm. If placed higher than this, it is likely to be excruciatingly painful at all times, and the animal's general health may be impaired. The hinged ring is then placed through the opening thus created and locked shut usually by means of a screw.

With small animals the method of control in stabling is not so much of a problem as several may be placed together in a common enclosure excepting at the time of parturition when a certain degree of isolation is necessary. (Figs. 25, 27, and 28.) Easily movable colony houses (Figs. 21 and 26) for hogs are very desirable. Sows that have recently farrowed **A guard** must be prevented from lying on their **rail to** young by a pig-guard rail (Fig. 28) eight **protect pigs** inches from the floor, and extending for an equal distance into the pen. Sloping the floors from the center towards the walls at the rate of one or one and one-half inches per foot will cause little pigs to gravitate under the guard rail and thus save lives.

Importance of avoiding crowding in the stabling of animals, especially swine and sheep, has already been stated, but is of sufficient importance to warrant emphasizing by repetition.

CHAPTER VIII

AIR AND VENTILATION FOR HOUSED ANIMALS

Ventilation is the act causing the movement of air through buildings with the objective of supplanting their foul air with fresh air. It is not **The need for ventilation** nearly so important a subject for consideration in the care and handling of animals as with human beings, for the simple reason that most of the animal's life is spent out of doors where nature maintains the proper balance of gaseous elements for respiration. It is only when the animal is housed and crowded in a small space with other animals that the problem assumes some of the significance correctly attached to it in the ventilation of human abodes. Animal houses are seldom if ever as well constructed as are dwellings intended for human occupation, and therefore a certain amount of natural ventilation always takes place in the structures occupied by animals.

In order that life may persist, the gaseous medium known as air is essential. Chemically, air consists largely of oxygen and nitrogen in the pro- **The composition of air** portion of one to five by volume, and in addition minute quantities of other gases. It is the oxygen of the air that is so important to life, since it is its combination with the food and tissues, through the medium of the blood in the body, that permits biological processes to continue; this action is known as oxidation. The nitrogen of the air does not enter into these activities, its principal function being that of an inert gas serving as a diluting agent for the more important oxygen.

When the cells of the body do not get enough oxygen the condition is designated anoxia. If this is

Not
enough
oxygen

prolonged the cells may be damaged beyond repair. It is not intended here to create the impression that anoxia—probably the words hypoxia or anoxemia (page 480) more correctly state the condition of oxygen deficiency—is always due to poor ventilation but it is a contributing factor. Anoxia for example may also be caused by habitation in high altitudes (aviator sickness); by decrease in hemoglobin; by the consumption of large amounts of nitrate of potash (page 479) by circulatory faults such as persistence of the fetal ductus arteriosus; in carbon monoxide poisoning, because this gas combines firmly with the hemoglobin, and others. In general it may be said that if the quantity of oxygen in the immediately surrounding air is adequate some of the other factors responsible for anoxia are not operative.

After the oxygen has entered the body and oxidized with the tissues and food, there is a gaseous waste consisting of a chemical combination of oxygen and carbon known as carbon dioxide, it being the major portion of the exhalation in breathing. The exchange in the blood is eight parts of oxygen for five parts of carbon dioxide. There existed for a long time the belief that so-called impure air acquired this impurity because of the presence of carbon dioxide, but more careful research has demonstrated that carbon dioxide in itself is not poisonous, though its presence in the air to the extent of more than eight per cent does replace that much oxygen and, therefore, when the air is "impure" and when a feeling of malaise is noticed, it is the result of oxygen starvation rather than carbon dioxide poisoning. From the practical standpoint, high carbon dioxide content in the air is evidence that there is improper or insufficient ventilation.

Impure
air

Under certain housing conditions the air supplied animals may become the carrier of harm in actually

Moisture in air and its effect

becoming a bearer of disease-producing agencies, or by interfering with certain physiological processes such as heat elimination. For example, it is well known that air always carries with it a certain amount of moisture. In the air it is spoken of as humidity. The degree of humidity varies with the temperature of the atmosphere, and it increases when improper ventilation prevents its evaporation. Even out of doors the humidity occasionally is so high as to interfere seriously with animal heat elimination so that death may result from heat stroke (page 521). This is especially true when at the same time there is increased heat production from muscular exertion or heavy food consumption. When buildings housing animals have the humidity raised as high as ninety per cent, health suffers from the presence of the moisture. Depending upon the general temperature of the atmosphere, the moisture content in the air agreeable to well being may vary from thirty to seventy per cent. The higher the general temperature, the lower should be the humidity, and vice versa.

It is estimated that a Holstein cow producing 30 pounds of milk a day will exhale 18½ pounds of water

Moisture from the animal

into the air during a 24 hour period; in an equivalent period a Jersey cow producing 20 pounds of milk a day will exhale 15 pounds of water.

Another factor of importance in connection with humidity is that moist air is in general a more favorable medium for the existence of germs, and therefore the transmission of contagious diseases is more likely to take place under this condition. It is not improbable, therefore, if one member of closely housed and grouped animals is affected with a contagious disease, that others will also contract the trouble simply because the two conditions of low vitality of the animal as induced by living in unwholesome surroundings, and livable conditions for germs are both present in humid atmosphere. Tuberculosis (page 595) may be cited as an example of a disease that thrives in damp, dark surroundings.

In improperly ventilated, animal-containing buildings, the air also soon becomes charged with more-or-less noxious gases. Ammonia is one of these. It is formed as a product of decomposing urine. When present in sufficient amounts, it is irritating to the delicate mucous membranes lining the eyes, throat, wind-pipe and lungs, the degree of irritation depending upon the extent of ammonia concentration in the atmosphere and the duration of time the animal

Harmful gases in the air

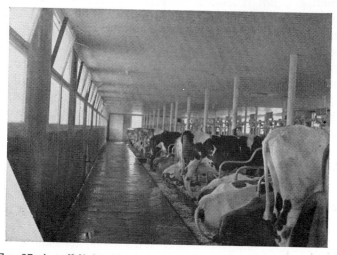

FIG. 37. A well-lighted and ventilated dairy barn. Lights are at the rear and provision is made for hinged windows and ventilator openings.

is exposed to it. Whenever it is noticeably present, it is indicative of the poor circulation in the air and its communication with the outside.

In the vicinity of some smelters and other industrial activities involving the use of copper, lead, arsenic and other poisonous chemicals, the air may under certain conditions become the means of conveyance of such chemical substances to deposit them on the vegetation where if consumed by animals in sufficient amounts they may result in harm.

The amount of air space to be allotted to each animal is subject to considerable variation because of conditions beyond control. When the outside air is not in a state of high motion, and when the barn is of average construction so that doors and windows do not fit snugly, a good general rule is to set aside approximately fifty cubic feet of space for each one hundred pounds of live weight of most domesticated animals, though sheep require one-half more than this, and poultry one-half less. The ventilating forces should be sufficient to permit a renewal of the air in the designated space (page 126) at the rate of eight times per hour. Though faults in housing construction usually permit this ventilation to take place, under abnormal out-of-door conditions the exchange of air in the building may be too violent, resulting in undesirable and frequently harmful drafts. It is difficult to guard against this, unless the barn has been provided with openings intended specifically for the entrance and exit of air which may be opened or closed as the out-of-doors weather conditions change.

Amount of air space needed

Sufficient heat in a barn is necessary for good ventilation—this is supplied by the cattle—or a 1000 pound cow should be available for every 550 to 650 cubic feet of space. Fewer cows leave the barn cold, more make the place hot and stuffy, and difficult to ventilate. In general, excess heat makes it easier to ventilate than a cold barn. Drafts are harmful. A temperature of 40° F. in a dairy barn will not reduce milk production if the animal is accustomed to it, but dairy workers prefer a higher temperature for their own comfort, and this is not harmful to their charges.

Heat and ventilation

There are numbers of excellent animal housing ventilators. There is the half-window hinged at the

Methods of ventilation
bottom so that it may be opened inwardly against a supporting frame work. During cold days, most of the windows on the windy side of the building may be kept closed, and the process to be reversed as the direction of the outside wind shifts (Fig. 37).

Another system of ventilation applicable in the better constructed barns with both outside and inside covering of the studding utilizes the space between some of the studding to serve as air-shafts. It provides for the admission of air by constructing a series of openings, each four by twelve inches through the outer wall, and a short distance above the foundation. The inrushing air passes through these openings, then in an upward direction between two adjacent studdings and gains admission to the building through another series of openings made through the inner wall and immediately below the ceiling. In this way the air enters the room from above, circulating in it without direct drafts, and after being warmed by contact with the animals and at the same time supplying them with fresh air, it leaves the building through large conduits having their openings on the inside of the building near the floor, and their exit in a special ventilator (a ventilator so constructed as to prevent entry of rain or snow but permitting free egress of air), placed outside on the highest portion of the roof. These long conduits take advantage of the physical law that warm air tends to rise as does smoke through a chimney. In the system of ventilation just described, an additional safeguard against undesirable drafts exists in shutters built in the inside entrance openings which may be closed during very inclement weather. If the barn,

Average barn permits outside air to infiltrate
including doors and windows, is of airtight construction this system of ventilation will be measurably helpful, but such air-tight construction is rare even in human dwellings. An analysis of several

barns showed that in most cases only a small percentage of incoming fresh air actually enters through planned inlets. Nearly all incoming air is by filtration.

The amount of air which is admitted through common types of fresh air inlets was carefully determined. Common inlets have a cross-sectional area of about 60 square inches and are built into the stable wall in such a manner as to deflect incoming air toward the ceiling. Under usual operating conditions, with still outside air, such inlets admit about 100 cubic feet of air per minute. Under the same conditions, the same amount of air will pass through 70 square feet of siding made of 8-inch boards nailed tightly together.

Wind pressure was found to greatly increase the flow of air through the common inlets. Wind at velocities of 5, 10, 15, and 20 miles per hour directed against the outside of inlets increased their discharge rate from 100 to 130, 190, 260, and 340 cubic feet per minute respectively. This explains why it is common practice to close inlets on the windward side of barns during cold weather. Too much cold air entering at one place creates drafts. Some manufactured inlets have built-in regulating dampers which are closed automatically by wind pressure; thus the flow of air through them is nearly constant at higher wind velocities.

Wind pressure also increases the amount of air which enters a stable by infiltration. This increased infiltration does not constitute a draft, if cracks through which the air enters are small and well distributed. Air entering through such cracks quickly mixes with stable air. Harmful velocities and chilly temperatures are quickly dissipated. Large cracks and openings must be closed for they admit excessive amounts of air at one point thus causing undesirable drafts and cold areas.

During recent years, because of the extension of high power electrical transmission lines into rural communities, an opportunity is afforded to equip farm buildings with electrically energized ventilator fans.

If only one fan is used it should be located at or near the cold end of the barn. This is usually the calf-pen section where less heat is given off. When two fans are used they are generally placed at or near opposite ends of the barn. If the barn is a very large one additional fans should be placed at intervals (Fig. 38) along the barn wall. When two fans are used the thermostat for a given fan should be at the opposite end of the barn so as to control and balance the temperatures. Two-speed fans are desirable because less ventilation is required during the colder weather and the lower speed is sufficient. A fan capacity of 50 cubic feet per minute per cow, supplemented with windows for ventilation in mild weather, will keep cattle barns dry in the colder months of the year. Automatic thermostatic temperature controlled fans, or a moisture operated humidostic one is to be recommended. Dairy cattle do as well at temperatures of 45° to 50° F. as at higher temperatures; in fact in the cold "loose housing system" (page 130) a low temperature has but little effect on production.

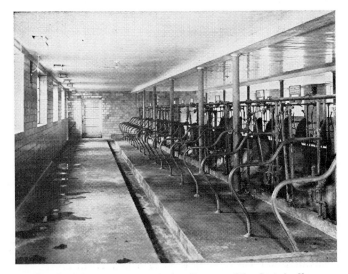

Fig. 38. A sanitary modern dairy barn, with electrically energized ventilation.

To prevent condensation in milk houses ventilation and heat are needed. The silo room may be kept dry by ventilation and by keeping it shut off from the rest of the barn. Hay-lofts frequently become wet when the hay-chute doors are not tight or if not closed when not in use. Roof ventilation and ventilators at each end of the ridge are good in tight hay lofts. Wide siding boards with spaces between them will allow enough air circulation without permitting rain or snow to enter.*

For the open front laying house either muslin or old burlap sacks, provided they have been sterilized, may be used for covering the open front (page 134). Ventilation through such coverings is adequate without contributing to drafts, and dampness is much better controlled than when window glass or substitutes are used (page 71). Fish-liver oils added to the ration during the low sun of winter are valuable in providing vitamins (page 80).

---

*For detailed information about ventilation consult Extension Bulletin 310 entitled "Ventilation for the Modern Barn," Michigan State University, East Lansing, Mich.

"Fan Ventilation of Poultry Houses" is Special Circular 13, Pennsylvania State University, University Park, Pa.

CHAPTER IX

ANIMAL SURROUNDINGS AND MANURE DISPOSAL

There are many factors responsible for insanitation or conditions injurious to physical well-being, but the situation which compels animals to live in their own bodily excreta is the most glaring one (Fig. 39). The intestinal and urinary discharges, as well as the exhalations from the lungs are seldom devoid of disease-producing elements.

Animals living in insanitary surroundings

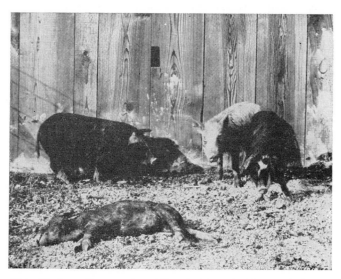

FIG. 39. Insanitary surroundings and unthrifty animals go hand-in-hand.

To impress this point, imagine a group of human beings residing in a small enclosure from which they cannot escape, with none of the usual toilet facilities, and their food given to them on the ground where it would be subject to almost instantaneous contamination by their discharges; no sunlight on or near the habitation; with poor drainage and all the other conditions that make surroundings insanitary. How long will it be till all the members of the colony are in a state of ill health? Almost identical conditions are imposed on many groups of animals to the detriment of their general health. As evidence of this it is only necessary to point out that when animals from such insanitary surroundings are transferred to more healthful conditions, such as good natural pasture, the almost miraculous recovery or return to "bloom" is noted of those not too seriously affected by their previous insanitary treatment.

No single step is so important to the health of housed animals or those confined in small enclosed **Frequent** spaces as the frequent—certainly not less **removal of** often than daily — removal from the **excrement** houses or spaces of their excrement. If **essential** there is any difference in the degree of importance of this step it should be to give the greater care to the surroundings of those animals that naturally prefer to take their food from the ground, such as swine. However, experience seems to indicate that in the "loose-housing barn" (page 130), and the "built-up-litter" in poultry houses (page 170) in which the manure is kept compacted and the droppings dry and aerated, there are advantages that must be weighed against daily removal of the excreta. There seems to be foundation for the belief that in these almost dry compacted manures there are sufficient heating and chemical changes to exert a deleterious action on the living forms contained in them.

In many urban communities where the keeping of animals is not prohibited by town or city enactments, though they must be kept confined, the greatest offenses are committed. Walk down the alleys of these small towns and note the immeasurably insanitary pig

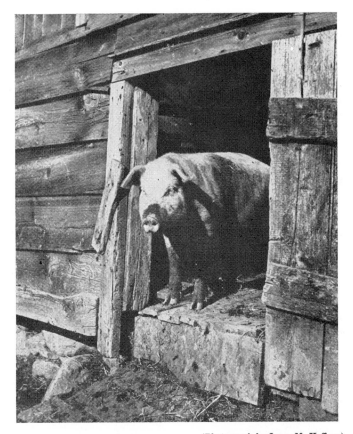

(Photograph by Irene M. Heffner)

FIG. 40. This porker deserves better sanitary surroundings.

stys (Fig. 40) and poultry yards, their occupants reeking in filth and being compelled to ingest more of the same daily, with their allowance of table scraps and other garbage (Figs. 41 and 42).

It is useless to compel the keeping of table refuse in closed garbage receptacles, when flies and other insects may develop without restraint in these filthy animal surroundings, nor do their foul gaseous emanations add to the comfort of nearby human residents. In rural communities the situation is seldom as bad, because animals from the sanitary standpoint practically run at large, though in small feed yards, inside barns and comparable places the situation leaves much to be desired. Those unfortunate animals that have become infected with a contagious disease so that they must be kept segregated or individually isolated are usually badly offended against from a violation of sanitary laws. In addition to the daily removal of ani-

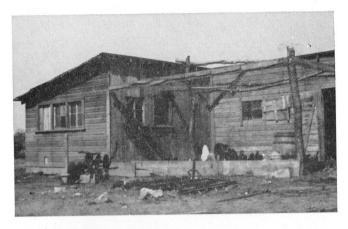

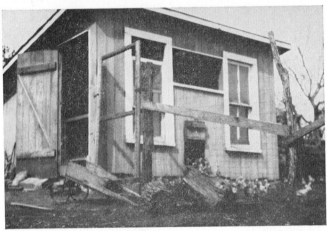

(Courtesy Dr. J. W. Lumb, Kansas State University)

FIGS. 41 and 42. Both illustrations indicate very insanitary surroundings—disease breeders.

mal excrement from small enclosures, there are other points to be considered in order that healthful, wholesome surroundings may be maintained.

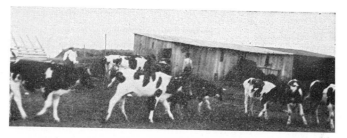

FIG. 43. Insanitary, disease-breeding surroundings.

Storage and final disposal of solid and liquid manure is a matter of considerable sanitary importance.

Methods of handling manure These substances always have a rather rich intermixture of parasites and their eggs, and at times the specific germs of well known diseases are present, such as those of tuberculosis (page 595), hog cholera (page 616), Bang's disease (page 578), blackleg (page 551), anthrax (page 591), and others. The eggs of parasites live for a long time in such surroundings (Fig. 39), and if animals are kept continuously and in crowded conditions on such places, it practically means that there will not be a break in the life cycles of many generations of parasites, to the detriment of the animals compelled to live therein.

The soil undoubtedly has the ability to react destructively to many forms of biological life if it is given an opportunity, but continuous or frequent pollution by excessively large numbers of animals on a very limited area soon exhausts nature's ability in this respect. A good recommendation in this connection is to change animals to new lots each year and not returning them to the original lot until the elapse of at least two years. The "resting" lots may be utilized for the growing of crops. When those manures that are gathered daily (Fig. 44) can be spread as they are gathered on arable land, a desirable method of handling is provided because on the land the purifying action of natural elements such as sunshine, heavy rains, and the processes of the soil and vegetation will soon render them sanitary. If, however, manure is believed to contain the specific infectious material or germs that are responsible for such diseases as tuberculosis, Bang's abortion disease, hog cholera, swamp fever, blackleg, foot-and-mouth disease, anthrax and comparable conditions, it is better to avoid danger by storing the manure until the heat generated by it, and fermentation processes or products shall have destroyed these infections. This can be accomplished in approximately two weeks in manure piles at least a cubic yard in volume in which the temperature reaches 180° F.

Manure as a disease factor

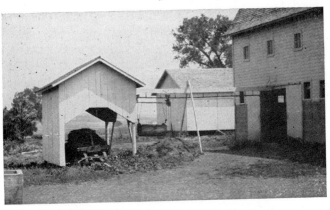

(Courtesy Dept. of Agricultural Engineering, Kansas State University)

FIG. 44. A litter carrier.

If the manure must be stored, it should be far enough away from buildings so that danger of contamination of the immediate surroundings of the animals is reduced to a minimum. Manure pits or sheds should be floored to control seepage, covered to prevent leaching (Figs. 45 and 46), and animals should not have

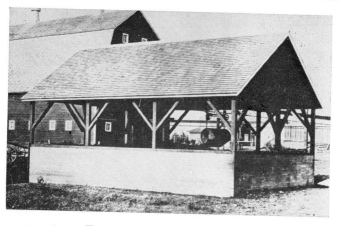

Fig. 45. A covered manure pit.

access to such enclosures. It is very desirable, though admittedly impractical, to fly-proof enclosures used for the storage of manure. DDT (dichloro-diphenyl-trichlorethane) (page 291) on manure piles has not proven to be entirely satisfactory. The heavier the numbers of larvae in the manure the greater will be the development of DDT fly-resistant strains. Try to keep DDT and comparable spray materials off manure piles and other fly breeding places unless there are only few larvae. The suggestion is to permit poultry to have access to manure accumulations so that they may pick out the fly maggots. But the more deeply lodged maggots are not reached by the birds, and neither is this sanitary, as it is well known that the immature form of a dangerous tape worm (page 668) is harbored by maggots and flies, and that these will later develop into the mature tape worms in the poultry consuming the maggots. Superphosphate (page 257) is also added at times to manure as an odor control.

Chemical treatment of manure and its value

A practical method assuring a fair degree of fly control, where the manure cannot be spread daily or

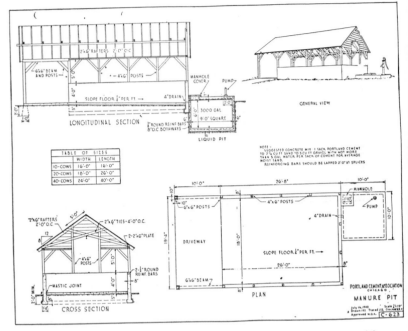

FIG. 46. Manure pit for the sanitary handling of manure, with full conservation of its fertilizing value.

Fly control in manure

when it cannot be stored in fly-proof enclosures, is to compact it ("loose-housing" and compacting, page 130). This is accomplished by *long narrow piles* with *straight sides*. The sides soon dry out and the deeper portions of the pile generate enough heat to destroy the developing flies. After the compact pile is once established, daily accumulations of manure should be buried in the center of the pile and covered with the dried outside layer. This seals the deeper portion of the pile so as to prevent escape to a considerable extent of the valuable ammonias and other fertilizing compounds.

The "deep or built-up litter" used in the poultry house where droppings are permitted to accumulate

Built-up litter in poultry houses

has much in its favor. At the least it is a labor saver. The litter used may be shavings, sawdust, cut straw, peat moss, ground corncobs, or sugar cane bagasse.

Any of the foregoing are placed on the floor to a depth of six inches and mixed with hydrated lime or superphosphate at the rate of 25 pounds for each 400 square feet of floor space. More recently pulverized lime or quicklime are also recommended; both will burn the feet of the chicks if not well mixed with the litter.

The fowl are placed on this litter and their droppings are not removed. In about four weeks, or sooner if there is compacting or moisture, an additional inch or two of litter is added together with another 25 pounds of hydrated lime or superphosphate, both being worked into the old litter. Additional lime and new litter are mixed with the accumulating mass at intervals of two to four weeks, or longer depending on the presence of excessive moisture. Frequent stirring and occasional lime applications aid in keeping the litter dry. This also controls embryonation of ascarid eggs (pages 670 and 690).

Lime fixes the nitrogen of the droppings thus stopping ammonia odors. It also absorbs moisture so as to aid in keeping the litter dry. However, general experience indicates that no known method of litter treatment will keep it dry if ventilation of the henhouse is inadequate (page 162).

The Ohio Agricultural Experiment Station has done research on these problems. It is claimed that young chicks kept on "deep" or "built-up litter" had less coccidiosis (page 735) even though several broods were raised on the same litter. Never-the-less a highly contagious disease, such as tuberculosis for example, can be perpetuated by litter that has had on it infected fowl. Removal of such litter together with general disinfection in cases of this kind is recommended. In fact, rather than permitting disease to make its appearance

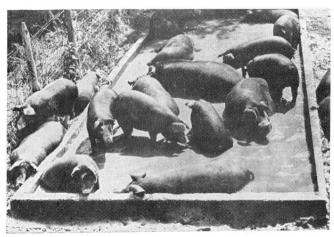

FIG. 47. Hog wallows of this type can be cleaned and kept more sanitary than the mud wallow.

it is recommended that deep litter houses be thoroughly cleaned and disinfected at the end of each season. It is even hinted that "built-up or deep" litter has in it the "unidentified factors" (vitamin B_{12}) (pages 44 and 69) that promote good hatchability when the rations are otherwise deficient. Chicks over ten weeks old were raised on "built-up or deep litter," even though on an inadequate ration. In fact, these chicks made the same rate of growth as those receiving a complete ration.

If the litter becomes wet in the vicinity of eating or drinking devices it is removed to another part of the floor and dry "built-up" litter used to replace it. Otherwise, "built-up or deep litter," if it remains dry, is removed only in the springtime. The more conservative poultry producers remove old litter for each new brood of broilers or at the end of each 10 to 12 weeks period, though others use the same batch of litter for two or three broods of broilers. Always change the litter when there are symptoms of coccidiosis, excessive parasitism, inflamed eyes, etc. If the litter is not kept dry there is potential trouble. (Penn. Agr. Exp. Sta., University Park, Penn., has is-

Change litter at the first sign of ill-health

sued "Reducing Wet Litter and Dirty Eggs by Feeding, Watering and Roosting Layers over Pit.")

Contagious material can be spread through the use of the itinerant manure spreading equipment. **The manure spreader as a source of danger** Usually manures are gathered directly from the stalls to be placed in the spreader. In some instances the stalls contain infected animals. The spreaders must

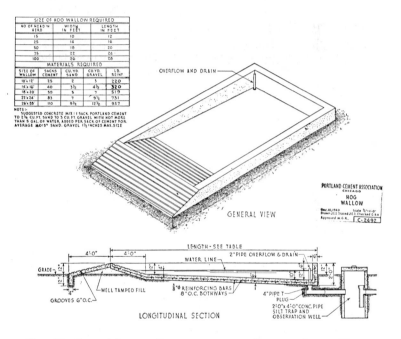

FIG. 48. Cement hog wallows are easy to keep sanitary. They assist in keeping animals free from parasites, and the filth-borne diseases of the old mud wallow.

not pass from these infected quarters through disinfected or cleaned places, or through yards or corrals harboring disease-free animals. The manure spreader and its contents should remain outside of all yards and corrals, otherwise it will spread infection to them, and thus to non-infected animals.

Neither can the possibility of the transmission of
diseases by fecal contamination of food and especially

**Contamina-
tion of food
and water
by manure**
drinking water be too strongly stressed
(pages 109). In the case of human beings,
our esthetic sense is violated by a possibility that the water supply may be fecal
contaminated, and it has therefore been a simple matter for human sanitarians to capitalize on this so that
there is almost universal insistence on clean water. In
the case of animals, however, there is not this same
urge, with the result that the problem is almost universally neglected. (Reference is made to page 109 regarding the influence of water in disease transmission,
to page 141 on droppings boards in poultry houses, to
page 163, concerning disposal of manure, to this page
on sanitary graveled poultry yards (page 174), and to
page 630 about sanitary drinking troughs; also to later
pages under the discussion of specific diseases and their
mode of transmission.) *Concrete* hog wallows are excellent (Figs. 47 and 48).

In the construction of yards for animals kept under
crowded conditions, hard surfacing, especially with

**Sanitary
yards for
animals**
concrete (Fig. 2) and with appropriate
drainage facilities, is undoubtedly a most
sanitary method. Such equipment is not
perfect from other standpoints in animal
production, as indicated by the development of pig
anemia (page 494) in suckling pigs not given access to
soil which naturally contains small amounts of essential iron and copper. Another method of good construction recommended in particular for the keeping
of poultry, is to gravel the yard. First the ground of
the yard is sloped so that the drainage will be toward
the middle of the yard, where a tile drain is placed on
the ground with its exit outside the yard at some point
where the effluvia may be safely discharged. The yard
is then enclosed by boards or other suitable building
material to a height of one foot, and the space thus
created is filled with a gravel so coarse that it will not

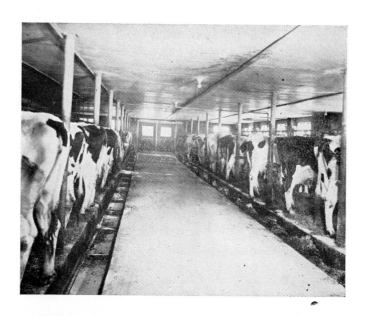

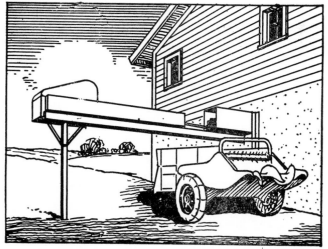

(Courtesy James Mfg. Co.)

FIGS. 49 and 50. An electrically operated cattle-gutter cleaner,
and an out-of-doors loader; sanitary and labor saving.

pass through a half-inch meshed screen. Rains or occasional flushing with a hose will carry animal excreta to the soil below, where it disintegrates, and the fluid portions are carried away by the drain.

(U. S. Dept. of Agriculture's Farmers Bulletin No. 1584 entitled "Feed Lot and Ranch Equipment for Beef Cattle" is excellent. It is for sale by the Superintendent of Documents, Washington, D. C. for 5 cents.) The daily or oftener removal of manure, manually, from gutters is a heavy and disagreeable task which probably is one reason for its neglect at times. An electrically energized "barn cleaner" (Figs. 49 and 50) is now available. For those so fortunate as to have this equipment life should be pleasanter, the barn more sanitary, and milk produced with a low bacterial count.

A new barn cleaner

PART TWO

Some Animal Disease Factors

⚜⚜⚜⚜

CHAPTER X

HEREDITARY FACTORS AND ABNORMALITIES

The importance of alleged hereditary influences in causing abnormalities, or at least their significance as predisposing disease factors, cannot be ignored in the light of convincing evidence.

Disease and heredity It is exceedingly questionable whether a disease, as this word is generally understood, can be inherited, though there is no question that the predisposition to certain diseases is heritable, and that the young may even become infected with a disease as acquired from its maternal parent at a very early period in its intra-uterine existence. For example, there is a reasonable foundation for the belief that certain bony growths in horses, such as the spavin, are most prolific when the structure of the involved bone has the correct texture as inherited, and when the conformation of the animal is such as to favor undue strain upon this specially textured bone. When bones and joints are distorted to a greater or less degree, or when joints are small as compared with a well developed musculature, then the correct basis is present for spavin formation. Or, as another example, when a horse has a naturally weak conformation as shown in the "curby" hock in which the normally straight line extending downward from the point of the hock is bowed backward. The animal is then predisposed to curb formation because the bowed or partially backward-broken hock is more likely to have this condition accentuated by severe exertion, with the formation of a true curb, than is the animal with a normal straight or unbowed condition of the region in question.

Congenital deformities or monstrosities are probably not in this class (Fig. 51).

Possibly it is permissible to extend the question of inheritance of conformation to such conditions as failure of the testes to descend into the scrotum, constituting the cryptorchid or "ridgling," the transmissibility of "rupture" in pigs, the undershot or overshot jaws of some animals, the presence of extra toes or the reverse, and comparable malformations. Also, there appears to be a reasonable basis for assuming that there may be heritable factors for the transmission of certain malignant growths, notably some cancers. (Figs. 112 and 113.) Furthermore, inheritance of certain characteristics also render species of animals so resistant to

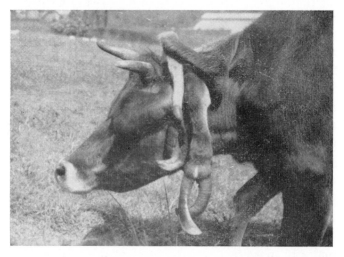

Fig. 51. Some congenital deformities—not hereditary. Legs and claws on the neck.

some disease-producing agencies as to make them "species" immune or resistant, as witnessed by the failure of many species such as horses, cattle, sheep, and poultry to contract hog cholera when inoculated with it, or the resistance of horses to that common disease of cattle, "blackleg," or the nonreaction of domesticated animals other than the dog to dog-distemper, or of cattle to glanders of horses, as well as a host of others. Whether these resistances are true hereditary influences as the geneticist interprets that condition is debatable. More likely, "species" resistance represents an unfavorable tissue reaction or environment to the invading disease-producing factor.

In each sperm of the male and in each egg or ovum of the female of all animals there are bodies known as chromosomes. The number, size, Chromo- shape and relative positions of the chrom- somes and osomes are the same in all the cells of a genes given species, though there is a good deal of variation in the different species. Thus, in man each individual has received 24 chromosomes from each of his parents, a total of 48, but in each generation the 24 received from the male ancestor may actually be 12 from each of the grandparents, with an average of six from each great-grandparent and an average of three from each great-great-grandparent, the number of each ancestor being halved with each generation back. However, probably about 20 generations back the ancestry extends almost to a "common brotherhood." The foregoing statement about chromosomes from the male is also correct for females.

If now the 48 chromosomes in each cell of the male and female bodies were transmitted to the offspring that would make a total of 96 in the first generation, and still more in following generations. Nature takes care of this problem during the so-called "maturation

period" just before the fertilization of the
Sex cells and ovum or female egg takes place. During
division of this period "reduction divisions" take
numbers of place so that each male and each female
chromo-
somes sex cell contain only 24 instead of the
usual 48 human chromosomes. Now the
male and female sex cells unite so that in the united
cell there are the normal 48 chromosomes, and this
number persists in all the cells of the offspring until
the sex cells of the latter at the maturation period are
divided by one-half.

In the chromosomes there are hereditary germinal
"factors" or units, their number is not known, that
carry the transmissible characters. These are the
genes. Each gene or factor determines a certain character in the fertilized ovum such as hairlessness, milk
production, speed, body type, blood type, color, sex,
lethals, longevity, and many others.

Gregor Johann Mendel, an Austrian monk and
naturalist (1822 to 1884) enunciated the law that some
traits and characteristics of plants and
Mendel's animals are transmissible or hereditary
law from parents to offspring in a definite
ratio. Mendel did his research work with peas and it
was determined, for example, that if a pea plant with
the factor of tallness (designated TT) is mated with
one which has the factor of shortness (designated SS)
then one-fourth of the offspring will be tall, one-fourth
short, and one-half will have a combination of the
two "factors" or genes. This means the resemblance
will be in the direction of the parent carrying the
dominant of the two characters—tallness and shortness. The other factors not outwardly noticeable though
present are recessive. In other words TT's mated with
TT's breed pure, as do the SS's with SS's. The TS's
mated with TS's will produce TT's, TS's and SS's according to the Mendelian ration. TS's mated with TT's

or SS's give the same combinations but in a different ratio.

In a consideration of heredity certain technical words must be understood and are used as follows:

Homozygous refers to an individual formed from the union of like germ cells as a TT with a TT, or such individuals are said to breed true. They are the homozygotes.

Heterozygous refers to individuals that result from the union of unlike germ cells as the TT with the SS. Such progeny will not breed true. These individuals are designated heterozygotes. (Hybrids are examples.)

Dominant is the condition in which a gene (this is the unit of inheritance much as the atom is the basic unit in chemistry) covers up its alternate partner in inheritance. As an example the normal covers up the hairless gene.

Recessive is the gene that is present though hidden such as the "normal" hiding the hairless—the latter being the recessive gene.

Lethal is the factor which is deadly in the homozygous condition or it brings about the early death of the individual—usually during gestation or shortly after birth. It is perpetuated by individuals apparently normal in every respect though "carriers" of the lethal factor. When two such homozygous "carriers" are mated together the offspring receives a gene for the lethal character from both sire and dam and therefore in conformity with Mendels law approximately one-fourth will die, while most of the remainder appear normal though "carriers" of the lethal gene which they in turn transmit to the next generation. Offspring of heterozygous parents receive the lethal gene from only one parent, almost always it is recessive, and therefore exerts no noticeable effect.

Some of the lethal characters observed in cattle resulting in early death are:

1. The "bull-dog" calf has a round vaulted skull, flattened nose, protruding lower jaw, cleft upper lip and swollen tongue. The legs are short and the body swollen. The gene for this trait is dominant in Dexter cattle and therefore one-fourth of the calves are born dead. If the short-legged, broad headed Dexter cattle are crossed with the long legged, narrower headed Kerry cattle— Dexter cattle originated from the Kerry type—no "bull-dog" calves result. There are some "bull-dog" degrees so that occasionally the affected calf is alive at birth but lives only a few days.

2. Hairlessness in which the skin at birth is devoid of hair though there may be some hair in the vicinity of the natural body openings and at the extremity of the tail. Sometimes there is no skin below the knees, on the ears and other parts of the body. This condition has been observed in Holstein cattle in Wisconsin and in Jersey cattle in California.

3. "Amputated limb" calves observed in Swedish Holsteins all trace back to a famous bull. The outstanding deformity is that the forelegs terminate at the carpal joint and the hind ones at the hock. There are additional minor head deformities. Death takes place a few hours after birth.

4. "Short spine" are the words descriptive of another abnormality. The back bone is so short-ened—because of fewer vertebrae—that the animal appears neckless, and the tail is very short and is attached high up. This condition occurs in Norwegian Mountain cattle. Death occurs shortly after birth.

5. Mummification usually means the drying up and shriveling of the unborn young. It has been observed in Red Danish cattle produced by

daughters of the bull Oluf Godthaab when mated to three descendants of the same bull. When mated to other bulls the offspring was normal, or the bulls mated to other cows brought normal calves. The calves died about the eighth month of gestation though carried full term. Excessive fluids in the foetal membranes (hydrops amnii) were a constant feature. Usually the neck was short, the joints prominent and the legs stiff.

6. Other lethals are lameness in the hind limbs observed in Red Danish cattle: muscle contractions of the limbs so that these members are almost wrapped around the body at birth; short legs and underdeveloped claws or more or less complete fusion of the claws observed in a Swiss breed of cattle domiciled in Russia; and a condition in which the lower jaw is shortened and immobile probably because of fusion—ankylosis of the joint.

Lethals observed in sheep include: Muscle contractions of the limbs; rigid bent fetlocks with a short thick body, large skull and straight wool; **Death of lambs at birth** paralysis of the hind limbs; amputations at the fetlocks; shortened immovable jaw; homozygous grey. All of the lethal traits of sheep quite closely resemble similarly named conditions in cattle.

Lethal hereditary traits noticed in swine that are mentioned in treatises on animal genetics are: Paralysis of the hind limbs; thick or greatly **Deadly inherited traits in swine** swollen fore limbs, these being born in the same litter with normal pigs; muscle contractions; atresia ani in which the anus is imperforate—it can be surgically corrected though if the condition also involves the rectum surgery in general is unavailing.

In horses, literature has only a slight reference to lethal hereditary traits. Probably the most important one is that in which the left dorsal colon **Horse inherited deadly traits** near its pelvic flexure is completely closed. The principal recording of this condition relates to the offspring of the Percheron stallion, Superd sent from Ohio to Japan. The condition is probably a recessive. Veterinary anatomists, however, state that in many horses used for dissection purposes the lumen of the left dorsal colon is frequently very small though patent.

Dogs are said to have a recessive lethal in the cleft palate of a strain of bull-dogs. With such a handicap nursing is impossible and death results **Lethals in other animals** from starvation. Hairlessness in homozygous puppies, together with a lack of external ears, and complete closure of the posterior part of the oesophagus results in death at birth. Poultry also have lethal characteristics such as color lethals (excessive white); "loco" or inability to stand, with head drawn backward, and rolling over; "creepers" or short-legged fowl—their progeny consists of both short-legged and normal birds—the condition is heterozygous being due to a dominant gene; therefore all affected homozygotes die about the fourth day of incubation.

Inherited conditions in livestock that are not necessarily associated with or result in death of the individual are quite numerous. However, **Inherited traits that are not deadly** conditions do result in economic loss to the producer.

In cattle, especially in males, there is the dominant responsible for rupture at the navel—mostly in Holsteins; Guernseys—both male and female may be three teated; extra or rudimentary teats in all breeds; blindness due to congenital cataract noticed in California Jerseys; defects in hair and teeth; extra digits in Holsteins; lack of pigment as in albinos; "screwtail;" syndactalism or single toes; fused teats; flexed pasterns; curly hair; notched ears; or blindness; and "cross-eye" the latter appearing at about one year of age, and "epilepsy" in Brown Swiss cattle as an autosomal dominant. Most frequently in White Short-

White heifer disease

horns, much more rare in animals of other color and breeds, the vagina is very small or contracted and the uterus distended or "ballooned" so that conception, or in fact breeding is not possible; this condition is probably of genetic causation and such animals are hopelessly barren ("white heifer disease") (page 186).

Dwarfism in cattle is a hereditary condition in which a calf is of average size and appearance at birth though it fails to develop to normal size, and there is some deformity except in the case of "proportionate dwarfism." Either the sire or dam may be the carrier of the causative gene. The long headed dwarfs are also known as the "snorter" type, as distinguished from "proportionate dwarfism" (dwarfs that are small but normally proportioned).

The important point is to diagnose the condition or the hereditary taint as early as possible in the dam or sire. Several methods are under investigation, but none are final—they are as follows:

1. The insulin test: A blood specimen is collected before making an intravenous injection of insulin, then one hour and two hours after the injection additional samples are taken—a total of three. Clean animals have a swift increase in the number of white blood cells, while in carrier animals there is very little increase and at a slow rate. The best dosage of insulin is undetermined.

2. X-ray examination of the loin vertebrae of carrier and non-carrier calves is based on the assumption that these anatomical structures in non-carriers are normal, though in carriers there is extreme abnormality. Suspected calves are X-rayed when they are one week old. At an older age the abnormality is not so pronounced,

and then there are borderline cases. Research is still in progress (1958).

3. Progeny test or genetic rating: This is a certain method, but it is unsatisfactory because the test has to be spread over several years owing to the necessity of producing several calves.

There is no cure for dwarfism.

Sometimes it is erroneously asserted that artificial breeding or insemination causes a different sex ratio.

Artificial insemination and heredity This is an error because the normal sex ratio of approximately 51 per cent calves born are bulls and 49 per cent are heifers —almost a 50-50 sex ratio. Stated otherwise it makes no difference to the male sperm whether it gets to the female ovum by natural or artificial means—the sex ratio remains the same.

In both "white heifer disease," and in the freemartin heifer (page 790) the vagina almost from the day of birth has a very small caliber.

A test for the early determination of white heifer disease and for free-martins Therefore, an ordinary six-inch test tube as generally used in chemistry or bacteriology laboratories, lubricated with mineral oil or vaseline, is inserted into the vagina. If it cannot be inserted full length the vagina is too small. By this simple test the expense of raising sterile heifers is avoided.

In sheep non-lethals include nakedness, and turning in of the eyelids and lashes so as to irritate the eyeball. (See entropion page 417.)

Swine may have non-lethal traits such as rupture—hernia—into the scrotum (page 428) or at the navel, the former probably a double recessive and the latter may be either a dominant or a recessive gene.

In horses osteoporosis—enlargement of the head appearing at about one to five years of age—is observed as a predisposition due to a dominant gene; the tendency to have "summer sores"—bursattae is inherited. Also "roaring," certain conformations, multiple digits, and tendency to nasal bleeding are related to inheritance.

To the practical livestock producer these inherited characteristics are of importance because of the reduction in reproductive efficiency, and consequent economic loss. The detection of the presence of these undesirable genes depends upon breeding tests, and since the lethal traits may appear late in the tests, the breeding efficiency of the sire or dam may have passed its maximum. If several undesirable characteristics appear in breeding flocks and herds the attending veterinarian should be consulted for his professional opinion so that future losses may be held to a minimum.

It is interesting and of value to the practical livestock breeder that the polled condition in cattle is a dominant genetic factor and the horned condition is a recessive one. Thus, if two animals are mated—one from an established polled breed and the other from a horned breed—the progeny will be polled. If two members of this second generation are in turn mated the hornless and horned condition will appear in the offspring in accordance with the usual genetic ratio of three to one.

Only by careful methods of inbreeding so as to preserve the entirely fit, and excluding the misfit by slaughter or emasculation can the animal husbandman build up a race of animals satisfying to his greatest utilitarian need.

Methods of improving breeds

Inbreeding, or the mating of closely related individuals is the supreme test which determines through the offspring the presence or absence of desirable or undesirable characteristics. Inbreeding and line breeding are reasonably well established as a means for the transmission of desirable physical attributes, and for increasing the prepotency of a herd in all of the distinct breeds of livestock, and also for the elimination of weak and undesirable conformations; they may yet be potential factors in "breeding out" disease.

The foregoing is well illustrated in the production of hybrid chicks which are the offspring of parents from different highly inbred strains of chickens until they breed true for such good characteristics as vigor, better egg and meat production etc., and at the same time breed out such undesirable characteristics as partial nakedness, spraddle legs, cross-beak and other deformities—these undesirable factors being eliminated by close culling. It usually requires at least four years to produce hybrids that have the desirable characteristics, and at the same time cull out the weaknesses.

Hybrid Chicks: Why and how

CHAPTER XI

ANIMAL CARE AND DISEASE

Approved care of domesticated animals implies that they shall be kept clean, have wholesome feed and water, and comfortable, healthful surroundings. Under native conditions, natural processes together with the animal's instinct in the matter tend to preserve comfort and health, but all this has been sadly disturbed by environment, use, and domestication.

Cleanliness desirable

All farm animals if given an opportunity prefer clean to filthy, dirty surroundings. Heavy dashing rains and sunshine, together with rubbing against posts and trees, as well as rolling on the ground in grass, sand or dust will remove loose hair and other skin debris, and many parasites. When denied these conditions by stabling, man must assume the task of regular grooming if he wants his charges to maintain health and vigor together with physical comfort. Grooming signifies (a) care of the skin and hair coat; (b) care of the feet; and (c) care of the genitals and external orifices of the body.

Natural methods of cleaning

Resistance to disease may be lowered considerably by a filthy body surface, this being especially true in relation to parasitic skin diseases. The skin of all animals, even more so than in the case of man because of the extreme hairiness in the former, becomes filthy as a result of accumulated exfoliated parts of its superficial layer, the secretion of fatty material, and sweating. When these natural processes are combined with a deposit of dust from fields in which the animals are compelled to live and work, and accumulations of filth

Resistance to disease lowered by a dirty skin

on the skin consisting of their own intestinal discharges, it becomes evident that conditions are not wholesome and tending towards well-being. Seal up the skin with dirt, and at once one of its functions is stopped as it is one of the important organs of the body in the elimination of waste products through the sweat glands. This is especially true in horses. Sweat glands in the horse are present in all of the skin of the general body surface, and to a less extent this is also true for sheep. In other animals the sweat glands are confined to certain skin areas such as the foot pads in the dog and cat, the snout in pigs, and mainly in the muzzle of the ox. Occasionally in this latter animal, as well as in the dog, sweating is observed from all haired portions of the body. If the openings of the sweat glands become clogged with dirt, either from the skin itself or deposited thereon, their action is interfered with. The goat, rabbit, and fowl do not sweat.

Sweat glands in animals

Sick animals are frequently offended against by failure to groom them properly. Animal owners will spend money for condition powders and tonics, forgetting that a brush and curry comb regularly and judiciously used are better conditioners and tonics than most of the patent medicines sold in bottles or other containers. It is surprising to the owner how a chronically unthrifty animal is stimulated and improved by the cleansing of its skin when presented to a veterinarian for treatment. In a natural state, animals may be trusted to keep themselves reasonably clean, provided their surroundings permit this.

Grooming for sick animals

Grooming, in general, needs but little explanation, though there are certain special features that are frequently overlooked. Horses wet with sweat should have this removed by means of a specially formed scraper made of either wood or metal such as aluminum. For animals with short hair, the brush is the best instrument to use, but should be supplemented by the curry comb, especially in those parts where the hair is long, where it has become matted, or when badly soiled by adhering mud and manure. Washing with tepid water and a mild non-irritating soap is helpful when the long-haired regions in the vicinity of the fetlocks need cleansing but the parts must be thoroughly dried afterwards, by means of sawdust or other absorbing material, because if left wet a form of eczema known as "scratches" may be a sequel. If washing of the entire body becomes advisable, it should be done only on warm days, free from exposure to cold winds or drafts, and preferably with exposure to the direct action of the sun.

The external orifices and genitals of the body need frequent attention. According to one author, 70 per **Parasites in the orifices of the body** cent of cats are infested with a mite in the ear that causes considerable irritation; in cattle there is the spinose ear tick (page 716); still others could also be named. In horses, types of the bot flies (page 705) deposit their eggs near the nostrils and mouth; the larvae of the flesh-flies (page 702) and of screw-worm flies (page 702) are not uncommonly found in the sheath of horses and ruminants, and occasionally in the genitalia of females.

Washing the sheath and genitals of stallions and geldings is to be recommended for the removal of an accumulated, dried and hardened fatty secretion of those parts known as smegma. If this is not done, the hardened mass colloquially known as a "bean" may effectually shut off the urinary passageway so as to inhibit this act, with the result that straining and severe pain are manifested as one type of so-called "colic." Also some misinformed people seem to believe that the site of many other forms of painful colic in **A pernicious practice** the horse is in reality in the genital organs with the harmful practice of injecting or otherwise introducing into these organs strong drugs, onions, syringe bulbs, and other substances. Furthermore, the severe tail rubbing of geldings is frequently the result of filth in the sheath, and may sometimes be overcome by thorough washing of this latter organ. In male hogs a collection of urine and even concrements (stones) have been found in the sack in the dorsal wall of the sheath near its opening (page 377). Inanimate foreign bodies such as sticks, splinters and hard vegetable burrs occasionally find lodgement within some of the natural bodily orifices.

In dogs and cats of the domesticated animals there are on each side of the rectum a gland and a communi-

Accumulations in anal sacs in dogs and cats cating sac to receive the secretion from the former. These are the anal sacs. Their excretory ducts open into the rectum just in front of the anus, one on each side. Quite frequently in the dog, less so in the cat, these anal sacs with their excretory ducts become inflamed and swollen so that the sac contents cannot be discharged normally into the rectum. The affected animal indicates that this is a source of irritation and discomfort by sliding on the floor, and in the later stages by difficult defecation, and moans and cries. An examination of the parts frequently discloses a painful swelling on each side of the anus. Sometimes in mild attacks the trouble may be overcome by lubricating the parts with vaseline and then compressing the swollen parts between thumb and fingers until the contents are discharged into the rectum through their excretory ducts, but more frequently the services of a veterinarian are required to correct it.

Possibly no part of the grooming is more important than care of the feet in horses since this

Care of the feet is so frequently neglected. Out in the open, if the soil is not excessively stony, growth and wear of the hoofs usually balance each other, and at the same time soil moisture keeps the horn of the hoofs in a good condition. When kept in confinement, conditions are reversed, so that growth soon exceeds the wear (Fig. 52), resulting in

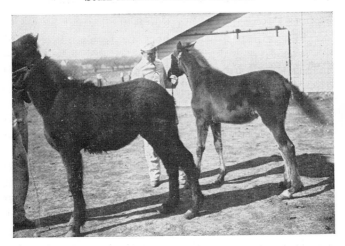

Fig. 52. Badly neglected feet.

distortion of the limbs. It is essential, therefore, to trim the hoofs to bring them back to a normal shape and position. The outstanding evil of stabling as it affects the feet is due to the animal standing in its own manure. Stabled stallions during winter months are terribly neglected in this respect so that the sole, and especially the horny frog and its deeper counterpart, the fleshly frog, become badly diseased. All of this may be prevented by clean stabling and occasional trimming away of excess parts. A fault in the grooming of the feet of horses or other hoofed animals is to rasp the outer surface and thus remove a "varnish" which nature has placed there to prevent evaporation of the hoof's moisture. If repeatedly done, dryness sets in followed by contraction and pain as manifested by lameness. When this dryness has taken **Soaking to** place the hoofs must be subjected to soak-**overcome** ing, which is correctly done by first wash-**dryness** ing away all dirt with soap and water and a stiff brush, and then placing the feet in water not quite reaching the hairline for twelve hours a day; when not soaking, the feet should be anointed with fish oil or other suitable material to prevent evaporation.

Before the next soaking the fish oil must be washed off to again permit the hoof to freely absorb fluid. In season, and during the hours between soakings, it is an excellent plan to permit the animal to have the run of pasture, especially during the wet, dewy hours of the night and morning.

Whenever the hoofs due to growth, lack of wear, or excessive wear become unbalanced or dispropor-

Methods of trimming a horse's foot

tionate in some part, an attempt should be made by hoof trimming to restore normal configuration as nearly as possible, and in order to obtain the correct direction of the setting down of the feet upon the ground. By examining the *bottom* of the hoof of the horse an experienced person can usually outline: (a) the lower border of the wall; (b) the sole proper; (c) the white line which is the boundary line between (a) and (b); (d) the horny frog bordered by two grooves, the lateral lacunae; and these in turn by (e) the bars which meet in an apex at the point of the frog and which join the wall behind. In a well formed straight limb the inner and outer

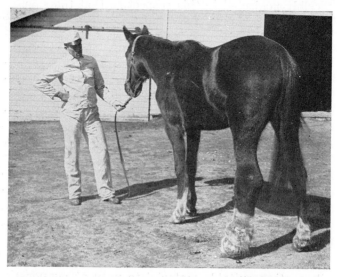

FIG. 53. The result of neglecting wire-cuts and rope-burns.

walls of the hoof should be of equal height and the foot should be trimmed to obtain this. The following parts of the under surface of the hoof should be in contact with any level hard surface upon which it is set: all of the lower border of the wall, the white line, about one-fourth inch of the lower surface of the periphery of the sole proper and the frog.

As viewed from the side with the animal in the standing position that portion of the limb below the fetlocks should incline in a downward and forward direction so as to form an angle of approximately 45 degrees in the front limb, and 50 to 55 degrees in the hind limb, the latter being somewhat more upright than the former. The hoofs of cattle and other animals and the claws of dogs and cats must occasionally be trimmed because of inhibited use and wear they become excessively long. After field and race-track competition the pads of the feet of dogs may be so sore as to require the wearing of soft leather boots.

Shoeing of the horse must be considered a necessary evil, though less of an evil than the excessive wear and tenderness of the unshod foot when **Horse-** the animal is compelled to work on paved **shoeing a** streets. Horses used only for farm labor **necessary** in comparatively soft ground seldom need **evil** be shod. An even greater evil than common shoeing, though still a necessary one under conditions imposed upon many horses, is the application of shoes with sharp calkins to prevent slipping on smooth or icy streets. The calkins elevate the sole of the foot away from the ground so that there is no counter pressure from below thus stopping the necessary expansion and contraction of the hoof, a movement which is essential to circulation within it and its proper nutrition. This abuse terminates ultimately in contracted, narrowed, and painful feet.

In utilitarian animals other than horses, grooming is not so generally a custom, though brushing and cur-

Grooming of animals other than horses

rying must be applied to dairy cattle, as well as moistening the udder, lower abdomen and flanks with a damp cloth to prevent contamination of the milk (page 573). Trimming the claws of cattle is frequently a necessity.* These animals, as well as sheep and swine, sometimes become so badly infested with ticks, lice, or mites that they must be dipped (Chapter XIX) in a medicated solution to overcome these pests. Providing hogs with rubbing posts or bars covered with oil-soaked sacking is recommended to limit insect infestation. An oil high in sulphur content such as Beaumont crude oil and the like is best.

Grooming of pet animals in large centers of population has almost become a refined art, dictated in a

Grooming dogs and cats

measure by a desire to make the animal comfortable and clean for human association, and for dwelling in human habitations. All too frequently it is also done to satisfy the dictates of fashion as shown by the fantastic hair trims at dog shows. Dogs may be bathed and brushed to clean the skin though cats, because of an inherent aversion to bathing, are best kept clean by brushing and combing. Bathing in tepid water and mild soap is not harmful to cats, at times may be positively necessary. Cats usually resent it so seriously, however, that under ordinary circumstances it is best omitted. "Plucking" dogs is a common practice, and a commendable one to remove the heating under-coat during the warmer days of the year.

Clipping animals is generally practiced. It is primarily done in the case of sheep for the purpose

Clipping animals and its advantages

of obtaining the fleece, but is followed to some extent with other animals. In all animals removal of the skin covering whether hair, wool, fur or bristles is a dis-

*Care and Management of Dairy Bulls (Farmers Bulletin No. 1412) U.S.D.A.—Price 15 cents, is recommended.

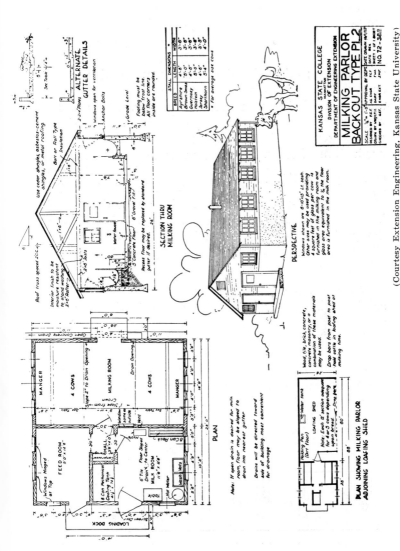

(Courtesy Extension Engineering, Kansas State University)

FIG. 54. Plans for a milking parlor, and loafing shed.

tinct aid in the treatment of skin diseases, and for the removal of skin parasites.

The greatest advantage of clipping is that it is an aid in keeping the animal clean, and that after perspiring, drying takes place more quickly. Cattle are not as a general rule subjected to clipping when the skin is in good health; otherwise it offers the same advantages as in sheep and horses in the treatment of parasites and other skin affections. In many dairies (page 573) it is a regular practice to clip the hairs of the udder as well as adjoining parts of the body to assist in the sanitary production of milk. It has been demonstrated that if during the winter months cattle are **Lice control by clipping** clipped every six weeks infestation with lice will be controlled without the use of insecticides. Lice cannot persist when they do not have the protection of the host's heavy hair coat. These clipped animals must have artificial protection against cold, wet weather.

No milking on the floor or ground is permissible, as this will simply be a source of infection for the

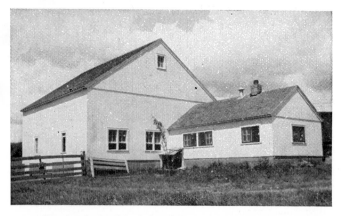

(Courtesy Dept. of Agricultural Engineering, Kansas State University)

Fig. 55. Dairy parlor in which cows are housed and cleaned in the larger unit, milked in one-half of the smaller unit, and the handling of milk limited to the remaining half of the smaller unit.

Floors will become contaminated if milked upon

udders of healthy cows later occupying the same place. If milk from diseased udders is to be used for animal feed, it should be boiled before use. If the milk is badly altered because of an udder disease, it should be discarded, though some antiseptic should first be mixed with it.

From a sanitary standpoint it is reprehensible to resort to wet-hand milking. If lubrication of the teats

Wet-hand milking is insanitary

is absolutely necessary, then this may be done with some bland substance, such as olive oil or vaseline.

Each day before it is swept, the floor should be sprinkled with hydrated lime (page 255), and if manure from udder-infected, as well as Bang's disease infected, animals is not spread on sun-exposed ground daily, it should have some superphosphate of calcium mixed with it.

A few days before the time of calving, or for that matter during parturition, in any of the domesticated animals it is preferable to segregate the mother in a maternity stall or isolated place. This is emphasized for cattle because it has been determined that at the

Care of cows and calves at the time of calving is recommended

time of calving, if the cow is Bang's disease (page 578) infected, she becomes a most prolific spreader of the infection. If confined in a maternity stall it is comparatively simple to destroy the afterbirth without excessive contamination of the surroundings, to disinfect all surroundings that

have become contaminated, and to keep these sanitary. The cow is to be kept in the maternity stall until there no longer is an abnormal discharge from her genitals. Her milk is not suitable for human consumption, nor for animal use until after it has been sterilized by boiling it, or at least pasteurizing it (page 235), until all such abnormal discharges have ceased. The navels of the newly-born should be disinfected immediately after their birth (pages 354 and 355) and daily thereafter until the navel cord has become desiccated, after which it is not likely to become infected. Several diseases of the newly born may be prevented by these comparatively simple sanitary precautions.

Long-haired dogs are made much more comfortable during the warm days of the year by being clipped.

Wire cuts and rope burns if neglected frequently result in permanent and serious deformities of the limbs (Fig. 53). Bandaging and appropriate wound treatment will prevent this if started at the beginning of the injury.

Neglected wire cuts cause deformity

The McLean County system of Swine Sanitation, (page 672) though primarily developed for the prevention of round-worm infestation, is remarkably effective in aiding in the control of filth borne diseases of swine such as cholera (page 616), erysipelas (page 620), the various dysenteries and others.

CHAPTER XII

COMMUNITY SALES, COMMUNITY SIRES, AND TRANSIT LOSSES

Community sales as they have recently been developed are potential sources of danger to livestock health.

Community sales are potential centers of danger to livestock health
The popularity and growth of these sales have been so rapid that state veterinarians have not been able to formulate fair regulations rapidly enough to safeguard the buyers in these markets. Steps are now being taken, however, in most states to afford a measure of sanitary control. The first and probably the most important step is the appointment of a qualified veterinarian to serve as the local inspector of health in so far as it relates to the animals that are bought and sold in these markets. He is also charged with the control of the general sanitation of the buildings, many of which are old and dilapidated. If they have inadequate drainage, poor lighting and ventilation and no screening they serve as harbingers for rodents and vermin. Surroundings such as these inspire no sense of sanitation and, therefore, they must be corrected.

Once clean, the building is to be kept so by thorough disinfection after each sale, as it is not improbable that some of the animals sold originated in diseased herds or flocks. If the inspector is not certain of the origin of the livestock offered, then to prevent the possible spread of disease he should insist that such livestock be kept in quarantine in the sales barn or on the new owner's premises for at least twenty-one days. If at the end of this time no recognizable evidence of disease has made its appearance, it is then reasonable to assume that it will be safe to place the animals with others on the farm.

All conveyances used in bringing animals to the sales must be cleaned by having all bedding, manure and litter removed and safely stored on the grounds of the sales building. Then the conveyance must be thoroughly disinfected, the last step of which should be the wheels as it has been proved that the wheels of vehicles are capable of transferring many animal disease infections from potential centers of infection, such as community sales, to the surrounding farms and territory; notable among these is hog cholera. Furthermore, it would be an excellent regulation if those people that attend these affairs were compelled as they are leaving the premises to walk over mats saturated with a reliable non-odorous disinfectant in order to prevent their footwear from serving as mechanical spreaders of disease-producing germs and parasite eggs. In the very scrupulous person, the hands also should be well washed with good soap (page 252), which is an excellent cleanser, and warm water, especially if they have handled any of the animals offered for sale.

In order that those not familiar with the seriousness of this problem and possibly somewhat skeptical about the necessity of all these steps, an example may be cited with the germs or rather virus, for such it is, of hog cholera (page 616) as the criminal. The virus of hog cholera is contained especially in the blood, though also during the fever in the urine, bile, tears and other secretions of ailing animals. Many times it is impossible to recognize that a hog has cholera, though it is a carrier of the virus because of an early stage of the disease and this would probably be the stage in which it is offered for barter at a community sale. The potency or power of the virus is exemplified by mixing one drop of the virus-containing blood with 50,000 drops of water; bio-chemists state this as a 1 to 50,000 dilution. Very roughly estimated this is approximately one drop of the blood mixed with one gallon of water. If, now, one drop of this dilution is placed within the eyelids of a young hog, a "susceptible" that has neither had cholera nor been protected against it by vaccination, it is likely to result in the development of cholera in the eye-inoculated subject. It would most certainly be possible for the same amount of virus, one fifty-thousandth of a drop, to be carried on the hands or shoes of a person, on the wheels of trucks, or on the feet of animals, and thus to be disseminated to surrounding premises. Similar examples can be cited for diseases other than hog cholera. The great importance of thorough sanitation in and around sales-barns and pavilions, and everything exposed to contact with it or its products cannot be over-emphasized.

Occasionally livestock owners expose their animals to almost the same disease dangers as those encountered in community sales by the use of a common sire for their breeding herds and flocks. Undoubtedly, the stallion is most generally used in this manner but fortunately the most serious equine breeding diseases have been stamped out or they are well under control. This is not the case, however, as it relates to the use of a community bull, and particularly the spread of Bang's disease infection.

Community sires as spreaders of cattle diseases

If the bull is not frequently blood-tested (page 758) to determine his freedom from this infection, he is a possible source of danger. Though it has been reasonably well demonstrated that a bull is not a mechanical carrier of the germs of Bang's disease from an infected female served by him to the next animal submitted to him for service, it is good sanitary practice to always keep the tuft of long hairs trimmed away from the entrance to the bull's sheath because these are habitations for infections, and also immediately after each copulation disinfecting the penis and its sheath. Usually this is done by flowing an antiseptic solution, such as that made by adding one large tablespoonful of carbolic acid to a gallon of lukewarm soft water, by means of a gravity apparatus such as a fountain syringe, into the sheath, at the same time grasping the end of the sheath with the hand so as to close it, and then with the other hand manipulating the sheath

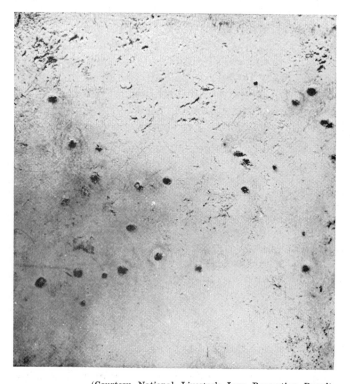

FIG. 56. Hide injuries following the use of sharp prod poles. Somewhat comparable injuries are observed following an infestation with ox warbles. (Page 706.)

so as to cause the carbolic acid water to reach all parts of it. A clean funnel and a piece of soft rubber tubing is satisfactory for this purpose.

The bull if he is Bang's-disease-infected and not simply mechanically germ-contaminated, but carrying the germ in his tissues, frequently has the germs lodged in his testicles to be carried out with the male element at the time of copulation, thus infecting all the females bred to him. Furthermore, some of the semen may drop on the ground contaminating it, later to be picked up by a susceptible female.

The use of a bull known to harbor in his tissues the germ of Bang's disease should not be tolerated, but sometimes this is not known and diagnostic attempts to disclose it are not perfect; therefore, in the use of a community bull, or in the use of any bull excepting under range or semi- range conditions where it is almost impractical, breeding should take place in a small fenced-off plot used for no other purpose which is the so-called neutral breeding ground. Contact between the sire and dam should be no longer than is necessary. Immediately after the completion of the service the outer surface of the female genitals should be disinfected, as well as those of the bull in the manner already described.

There is a relatively enormous preventable annual *loss amongst animals in transit,* particularly during the period involving transfer from the farms to the central livestock markets. In a recent survey 163,444 head of cattle and 775,332 hogs were checked at 70 processing plants:

Preventable injuries to animals in transit result in large losses

The following is a breakdown of a representative sample of cattle and hog reports indicating the frequency and proportionate distribution of bruises:

Cattle	
Loin	45.0%
Rib	17.0%
Rounds	11.8%
Chuck	10.8%
Plate	8.5%
Rump	6.9%

Hogs	
Ham	51.3%
Belly	18.0%
Fatbacks	13.0%
Loins	9.0%
Shoulder	8.7%

A quick glance at the above percentages would indicate that the loin, rib and round of cattle and the ham and belly of a hog are the most vulnerable spots for bruises. It is difficult to picture these bruises occurring without the careless assistance of man.

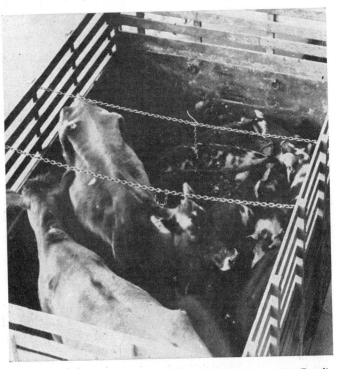

(Courtesy National Livestock Loss Prevention Board)

FIG. 57. Mixed shipments of livestock without partitions in the vehicle mean costly injuries that reduce profits.

A downward dollar loss trend was evidenced in the latest audit. Of the 163,444 head of cattle, 10,414 were bruised (6.37%) with a monetary loss of $5.71 per bruised animal. The figures on the 775,332 head of hogs show 65,829 were bruised (8.49%) with a monetary loss of $.95 per bruised hog.

The principal causes of losses in transit as given by the National Live Stock Loss Prevention Board are:

Some causes of losses in transit (1) overcrowding in trucks or cars; (2) mixed shipments (Fig. 57) without partitions; (3) poor footing and inadequate or improper bedding; (4) weak poorly constructed partitions of the wrong type, which are broken in transit; (5) low vitality and diseased conditions; (6) rough handling (Fig. 58) in cars and trucks by railroad, stockyard, and meat packer employees or other caretakers; (7) excessive feeding and watering before loading in cars or trucks; (8) exposure in extremely cold weather, and lack of ventilation in hot weather; (9) fighting by strange animals; (10) sharp corners on gates and post; and (11) protruding nails

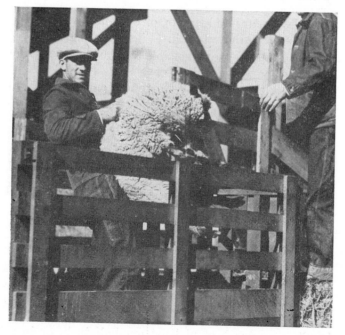

(Courtesy National Livestock Loss Prevention Board)

Fig. 58. Picking up sheep by the wool causes flesh bruises.

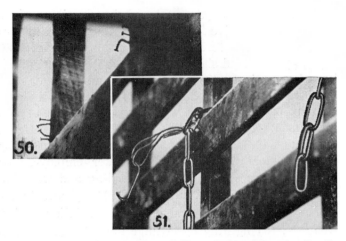

(Courtesy National Livestock Loss Prevention Board)

FIGS. 59 and 60. Inside of truck showing projecting wires and chains. These are frequent causes of injury to animals.

and bolts in cars and trucks, or on fences which gouge and tear the skin and flesh. (Figs. 59 and 60.)

If those persons responsible for the welfare of their livestock charges could observe these animals shortly after their slaughter to note the extent of the injury caused by kicking or striking; prodding with poles and end-gate rods; (Fig. 56) the effect of clubs and whips; and extensive muscle bruising (Figs. 61 and 62), let alone hide injuries, they would be more humane in their treatment. Furthermore, in the feed lot better gains are made and a source of loss is eliminated when horns are removed.

Some of the remedies recommended to reduce the large annual loss among livestock in transit are: use canvas slappers with wide surfaces; electric prodders instead of poles, clubs, whips, and end-gate rods; canvas or other roofs on trucks to protect from excessive cold; **Means of** cleating the floors of trucks, possibly with **preventing** a false bottom; a covering of sand to a **transit** depth of at least one-half inch, or in cold **losses** weather the use of straw bedding; proper

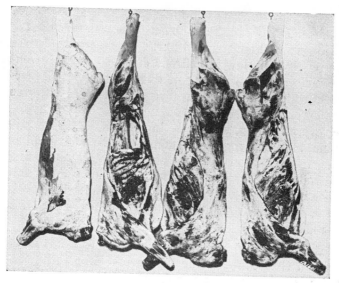

(Courtesy National Livestock Loss Prevention Board)

FIG. 61. Beef carcasses trimmed in order to remove bruised flesh.

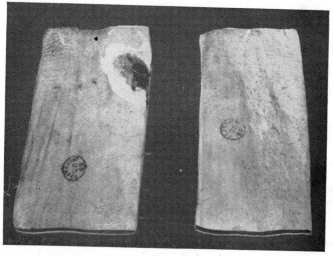

(Courtesy National Livestock Loss Prevention Board)

FIG. 62. Trimmed out bruise in the side of bacon on the left; undamaged side on the right.

construction of trucks so as to be without low cross-rods and low narrow end-gates; sideboards so spaced that animals are not likely to get their legs through the openings; well constructed partitions in trucks (these are required by law in railroad cars) so as to prevent the indiscriminate mixing of different species of live-stock which almost always results in injury to the smaller ones; good loading and unloading chutes; avoiding overcrowding, especially in the case of sheep and swine; and allowing the animals a good rest as well as some food and water before shipment. Heavy feeding and watering should always be avoided since a fat animal with full or overloaded stomach results in crowding of the lungs and heart, which is a poor risk for a long shipment.

Even on the farm where livestock originates there is much that can be done to prevent unnecessary injuries. Farm facilities for reducing these losses consist of corrals to serve as sorting and holding pens; loading chute of the all-purpose type—width 32 inches, length of ramp about 12 feet or more, with smooth sides the lower two feet of which are tight, and the ramp flooring should be cleated, or have low "stair steps"; and trucks should have wide open end gates to prevent cattle from getting jammed and bruised.

Carriers (pages 214 and 220). Another closely related factor in disease dissemination must not be over-looked, that of the aged animal "carrier."
The "carrier" of animal diseases It is not uncommon for one or more older animals to have apparently recovered from a disease, though actually they still harbor the contagion to which they have become resistant, but which they still are capable of passing on to less resistant or more susceptible and usually younger members of the same species. For the purpose of illustration mention is here made to Bang's disease and leptospirosis in cattle, anaplasmosis in cattle, swamp fever in horses, hog cholera in swine, and

a host of others. These outwardly harmless "carriers" of disease are sources of potential danger, especially to the younger and recently introduced members of herds and flocks. It is always best to eliminate these "carriers" by establishing their identity through suitable physical or biological tests. A further safeguard against the introduction of disease into a group of known healthiness by a newly obtained animal that may be in either the incipient stage or the "carrier" stage is to keep such animals in quarantine (page 212) for periods varying in duration from two weeks to three months. Neglect of these precautions may be the source of severe economic loss.

PART THREE

Some Methods of Disease Control

⚜⚜⚜⚜

CHAPTER XIII

(A) THE QUARANTINE

Quarantine (page 825). The word quarantine is derived from the Italian "quaranta" meaning "forty," because originally ships and their passengers coming from a port where smallpox or other infectious diseases prevailed were detained for a period of forty days. Today the word in general means the *isolation* of a person or an animal sick with a contagious disease, or it also refers to a place where the sick are detained away from other animals until the danger of spread of a contagious disease has disappeared. In its wider application, the quarantine may be enforced against an individual animal, against all the animals, or all animals of the same species, in a township, county, or state, and against those in a foreign country. There are legal provisions for the enforcement of a quarantine usually by the sheriff, and occasionally aided by the militia, though in regard to animals original authority in a state has been placed in the hands of the state veterinarian, or for interstate or foreign quarantines the authority has been delegated to the Secretary of Agriculture, the Secretary acting upon the advice of the veterinarians and Chief of the federal veterinary forces. Livestock owners on their

Quarantine means the isolation of animals affected with contagious diseases

Legal quarantine

own initiative very frequently place in quarantine an individual animal or groups of their animals for the purpose of controlling the spread of a contagious disease. They do this especially when their herds and flocks are already free from disease and they desire to add to them by the acquisition of new animals. These new animals are kept in isolation for so long as ninety days in extreme instances, or until persons concerned are satisfied after a conference with their veterinarian that there is no longer any danger of contaminating their original animals with a contagious ailment.

The principles governing an effective quarantine are similar in general for individuals or for groups of animals. *There must be no direct or indirect contact between the animal in quarantine and those not so restrained.* It has its variations depending upon contagiousness of a disease or upon the volatility of its causative factor. For example, many parasitic diseases of the skin, including mange, are not nearly so easily spread as is hog cholera. A quarantine does mean that an animal affected with any one of the very large numbers of external parasitic and contagious diseases must be kept segregated in a separate barn or yard away from other animals.

Theoretically the quarantined animals should have separate attendants, their own drinking vessels and other utensils, as well as the usual barn equipment. If a separate attendant is not available, then the common attendant should take care of the sick group last and when he is through with them he must clean his footwear by thoroughly rubbing them on a mat saturated with a disinfectant, as well as washing his hands. Soap (page 252) in warm water is a mechanical remover of infection and in a limited manner is an antiseptic. In very highly volatile diseases, such as foot-and-mouth disease of cattle, fumigation of clothing or protection of the usual clothing by wearing of rubber outer garments may be necessary.

Whenever certain animals of a group contract a contagious disease, though other animals of the same group are still apparently free from it, the healthy are to be moved to clean surroundings and the diseased should remain in the old, contaminated yards and buildings. The usual practice of removing the sick and leaving the healthy in disease-contaminated surroundings is an unsound one. If it is not practical to follow the foregoing procedure, that is, if the healthy must be retained in the yards or buildings in which the disease originated, then such places must be disinfected in a most thorough manner (page 216). Furthermore, yards and buildings housing diseased animals must have drainage away from places occupied by the healthy ones.

Unsound to remove the sick from the healthy

It is by means of the quarantine, aided by other steps, that the spread of communicable animal ailments have been controlled. It is much more effective for such conditions as Southern cattle fever than for foot-and-mouth disease because the latter is due to a highly volatile contagion while the former is almost stationary in its nature. The quarantine has not effected the high hopes held out for it at one time, it is nevertheless a disease control measure of some value.

Possibly one of the reasons for its lack of effectiveness is that all animals infected in a herd or flock in all instances do not show symptoms of the infection with the result that these sub-chronic individuals perpetuate the disease in the healthy herd. "Carriers" (page 220) offer a similar problem—anaplasmosis (page 745) for example.

Another factor is that to prevent the spread of an infection the person delegated to apply the principles of isolation must have enough reasonably good knowledge about the nature of these invisible disease producing elements. At least the veterinarian in general charge of the attempt to control the spread of the disease should regard it as his duty to specifically instruct the attendant of the animals about the intelligent application of the principles involved in the quarantine.

Finally officers—usually state or federal veterinarians—must recognize that in establishing a quarantine they are acting for the public good. This imposes great restrictions, and usually heavy financial loss, upon the owners of the livestock. Possibly with the single exception of restricting the freedom of an innocent person in the jury of an established court there is no other procedure where an entirely innocent individual has such a severe "penalty" imposed by legal authority. It has been stated that in establishing the restrictions of a more or less general quarantine the state livestock sanitary officer is acting as prosecuting attorney, jury and judge. America has been fortunate in having in these officers men of sound judgment and high professional standards and training.

In a measure the quarantine includes, in most states, animals that have died of infectious and contagious diseases in that carcasses may not be placed in or near flowing streams—such an act would endanger down-stream livestock, nor may such carcasses be transported over public highways. The only exception to this latter regulation, in those states having such a regulation, is that bonded rendering establishments that have approved safe-guards may move or transport carcasses of animals dead of communicable ailments.

By means of the quarantine, sanitary officials in America have controlled contagious pleuropneumonia, foot-and-mouth disease, tuberculosis, fowl plague and many other diseases. Rabies of dogs and other animals could be so controlled. The quarantine is one of the most effective measures to prevent the spread of many ailments.

(B)   DISINFECTING PREMISES

Cleaning premises must precede all other steps to again make them safe for animal occupation after an outbreak of a contagious disease. It is spoken of as "disinfecting" the premises. It includes the removal of all litter and refuse, and then disinfection. The latter implies the destruction of all disease-producing germs; in a broader sense it may also include the destruction of parasitic factors. However, it must be emphasized that many animal diseases are contracted because of close contact between the ailing and the well animal, or stated another way the premises may be no more than of secondary importance in a matter of this nature.

Disinfection of premises will make animal quarters reasonably sanitary, but the value of such a step is limited strictly to an attempt at preventing the premises from spreading disease, and does not in any way control the disease due to the presence of the sub-chronically infected animal or "carriers" in a group.

On the other hand infected animals do contaminate premises with disease-producing factors that are in their urine, manure, and occasionally in their secretions and exhalations. Since the number and vigor of germs are the greatest in the immediate area and vicinity occupied by the ailing animal therefore disinfection should be concentrated in such places.

The suggested steps in premises disinfection are as follows:

1. Since organic material such as manure and the usual animal habitation refuse protect germs and limit the action of disinfectants, such material must be removed. First, moisten with water or a disinfectant so as to control dust and air-borne infections. This moistening should include all woodwork, and is to be followed by litter removal from night barns, night lots, feed sheds, small pastures and yards, and fences, especially those of wood construction, and around hay and feed racks even though they have not been in use for some time. The walls and ceilings and other woodwork in barns and sheds must be thoroughly

brushed or broom swept to remove cobwebs, old scaled whitewash, and other objectionable material. All burnable material removed by these steps is to be so destroyed, and the remainder may be spread out on arable land at some distance away, so that it will be fully exposed to the sun's action. Old sacks may later be disinfected (page 262). If buildings have dirt floors, at least three inches of this is to be removed, then apply a disinfectant to the exposed surface, and finally cover it with clean material such as fresh dirt, sand, gravel, or cinders.

2. If there are pools of water on the premises, these are either to be drained, or fenced off so that they will not be accessible to animals.

3. All feed in mangers and feed boxes in the rooms that are to be disinfected is to be removed and burned, or it may be fed to livestock not susceptible to the disease against which the disinfection is being applied.

4. If water under pressure is available, it is an excellent plan to hose off everything that has previously had litter and other material removed from it. To follow this by a thorough scrubbing with scalding hot water to which some lye has been added (page 253) will dissolve off a good deal of the dirt, and besides, the hot water will kill worm eggs and the lye will destroy many types of germs. Use one pound of lye to 20 gallons of water.

5. Water troughs and feeding boxes and racks should be scrubbed with the lye solution (page 253) in readiness for effective treatment with a disinfectant solution. Since there is a valid objection to the use of odorous disinfectants in the treatment of many utensils those constructed of metal may be satisfactorily handled by cleaning with hot water and soap, and then immersed in boiling water. Special attention should be paid to the surface and ground about and underneath water troughs. The muddy or moist soil under water troughs has been known to harbor some

disease-producing germs for over a year after surface disinfection has been applied. If on low ground, water troughs should be moved to a part of the yard or corral where good drainage may be established.

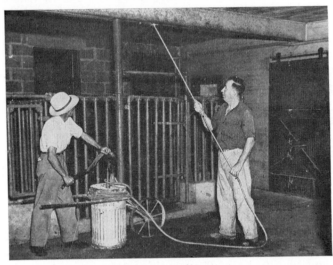

(Courtesy U.S.D.A., Bureau of Animal Industry, 110.62-A)

FIG. 63. Disinfecting a barn. About the same technic may be used to spray for lice on animals.

7. The application of the disinfectant solution is best done by means of a (page 285) spray pump (Fig. 63) so as to force it into all cracks and crevices in the woodwork. Applying it with a broom is a good method but this does not force it into the wood. The addition of some whitewash (this must be fresh water-slaked lime) to the disinfectant solution is of value, as it can then better be seen where the material has been applied. Blankets, robes, harness and other loose paraphernalia may be disinfected by immersing them for at least several hours in the disinfectant.

The choice of a disinfectant varies somewhat, depending upon the nature of the infection. Different types of germs do not all react similarly to the same disinfectants. This is discussed more fully in the chapter relating to disinfectants. In general it may be said that disinfectants are more effective when used as hot solutions, and that a disinfectant having "a phenol coefficient" (page 251) of at least six should be used. Usually the better disinfectants have a printed statement on the label indicating their "phenol coefficient." A phenol coefficient of six means that the disinfectant in question is six times as effective in its action upon typhoid germs as is phenol (carbolic acid). (Consult page 260.)

For the disinfection of all woodwork Saponated Cresol Solution (Compound Solution of Cresol) (page 263) made in accordance with the United States pharmacopoeia, and diluted with hot water so as to make a three per cent solution is effective, but its odor is objectionable in dairy barns. For outside woodwork, a cheaper and very effective disinfective is a five per cent water solution of chlorinated lime, but it must be used in the open, as it is very irritating to people inhaling its fumes inside of buildings. If formaldehyde solution (page 266) is used for inside disinfection, it should be in four per cent strength, though for use in previously cleaned water troughs it should be painted on full strength over the inside and outside of the trough, and permitted to dry, after which drinking water may again safely be placed in the trough. A full strength solution of the gas formaldehyde in water is known as formalin—in it there is thirty-seven per cent of the gas in the water.

Dirt floors or corrals are best disinfected, though not perfectly, by saturating them with oil and burning this, and then turning under the top soil by means of a plow. Whenever an infection is very severe, it is an excellent plan to repeat the disinfection at the end of twenty-four hours. Always remember that the direct action of the sun's rays is a most efficient destroyer of germs, provided the germs are not hidden under rubbish or in darkened places. If disinfection is not done thoroughly we accomplish little more, as stated by an eminent authority, than to create a bad smell.

In this connection, when disinfection of buildings is under discussion, it is appropriate to mention the importance of disinfecting hypodermic needles. The use of these needles has become so very general in obtaining blood samples from animals for laboratory diagnostic purposes, as well as in the injection of vaccines that without disinfection or sterilization there is grave danger of spreading from infected and "carrier" (pages 210 and 553) animals the infections of anaplasmosis (page 745) and others. The needle should be disinfected after each use by placing it in a reliable disinfectant, and rinsing it in clean water before it is inserted into the next animal. Storing the needles in grain alcohol during intervals when they are not in use is an excellent expedient. Sterilizing needles over a flame softens the metal. Boiling water will sterilize needles in a few minutes but if a stilet is not kept in them rusting is a problem.

Disinfecting needles

Care must be exercised in the use of the hypodermic needle and syringe

In conclusion attention must again be called to the close relationship existing between cleanliness in the care of animals and disinfection. When premises and animals are kept clean it means frequent removal of animal excretions and debris as well as grooming. These steps mechanically remove many germs and their hiding places—the latter protect them. The exposure of germs not mechanically removed by cleaning processes nevertheless weakens them and makes them more susceptible to natural destructive agencies, and also in most cases renders them incapable of causing disease in their weakened condition.

(C)   PASTURE ROTATION AND SANITATION

This is a practical and important method of control, not only for some of the communicable diseases, but for the prevention of parasite infestations as well. (Consult page 715 on control of Southern fever ticks.)

Some disease-producing germs go into a resting or seed stage during which they are designated as "spores." These are much more resistant to destruction by the elements or by man-made and applied agents than are the parent germs, so that yards and pastures once contaminated by them will remain so for an indefinite number of years. Anthrax (page 591), that highly fatal disease of cattle, horses, sheep, and swine, is an outstanding example of this type of ailment. Whenever diseases of this kind become established on premises, then these may no longer be used for livestock production, excepting animals protected by specific vaccination. Some times it is necessary to fence off such regions for a number of years, provided their drainage is not in the direction of occupied livestock pastures, in which event the drained into area must also be fenced off. In other instances it is simply necessary to keep off from those pastures that species of animal that is susceptible to the infection, though non-susceptibles may be safely placed thereon. This advice is in line with the often repeated injunction not to permit healthy animals to congregate in places that may have been contaminated with disease producing factors. Common watering places are to be regarded with suspicion.

Spores and their nature

Protection against parasites (page 663) is an important problem in animal husbandry. Those comparatively few persons, trained observers, that have noticed the almost universal and many times intensely severe parasitic infestation of all animals, including the domesticated ones, can testify to the correctness of this statement. To the average layman it is an astounding revelation that animals are so generally parasitized. Theoretically, all of it is controllable by sanitation, and all efforts devoted to this cause will repay many fold in better health and vigor of the hosts.

The severity of parasitism

A parasite may be defined as an organism that lives in or on another organism known as the host and usu-

Injuries to the host by parasites
ally with some degree of harmful results to the latter. The parasite abstracts nourishment from the tissues of the host or it may appropriate for its own use food intended for the host and at the same time be deriving shelter and warmth from the latter. Incidentally the parasite produces mechanical injuries by bites; not infrequently it injects irritant poisons at the time of the bite. It may mechanically obstruct certain organs, as for example hog worms invading and lodging in the bile duct or stomach bots of horses filling that organ. When crushed within the tissues of the host the parasite may set up certain reactions (anaphylaxis) resulting seriously and even fatally to the host.

Those parasites that live on the outside of the host are the most readily controlled by the use of poisonous agents such as dips, and by mechanically acting substances such as dry insect powders which frequently act by sealing up the breathing pores in the skin of the parasite, and by the cleaning of the premises (for details refer to pages 288 to 323, inclusive).

Those that live within the host are most difficult to contend with successfully. Sanitary preventive methods are outstandingly of the greatest importance. How well is this exemplified in the little or total absence of infestation in humans living in sanitary surroundings as compared with the universal heavy infestation in animals living under insanitary conditions. In animals, however, the problem usually resolves itself into the economic question of whether it is more profitable to control the parasites or to permit infestation, the answer probably lying somewhere midway between the two points of view. There can be no question, however, that within the limitations prescribed prevention is of greater importance than cure, though the average

livestock owner is inclined to favor the latter, forgetting that after an animal has once become
Many infested, the parasite has frequently in-
parasite- flicted such severe damage upon its tissues
infested that elimination or cure does not restore
animals are the animal to normal. Witness, for ex-
irreparably ample, the droves or bands of perma-
injured
nently runty hogs and unthrifty sheep or other animals,
following the elimination of their parasites.

A general rule in relation to parasites that live
within the host is that the young animals are much
Young more susceptible to parasite invasion than
animals most are the mature. This fact is taken advan-
susceptible tage of in their attempted prevention by
to parasites the so-called creep-feeding of lambs and
calves, in the McLean County sanitary system (page
672) against intestinal round worms in hogs, the raising of young poultry on sanitary runways (page 144)
to prevent coccidiosis (page 735) and other means.
All these and other methods are discussed more in detail in later pages of this publication.

Most intestinal worm parasites need moisture for
either the hatching of their eggs, or for the immature
worm (larva) to reach a favorable location on vegetation prior to animal consumption. If therefore infested
pastures must be grazed by susceptible hosts—especially the highly susceptible young ones—keep them out
of such pastures until the wetness of dew and rains
has evaporated.

Deep plowing of infected and parasite infested
land as well as draining all low places is very helpful
in control practices. Most parasite eggs and larvae
rarely reach the surface again after having been
plowed under several inches of soil. If such land can
be applied for a season to the growing of crops it will
be practically free from parasite contaminants at the
end of this period.

The Florida Agricultural Experiment Station reports that "sulphured" soil is of assistance in the con-

trol of diseases on premises in which poultry must be confined in the same yard continuously. Commercial flour sulphur is broadcast over the surface of the soil at the rate of 800 pounds to the acre, and mixed with a spade into the top six inches of soil. Sulphuric acid was produced in the soil and at the end of one year was still at a maximum acidity. The development and growth of many parasites and bacteria were retarded or inhibited.

Parasitic infestations of livestock may very generally be controlled by a system of *pasture rotation*. Burning off pastures has some merit, but does not possess the efficiency with which it is usually credited as those parasites and their eggs that are in or close to the ground may escape destruction. In general, permanent pastures used regularly by recognized host species are to be regarded as highly dangerous for profitable livestock production and a system of change of land areas from pasturage to crop production is

Parasites are frequently host specific

commendable. In the case of parasites, as well as for germs, it is fortunate that some of them are specific for certain hosts. For example, some of the round worms (the strongyles) of horses will not infest cattle, sheep, and swine, and the stomach worms of sheep are not dangerous to swine and horses, though in general sheep, goats and cattle are susceptible to the same parasites. This fact suggests the safe use of pastures for some species, though unsafe for others.

Pastures that have been freed of parasites are again soon contaminated when the mature animals— these are almost invariably heavily parasitized—are again placed on them. If the surrounding daily temperature reaches 95° F., and when moisture conditions are favorable, the invading stage of the parasite will be reached in three to four days; at 70° F. it requires six to ten days; at 50° F. three to four weeks. In those portions of the United States where hard freezes are common both parasitized and non-parasitized sheep may safely be placed in a common pasture for the period extending from late October to early March, and then if transferred to a clean pasture they may be safely kept there for another month.

Such a procedure is safe for all parasitic diseases in which the eggs hatch outside of the host—stomach worms of ruminants—but not when the eggs hatch inside the host—round-worms of swine. When the weather warms parasite development gains momentum and therefore hosts comparatively free of intestinal parasites must be moved to clean pastures every two weeks. As the cooler weather sets in the time permitted on such pastures may again be lengthened.

The consumption by animals of forage or roughages grown on parasite infested land is not an entirely safe method as such vegetation may have on it the eggs or larvae.

Insofar as the contaminants of soil are bacterial spores—anthrax and blackleg are examples—such pastures remain unsafe for many years for susceptible animals. Frequently protective vaccination is the control method adopted. This protects the vaccinated animal, though the pasture retains its infective potentialities for a long time. In fact, pastures on lower ground may become dangerous because of drainage. Plowing such land has some merit but it does not prevent earthworms and other forms of subterranean life from conveying the highly destruction resistant spores to the surface.

To summarize the control of livestock diseases by pasture rotation the following steps are emphasized:—

1. Select well drained pastures.

2. Avoid overstocking of pastures.

3. Separate the young from the old as soon as possible, and raise the former on a dry pasture or rotate pastures.

4. Use clean water and feed in raised troughs or racks.

It must not be inferred that the foregoing steps will invariably control all contagious and parasitic diseases. As an example it may be cited that the life history of certain parasites is unknown as is evidenced in that frequently occurring tapeworm of sheep. The *Thysanosoma actinoides*—also known as the "fringed tapeworm" or the "liver tapeworm"—undoubtedly requires an intermediate host for its development (page 665). Usually grass mites are the intermediate host, but an examination of thousands of these mites has failed to incriminate a single one as the intermediate host of the "fringed tapeworm." Moreover the direct association of infested sheep with those free from infestation has not resulted in the contamination of the latter. At this writing, the intermediate host of the *fringed tapeworm was still unknown.*

(D) DESTROYING AILING ANIMALS, AND DISPOSAL OF CARCASSES

Destroying diseased animals having a low value, or those chronically and incurably ill is a sanitary precaution worthy of the widest application. Fowls, especially, have such a comparatively low value that it is good insurance to get rid of ailing birds rather than to jeopardize the health of the remainder of the flock by permitting what may possibly be a "living reservoir" of disease to associate with others. In the larger and more valuable animals this principle does not have such a wide application, and it may be necessary to limit the sanitary steps to a quarantine of the ailing.

A good plan to destroy the ailing fowl in a flock

Even after the death of animals from contagious diseases their carcasses remain as reservoirs of disease-producing factors. For example it has been found that the virus of hog cholera (page 616) will remain virulent during the winter months in a body buried in the

Carcasses reservoirs of infection

fall. (Page 616.) When not buried the hog cholera virus in the body of the dead animal is more accessible than in the buried one. It has been found to be infective for as long as eleven weeks, though sooner reaching the non-infective stage because of being subjected to the higher above-ground temperature. Mid-summer direct sunlight will kill the unprotected cholera virus in less than 24 hours, though during the cold of winter it may remain virulent for as long as a month. In this connection it is well to reiterate that cold makes infective material dormant, heat hastens its metabolic processes and earlier death in unfavorable surroundings, usually outside the body.

Putrefaction in dead bodies also results in the early destruction of the virus of hog cholera, and of others. Statements regarding the infectivity of cholera carcasses apply also to anthrax, swine erysipelas and in general to most communicable diseases. Whenever in doubt as to the cause of death treat the carcass as a potential source of danger, and dispose of it in a proper manner. This is an important step in animal disease prevention; other suggested steps are:

1. Don't dispose of a carcass by depositing it in or near a stream of flowing water, because this will carry infections to points down-stream.

2. Don't use carcasses for animal feeds because there is too much danger that an infection is responsible for the death and by using it for animal food it may infect the latter. They may carry infected parts to distant places, thus setting up new centers of infection and, furthermore, the consuming animal may contract a serious indigestion from gorging.

3. Don't permit an animal dead of a contagious disease to remain so that biting insects can reach it as these dead animals are usually loaded with infection. It is best to cover the dead animal with a tarpaulin or screen until permanent disposal (page 826).

4. Don't open a carcass (page 764) for an autopsy or other purpose unless this has the approval of a graduate veterinarian. The blood or other tissues of animals dead of such diseases as anthrax, blackleg and others are rich in the causative germ, and as these are spore-formers (see page 221), the opening of the carcass would likely result in a more or less permanent infection of the premises. Even the opening of carcasses of hogs is dangerous because the premises may thus become infected with the virus of hog cholera and, though it is not a spore former and will in the course of time become devitalized, during the period of its vitality it may still be carried from infected premises through the agency of predatory animals and birds to surrounding territory. Therefore, unless approved by a veterinarian, and then only in an easily disinfected place, it is not safe to open carcasses of animals that have died as the result of disease.

5. Undoubtedly the most sanitary method of destroying carcasses is to burn them, preferably close to the site of their death, without dragging them any more than is absolutely necessary and then only on a wheeled vehicle or on a sled, because of the danger of ground contamination. The site having been decided upon, a trench should be dug. The trench should be at least eighteen inches deep, shallower towards the ends, and comparing in width and length to the extent of the animal's width and length. The general direction of the trench should be that of the prevailing air current. The trench is then filled with wood, some iron bars or an iron cultivator wheel placed across it and the carcass placed thereon. By firing the wood, the carcass will be completely consumed and with it all infectious material.

A method of burning a carcass

6. In the larger centers of population the so-called rendering plant is usually available for the industrial utilization of dead animals. In these the hides are re-

moved with proper regard for the dangers of disease dissemination. The hides after removal are usually disinfected by immersion in a disinfecting solution and the remainder of the carcass "fried out" for its fat content, the latter being used in the manufacture of soap.

7. Probably the most common method of carcass disposal is by burial. This is a reasonably safe method

A safe way to bury a dead animal if done deeply enough and in soil from which there is no drainage to neighboring places. Deep burial is necessary to prevent worms from carrying spores (page 221) to the surface. The highest part of the carcass must be at least four feet below the level of the surrounding terrain. Drainage is best safeguarded by seeing to it that the burial ground is in an area where the general water level is at least eight feet beneath the ground. After the carcass is in its grave, and in order to make it unpalatable to marauding animals, it may be "denatured" by drenching it with kerosene, crude carbolic acid or a comparable odorous and bad tasting substance. Covering the carcass with freshly burned quicklime is also an excellent procedure. The grave is then filled with dirt and topped with some rocks to still further circumvent marauders.

A DISPOSAL PIT FOR DEAD CHICKENS AND TURKEYS*

"The disposal of dead birds on the average specialized poultry farm often becomes a burdensome problem that is not satisfactorily handled. The average annual mortality of poultry in the United States is about 20 per cent. On a poultry farm with 2,000 laying birds, therefore, one may expect to lose about 400 birds during the year. Incineration is the preferred method

---

*The following material is a reproduction of the Circular of Information No. 444 of the Oregon Agricultural Experiment Station. The writer of the Circular is E. M. Dickinson of the Department of Veterinary Medicine. It is reproduced here by permission of the Director of the Oregon Agricultural Experiment Station, Corvallis, Oregon.

of disposal, provided the carcasses are completely burned. Carcasses that merely have the feathers burned off and the skin scorched may be left as a serious source of disease. The disposal pit is an effective convenient means for disposal of dead birds that is within the means of all poultry raisers."

"SELECTING THE LOCATION"

"The location of the pit should be selected with care. Some points to consider in selecting the location are as follows:

"1. The pit should be kept a reasonable distance (at least 150 feet) from the poultry houses or other buildings and the well or spring that provides the water supply."

"2. The area selected should have reasonably good drainage. Any area that might flood and fill the pit with water should be avoided."

"CONSTRUCTING THE PIT"

"The most practical size is about 6 feet square by 7 to 8 feet deep. The first foot of earth removed should be over an area 10 feet long by 7 feet wide. The 6-foot square pit is dug in the center of the 10-foot length, thus leaving a 2-foot shelf on each end on which to lay planks for covering the pit (see figure). Seven planks of 2" x 12", 10 feet long, should cover the pit. In the center of the middle plank a hole is cut and framed so that a tube made of 2" x 12" planks 3 or 4 feet long may be fitted, through which the dead birds may be dropped into the pit. For turkey the tube must be made larger and the hole cut through the two center planks. A tight fitting lid should be made for the upper end of the tube to prevent the escape of odors and the entrance of flies. If the lid and that part of the tube above the ground are given several coats of paint the lid and tubes will not be so readily affected by drying and moisture and the lid will fit into the tube more evenly. The tube should extend 1 or 2 feet above the ground and at least 1 foot of earth should be filled in over the planking and banked around the tube so that water will drain away from the tube."

"If the soil is firm and well bound together, retaining planks to keep the edge of the pit from crumbling may not be necessary. However, the surest procedure is to provide retaining planks to keep the earth walls from crumbling. To kill flies that may drop in the pit spray the underside of the lid and the inside walls of the drop tube with a fly killing agent, such as DDT, at frequent intervals. When the pit is filled with dead birds the pit should be sealed by filling the rest of the pit and the drop tube with earth."

"A pit of this size should provide suitable disposal facilities for dead birds for several years on the average poultry farm.

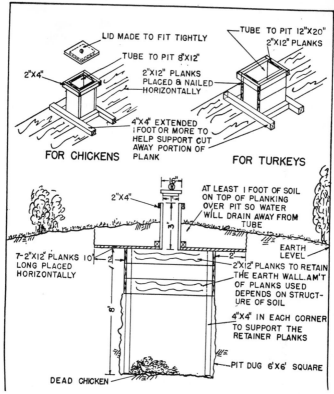

LID MADE TO FIT TIGHTLY

TUBE TO PIT 8"X12"

2"X4"

2"X12" PLANKS PLACED & NAILED HORIZONTALLY

TUBE TO PIT 12"X20"
2"X12" PLANKS

4"X4" EXTENDED 1 FOOT OR MORE TO HELP SUPPORT CUT AWAY PORTION OF PLANK

FOR CHICKENS

FOR TURKEYS

2"X4"

AT LEAST 1 FOOT OF SOIL ON TOP OF PLANKING OVER PIT SO WATER WILL DRAIN AWAY FROM TUBE

7-2"X12" PLANKS 10' LONG PLACED HORIZONTALLY

EARTH LEVEL

2"X12" PLANKS TO RETAIN THE EARTH WALL. AM'T OF PLANKS USED DEPENDS ON STRUCTURE OF SOIL

4"X4" IN EACH CORNER TO SUPPORT THE RETAINER PLANKS

PIT DUG 6'X6' SQUARE

DEAD CHICKEN

Fig. 64. A disposal pit for dead chickens and turkeys.

The success of the pit will depend on its careful and tight construction. A pit that is not tightly covered with at least one foot of soil and with a tight fitting lid on the drop tube will soon be a detriment rather than an asset."

Again, in the handling of carcasses, including the sick as well, assume that the condition is the result of infection and adopt the proper sanitary precautions to prevent disease dissemination. If later the diagnosis or the autopsy findings do not demonstrate the presence of an infection, only a little labor will have been lost. If findings indicate a disease of infectious nature, the health of the remaining animals will have been safeguarded. Violation or disregard of the foregoing general principle of sanitation, or its adoption after it is too late, has been an expensive experience for many livestock producers.

So potentially dangerous, from the standpoint of animal disease spread, are carcasses, that most states have livestock sanitary laws prohibiting their transportation over public highways, and by common carriers, excepting under most rigid prescribed regulation. Usually transportation requests are rightfully denied as a protection to livestock, welfare and health.

PART FOUR

Infections and Their Handling

CHAPTER XIV

HISTORICAL, AND DEFINITIONS

In ancient times there was no rational knowledge regarding decomposition and decay, nor of the action of preservatives, but the people of those days were aware of the fact that salting, smoking, the use of aromatic oils and spices, and wines and vinegars did in some manner inhibit the natural destructive processes in animal and vegetable tissues. Disease was felt to disclose the displeasure of the gods and of malign spirits, and attempts were made to propitiate the former with aromatics, and to dislodge the latter with incantations and acrid, malodorous substances. It is not improbable that any favorable results observed following these practices rested in the fact that the agents used possessed some action destructive to germs. Also, ancients advised their people to remain away from places where evil spirits had evidently taken up their abode. This was always where disease was rampant and thus a measure of quarantine was imposed. This was manifested in still another manner by labeling as "unclean" the unfortunate victims of leprosy, and compelling them to practice some degree of isolation.

Ancient practices

Unconscious isolation

At the beginning of the nineteenth century, and without knowing that living germs cause many diseases, there was the beginning of a somewhat more rational use of disinfectants. Observations had determined that disease was, in a measure, controlled by whitewashing living quarters; by the addition of quicklime to drinking water; by the cauterizing of fresh wounds with nitrate of silver; in the use of chlorine gas for fumigation; and in other procedures. Several years after the middle of this century, Joseph Lister, the

Lister as a pioneer Englishman, who was father of clean surgery, and his contemporaries demonstrated the practical importance of the use of wound dressings impregnated with such agents as carbolic acid. Undoubtedly the practices of Lister were based on the

Pasteur and his work shortly previous discovery made by the great French chemist and bacteriologist, Pasteur, who found that the air was full of living germs, and that these particles could be filtered off by cotton wool, and that they could be destroyed by

The discovery of the microscope heat. Many years before this, Antony Van Leuwenhoek of Delft, Holland, the discoverer of the microscope, had observed by its use certain "living animalcules," though this knowledge remained without practical application until 1850 when Davaine and Rayer demonstrated the causative relationship between the anthrax germ (page 591) and anthrax. From this time on, and during the earlier days of this period, the inspirational work and progress of Louis Pasteur, the Frenchman, and Robert Koch, the German, in establishing the direct relationship between specific germs and many diseases was very rapid; they were laboring in a virgin field.

The new knowledge thus gained at once gave rise to the matter of controlling and possibly destroying these agents of disease. It may be well to explain here that most germs are harmless to human and animal welfare. In fact, life cannot exist without their aid but at times and under conditions not well understood benign germs may assume malignancy, while still others have these baneful qualities at all times. To destroy the malignant germs and thus stamp out or at least control many human and animal diseases is one of the goals of sanitarians. This in turn has given rise to a study of methods of accomplishing these results.

DEFINITIONS:

Disinfectants are agents that destroy the germs of putrefaction or disease, as well as the poisons elaborated by these germs, and also vectors, thus inhibiting disease development. More especially disinfection refers to the destruction of one kind of a germ only, such as the germ of tuberculosis, or the germ of anthrax, or that of blackleg, and so on, though the disinfectant need not necessarily affect other germs that may be present. Disinfectants attempt the destruction of these specific germs after their invasion of tissues and places. Disinfestant is a comparable term used in relation to vectors and other forms of biological life.

Antiseptics are agents that seek to prevent infection by destroying germs in general before they gain entrance to tissues and places. The word is derived from the Greek, meaning "against putrefaction." A surgeon, for example, uses an antiseptic on an operative area, and in a surgery so that there will be no germs to invade the tissues that he intends to incise.

Germicide, bactericide, viricide, and other such words mean virtually the same as disinfectant, excepting that they apply respectively to the destruction of germs, bacteria, and viruses. For practical purposes this fine distinction is without value.

Sterilization is a very broad term. In general it means the destruction of all forms of animal or vegetable life. It may be accomplished by the use of a flame, by means of steam under pressure, by immersion in boiling water for a definite period of time, and by some very powerful chemical agents.

Pasteurization by the application of heat seeks to destroy certain kinds of germs contained in heat-stable products, or to materially reduce the total number of germs in such products without actually resulting in sterilization. Milk is a good example. All of this must be accomplished without at the same time harming the product. In the case of milk-pasteurization rapid cooling must be practiced when the pasteurization is completed to prevent the growth and multiplication of those germs that have not been destroyed.

At least two standard types of pasteurization are recognized, i.e., "the holding method," and "the high-temperature short-time" method.

The "holding method" is in most general use. It consists in heating the product for the duration of thirty minutes to a temperature of between 140° to 148° Fahrenheit, or an average temperature of 143.5° Fahrenheit.

The "high-temperature short-time" method, also known as the "flash" method, is a process so developed that milk may quickly be heated to a high temperature, and holding it there under perfect control without either insufficient pasteurization or scorching. It is accomplished by passing a high-frequency alternating electrical current of 2500 to 6000 volts through milk, for approximately ten seconds, the final temperature reached being 161° to 163° Fahrenheit, or holding the temperature at 161° F. for 15 seconds.

Deodorants are agents that destroy or mask foul odors. They do this by effecting a chemical combination with the odorous substance, thus changing it into a new non-odorous compound. This takes place when formaldehyde (page 266) destroys fecal odors almost instantaneously or the deodorant used has its own strong, though usually not unpleasant, odor which supplants that of the unpleasant odorus substance.

Detergents are chemical agents of very limited value for animal disease use. They act by altering surfaces and interfaces and are therefore anti-infectives.

They are weak against gram-negative germs as well as against acid-fasts, spores and viruses. This action is reduced by organic matter—i.e., blood serum, pus, manure, etc.

Chapter XV

GUIDES IN THE SELECTION OF CHEMICAL DISINFECTANTS, AND THEIR MODES OF ACTION

If disinfection must be accomplished during cold weather, it is best to use warmed solutions. Gradually,

The influence of cold on disinfectants as the surrounding temperature approaches the freezing point, most disinfectants used under these conditions become practically inactive, and inversely as the temperature rises, the disinfecting properties are very much enhanced.

It is always an excellent plan to disinfect daily the surroundings as well as intestinal and other discharges

Sanitation and sick animals of animals having an infectious disease. Permitting such materials to accumulate without disinfection invites the spread of disease.

Blankets and clothing, including boots and shoes used in stables, may be disinfected by keeping them

Disinfect clothing immersed in a strong disinfecting solution for a day or longer. Leather goods may be thoroughly wiped off with the disinfectant, and in addition, if necessary, hard leather may be submitted to formaldehyde fumigation (page 266).

Contaminated drinking water, before being dumped on the premises, should have disinfectant mixed with it.

Drinking water a source of danger Chlorinated lime (page 257) at the rate of one pound to each five gallons of water and left for one-half day has been recommended; the vessel to be later painted inside and outside with undiluted formalin (page 266).

Contaminated feeds are best destroyed. If for economical reasons they must be used, it is best to submit them to drying by spreading them out so **Contaminated feeds to be treated** that full exposure to the sun's action may be obtained, or they may be fumigated with formaldehyde in emergencies (page 266). Then their safeness may be tested by first feeding them to one of the less valuable animals. If the nature of the specific germ-contamination of animal foods is known, they may sometimes be fed to animals not susceptible to the germ in question. Fumigation with gaseous formaldehyde is not dependable, though formaldehyde was formerly extensively used for this purpose. To destroy viruses, formaldehyde fumigation may be used if other, more reliable methods are not applicable.

The ideal disinfectant has not yet been discovered and probably never will be, because of the varying conditions under which they are asked to operate. Some of the desirable features of a disinfectant and an antiseptic in livestock sanitation are as follows:

1. It must be reasonably low priced; otherwise, the large quantities needed make it economically unprofitable.

Desirable qualities in disinfectants 2. It must be free from strong or objectionable odors, especially in dairies; otherwise, their products will become tainted.

3. It must not be excessively destructive to materials or tissues other than the agent disinfected against. As an extreme example the flame will destroy all germs, but if the germs happen to be on combustible material it will also burn the material. Undiluted carbolic acid will destroy many infections but at the same time it destroys the tissues in which the germs are lodged.

4. It must not remain strongly poisonous after its application because of the danger to the life of those animals that graze over areas that have been disin-

fected, or that are likely to obtain it by drinking, or by licking one another.

5. It must not combine chemically so as to become inert with materials, utensils, blood, and the like the moment it establishes a contact with them. This is true of some of the mercury compounds such as "bichloride" (page 274), which combine with the tannin in wood to form the tannate of mercury, with metals to form amalgams, and with albumen in blood to form the albuminate. All are conditions that effectively stop the disinfecting action of the "bichloride."

6. It must be neither excessively irritating nor poisonous when inhaled. Some of the gaseous disinfectants, such as chlorine (pages 116 and 257), formaldehyde (page 266) and others are unbearably irritating to the mucous membranes lining the air passages, and if in sufficiently high concentration they may even be destructive to life other than the germs alone.

7. The disinfectant used must be effective at ordinary temperatures, and it must not lose an appreciable amount of this effectiveness when the general surrounding temperature drops considerably below that of the usual "mild" day.

8. It must be effective after it has been diluted with water, in other words, it must not be effective only when in concentration.

9. It must mix readily and uniformly with water. To illustrate this point, carbolic acid may be cited as an example, in certain dilutions when added to water, droplets of the practically pure acid will remain on the surface of the water and when used on living tissues may result in severe injury.

10. It must be in such concentration, and in such form that it may be readily and economically transported from its place of manufacture to its place of ultimate utilization.

Modes of action of disinfectants vary. In grouping these actions in a general way, it may be asserted they exert their action:

1. By *oxidation,* which means that the oxygen of the disinfectant or the oxygen derived from other sources, because of the action of the disinfectant, combines chemically with the germ or actually oxidizes or burns it.

How disinfectants exert their action

2. By the *removal of water,* or at least the elements that form water. Some disinfectants have a very great affinity for water and withdraw this from all sources including germs and the media in which the latter lives, so that death results, or the surroundings become untenable.

3. By *coagulation* in which the fluid state of a substance is changed to a soft jellylike solid, with the resulting inhibition of life processes.

4. By *chemical reactions* with germs so as to form new complex compounds which are free from harmful qualities.

There are many factors that affect the action of disinfectants, most of them imperfectly understood. The disinfectants made out of coal tar, which includes carbolic acid, though in general effective against germs have practically no effect on viruses. (This latter is taken advantage of in the preserving of hog cholera virus. A small amount of carbolic acid is added to all the hog cholera virus used in the serum-virus method of vaccination against hog cholera, so that any contaminating germs in the virus are killed, though the virus itself maintains its full potency.) Furthermore, the action of the alkali disinfectants, such as lye (page 253), which is very active against viruses (page 253), is resisted by gram-positive germs, though the gram-negative ones are susceptible to its action. (Gram's stain, page 248). Also, the pres-

Carbolic acid not effective against viruses

Manure limits the action of disinfectants

ence of organic matter which includes blood, intestinal discharges and vaginal discharges always present in greater or less amounts in living quarters of animals, prevents disinfectants from exerting their full action either by being diluted or neutralizing them, or because the organic matter affords a measure of protection to the germ. Furthermore, some germs have coatings, sometimes of a waxy nature, which seem to protect them.

Many disinfectants are more effective when their temperature is raised. Another important point to remember is that some germs acquire a degree of resistance or tolerance to a certain disinfectant if they are repeatedly exposed to it, and this is guarded against in the treatment of infected wounds by frequent changes from one disinfectant to another. A final point is that some disinfectants actually have a more intense action on certain strains of almost identical germs than they do on others. For example, certain dye-disinfectants which will stop the growth of some members of the Brucella group (the generally best known member of this group is the germ that causes Bang's disease (page 578) in cattle) though without action on others, each strain showing greater susceptibility to specific dye-disinfectants so that it is possible to easily distinguish the various strains on the basis of their susceptibility or non-susceptibility to the action of these agents.

It is on the foregoing premises that it must be stated that there is no strictly "general" or all-purpose disinfectant. In so far as it is possible, a disinfectant should be selected on the basis of its efficiency against the specific germs of a disease, and its suitability for use where it is to be applied (page 283).

CHAPTER XVI

NON-CHEMICAL DISINFECTION

At least two non-chemical methods are recognized as aids to disinfection, or as having disinfecting action of their own. These are: (1) mechanical agencies, and (2) natural agencies. The latter frequently closely approaches the chemical disinfectants in their action.

MECHANICAL AGENCIES. Taken as a whole, their value depends upon the removal of superficial dirt and infectious material, so that the remaining germs may be made more accessible to the action of chemical antiseptics. The mechanical agencies include such processes as sweeping, brushing, scraping, scrubbing, and the use of water under pressure.

Probably the best method is to dampen all material that may be removed by mechanical means, transport-

Dampen material before removal ing this to some area where it may be safely rendered harmless either by burning, burial, or spreading on sun-exposed arable land. The preliminary dampening prevents germs from being transported with dust from infected to clean areas. Dampening is also better than to resort to the use of water under pressure during the mechanical cleaning because with the latter the great volume of water used is likely to flush germs to clean areas.

In view of the fact that the very best that may be anticipated following the use of mechanical agencies

Some germs are removed mechanically is the removal of dirt *and some of the germs*, it necessarily follows that many other germs remain upon the completion of these processes. Therefore, the disinfection is incomplete and in order to be

243

thorough, it must be followed by such more potent methods due to natural forces, or by chemical means.

NATURAL AGENCIES:

Sunlight is deadly to germs and their spores if it can reach them. Its germ-destroying ability which is the ultraviolet ray is not passed through ordinary win-

Window-glass stops the germicidal action of sunlight passing through it

dow-glass, only to a very limited extent through smoky atmosphere or haze, and it is practically ineffective during the earlier morning and late afternoon hours. The germ-destroying rays of the sun are effective only against surface infections since they do not penetrate material *behind* which germs may be screened such as mucus, stable manure, dirt, and comparable material. Neither is it to be overlooked that virtually all disease-producing germs multiply and grow only in the bodies of their host, so that exposure to sunlight can have no effect in the control of this phase of disease. Sunlight as a disinfectant is too slow to serve the purpose of controlling or stamping out any specific infectious disease, though it serves an admirable purpose as a surface disinfectant when the action of its rays is neither impeded nor obstructed by glass or foreign material. Exposure to bright sunlight is to be encouraged on the basis of its lethal action against germs.

Heat is deadly to all forms of life, including that of animal parasites and germs, if applied in sufficient con-

Heat, in a sufficient degree, is destructive to germs

centration such as that produced by fire. It is also highly effective in the form of steam under pressure, and scalding water. It is still surprisingly effective as generated in heating packed manure piles. There is a decrease in its effectiveness correspondingly as its heat decreases, so that the heat of the sun as expressed through its infra-red rays has no germ-destroying qualities.

Heat is utilized because of its germ-killing powers in the process of pasteurization (page 235), in the burning of carcasses and barnyard refuse, and occasionally in the destruction of badly disease-contaminated frame buildings of low value. A powerful jet of fire as generated in a large torch and applied to concrete or other non-combustible material for a long enough period, several seconds at least, so as to heat or deeply penetrate this, will destroy all germ and parasite life contacted by it. In the barnyard

Burning substances on germ-contaminated ground of some value

the saturation of the ground with oil or kerosene, and to a less extent covering it with straw or other highly combustible material, and firing this is a practical method of producing a degree of surface sanitation, though it is not to be depended upon for any penetrating effect.

The addition of one per cent of sal soda to the water will prevent the rusting of iron or steel during the disinfecting process.

Steam disinfection shrinks wool, ruins leather, fur and all kinds of skins, rubber shoes, and articles containing varnish and glue.

Refrigeration is of no value as a sanitary measure, excepting that germs active during warm weather may become inactive during the colder seasons,

Cold slows germs

and during this time other destructive agencies may prove lethal to them. During cold temperatures most germs live longer, simply because the life processes are so retarded that the surroundings do not become saturated with the germ's own poisonous products. If enough moisture is present they survive terrifically low temperatures so that they are as capable as ever of causing disease. Germs cannot live in dry surroundings. Refrigeration for a continuous period of not less than twenty days at a temperature not higher than five degrees Fahrenheit will destroy the small parasite trichina (page 681) in pork so that it is safe for human food purposes.

Filtration is of minor importance in animal disease prevention. Insofar as it is applicable, it probably exerts its greatest influence in animal disease control on deep waters (see page 112) that are intended for ultimate animal consumption. If in becoming a "deep" water it has filtered for some distance through sand or gravel, it becomes reasonably free from germs, but if it is simply surface water, which is always badly contaminated, that has reached a deep location by passing through cracks in limestone or comparable material it is not improved thereby from a sanitary standpoint.

Filtered water is better   Properly filtered waters are safer from the standpoint of disease production than are flowing stream waters, or than surface waters. For human consumption, in addition to filtration they should be chemically treated before they may be considered entirely safe.

Sedimentation is one of nature's methods of purifying water that is not in motion. Animal disease germs contaminating water under this condition settle to the bottom where in the course of time they die. This process must not be depended upon in the small pools or ponds which are repeatedly reinfected or reinfested from surface contamination, and that are frequently agitated by various animate or inanimate forces.

Time will gradually result in the death of all living things, including germs and parasite eggs. The rate **All life destroyed in time** at which dissolution takes place is extremely variable, and may in some instances require several years. It is always considerably retarded by cold, when life's processes are slow. The germ responsible for Bang's disease (page 578) will live in pastures for several months during freezing weather, though only for a comparatively brief period during the warmer months. In general, this is also true for other germs. A combination of time, bright sunshine and low optimum conditions for the evolution of life's processes will free pastures of specific infections in due course. Extreme dryness accounts for the death of many more germs.

Electricity, bodily juices, and germ antagonisms are known to have some influence on germ life. Electricity, by its heat-generating ability or by its powers to free elements from chemical combinations such as chlorine, which is strongly disinfectant, from common salt (chloride of soda), or possibly from the direct action of the electrical current, is in a measure destructive to germ life.

The bodily juices here considered are the blood, its serum, and white (phagocytes) and red cells, and the gastric juice. Blood serum can kill germs, **Blood and gastric juice germicidal** and this ability may be increased by injecting limited, though gradually increasing, doses of germs or their poisons into the blood stream of living animals so as to produce in that animal a hyperimmune serum. This serum when withdrawn and later injected into another animal, confers upon the latter a degree of resistance against a specific infection. This fact is used in the immunization of swine against hog cholera (page 618), as well as in other disease-control measures.

The white blood cells actually "eat" or ingest germs that get into the blood stream, by gradually growing around them and finally completely disposing of them. Technically this process is known as phagocytosis. If the white cells win the victory, that animal is said to have resisted an infection; if the germs gain the upper hand, disease sets in.

Another of the bodily juices having germ-destroying ability is that secreted by the normal stomach, the gastric juice. It is acid in character as a result of which it is destructive to germ life.

It is an observed bacteriological phenomenon that many germs are antagonistic to each other. For exam-

Germs destructive to each other ple, many of the specific disease-producing germs get out of their natural element when they leave the animal body to get into the soil, and in the latter they are destroyed in the course of time by the germs that have their normal abode in the soil, or in other instances the intruders cannot compete successfully for a food supply with the natural inhabitants. This antagonism is at times shown in the growth of germs in their artificial food supplies in the laboratory. It is even taken advantage of in the handling of certain infectious diseases by adding antagonistic organisms to the surroundings. The antagonism between bacteria is known as antibiosis. *Antibiotics* are antibacterial substances of biologic orgin derived from 1. bacteria— these include pyocyanese, tyrothricin, and bacitracin (page 249) ; 2. from actinomyces—including actinomycin, and streptomycin; 3. from molds and fungi— including penicillin, and flavicin.

From natural substances other than bacteria there are obtained such antibiotics as allicin from common garlic; canavalin from soy bean flour; chlorellin from a fresh water-seaweed; lysozyme from saliva, tears, egg white and from many animal fluids.

Probably the best known antibiotic is penicillin derived from the mold Penicillium notatum. Commercially it is usually in chemical combination as either the sodium or calcium salt. It is used with a high degree of efficiency in infections due to staphylococci, streptococci, pneumococci and gram positives (page 248). With animals it is extensively used in mastitis (page 569). Another antibiotic that is coming into greater use is streptomycin derived from Actinomyces (Streptomyces) riseus. It is most highly effective against conditions resulting from gram-negative organisms (page 248)—it is not as effective as penicillin in the handling of gram-positive organisms (Gram's method of staining germs so that the organism may be identified is the same for all bacteria. However, when the stain can be washed away with alcohol the germ is said to be gram-negative, while those that do not decolorize are gram-positive.) In the treatment of tularemia (page 561) in both animals and man it is a most effective agent.

Current medical literature also records with increasing frequency the comparatively favorable results obtained in the handling of human brucellosis (Bang's disease) (page 588) from the use of dihydro-streptomycin in the form of the sulphate. It may be administered safely by the intramuscular route. Recent researches indicate that both penicillin and streptomycin are of value in limiting the infections so commonly present in the semen used in artificial insemination (page 808).

Another antibiotic is aureomycin—derived from a strain of Actinomyces aureofaciens. In humans it is said to be more than ordinarily effective **Recent antibiotics** in the handling of Rocky Mountain Spotted Fever (page 714). It is in frequent use as a cattle feed additive.

Bacitracin is an antibiotic substance produced by the growth of "Tracy 1" strain of Bacillus subtilis. It is chiefly effective against gram positive organisms (this page). It is more effective than penicillin (page 249) for local (topical) application, and its effectiveness is apparently not interfered with by wound exudates. As a dry powder it is commercially handled under the name of "Bacitracin Topical."

Another recently reported "antibiotic" of interest in animal disease control is *hygromycin B*. It is under test at three Agricultural Experiment Stations for its possible value as an agent to remove intestinal parasites in swine. (Consult page 670.)

Under conditions of nature, what are believed to be certain extremely minute forms of life are present in many streams, the bacteriophage. These are known to be destructive to some specific disease germs. This is true in the Ganges river of India, which at times becomes badly polluted from sewage with the germ-causing human cholera, but these are promptly destroyed by the bacteriophage so that healthy cholera-susceptible humans bathe in this so-called "sacred" river without contracting the disease.

Most of the forces and agencies included under the general caption of "natural agencies" certainly exert an immense collective action in holding disease under control. With the exception of "heat" (page 244), the antibiotics (page 249) and specific immunizing blood serums, however, their influence in attempts to immediately or quickly control outbreaks of specific infectious diseases is altogether too slow for practical application.

CHAPTER XVII

IMPORTANT CHEMICAL DISINFECTANTS AND BACTERIOSTATS

Before starting the description of chemical disinfectants, it is well to review briefly some of the statements made about their properties and actions, as well as listing additional facts.

Use only disinfectants of established value It is not intended to list all chemical disinfectants and antiseptics but instead simply those that are believed to have value in the control and prevention of animal diseases. The average live stock owner will do well to limit his purchase of disinfectants to reliable, well known agents of an established reputation and when commercially economical. Many of the newer, highly refined preparations are valuable but they are intended primarily for human use only.

Again it must be emphasized that the first requirement in disinfection is to start with clean surroundings and surface. There is no substitute for this. No disinfectant applied to a dirty surface will destroy all germs.

An additional brief statement about the term "phenol coefficient" (page 251) may be of interest. It is used to designate the value of a disinfectant. Since phenol (its common name is carbolic acid) is a well known disinfectant, its value is taken as unity, and the value of any other disinfectant similarly used can be expressed by a number called its "coefficient." This indicates how many times more, or in some instances less, the disinfectant can be diluted than

The significance of the "phenol coefficient" phenol and retain an equal disinfecting value. The "phenol coefficient" is usually determined by comparing the disinfectant to be tested with phenol in its action on

251

the typhoid fever germ, thus determining the dilutions of the samples that are as efficient as given dilutions of phenol. That a low "phenol coefficient" definitely indicates inferiority of that product is accepted, but it cannot be correctly asserted that a high "phenol coefficient" always indicates the rated superiority because the test has been under carefully controlled conditions in a laboratory which are not duplicated in the actual practical application of the disinfectant. The "phenol coefficient" of a disinfectant is nevertheless a useful base to evaluate disinfectants, and should be determined and stated on the label of all disinfectants offered for sale to the public.

Soap is cleansing and tends to dissolve the natural, protective, greasy coating of the skin, and of other surfaces. This permits a more penetrating action by subsequently applied antiseptic agents.

Soap and its limitations Soap should be looked upon as a cleansing substance rather than as a disinfectant. It is true that some germs are killed by soapsuds if they are permitted to remain in contact with them long enough, five to fifteen minutes, which is seldom practical. The compositions of soaps vary so greatly that no uniform action by them on germs may be expected.

Frequent attempts are made to increase the slight antiseptic action of soap by adding to it such a substance as carbolic acid and other substances, but carefully conducted tests indicate that, in general, such a procedure is of no value. However, a soap of the proper composition with a certain amount of red iodide of mercury added for its antiseptic qualities has some merit.

To sum up the situation, soap must be considered a cleanser rather than a disinfectant. As a cleanser it removes grease and dirt so that a subsequent application of a disinfectant penetrates more deeply. Soapsuds enmesh many surface germs that in the rinsing process are carried away. This is a very important point, since the total amount of infection on the washed area is reduced very much.

"*Wetting Agents*" or soapless detergents though they have the physical appearance of soap powder should not be confused with soap powder. An outstanding characteristic of a "wetting agent" is that it reduces surface tension of water and other liquids.

In the meantime these soapless powders—now available commercially in grocery stores—have an established value as cleansing agents for cream separators, milkers, kitchen utensils and the like.

Lye (page 241) : Chemically this is hydroxide of soda, or hydroxide of potash, or a mixture of the two.

Lye effective against viruses It is usually used in the form of household lye. It is rated highly as a disinfectant against all viruses including hog cholera, foot and mouth disease of cattle, fowl-pox, and dog distemper; also against some germs such as the anthrax and its highly resistant spore, and against the germ causing Bang's disease in cattle. It is of no practical disinfecting value against the group of germs

Lye valueless against tuberculosis known as "acid-fasts" which includes the germ of tuberculosis and that of Johne's disease, nor against that group known collectively as "gram-positives" (page 248). A very important point in its action as a germ destroyer is that it is more effective when its solution is used cold rather than hot, and this obviates the necessity of heating water for dissolving it. However, this action of a cold solution is only against germs, and must not be interpreted to mean that a cold lye solution is to be used in the cleaning of hog houses infested with worm eggs. In this latter event the lye serves principally to dissolve the dirt, and it should be in scalding hot solution in water; it is the hot water that is destructive to the worm eggs. (Page 672.) An additional advantage of lye as a disinfectant is that it dissolves dirt, manure and comparable filth so that it will effectively disinfect these.

For stable disinfection against virus diseases, such as foot-and-mouth disease and vesicular exanthema, one 13½ ounce can of lye should be dissolved in five gallons of water; this is active against Bang's disease, and gram-negative diseases but not against tuberculosis and other "acid-fasts" nor against "gram-positives," household lye may be used by previously dissolving it in cold water to the extent of making a two per cent solution. Roughly estimated, this means two and one-fourth ounces of lye to each gallon of water or one pound to seven gallons. Ordinarily an exposure of ten minutes duration is sufficient, though in the case of highly resistant spores, such as that of anthrax and blackleg, the exposure must be for ten hours when the lye solution is in at least a five per cent concentration.

How to use lye as a disinfectant

Lye (hydroxide of soda) alone or in mixtures with carbonate of soda (washing soda or sal soda) has a **relatively** high germicidal efficiency including the spores of anthrax and other spores. It was found to be effective even in the presence of organic matter such as chicken droppings, skim milk or defibrinated horse blood. However, solutions containing two per cent of lye and ten per cent of hydroxide of lime (milk of lime or hydrated lime) failed to kill the germ of tuberculosis, not protected by organic matter, after two hours of exposure. For foot-and-mouth disease disinfection of wood work and premises the U. S., B.A.I. uses two pounds of lye in ten gallons of water applied with a power spray.

Lye solutions are harmful to aluminum and must not be used on this metal. Rubber is benefited by periodical hot lye solution immersion.

Washing soda (carbonate of soda) has only very slight germicidal value at ordinary temperatures though the germicidal efficiency of it alone, or a solution containing both washing soda and lye is greatly increased by heat. However, since alkalies (carbonate of soda is one of these) are strongly destructive to viruses including that of foot-and-mouth disease of cattle the use of four per cent mixtures of sawdust and soda-ash (commercial anhydrous carbonate of soda), or of a four per cent water solution is justified.

Lime. Chemically this is oxide of lime. It has various other designations such as burned lime, stone lime, quicklime, and others.

Lime and its uses as a disinfectant   When quicklime is freshly water-slaked, it forms true hydrated or hydroxide of lime, or "milk of lime." The lime is first slaked by adding water at the rate of one pint to two pounds of quicklime. A good deal of heat is generated and the product formed is hydrate of lime or water-slaked lime. The development of heat and the crumbling of the hard lumps of quicklime are signs that it is of good quality and will make a good water-slaked lime or "milk of lime" which must be stored in tightly closed containers because exposure to the air makes it inert as a disinfectant. This fresh product is that of greatest disinfecting efficiency. Lime loses this efficiency when it becomes "air-slaked," because it is an entirely different chemical compound having no ability to destroy germs.

Fresh water-slaked lime has a "phenol coefficient" of about 20, and theoretically it is highly efficient as a disinfectant, but practically this is limited because the fresh lime changes so easily in the air to a valueless compound. Also, it is not entirely soluble in water and, therefore, wherever it is applied it leaves a residue which is not always as desirable as it is following whitewashing. When it is added to such a reliable disinfectant as saponated cresol solution (page 263) to make visible where application is completed the lime, if it is not freshly water-slaked (page 255), will render the basic disinfectant less effective.

For disinfecting floors, stanchions, walls, fences, and other objects that may have been contaminated

White wash for foot-and-mouth disease infection with the virus of foot-and-mouth disease, the U. S. Bureau of Animal Industry uses a whitewash made of five pounds of water-slaked lime, one pound of concentrated lye or caustic soda and ten gallons of hot water. Apply with power spray.

Quicklime scattered as a dry powder has value as a disinfectant on moist surfaces. It is a good disinfectant on manure and other animal discharges. If there is no objection to its residue, it may be used as a disinfectant in the form of "milk of lime" in dairies and animal yards, and in these places if properly applied it has the advantage over chlorine disinfectants in its lack of noticeable odor.

Lime in the form of whitewash freshly prepared is too weak to exert any great influence as an antiseptic, **Whitewash seals up cracks in wood and thus imprisons germs** but it does seal up the smaller cracks in wood so as to imprison infectious material, thus rendering such materials more sanitary as well as more attractive in appearance. In Farmers' Bulletin 1452 issued by U. S. Department of Agriculture the following whitewash formulas are given:

"Whitewash No. 1 (for sheds, etc.)—Carefully slake half a bushel (38 pounds) of good quicklime; strain the paste, while still thick, through wire fly screen and add it to a solution made by dissolving 15 pounds of common salt in 7½ gallons of water, mixing thoroughly. Thin with more water."

"Whitewash No. 2 (for sheds, etc.)—Carefully slake half a bushel (38 pounds) of good quicklime; strain the paste, while still thick, through wire fly screen and add about 4 gallons of hot water. While stirring vigorously pour into the lime mixture a solution made by first dissolving 12 pounds of salt and 6 ounces of alum in about 4 gallons of hot water and then adding 1 quart of molasses. Thin with water."

Because of its use in the building trades, lime is quite readily available, and it is comparatively cheap.

It lacks reliability as a disinfectant against resistant forms of germ life.

"Superphosphate" as marketed for fertilizing purposes is a calcium salt or it is a mixture of gypsum (sulphate of calcium) and calcium superphosphate—the latter having the chemical formula $CaH_4 (PO_4)_2$.

A calcium salt or compound The question is occasionally raised as to the germicidal value of this compound, as well as of the double superphosphate and the concentrated or triple superphosphate. If these compounds have any germicidal value at all it is of such a low order as to be practically negligible. Added from time to time to manure accumulations it serves as a deodorant and fixes the ammonia nitrogen so as to prevent its escape, and thus leaves the manure as a more valuable fertilizer (page 171).

Tribasic Phosphate of Soda: This sodium salt, also known as trisodium phosphate, in contradistinction to the calcium salt, has appreciable disinfecting value. In a hot solution having a two and one-half (2.5) per cent strength it is of marked value. When it is to be used cold it should be reinforced by the addition of one-half (0.5) per cent hydroxide of soda (lye).

A sodium salt or compound

Chlorinated lime (also known as bleaching powder, or simply as "bleach" and sometimes incorrectly designated as chloride of lime or calcium chloride), is a powerful disinfectant because of the large amount of chlorine gas incorporated in it. It is also an effective deodorant. Chlorinated lime is made by passing chlorine gas into hydrate of lime to the extent of from twenty-four to thirty-five per cent. Commercial chlorinated lime usually is said to contain at least twenty-four per cent of available chlorine. The chlorine is in loose combination with the lime so that in the presence of organic material such as germs and stable refuse, it is liberated as a gas to

Chlorinated lime a good source of the gas chlorine

combine with the organic material. It is because of this feature that large amounts of chlorinated lime must be used as a disinfectant, so that there will be an excess for action against infection. This is always done in the treatment of public water supplies with chlorine gas and accounts for the frequently noticeable taste of chlorine in it. (Page 116.) Also, because of the loose combination it should be stored in tightly closed containers to prevent the escape of the chlorine gas; otherwise it may lose as much as one per cent a month. "Bleach" is one of the few substances that spontaneously evolves an efficient disinfecting vapor in the form of chlorine gas which will kill germs if there are at least five parts per 1000 in dry air, or one-eighteenth of this amount is equally effective in moist air.

The disadvantages of chlorinated lime for stable disinfection are the expense due to the comparatively large amounts that must be used, the fact that it is a very powerful bleaching agent, removing colors from fabrics and leather, its corrosion of metal, irritation to the mucous membrane of the nose and throat, imparting its odor to foods such as milk and meat, and the fact that it is so unstable that it is practically impossible to estimate the exact chlorine content.

As a disinfectant it has a "phenol coefficient" (page 251) of twenty-one when there is ten per cent of available chlorine, but it quickly loses this in the presence of organic matter. There is **Chlorinated lime without value against tuberculosis** evidence to indicate that it is a destroyer of viruses, such as that of hog cholera, foot and mouth disease, and other diseases, it is quickly lethal against most germs, but the "acid-fast" germs, including that of tuberculosis, are so resistant to its action that from a practical standpoint it is valueless against them.

For disinfecting purposes, chlorinated lime may be used either in powder form or dissolved in water. Six ounces of it in one gallon of water is recommended for

general household and farm use in the dis-
A good household disinfectant infection of drains and sewers. For the disinfection of teats of dairy cows and of
dairy utensils, a solution containing 200
parts of chlorine gas in each one million parts of water
may be used.

A method employed in the disinfection of the teat
cups of milking machines is to first free them
A method of disinfecting milking machines of milk by dropping in clean water
while the suction is still operative. A stock
solution of lye (page 253) is made by dissolving one pound of it in a gallon of water. Six ounces of this stock solution is added to one
gallon of water, and this latter is used to remove the
fat by drawing it through the milking machine, provided there are no aluminum parts. Finally, the milking parts are stored until the next milking in a solution
containing two hundred parts of chlorine in one million parts of water (page 116). (Consult "Milking
Machine Care," Leaflet 134 of Pennsylvania State University, at University Park, Penn.)

In the cleansing and disinfection of wounds, a reliable agent (Carrel-Dakin) may be made by mixing to-
How to make a wound disinfectant gether one and one-half ounces each of
powdered boric acid and chlorinated lime.
This powder is placed on top of a piece of
absorbent cotton contained in a glass fun-
nel. One gallon of hot water is then poured on, to filter
through the powder and cotton. It is ready for use without additional dilution, as soon as it has cooled.

For the disinfection of drinking water for poultry,
(page 116), which is limited in its value because of its
A water of limited disinfectant value negligible action on the germs of tuberculosis and other "acid-fasts," make a
stock solution by dissolving one-fourth
ounce of chlorinated lime (about a teaspoonful) in a pint of water. Of this stock
solution add one-half ounce (a large tablespoonful) to
five gallons of water. This will destroy the infections

of fowl typhoid, fowl cholera, and others to the extent of probably ninety per cent, though it will not be harmful to the fowl drinking it.

As a deodorizer and disinfectant, the dry powder may be sprinkled lightly on stable manure, and decaying animal and vegetable matter. This should be repeated frequently.

An excellent deodorizer

As a very strong disinfectant, one pound of chlorinated lime may be mixed with two gallons of water. After permitting it to stand for an hour, pour off the clear solution. This may be used in stables and hog houses, but not in dairies or near food supplies as it will taint them. Neither should it be used near colored goods as it will bleach them, or in closed rooms containing people or animals, as it is too irritating to the mucous membranes lining the eyelids and air passages.

Sodium hypochlorite has appeared on the market under various trade names. It is usually sold in solution or liquid form. The chlorine content varies from two (2) per cent to twenty (20) per cent. The original container indicates the percentage of available chlorine. The sodium hypochlorite alone in solution, or in combination with calcium hypochlorite, has high value in the disinfection of dairy equipment, and as a household disinfectant. However, like all chlorine preparations its value as a disinfectant is greatly reduced in the presence of organic material—manure, milk, blood, etc., or in other words it is a clean surface, though germ contaminated, disinfectant. Also because the chlorine odor is penetrating these compounds are not to be used in places where human food is stored.

Another chlorine preparation

All containers of chlorine solutions should be porcelain, enamel, glass, wood or granite ware; never use tin, galvanized iron, or aluminum as chlorine is corrosive to these.

Carbolic acid or phenol is derived from coal-tar oils. In its pure form it occurs at ordinary temperatures as closely welded needle-like crystals. It is kept liquid in a saleable condition in drug stores by first liquefying it through exposure to heat, and then adding either ten per cent of water or glycerin.

It is one of the oldest known disinfectants, probably because its first practical use for this purpose was by Lister, the pioneer surgeon, when he demonstrated its value in keeping wounds free from infections, and he lauded it very highly.

It is still a standard today for measuring the efficiency of other disinfectants. The term "phenol coefficient" is indicative of this. (Page 251.)

Carbolic acid has certain decided advantages as well as disadvantages as a disinfectant. Some of its **Carbolic** advantages are that it is a very stable com- **acid has** pound, in that it appears to suffer no de- **many advan-** terioration from exposure to air or light. **tages** It does not injure fabrics immersed in a sufficiently strong solution of it for a period of time necessary for their disinfection. It does not corrode metals. It is reasonably effective against germs in the presence of organic matter such as stable and barnyard refuse. It is available in all drug stores. It is effective as a disinfectant against all germs, and if permitted to act long enough (at least twenty-four hours) against the highly resistant spores.

Its disadvantages are that it is extremely poisonous and it is therefore an unsafe agent to have on the prem- **Some disad-** ises. It has a penetrating odor which is **vantages of** readily absorbed by milk, meat and other **carbolic** food products. It is of very low efficiency **acid** as a germ destroyer when it is in cold solution, or when used on a cold surface, though dissolved in hot water it is a very effective disinfectant. It is apparently without destructive action against the viruses of such diseases as hog cholera (page 616), foot and mouth disease, fowl-pox and others. It is not soluble in water above seven per cent, though in many instances the use of a stronger dilution is very desirable. When its dilutions approach seven per cent, or when the diluting water is cold, droplets of the carbolic acid may float on the surface, and these are dangerously destructive to animal or human tissues. Applying ordinary grain alcohol controls its action.

Of the domesticated animals, cats are notoriously susceptible to the poisonous action of carbolic acid, as well as to that of other disinfecting agencies derived from coal-tar oil, even in its external application. Carbolic acid even in the weaker dilutions is numbing to the hands of operators, and interferes seriously with their touch perception. For the purpose of disinfecting stables and barnyards, the quantity of a disinfectant required is so relatively large that it makes carbolic acid prohibitively expensive; its place for this purpose has, therefore, largely been taken by other, cheaper agents derived from coal-tar oil.

When it is desired to disinfect fabrics, they may be immersed in a warm or hot five per cent water solution of carbolic acid for a period of one hour, providing the fabrics are not contaminated with any one of the viruses against which it is ineffective.

For stable and barnyard disinfection, as well as for the disinfection of discharges from diseased animals, it may be used in warmed five per cent solution.

For the disinfection of badly contaminated wounds, a solution containing from one to two per cent of carbolic acid is strong enough, and for the disinfection of the sheath in bulls and other male animals, and the genitals in females, a one-half per cent solution is strong enough.

Because of its anaesthetic or numbing action it is frequently employed as a douche in one-half per cent strength to overcome not only the infection in the genitalia of animals incidental to parturition, but the subsequent straining as well.

For the purpose of destroying spores, a hot five per cent solution of carbolic acid must be applied for at least twenty-four hours.

Crude Carbolic acid is really not carbolic acid in the same sense as phenol, in that it contains impurities

Crude carbolic acid of uncertain strength, and therefore not reliable

which may make it more powerful as a general disinfectant; in fact, it may contain no pure carbolic acid at all. It has a "phenol coefficient" of approximately two and three-fourths, when it contains at least fifty per cent of tar acid (cresylic acid). It is a dark, oily fluid having a disagreeable odor, and staining almost everything with which it comes in contact. Its principal disadvantage is that it has no definite composition and therefore lacks definite action as a disinfectant. It is not freely mixable with water but it floats on it and, therefore, it must be continuously agitated during the process of application.

If it is to be used as a disinfectant, it is well to first ascertain from the label its content of tar-acid (cresylic acid), and then make a solution containing two per cent of the latter. If, for example, the label states that the contents have fifty per cent of tar-acids, then this particular product should be diluted with twenty-five parts of water to make a two per cent solution. It must be used hot.

In view of the fact that there are more reliable, though no more expensive disinfectants, crude carbolic acid is not recommended.

Saponated Cresol Solution (compound solution of cresol liquor cresolis saponatus) is an emulsion of

Compound solution of cresol is one of the best all-round disinfectants

cresol made by the addition of raw linseed oil and lye. It is necessary to have this in the form of an emulsion in order that it may be mixable with water, pure cresol simply floating on top of it.

Cresol, the basic portion of the compound, is derived from coal-tar. It is one of hundreds of coal-tar disinfectants. The cresols are liquid at ordinary temperatures.

Saponated Cresol Solution makes a clear preparation when mixed with soft water in any proportion. This is a decided advantage over carbolic acid, as the latter is limited to seven per cent of solubility in water, and limited solubility means that carbolic acid is of no use when a solution exceeding seven per cent in strength is needed. If soft water is not available for diluting compound solution of cresol, then hard water that has previously been softened with lye or washing soda may be used. Non-softened hard waters interfere with the efficiency of this compound.

Other advantages of compound solution of cresol are that metals such as those of surgical instruments are not corroded by it and when immersed in it will keep a sharp edge; it is almost non-irritant to the skin when used in the usual recommended strength; it is soapy, which aids in its penetration; it is as efficient, though somewhat slower in its action than carbolic acid when organic matter is interposed between it and the germs to be destroyed; it is less affected than most other disinfectants by factors which tend to inhibit the action of germicides; it is less poisonous and more germicidal than carbolic acid due to the fact that its phenol coefficient is approximately two; as a deodorant it destroys putrefactive germs, and it replaces bad odors; it is less poisonous than carbolic acid on the basis of its efficiency; and its cost based on the unit of efficiency is low.

Saponated Cresol Solution is effective against the virus of hog cholera. Carbolic acid is not. There are more effective disinfectants than it against other virus diseases. It is the disinfectant of choice against acid-fast germs as represented by the germ of tuberculosis. In a strength of four per cent—cupful to two

Cresol effective against viruses and tuberculosis

gallons of water—it is effective against the infection of such diseases as hog cholera, brucellosis, shipping fever, and swine erysipelas.

The principal disadvantage of Saponated Cresol Solution are that it will taint with its odor all foods in the same room with it, and on exposure to light it loses some of its efficiency as a disinfectant though the loss is almost negligible. It is best guarded against by storing it in dark colored bottles.

For the disinfection of barns, fences, and other animal enclosures, and the discharges of diseased animals, **Cresol must** it is used by mixing it with soft or lye-**be diluted** softened water to the extent of from two to **with soft** three per cent—usually about four ounces **water** of the compound solution of cresol in a gallon of water.

When it is desired to make clearly visible where the cresol compound has been applied to woodwork, one and one-half pounds of freshly water-slaked lime (page 255) may be added to each gallon.

Saponated Cresol Solution made in accordance with recognized methods is superior to carbolic acid under all conditions, and surpasses all other disinfectants aside from the purpose for which the latter are peculiarly adapted.

Pine Oil Disinfectant is widely used in animal sanitary procedures as a substitute for the cresol preparations because of its pleasing aromatic odor and its relatively good germicidal efficiency—it has a phenol coefficient (page 251) varying from one and one-half ($1\frac{1}{2}$) to four (4). The usual emulsified preparation consists of 70 per cent steam-distilled pine oil, **21 per** cent rosin soap, and not over nine (9) per cent of **water** and other extraneous inert substances. As a matter of general interest it may be recorded that many aromatic oils and spices have some germicidal value. These include such agents as thymol derived from oil of thyme; oil of cinnamon, and oil of cloves.

Sodium Ortho-phenyl-phenate is available under several trade names. It occurs in the form of grayish, brownish, or white powder which must be kept in a tightly closed container in order to avoid deterioration. In one per cent strength it is as effective as Saponated Cresol Solution provided it is applied hot. It is free from objectionable odor and its use is approved for disinfection in tuberculosis eradication work.

Formaldehyde is a gas. When the gas is dissolved in water, the latter will take up approximately thirty-seven to forty per cent of it; the water solution of the gas is known as formalin, or as "solution of formaldehyde."

Formaldehyde is a powerful disinfectant when used under proper conditions of heat and moisture. It is probably the only generally applicable fumigant. It is also an excellent deodorant, destroying the odor of intestinal discharges almost instantaneously after its application (page 236), and it may be used for the purpose of disinfecting bodily discharges. It is very effective against the germ of tuberculosis. It is occasionally used to disinfect small areas in stables, as well as for the purpose of sterilizing surgical gloves and instruments by immersing these latter in a four to ten per cent water solution of formaldehyde. In view of the fact that many of the cheaper shaving brushes are not at all times sterilized previous to their initial use, and as the bristles may harbor spores of the anthrax germ which in turn get into small shaving wounds to result in the serious disease, anthrax (page 591), it is recommended that, previous to use, these brushes shall be sterilized by placing them for four hours in a ten per cent solution of formaldehyde at 110 degrees Fahrenheit.

Formalin, which is a water solution of formaldehyde gas, has many valuable properties

Fumigation with formaldehyde gas may be resorted to in the disinfection of hay, grain, and fabrics. Soft leather and furs are hardened by it, but it is not injurious to paint or metals. In the field of disinfection by fumigation no other preparation can replace formaldehyde, though even it fails to destroy insect life by this method. It is poisonous to household flies when they eat a mixture of one part of formalin in thirty parts of milk, and the same amount of water. One of the indications for use of the gas is when liquid disinfectants **Formalin is** would be injurious to the surroundings. **the best** In fumigation, all articles to be disinfected **gaseous** must be freely exposed and spread out **disinfectant** because the gas does not penetrate deeply **by means of** into closely packed material. Some au- **fumigation** thorities contend that it is possible but not practical to kill germs by fumigation with formaldehyde gas.

Several factors are essential for successful fumigation. The formaldehyde gas, which is in solution in water, must be rapidly liberated from its association with water as formalin though for its effective use it must again immediately combine with moisture (page 268) in the room, the latter in the form of high humidity obtained either by moistening the floor or by the use of steam, and this must be supplied at least fifteen minutes before actual fumigation begins, because dry formaldehyde gas is almost harmless to germs. The temperature of the room must at no time fall lower than sixty-five degrees Fahrenheit during the fumigation process, and it should preferably be considerably higher. The room to be fumigated must be tightly sealed to prevent the loss of the gas, and there may be no air-currents.

A four per cent solution is made by diluting the official "solution of formaldehyde" (formalin) with ten parts of water and is effective against all germs and viruses such as that of foot-and-mouth disease when on woodwork, blankets and ropes, as well as on germ spores, though it requires an exposure of at least two hours for the latter. It also inactivates germ poisons or toxins, and it is believed to do the same to viruses. Only in the stronger liquid dilutions, which is ten per cent or more, is it lethal to the eggs of animal parasites. The presence of three per cent of organic matter does not appreciably retard the action.

It is only mildly poisonous in its gaseous form, though very irritating to the mucous membranes of the nose, throat and eyes. In sufficient dilution it is sometimes administered by way of the mouth but not recommended as it is too irritant, for the purpose of controlling fermentation of the paunch of cattle. People have had the skin of the hands seriously hardened by repeated or unduly prolonged immersion in a ten per cent water solution of the gas.

If a room and its contents are to be disinfected by **A method** fumigation with formaldehyde gas, the **of disinfect-** first step is to tightly seal all the room **ing a room** openings with the exception of its exit, which is left until the evolution of the gas has actually started. About fifteen minutes before starting the gas, thoroughly moisten the floor or make arrangements for a continuous flow of steam into the room so as to get the air saturated with moisture; the dry gas is ineffective. See to it that the temperature of the room is maintained above sixty-five degrees Fahrenheit and that there are no air currents.

The simplest method—though the least effective—is to impregnate sheets with formalin and suspend them in the room. For each thousand cubic feet of space to be disinfected, at least ten ounces of formalin is to be used. The room should be kept sealed for at least eight hours. As a test for the control of Newcastle disease of poultry a causative-virus-contaminated room with brooders and incubators was handled by draping large pieces of cotton gauze wrung damp dry after immersion in ten per cent formaldehyde solution over each brooder, incubator and hatcher. Four gallons of 40 per cent formaldehyde were poured on the floor of the room, and an additional gallon on the floor in front of the fan of the forced draft ventilating system. The temperature of the room was raised to 100° F., and by the use of steam the humidity was raised to 100 per cent. Thus 5500 cubic feet of space were fumigated. Then all doors and exists were closed and sealed for 20 hours. Careful tests at the end of this period failed to disclose any evidence of the virus. Chicks were hatched in the incubator within two days and did not contract Newcastle disease, nor did it occur in this hatchery for that hatching season.

One method of disinfecting a hatchery house

The more complicated method, as well as the most effective, is to generate the gas from formalin by means of permanganate of potash crystals. For the disinfection of one thousand cubic feet of space, place 16⅔ ounces of permanganate of potash crystals in a wide-bottomed bucket or basin with flaring sides. Raise above the floor level by setting the receptacle on two bricks in order to protect the floor from the heat generated in the process. Also place some heavy paper on the floor surrounding the container, as there will be some sputtering and splashing from the chemicals. Then quickly pour 20 ounces of the "solution of formalde-hyde" (formalin) upon the permanganate of potash crystals, immediately leave the room, and complete its sealing by packing all the crevices around the doorway, as well as the keyhole. The room is to be kept sealed for at least eight hours, after which it may be aired. The gas is not poisonous, so there need be no fear of entering the room.

Fumigation of poultry incubators is one of the very important steps in preventing the spread of pullorum disease (bacillary white diarrhoea) (page 651). In this work, the humidity or moisture content of the air in

How to
disinfect
poultry
incubators

the incubator or room must be high, the temperature 65 degrees F. or higher, and the incubator or room must be sealed. The usual precautions in regard to preventing damage from heat or splashing of chemicals must be observed. The incubator, or the incubator and the room in which it is contained must first be mechanically cleaned so as to permit of more thorough penetration by the formaldehyde. For each one hundred cubic feet of space inside the incubator, place in it four and one-half drams of permanganate of potash crystals, and pour on this nine fluid drams of the "solution of formaldehyde" (formalin). Maintain a wet bulb reading of 90 to 92° Fahrenheit or even more. Low humidity tends to concentrate the action of the formaldehyde gas on the chicks with disastrous results, while with a wet bulb reading of 92° F. or higher the wet chicks are not injured. Immediately seal the incubator and keep it closed for ten minutes. In order to obtain maximum effects from fumigation, Kansas Experiment Station Bulletin No. 247 states that "the procedure may be carried out three times at eight-hour intervals during the time the hatch is coming off. By removing all dry chicks before the second and third fumigations, practically all chicks are exposed to one fumigation. Neither the very young chicks nor the eggs seem to be injured if the fumigation is carried out as recommended." Under no circumstances should the same chicks be fumigated twice. The method just described requires special attachments which many incubators have and without sealing the incubator—the regular ports being left open. If the foregoing described method is not applicable, the empty incubator may be placed in a room, opened, and the entire room and its contents fumigated as described in a preceding paragraph. (Detailed instructions, page 48, Jan., 1940 Vet. Med.)

Probably the chief disadvantages of formaldehyde are that it is ineffective when the temperature is below

Some disad-
vantages of
formaldehyde
sixty-five degrees Fahrenheit, that the gas is not effective in dry atmosphere, and that it requires a good deal of careful detailed work in the sealing of a room preliminary to fumigation.

Permanganate of potash occurs in the form of purplish-red, needle-like crystals. It is soluble to the extent of approximately six per cent in cold water or fifty per cent in hot water. The color of the solution varies from pink to deep wine, depending upon the amount of the crystals in solution.

It is an active disinfectant under certain favorable conditions in laboratory tests, but clinical experience

Permanga-
nate of
potash not
so effective
clinically
does not entirely substantiate these. It owes its germicidal action to the fact that in the presence of organic matter it rapidly releases oxygen, and the latter in the recently released state—so-called nascent state—is very active.

In laboratory tests, permanganate of potash in a four per cent solution kills the spores of anthrax germs in forty minutes, and a two per cent solution of it reinforced by the addition of nine-tenths of one per cent of hydrochloric acid will accomplish the same result in two minutes. The germ responsible for the animal disease known as glanders (page 614) is destroyed in two minutes by a two per cent solution.

It has one
decided
advantage in
being non-
irritating
In the weaker solutions, approximately one part of permanganate of potash in one thousand parts of water is used to aid in the disinfection of bodily cavities lined by mucous membrane such as the genitals, the eyes, mouth and nose. In contradistinction to many other disinfectants, it is not irritating to mucous membranes. In strengths up to four per cent it is a favorite of veterinarians for the disinfection of odorous wounds, especially those involving necrosis of bone-tissue, and decaying teeth.

It is a frequently used disinfectant of drinking water intended for poultry consumption (page 259) during epizootics. It is not recommended **It should not be used as a routine disinfectant of poultry drinking water** for this purpose for routine use during generally disease-free periods as it leaves in the water the residue manganate of potash which is not free from some poisonous effects. It also imparts an unpleasant taste to the water.

Occasionally there are remnants of water, badly contaminated with disease germs, left in drinking vessels. It is frequently essential to destroy this infectious water without contaminating the vessel containing it with the odor of a disinfectant so objectionable that animals refuse to take water from it in the future. For situations of this nature, permanganate of potash may be safely and effectively used.

Permanganate of potash is practically valueless as a disinfectant when there is much organic material present, as this neutralizes its action.

Another disadvantage is that it stains everything with which it comes in contact a walnut-brown color, including the hands of the operators ap- **It stains** plying it. Surgeons remove this stain from the hands by washing them in a solution of hyposulphite of soda to which a few drops of hydrochloric or sulphuric acids have been added.

Taken as a whole, permanganate of potash, excepting for a few specialized uses as mentioned in preceding paragraphs, is not suited for general disinfecting purposes. Another limitation is its expense.

Solution of hydrogen dioxide, also known as "solution of hydrogen peroxide," or colloquially simply as "peroxide" is in reality oxygenated water.

Hydrogen dioxide, the basic substance, is a syrupy, colorless liquid, heavier than water, and so very unstable chemically that it will keep only at a temperature several degrees below the freezing point.

The hydrogen dioxide described in the preceding paragraph is diluted with water so that the dilution represents approximately a three per cent solution of it. It is this three per cent solution that is sold in drug stores as either "solution of hydrogen dioxide," "solution of hydrogen peroxide," or as "peroxide."

The "solution of hydrogen dioxide" is still an unstable preparation in spite of its dilution. It should **"Peroxide" rapidly loses strength** therefore be kept in a cool place and in amber-colored well-corked bottles. If there is evidence of gas pressure when the cork is withdrawn, it means that the contents have lost strength.

Under laboratory conditions, the "solution of hydrogen dioxide" is a good disinfectant, but unfortunately clinical experience does not in many instances substantiate the laboratory findings. Its disinfecting properties are owing to the fact that in the presence of organic matter it releases oxygen in a nascent state which means the highly active, newly-born state.

This oxygen is supposed to actually oxidize or "burn up" the germs susceptible to its action. In this process there is very marked effervescence, so that when used on a wound it is common to hear the expression, "the poison is boiling out." Its action is always transitory and comparatively feeble, though it does assist in the removal of dead tissue from wounds. It is not irritating to tissues, though it must never be used in wound cavities where its complete effervescence is prevented.

Theoretically it seems that the "solution of hydrogen dioxide" should be more than ordinarily effective against those germs collectively designed as **anaerobes**, (obligates) which indicates that they thrive best in surroundings free from oxygen, but actual practice indicates that no more than ordinary germicidal power is exhibited. In other words, the "solution of hydrogen dioxide" is not a specific against anaerobic infections such as blackleg, gas-gangrene and others.

It has been found active against the virus of fowl-pox. It also seems to be highly effective against a group of very minute disease-producing animal organisms known as protozoa, and of this group the trypanosomes, and the tricho-monas abortus seem to be particularly vul-nerable. The former is not of great sig-nificance in American animal husbandry, though the latter is beginning to assume more importance as a cause of abortion in cattle.

Peroxide is effective against fowl-pox virus

Excepting, then as an agent for occasional use in the treatment of wounds and some protozoan infec-tions, "solution of hydrogen dioxide" may be disre-garded in the field of animal sanitation.

Bichloride of mercury (page 489) is also known as mercuric chloride, perchloride of mercury, sublimate of mercury, or simply as "bichloride," and "sublimate." It is in the form of masses, which for commercial purposes are re-duced to a white powder. Frequently the powder is compressed into tablets and in these it is not uncommon to add some chloride of ammonia to make them more readily soluble; in others there is tartaric acid, five parts to each part of bichloride of mercury. In view of the fact that it is decomposed by alkaline solutions such as hard water, it is best to add a little vinegar or acetic acid to the water before dissolving the bichloride of mercury in it. The uncombined bichloride of mercury is soluble in cold water to the extent of six per cent, and hot water will dissolve thirty-three per cent of it.

A very powerful disinfectant though having decided dis-advantages

It is a powerful disinfectant in solutions of one part of bichloride of mercury in a thousand parts of water. One part of it in five hundred parts of water will kill spores. For use on the mucous membranes in the mouth, eyes and genitals it is occasionally employed in solutions varying in strength from one part of it in from three thousand to five thousand parts of water.

The chief advantages of bichloride of mercury are its rather high germicidal action under favorable conditions, its lack of bulk so that a small quantity of it dissolved in water or alcohol makes a comparatively large amount of disinfectant, and its freedom from odor so that it imparts nothing of this nature to anything with which it comes in contact.

Its disadvantages are its intensely poisonous nature causing many human fatalities resulting from its accidental use, its reduced disinfectant power when applied to infections contained within or surrounded by organic matter such as barnyard filth, its incompatibility with hard water, and the fact that it combines with many substances to form inert compounds (page 240 "5").

Because of its many disadvantages, it is not recommended for general use as a disinfectant. In human practice it has been largely displaced by the safer organic mercury compounds, either phenylmercuric chloride or nitrate.

In order to prevent absorption of bichloride of mercury from the human stomach as a poisoning agent, a **How to deal with accidental bichloride poisoning** mixture of egg-white and water should be swallowed as quickly as possible after the bichloride has been taken; then call a physician. The egg-white combines with the bichloride in the stomach to form the insoluble albuminate of mercury, which should be removed by the physician with the aid of a stomach pump, or less satisfactorily by inducing vomiting by taking a mixture of mustard and water, or other emetic.

Copper Sulphate (page 490) or "blue vitriol" has at various times been lauded for its alleged disinfectant properties but careful research has failed to substantiate these claims. For example, a solution of almost 16 per cent strength of copper sulphate failed to kill anthrax spores after an exposure of ten days. For the destruction of algae, fresh water plants caus-

ing "green scum" on stagnant water, it is the outstandingly approved agent. (See pages 117 and 457.) Concentrations of one part of sulphate of copper in 500,-
000 parts of water will destroy most forms of algae.
This strength does not make the water unfit for animal consumption and it does rid ponds, water reservoirs and tanks of these noxious algae. The most practical method of use is to place a quantity of the copper
sulphate in a small cloth bag, and stir this through the
water so as to give the water a very slight bluish tint.
This copper sulphate treatment should not be used if
there are fish in the reservoir because copper sulphate
is detrimental to many forms of aquatic life.

Iodine (page 827) is a solid occurring usually as
blackish gray scales, the so-called resublimed iodine,
obtained from Chili saltpetre, and from
The origin   seaweeds. It is readily dissolved in alcohol,
of iodine   chloroform and other liquids, but only
very slightly so in water, though readily
soluble in water that has previously had some iodide of
potash dissolved in it.

Tincture of iodine is the preparation known to most
people. It is made by dissolving resublimed iodine
scales to the extent of seven per cent in a five per cent
alcoholic solution of iodide of potash. It is the most
extensively used of the iodine preparations. There is
also a two per cent tincture which is in general as
effective as the "stronger" seven per cent though less
irritating.

Lugol's solution of iodine (page 797) is also one
with which many are familiar. It is made by dissolving
resublimed iodine scales to the extent of five per cent
in a ten per cent water solution of iodide of potash. It
is cheaper than the tincture of iodine. It has approximately the same uses as the tincture of iodine, though
lacking the additional value conferred upon the latter
by the alcoholic solvent.

Resublimed iodine has a phenol coefficient (page
251) of from 170 to 235, though this is very much

reduced when it is in the form of the tincture or
Lugol's solution. Iodine in the form of any of its preparations, though especially the tincture, continues to
be the standard skin disinfectant. It is one of the few
agents that is almost immediately destructive to the
highly resistant bacterial spores. If it is used too often
it also acts as an irritant so that it finally lowers the
natural resistance of the skin to infections.

Not only is it useful as a skin disinfectant but at
times it is used as a water disinfectant (page 277). It is
also very efficient as a local or deep applica-
Iodine is tion against mold diseases such as the so-
highly called ringworm (page 567) and lumpy-
effective jaw in cattle (page 422). In the latter the
in the iodine is frequently administered intraven-
handling of ously in the form of iodide of soda, because
many dis- this drug contains a large amount of
eases iodine. For either surface or deep wounds
it is the agent of choice to destroy the germ causing
tetanus (lock-jaw).

Another compound of iodine is *iodoform* which is
frequently used as a wound dressing. It is said to liberate its iodine slowly when in contact with
Iodoform is wounds, and this is probably the reason
a valuable that it has received such extensive and fa-
iodine-con- vorable recognition by clinicians as one of
taining com- the best agents to use for the control of
pound wound infections. It is non-irritating and it is not
soluble in water. It may be held in suspension, however, in a heavy mineral oil, and in this manner is used
for disinfecting the female genitals. Its disadvantages
are its almost prohibitive price, and its exceedingly
pungent, penetrating, and to many people disagreeable
odor. It imparts this odor to everything with which it
comes in contact. If used over a prolonged period on
fat subjects, it may result in iodine poisoning, as the
fat will dissolve it so that it is an absorbable condition for the animal tissues.

Sulphuric acid is a powerful germicide.
In one to two per cent water solution it is
destructive to most germs in an hour,
though more time and greater strength
are required to exert a lethal action on
their spores. In a three per cent water dilution it is
destructive to coccidia (page 734), which is the parasite causing a bloody dysentery in many species of
animals. It is occasionally used for the disinfection of
yards, manure, and filth.

Sulphuric acid is too dangerous for general use

Sulphuric acid is destructive to most materials with
which it comes in contact, including paint, fabrics and
metals. It causes extensive sloughing of all animal
tissues. The reaction between it and water is explosive if the water is added to it, though if the sulphuric
acid is slowly added to a considerably larger volume of
water, the only noticeable reaction is the evolution of
heat. It is highly poisonous.

Because of its many dangerous and potentially destructive properties, it is seldom used as a disinfectant.

Boric acid in the form of the bland powder is very
generally applied either alone or in combination with
germicidally more potent substances such
as sulfanilamide, to wounds immediately
after an operation. Its value in this connection is based on the fact that many germs
do not grow well or develop in its presence,
or it has an influence in preventing infections rather
than destroying germs, because as a germicide its action is negligible. It is extensively used in solution in
water as an eyewash. For this latter purpose its action
is largely mechanical in washing away existing infections. It is virtually non-irritating and not at all
destructive to animal tissues.

Boric acid is very mild, but its presence controls germ growth

Vinegar of a good grade should have in it as its
active ingredient from five to six per cent of acetic

Vinegar
is a good
household
disinfectant
acid. It is mentioned here because in general it compares favorably with the official "diluted acetic acid," though the latter is preferable because it is colorless, is of greater purity, and of uniform strength which is exactly six per cent of acetic acid in distilled water. However, "diluted acetic acid" is not always available in the home, though vinegar is.

Vinegar, on the basis of six per cent of acetic acid, has decided value against many germs and it is for this purpose, as well as that of a relish, that it has been used for many years in preserving foods such as pickles. As an application to wounds it will free them from certain pus-producing germs. Many veterinarians consider its action to be almost specific during the earlier stages of so-called foot-rot (page 527) in animals in destroying the causative germs of this malady.

Quaternary Ammonium Compounds: (page 117). The chemical formulae of these compounds vary

A comparatively new
disinfectant
considerably. Many have already been produced or synthesized. Usually they are mixtures of related compounds in which the number of carbons in the fatty acid radical varies from C_8H_{17} to $C_{18}H_{37}$. They have the property of depressing the surface tension of liquids and in this respect they belong in the group of chemicals described as "wetting agents" (page 253). Some of the names applied to the "quats" are amicide, emulsept, hyamine, queseptic, phemerol, roccal, stericide, septo-sol, thoral, zephiran, cetavlon, etc.

The "phenol coefficient" (page 251) of the many preparations varies; therefore, for this information consult the label of the original container. Rather definite information in regard to the "quats" is that they are inactivated by organic material, especially if it is at all acid in its reaction. One advantage of the "quats" is that they are not corrosive to equipment so that clean instruments, when not in use, may be kept disinfected by placing them in a 1-1000 dilution of one of these compounds such as cetylrimethyl-ammonium bromide (cetavlon). Since these compounds are both detergent and antibacterial they play an important part in bringing about conditions of aseptsis. Un-fortunately the bactericidal effects of these compounds vary widely in their ef-ficiency for different organisms. In hu-man sanitation the "quats" have been urged for use in public eating and drink-ing establishments but for this purpose up to the present time, they have not received an unqualified en-dorsement—especially because they are not effective against the germ of tuberculosis. Their alleged ef-ficiency is influenced by such factors as temperature, organic matter, and the usual water mineral constitu-ents. In veterinary medicine they have been tried for udder infusion purposes in the handling of chronic mastitis (page 569), and in strengths of 1 to 1000 as twice weekly applications in the treatment of ringworm of cattle (page 567). They are also used in some poul-try ailments. They are not reliable.

Not equally effective against all bacteria

Sulfonamides: This group of chemicals is not prop-erly classed as either antiseptic, disinfectant or germi-cide, but they do influence bacterial development and are therefore grouped here.

The sulfonamides are chemotherapeutic agents that stop the growth of infecting germs in concentrations that are not poisonous to the host. They are appropri-ately classified as being *bacteriostatic* in their action. They prevent or arrest the growth of bacteria. It is not incorrect to state that the sulfonamides are antiseptics which prevent the growth or multiplication of bacteria in the body though not—within proper limits —being injurious to the host. Under improper condi-tions they may be injurious to the host in their re-ducing the white blood cells count; by crystallization in the urinary tract; and they inhibit thyroid function

Sulfonamides are bacterio-static

(page 96) by combining with its iodine (page 276).

The important basic principles to determine in the use of "sulfas" are (1) what blood levels do they produce; (2) how persistent is their action; (3) how active are they against the organisms causing the ailment. In a measure, answers to the foregoing questions depend on the rate of absorption by the tissues of the body and the rate of their excretion. The following are generally accepted.:

Questions bearing on the use of "sulfas"

Sulfanilamide—very good absorption and rapid excretion.

Sulfapyridine—moderate absorption and moderate excretion.

Sulfathiazole—poor absorption and rapid excretion.

Sulfamerazine—good absorption and slow excretion.

Sulfamethazine—formerly known as sulfamezathine—good absorption and slow excretion.

Sulfaquinoxaline—for fowl cholera (page 649).

The bacteriostatic action of sulfonamides is not the sole influence of these chemicals in controlling infections. During the time that the sulfonamides are checking the growth of the invading germs the host has time to develop antibodies—these are the specific bodies that make man or beast immune to diseases, and furthermore certain blood cells phagocytize—this means that the cells ingest invading germs and other substances—the disease producing germs.

The invading germs destroyed by the blood

In veterinary medicine the sulfonamides that at the time of this writing have found their greatest usefulness are sulfanilamide, sulfathiazole, sulfadiazine, sulfapyridine, sulfaguanadine, sulfamerazine, and sulfamethazine. Sulfanilamide is practically useless in enteric and septicemic disorders in foals as these are mostly due to gram negative organisms and these are not susceptible to sulfanilamide—sulfamerazine or sulfamethazine are better for this purpose. Since the pneumonias in cattle, sheep and pigs are usually associated with gram negatives, sulfamethezene or sulfamerazine are the "sulfas" of choice. Joint-ill in lambs is most responsive to sulfanilamide, and it is the only "sulfa" that is measurably of value in bovine mastitis though in the latter diseases 4:4 diaminodiphenylsulphone has potential value because of its more persistent action. Two solubilized derivatives of diaminodiphenylsulphone known as *diasone* and *promin* have experimentally been demonstrating some value in tuberculosis infection, though because of high toxicity for humans and because treatment of tuberculous cattle is not warranted their use for this purpose has not been developed.

Acridines: In the treatment of both human and animal ailments the acridine dyes such as acriflavine and its hydrochloride, proflavine dihydrochloride and proflavine sulphate have decided value in the handling of staphyloccic infections and suppurating wounds in general. These dyes are stable, non-irritant, easily applied, reasonably effective and not too expensive.

Chemo-
therapy
and
infections

Crystal Violet (hexamethylrosaniline) is a dye that has attained prominence through its action in attenuating disease producing viruses so that vaccines for immunizing purposes may be prepared. Probably the outstanding example is the so-called "crystal violet hog-cholera vaccine" that is now used, on the whole, with satisfactory results. Other dyes such as "gentian violet" (pyoktanin) and "methyl violet," are bactericidal to gram positive organisms though gram negatives, including the tuberculosis germ, are not affected. Other dyes having merit are brilliant green, isamine blue, trypan red, etc. It should be clear that the field of chemotherapeutics is an important one. The aid of the organic chemist and the biologist is needed in the development of these agents.

Nitrofuran Derivatives: These are substitution products of furan (which is a colorless liquid from wood tar). There are many of them now made chemically from wheat husks, corn cobs, oat hulls, etc. The nitrofurans are both bacteriostatic and bactericidal. In the test tube it is difficult to develop bacterial strains that are resistant to nitrofurans, though this resistance does occur with some of the sulfas, penicillin, streptomycin, etc. The nitrofurans most frequently reported on are:

1. *Nitrofurazone (N.F.Z.)* which has been used in the prevention of some animal ailments—coccidiosis in poultry, and those due to the Salmonella group of organisms such as pullorum disease or typhoid in chickens; blackhead and hexamitiasis in turkeys; and some forms of swine enteritis.

2. *Furazolidone nf. 180 (Furaxone),* which seems to be most effective in the handling and prevention of infections in the organs of digestion.

3. *Furadantin* as a urinary disinfectant.

As feed additives in amounts of two to four pounds per ton of feed the nitrofurans are establishing reports of success in the fields of their specialization. These agents are practically harmless in therapeutic doses. Veterinarians prescribe them as ointments for the relief of infectious eye and ear ailments.

The average user of antiseptics, disinfectants and bactericides has no means by which he can determine their value, his knowledge of them not infrequently being obtained from prejudiced sources. In the hands of many, their mode of application may be open to question, and if this is combined with the use of an agent of doubtful value, the practical usefulness of the "disinfection" may be nullified. The agents mentioned each have their sphere of usefulness, and some of them closely approach the ideal in that sphere. No single disinfectant is appropriate in all instances (page 241). Select the most appropriate for the results demanded of it, apply it liberally and give it plenty of time to exert its action. Of practically equal importance is the exactness, and the painstaking care of the person entrusted with the disinfection.

Chapter XVIII

METHODS OF APPLICATION OF CHEMICAL DISINFECTANTS

Methods of application of disinfectants (see page 215 and page 573) vary depending upon the region or area, as well as upon the material to be disinfected.

1. Woodwork is best treated by an application of a liquid disinfectant by means of a spray-pump (Fig. 63) (page 218). This not only results in **The spray pump in applying disinfectants** a surface treatment, but a good deal of the disinfectant is forced into cracks and crevices, this being a particularly desirable feature because these are harboring places for many germs. It also is an excellent plan to mix some whitewash with the disinfectant so as to more clearly indicate the places that have been treated, as well as imprisoning germs by sealing the wood.

2. A spray-pump (page 218) not being available, the disinfectant may be applied with a large whitewash brush, or a broom. This method lacks the efficiency of the spray-pump method, and in addition it is quite wasteful of material.

3. When wounds on animals are badly infected, and especially if these are deep, "continuous irrigation" may be found to be the desirable method of applying an antiseptic. Only the very mildest antiseptics may be used for this purpose. A quantity of it is placed in an overhead container and by means of a piece of rubber tubing suitably fastened to the container by one of its ends and to the wound area on the patient by the other end, the antiseptic is permitted to trickle slowly into all of the recesses of the wound. The length of time for this process depends upon the extent of the wound, the degree of infection and the vitality of the

patient. These are all factors that must at times be left to the judgment of the attending veterinarian.

4. Another excellent method of applying antiseptics to wounds is by means of a two-ounce capacity soft rubber bulb syringe having an eight-inch hard rubber nozzle. Rubber is not acted upon by most of the antiseptics, and a syringe made of it affords a safe, efficient and economical method of application.

5. Occasionally it is desirable to wipe off a badly infected wound. This must be done carefully to avoid unnecessary irritation, and without inducing bleeding as this especially indicates the opening of new avenues for the deeper penetration by infections. Long-fiber absorbent cotton is almost an ideal agent for this method of wound handling. It is soft, comparatively cheap, and it has spongelike action in absorbing large quantities of fluid antiseptic. When partially squeezed free from previously absorbed antiseptic, it may be used in a "patting" manner on a wound to absorb wound exudates and infections. Because of its cheapness, each pledget of it should be discarded as rapidly as it has been used. Instead of cotton, soft cloths of absorbent material are sometimes used for the purpose of applying antiseptics to wounds or bodily areas. Though they have the advantage when antiseptics are to be applied to such an area as the mammary gland, in general they do not compare favorably with absorbent cotton.

The treatment of wounds with disinfectants

6. Occasionally disinfectants, and antiseptics, are applied in the form of a dry powder. Examples are applying freshly-hydrated lime by scattering it on the floors of barns, though this is a practice having limited value, applying fluoride of soda as a disinfestant to lousy fowl, and applying veterinary antiseptic dusting powders to wounds. When wound secretions, or any kind of moisture dampens these dryly-applied disinfectants they are most efficient.

7. Both human and veterinary surgeons frequently resort to the use of antiseptic-impregnated gauzes. Usually this is sterilized cheesecloth which has in its meshes a definite percentage of a dry antiseptic. If it is desired to have a gauze antiseptic dressing somewhat moist, a small amount of glycerin is added. These antiseptic gauzes, either dry or moist, are very valuable as protective dressings on aseptic or only mildly infected wounds.

8. Gaseous disinfection of rooms and their contents is frequently attempted by means of the gas formaldehyde (page 266). This is effective provided that the moisture content (page 267)—humidity—of the room is high when formaldehyde is used. Since bacteria do not breathe so as to inhale a gaseous disinfectant, and as they absorb only substances that are in solution, fumigation with the objective of destroying germs is of very little if any value, excepting formaldehyde gas released in humid atmosphere.

PART FIVE

Some Insecticides, Larvicides and Their Use on Premises and on Hosts

⚹⚹⚹⚹

CHAPTER XIX

DISINFESTING BUILDINGS AND ANIMALS

An infestant is a parasite present so continuously or in such numbers as to be a source of annoyance, trouble **An infestant defined** or danger to the host. In a limited sense in this dissertation it refers particularly to the infestation for varying lengths of time of the outside of the bodies of domesticated animals with parasites that derive heat or sustenance, or both, from their host. Some of the parasites may infest the host only briefly to obtain food, retiring then to or into some of the surroundings such as rubbish, and cracks and crevices in buildings (page 726) ; others spend a certain phase of their biological development on a living host, the remaining phases being spent elsewhere; and still others maintain a permanent lifelong existence on the host.

A disinfestant is an agent that disturbs the parasite-host relationship usually by attempts to kill the parasite either on the host or in the surroundings. It concerns itself with the extermination or destruction of insects, rodents or other animal forms—usually visible to the unaided eye—these being a source of annoyance, and which might transmit infection or disease because of their presence on the host or from his surroundings. Some writers prefer to use the word *disinfectant* rather than *disinfestant* though in this text the former is limited to microscopic forms or the freeing from or destruction of infection.

A group of agents closely related to disinfestants, known as repellents, seek to prevent the establishment of intimate parasite-host relationships. **The nature of repellents** The result of their action is conducive to physical comfort, or probably it may be better stated that they insure a lesser degree of discomfort to the intended hosts by keeping hordes of irritating parasites away from them. It is because of their lack of complete efficiency, as well as the comparatively small numbers of parasites they affect as related to their total numbers that they influence that their use is based on expediency rather than on more complete control.

It is well to emphasize that true sanitation and disease control, insofar as insect pests are concerned, rests in the destruction of the offending agent, or even in preventing its development before the parasite-host relationship is established. Infestation of poultry **Prevention of poultry lice** with lice, for example, may be prevented on the average farm where usually no contact because of distance is established with neighboring flocks. Starting with clean houses and well fenced runs, the birds must be incubated and hatched on the premises. No fowls should be brought on the premises from other sources. Used crates must be disinfested and disinfected before being used. There is always the hazard that sparrows and other birds may infest the premises with their lice, but this is a rather remote possibility.

Pasture rotation will do much to prevent infestation with other parasites, notably ticks (page 220). A **Pasture rotation to control ticks** film of kerosene on ponds and other stagnant waters to control mosquitoes, proper and sanitary disposal of manure (page 163), controlling the breeding of insects from various sources (pages 697 to 732) inclusive, and clean drinking water in clean drinking vessels are all preferred steps in the ceaseless battle against the host of parasitic pests.

Mechanical agencies include tightly closed buildings to house the animals, or the buildings more appropriately equipped with window and door screening, the latter frequently charged with an electrical current of low voltage so as to electrocute flies and other parasites upon contact. It is a common practice to have burlap sacking, or strips of other fabrics suspended from doorways to mechanically brush flies and other pests from entering animals, or these may be hung from ceilings of animal stalls so that they by their motion induced by air currents keep these pests away from their intended host. Fly-nets and muslin covers are helpful. Inside of tightly closed or screened buildings mechanical traps (The reader is referred to U.S.D.A. Farmers Bulletin No. 1097 entitled "The Stable Fly, How to Prevent Its Annoyance and Its Losses to Live Stock.") are used. Sometimes these are baited with sweetened or other enticing agents. They are ingeniously contrived to permit flies to enter easily, though their escape is practically impossible. Another form of trapping is by sheets or strips of "sticky" papers.

Mechanical agencies to control insects

To an extent horses may be protected against the egg-depositing habits of the bot-fly (page 705) by the application of modified food bags that do not interfere with breathing and eating. (Consult Chapter XXXI, page 697, Insect Carriers and Their Role.)

It is practically useless to free animals of infestants if the buildings in which they are housed, together with the immediate surroundings are permitted to harbor obnoxious pests, and from the disease stand-point potentially dangerous, animal forms. Before, therefore, dis-

Building disinfestation

infested animals are returned to buildings and surroundings the latter must be disinfested.

Some disinfestants or insecticides that are frequently used in keeping animal habitations free from
insect and other pests are as follows:

1. *D.D.T.* (*dishloro-diphenyl-tri-chlorethane*) (pages
298, 299, 300). As a contact and stomach poison D.D.T.
is effective against house flies (page 697), stable flies
(page 698), horn flies (page 699), mosquitoes, gnats,
lice, fleas, sheep ticks or keds, wood ticks, the instar
(the larval stage of an insect between molts) stage
of other ticks including the brown dog ticks, bed bugs,
Insects roaches, ants, Japanese beetles, chiggers
controlled and others. Unfortunately it is also deadly
by D.D.T. against such beneficial insects as bees, lady
beetles, syrphus flies, and aphis lions.

D.D.T. is not effective against any of the flies which
D.D.T. not dart in to lay eggs on the hairs such as
effective screwworm flies, heel flies, bot flies, sheep
gad flies, and others.

D.D.T. is one of the most effective agents for fly
control because in less than twenty minutes after they
have had contact with it—either on the previously
sprayed animal or buildings—they are dead. Therefore
there usually is not enough time for egg laying. It is
both a contact and a stomach poison. It is not a repellent. It kills house flies, stable flies, and horn flies. Some
species of the horse-fly family are controlled by D.D.T.
but not as fast as other species of flies. One source of
information states that "some 3 days after treatment
of stock, the horseflies kept away altogether for several weeks." D.D.T. is relatively ineffective against the
heel-fly (page 706), and the screwworm fly because
these two have such a very brief contact with the
sprayed animal. Details regarding the application of
D.D.T. on page 293.

Nature provides many examples of the ability of

living organisms to adapt themselves to adverse conditions. The D.D.T.-resistant flies are quite common.
During the Korean engagement there was **Resistance to insecticides** found a D.D.T.-resistant louse. Benzine hexachloride (BHC) (see later pages) is no longer effective against a strain of Blue tick; in fact, before the days of the synthetic insecticides an arsenic-resistant "Blue" tick became established in South Africa. The simplest explanation of the development of resistant strains is that in the repeated application of insecticides the more susceptible individuals are removed so that a system of selective breeding results in producing resistant individuals.

Technically D.D.T. is a white waxy powder, containing 50 per cent of chlorine, the chemical formula is C_{14} H_9 Cl_5, non-volatile at ordinary tem- **D.D.T. not a repellent** peratures—it is therefore not an insect repellant. It is not soluble in water—therefore it must be combined with a wetting agent to hold it in suspension in water. It is freely soluble in most organic solvents including kerosene, distillate, crankcase oil, acetone, alcohol, xylene, naphthas and others.

A particularly valuable characteristic of D.D.T. is its residual effect. In this manner it protects against body lice—in humans these may be in **A valuable characteristic** clothing, even though the clothing is laundered weekly—and other insects. It will destroy flies alighting on the animal four months after cattle are sprayed with it. The residual characteristic is in a measure modified by the nature of the surface to which it is applied; thus rough surfaces as unplaned wood, wall-paper, wallboard, natural fabrics and pitted metals **Surface effect on D.D.T.** remain highly lethal for six months or more; smooth surfaces as glass and tile loose their film of D.D.T. much quicker; freshly painted surfaces, linoleum, cement, new metal screen and synthetic fabrics give very poor results.

The principal enemy of D.D.T. is alkali or alkali salts—lime, or calcium oxide is one of these alkalies.

D.D.T. and whitewash

Since lime is the principal ingredient of whitewash and as whitewash is weakly alkaline it follows that when D.D.T. is mixed with whitewash, or applied to a whitewashed surface at least 50 per cent of its original value is dissipated. Also it has been demonstrated that aluminum, chromium and certain iron-containing materials all cause a catalytic (dissolving reaction) decomposition of D.D.T.

D.D.T. may be removed from surfaces by dry-cleaning, with paste wallpaper cleaner, the hot flat-iron, and vigorous brushing; light sponging with soap and water does not have very much effect in its removal.

D.D.T. as a poison

D.D.T. if used with reasonable care may be considered to be non-poisonous; however, it is not entirely free from toxic properties. It must be kept out of animal or human foodstuffs, though in one research project cattle, horses and sheep were given D.D.T. in daily doses of from 100 to 200 milligrams for each kilogram of body weight—continued for three weeks, and succeeding in producing only loss of appetite, trembling, and excitability, all of which disappeared shortly after the dosing was discontinued. Also when used as a spray for the control of forest insects at the rate of one pound to the acre it was not dangerous to terrestrial wildlife, but dosages of five pounds to the acre were dangerous.

When used on domesticated animals as a powder or in water suspension there is relatively little danger,

D.D.T. in an oil solvent dangerous

though when the D.D.T. for external application to animals is in an oil or kerosene solvent there may be sufficient absorption to occasionally cause toxic manifestations. Humans should also avoid inhalation of the spray or the dry powder. Barbiturates are considered to be antidotes; intravenous calcium borogluconate is also given animals for this purpose. D.D.T. orally administered to two goats—0.68 grams to 1.25 grams for each pound of live weight—was eliminated in sufficient amount in the milk to produce poisonous symptoms and death of white rats fed this milk. Death occurred in 29 to 30 minutes.

In any plan of livestock insect control, the buildings and immediate surroundings should receive attention. In dairy barns, horse stables, hog and poultry houses, around the outside of entrance doors, and fence posts the standard rule is to use a spray of a five per cent solution of D.D.T. in an oil solvent—the water solution is just as effective but its results are not so lasting. Use one gallon of spray to each 1,000 square feet of surface. Try to obtain solid covering but avoid excess run-off. Cover ceilings, side walls, pipes, fixtures, etc., but avoid feed bins or containers as well as forage or other feed. One spraying will last from six to twelve weeks depending upon the roughness or smoothness of the sprayed surface. For hog and poultry houses five per cent D.D.T. in kerosene or distillate is preferred because of its action against mites as well as flies. (For manure treatment with D.D.T. consult page 169.)

Use of D.D.T. in buildings

For cattle, stable flies (page 698) and horn flies (page 699) are probably the most annoying pests. Spraying, not dairy cattle, with a one-half of one per cent D.D.T. preparation is effective if properly applied. (Page 293.)

Probably the most important thing is to have good pens for holding the cattle while they are being sprayed. The second necessary thing to do is to get the animals thoroughly wet with the spraying solution. The material should be applied with 400 to 450 pounds pressure, using eight pounds of the wettable 50 per cent D.D.T. powder in 100 gallons of water. The 100 gallons will treat 125 to 150 head of grown cattle. The third important thing to do is to get the first treatment applied before there are too many flies on the cattle. The number should not be more than 10 per animal for three successive days. The second treatment should follow when there appear about 10 flies per day, and the third treatment should be applied when the flies return.

Also remove piles of manure and decaying wet straw and other vegetation as they are breeding places for flies.

D.D.T. should not be used on dairy cattle nor on their surroundings such as buildings and other woodwork since ingestion or contact with it is **Not for dairy cattle** later evidenced in the milk, and this latter if consumed by humans might be harmful. It is still recommended for fly control or others such as lice on beef animals or for other places on the farm excepting inside dairy barns, milk rooms, and on feed.

Ticks on sheep controlled by spraying Spraying sheep by means of a power sprayer with a 0.25 per cent D.D.T. water suspension controlled both sheep ticks (keds) and wood ticks. On full fleeced sheep the power sprayer is directed along the neck and back, though in shorn sheep the sides and under surfaces also should be sprayed.

An emulsion of D.D.T. is made by dissolving the powdered drug in an oil solvent, and then by means of an emulsifying agent converting the preparation into an emulsion or in other words a preparation in which the D.D.T. is held in reasonably permanent suspension, and so that it will mix—usually to form a cream-like preparation—with water. For dipping purposes many consider an emulsion of D.D.T. best. In experimental trials, dipping sheep once in a 0.1 per cent emulsion is said to have destroyed at least 99 per cent of sheep keds. Hog lice were destroyed by dipping the hogs once in a kerosene emulsion containing 0.75 per cent D.D.T. when the quarters were sprayed at the same time. Cattle lice required a 0.25 per cent D.D.T. emulsion and died off slowly over a period of 48 hours or more. Even though the nits of lice may not be killed, there is usually enough D.D.T. left in the coats of animals to kill any newly hatched lice.

In the control of lice by dusting with D.D.T. Twinn in Contribution No. 2463, Division of Entomology, Science Service, Department of Agriculture, Ottawa, Canada reports as follows:

Dusting with D.D.T. for lice control "Lice spend their entire life cycle as ectoparasites of mammals and birds. The sucking lice (Anoplura) are found only on mammals, but biting lice (Mallophaga) occur on both mammals and birds.

"D.D.T. is a very efficient insecticide for controlling both forms of lice, and was widely used during the second World War in protecting armed forces' personnel and, in some instances, civilian populations from infestation by Pediculus humanus L., the vector of typhus fever. Since the war the value of D.D.T. for delousing livestock and poultry has been demonstrated, and its use for this purpose is likely to become increasingly widespread and popular.

Chicken Lice: (Consult pages 291 and 723).

Cattle Lice: (Consult page 721).

Commercial D.D.T. preparations Commercially D.D.T. is available in (1) solution in kerosene or other solvent; (2) dusting powders; (3) wettable powders—containing from 20 to 50 per cent D.D.T.—for mixing with water; (4) emulsion concentrates to be mixed with water; (5) aerosol bombs for space spraying. The concentrated wettable powder is most popular because it may be used for building treatment as well as for dipping or spraying animals. A refined five per cent hydrocarbon oil solution—practically non-staining and odorless—is used for spraying walls, and screens in homes, hospitals, kennels, dairies, and stables, but not on animals because of the danger of absorption and poisoning. The emulsion type of D.D.T. preparation is best used in building treatments, and as they contain oil only to very limited extent.

In the use of D.D.T. certain precautions should be observed:

Precautions in the use of D.D.T.

1. Do not inhale dusts or sprays containing D.D.T.

2. Avoid contaminating human and animal food.

3. Avoid getting D.D.T. on skin or clothing. If contaminated, wash with soap and warm water.

4. Do not apply D.D.T. to mature crops. Early in the season weathering reduces the level of the insecticide and the danger is correspondingly less.

5. Never use on dairy animals, this includes the non-lactating ones, D.D.T. preparations having an oil base. On non-lactating dairy animals and on other animals use suspensions of the wettable powder.

2. *Chlordane* is a chlorinated hydrocarbon containing 69 per cent of chlorine; its formula is $C_{10}H_6Cl_8$. It is a wartime discovery. In the highly refined state it is a viscous, nearly odorless liquid that occasionally shows a tendency to crystallize. Commercially, it is in the form of a wettable powder, dusts, emulsifiable concentrates, and oil solutions. It is completely soluble in the usual organic solvents, and it mixes completely with deodorized kerosene—this latter commonly used in insecticidal preparations.

Physical properties of chlordane

In the presence of alkali—whitewash, etc.—it reacts to form products of a low order of toxicity to insects.

In field and laboratory tests it has proven superior to D.D.T. against the German cockroach, American cockroach, chigger mites, the lone-star tick and certain species of ants. Indications are that it is more effective than D.D.T.

Compared with D.D.T.

against the body-louse in both duration of action and lower toxic concentration requirements, but when used on clothing it is less resistant than D.D.T. to laundering. As a residual spray it is generally inferior to D.D.T. against house-flies and mosquitoes, and it declines much more rapidly in effectiveness. To livestock owners and veterinarians it is of value because of its action against cattle and hog lice, sheep ticks, horn-flies, and poultry lice. Chlordane used at the rate of one pint of an emulsified preparation in 50 gallons of water applied to one acre gave an excellent kill of grasshoppers. Another use is against the American lawn ant—eight ounces of 50 per cent wettable chlordane powder in 50 gallons of water for 1,000 square feet of turf. It may be mixed with the weed killer 2 4-D as they are compatible.

Effective against animal parasites

Against ticks, mange mites, lice and fleas infesting dogs chlordane has given good results. Usually it is employed as a dip containing from 0.25 to 0.5 per cent chlordane. It is on the market in the form of a 40% wettable powder and as an emulsion. It is a non-crystalline chemical and leaves no noticeable residue on fur, hair, wool or feathers, nor does it discolor the animal. The fact that it is odorless makes it of greater usefulness than benzene hexachloride (page 300) on animals or their food products, or in the presence of foods. One report about the treatment of mange (scabies) of swine indicates that the use of a 0.25 per cent chlordane preparation, made by adding 500 cc of a 74 per cent emulsified concentrate to 500 gallons of water, was applied with a power sprayer, using from one to two quarts per head, and at from 50 to 250 pounds of nozzle pressure. Itching disappeared in less than a day, and all evidence of mange was gone in seventeen days.

Chlordane kills by contact, by its vapor, and by stomach ingestion. To humans and animals it is reported to be less toxic in general than D.D.T. However, chlordane has been shown to have marked toxicity for sheep and goats because when dipped at four day intervals in chlordane wettable powder and **Strong preparations kill sheep and goats** emulsion formations with 1.5 per cent active ingredients—this is much stronger than used in actual practice—several of the sheep and goats died after three dippings. The observed symptoms were vision impairment, incoordinated gait, convulsions, collapse and death.

No offensive odor Chlordane has no offensive odor and may therefore be used on meat producing animals and pets without the difficulty of contamination with odors. It has the same general uses—though in somewhat lower strengths than D.D.T.

Chlordane is hazardous though *acute* oral toxicity for rats is approximately half that of D.D.T. In liquid **Poisonous nature of chlordane** form it is readily absorbed through the skin and therefore rubber gloves and an organic-vapor-type respirator should always be worn when it is applied as a spray. Spillage should at once be cleaned up with soap and water. Young animals and presumably children are more susceptible than adults.

From the standpoint of *chronic* toxicity there is some evidence that it is more poisonous that D.D.T. As it is volatile its use in large quantities in closed structures is not recommended; the use for localized or "spot" treatment for fly and cockroach treatment is permissible. In general, follow the rules laid down for D.D.T. for the handling and applying of chlordane. The following is a release from the U. S. Dept. of Agriculture: "Studies have shown that chlordane, when present in insecticides, used on dairy animals or on forage fed to dairy animals, appears in the milk. It may also be found in milk following its ordinary use for fly control in dairy barns. Because of the vital importance of milk in the diet of infants, children, and people of all ages, it is essential that proper precautions be taken to protect the milk supply." It should therefore not be used as an insecticide spray in dairy barns or human dwellings.

3. *Benzene Hexachloride*—also known as 666, BHC and Gammexane having the empirical formula $C_6H_6Cl_6$, it contains 73 per cent of chlorine, is a complex of five known isomers (having the same number of atoms, but differing in the order in which the atoms are arranged in the molecule), alpha, beta, delta, epsilon and gamma. The gamma isomer is the principal insecticidal ingredient — commercials have about twelve per cent of this isomer.

Benzene hexachloride is a buff-to-tan colored powder having a persistent musty odor arising largely, though not entirely, from the presence of small amounts of manufacturing impurities. The odor makes its use objectionable in buildings and on pets.

It is insoluble in water but readily soluble in a wide range of common organic solvents. Its toxic action against insects may be as a contact poison, as a stomach poison, as a fumigant or as a combination of the three. The fact that it is insoluble in water is not a matter of concern because it is commercially combined with a wetting agent which holds it in suspension in water. It is not compatible with such alkali substances as whitewash, bordeaux mixture, calcium arsenate and others.

From the standpoint of *acute oral* toxicity the gamma isomer is twice that of D.D.T. However, it is not stored in the body and therefore the danger of *chronic* toxicity is low. It is reported as being only 1/15 as poisonous as D.D.T., and it has been used without adverse effects on domesticated **Not as poisonous as D.D.T.** animals as indicated by the fact that dipping them every four days in a benzene hexachloride (10 per cent gamma isomer) suspension having a 1½ per cent concentration—this dosage is higher than that used in actual practice—

produced no ill-effects. However, in the same concentration but will 50 per cent gamma isomer the cattle were killed.

It must be stressed that the strong musty odors will taint milk and foods, and even the flesh of animals if they are slaughtered shortly after having been treated with this compound. So persistent is this odor that a crop of potatoes was made unfit for human consumption following the earlier application of B.H.C. to the soil on which they were grown.

Musty odor objectionable

In general it may be said that it is active against the same insects as D.D.T., and in addition is much more effective against ticks, mites and lice. A single dipping of sheep in an aqueous suspension containing 0.5 per cent of wettable benzine hexachloride gamma isomer (0.0325 per cent) completely eradicated a simultaneously existing infestation with *Melophagus ovinus* (sheep ked) and *Linognathus pedalis* (the foot louse). The sheep ked pupae were not instantly killed but newly hatched keds were destroyed on contact with the wool of treated sheep. This also is true for new-hatched lice from the eggs of this parasite, in fact some of the eggs were rendered non-viable.

Highly effective against ticks, mites and lice

The residual durability of benzene hexachloride is limited as it is lost by evaporation. Even increasing the dosage did not extend its effectiveness beyond ten weeks.

If there is no objection to its musty odor it deserves a high rating as a disinfestant in the handling of animals infested with the mange mite (scabies) (page 725), or with lice, or ticks, especially the troublesome sheep tick or ked. In the handling of swine mange (scabies) the scabs should first be broken up by scrubbing with a stiff brush, and

B.H.C. has a musty odor but it's a good disinfestant

then sprayed with a 0.5 per cent wettable benzene hexachloride having a *gamma isomer* of 10 to 12 per cent. A single application is sufficient. Of course the surroundings must also be disinfested because many of these infestants spend some time off the host. The musty odor of the B.H.C. disappears in two or three weeks. B.H.C. is no longer recommended—lindane (page 303) has taken its place.

Cobbett in a project of the Zoological Division, Agricultural Research Service, U. S. D. A. (American Journ. of Veterinary Research No. 32, Vol. IX) has reported on the control of the cattle fever tick (Southern Cattle Fever) (pages 714 and 747) following the use of combinations of D.D.T. (pages 291 and 295), and benzene hexachloride (page 300).

The chemicals used were wettable powders that contained 50 per cent by weight of the D.D.T. and B.H.C.—the latter with 13 per cent *gamma isomer* content—and 50 per cent by weight of an inert wetting agent.

"One dipping in dips containing 1 per cent of D.D.T. combined with 0.33 per cent to 0.5 per cent of B.H.C. destroyed all existing ticks on grossly infested cattle in about five days and prevented their becoming reinfested during eleven to sixteen day periods of exposure in tick infested pastures. One or two additional dippings in such dips at five to twelve day intervals produced no injurious effects to the cattle. Such dips, therefore may be safely and effectively used to cleanse grossly tick-infested cattle without resorting to the use of tick-free premises during the process."

"Tick-free cattle that were susceptible to piroplasmosis (Southern cattle fever, page 747) were dipped once in a dip containing 0.66 per cent of D.D.T. alone just prior to leaving their tick-free range, and again in a tick dip upon a completion of a five day drive through heavily tick-infested country. The animals were apparently protected against the exposure to fever ticks and tick-borne piroplasmosis, as no symptoms of the disease occurred later among the animals."

Since benzene hexachloride in the form of wettable powder is marketed having a gamma isomer concen-

Sheep tick dipping

tration of 6, 10, or 12 per cent it is necessary to make varying concentrations in the dip. For sheep a gamma isomer concentration of 0.025 per cent is recommended. To obtain this degree of concentration with the wettable B.H.C. powder for each 100 gallons of water there should be used 3½ pounds of the 6 per cent powder, or 2 pounds of the 10 per cent powder, on 1¾ pounds of the 12 per cent powder. A single dipping is recommended for the eradication of the ticks.

4. *Lindane*: This is a pure gamma isomer of B.H.C. or it contains not less than 99 per cent of the

A purified BHC

gamma isomer of B.H.C. and thus the disadvantage found in B.H.C. has been overcome so that it is practically odorless. It is available as dusts, wettable powder, oil solutions, and emulsifiable concentrates. Its use in dairy barns for fly control has been approved, as well as low percentage dusts for only one application directly on livestock (not on milk producers) for the control of lice, scabies or mange, and similar parasites.

A one per cent dust of lindane applied either over poultry as with a hand duster as the birds are roosting or distributed by hand over litter has provided control of lice. For the destruction of sheep ticks it should be used in the same degree of dip concentration as B.H.C. —0.025 per cent. This means that in 100 gallons of water there should be placed 13 ounces of the 25 per cent wettable powder, 0.8 of the 25 per cent emulsifiable concentrate. Precautions in its handling are the same as for D.D.T.

Lindane is the principal ingredient of a smear recently announced by the U. S. Bureau of Entomology and Plant Quarantine. It is referred to as EI-335. Its ingredients consist of—by weight—three parts of lindane, 35 parts of pine oil, 42 parts of white mineral oil, 10 parts of an emulsifier, and 10 parts of silica gel. It is applied with a paint brush to the wound and a narrow strip one inch wide around the edges of the wound at 3 or 4 day intervals. It kills the maggots as rapidly as they are hatched, as well as the adult flies attracted to the wound to lay more eggs. (See page 317—for Smear #62.)

A new "smear" for screw-worm control

5. *Methoxychlor:* It is available in the same formulations so that it is closely related to D.D.T. though it is less toxic to higher animals—about 1/24 that of D.D.T. It is used in the same concentrations as D.D.T. and in general it is somewhat less effective. The same precautions in its handling should be followed as for D.D.T. It may be applied to dairy cattle (D.D.T. is not approved for use on dairy cattle by the Federal Agency, but on the other hand the Federal Agency has not forbidden its use for this purpose) and in reasonable amounts to edible crops. Dairy cattle may be sprayed with it every few days to control the small blood sucking flies. Do not get on feed, in drinking water, or in milk.

6. *Toxaphene* (chlorinated camphene). It is more effective in the control of sheep ticks than D.D.T. It is approximately four times as acutely toxic as D.D.T. and therefore the precautions in its handling should be even more rigorous than those recommended for D.D.T.

7. *Dieldrin and Aldrin:* These two synthetic insecticides have the property of diffusing along the wool fibers to a much greater extent than many of such chlorinated hydrocarbon insecticides as D.D.T., methoxychlor, chlordane, toxaphene, and B.H.C. Fielder and Du Toit in So. Africa conclude that against the mange mite *Psoroptes communis ovis*—a scab mite of sheep a single dipping to control sheep scab, using

Greater diffusion along wool fibers

a 0.003 concentration of dieldrin was highly effective. As a control measure against the sheep maggot fly (*Lucilia sericata*) a single dipping in a 0.05 per cent in a dieldrin emulsion, or water suspension, protected sheep for at least 12 to 16 weeks. Aldrin in wettable powder or emulsion form in a concentration of 0.05 is not considered effective to eradicate scab with a single dipping. The 1950 Report of the Chief of the U. S. Bureau of Animal Industry states "Dieldrin, a recently developed chlorinated hydrocarbon insecticide when applied in a 0.25 per cent concentration was toxic and in some instances fatal to 1- to 2-week-old Jersey calves; a concentration of 0.1 per cent failed to produce toxic reactions." "Suckling pigs tolerated 4.0 per cent, and suckling lambs were able to resist 2.0 per cent but were killed by 3.0 per cent." "In single applications, dieldrin was toxic to adult cattle at 2.0 per cent but not at 1.0 per cent concentration, and was toxic to sheep and goats at 4.0 per cent." "When applied three times at 2-week intervals, a 0.5 per cent concentration was toxic to adult cattle."

8. *Malathion* is an organic compound of comparatively low toxicity in mammals, but toxic to flies and mosquitoes, and to insect pests on vegetation. In its comparatively pure form, it is a liquid of a dark yellow to brown color but commercially it is marketed as a four per cent dust; 25 per cent wettable powder; poison bait, and as an aerosol. It may be used as a sugar bait in dairy barns at the same time that the wood work is sprayed with lindane, but care must be taken not to get it in the milk room. In poultry houses, on floor litter, roosts, nests and on droppings malathion may be used as a four per cent dust for the control of poultry mites, flies and mosquitoes, but care must be taken not to get it in the drinking water or on the feed. It was found to be toxic for baby calves in a concentration of 1 per cent, but not at 0.5 per cent.

In addition to the general precautions included in the discussion regarding D.D.T., unless otherwise in-

Some more precautions dicated under the various synthetic insecticides, the following points are to be borne in mind:

1. All synthetic insecticides are poisonous if used in sufficiently high concentration.

2. Do not use a dip or spray if the insecticide has not mixed smoothly and uniformly with the water, or if an oily layer appears after mixing.

3. D.D.T., toxaphene, chlordane, and benzine hexachloride, contaminate the milk of dairy animals —use methoxychlor instead, even though it is not quite as effective.

4. Keep in a dry place, and *out of the reach of children.*

5. In making dilutions use exactly the strength recommended—the statement "if a little is good, a lot is better" may result seriously.

6. Unused residues must not be discarded in streams or ponds as many are toxic to most forms of aquatic life. Neither should they be poured on the surface; rather dig a space in the ground for the residue and then cover it with clean soil.

7. Clean sprayers and dusters thoroughly after use.

8. D.D.T., Lindane and toxaphene should not be used on livestock within 30 days of slaughter, though malathion may be used right up to the time of slaughter, except for animals in lactation or calves less than one month of age. (Consult page 710 about the chemical "Trolene.")

SOME OTHER INSECTICIDES—NOT CHLORINATED HYDROCARBONS

1. *Carbon bisulphide* is also known as carbon disulphide, or colloquially in some of the southern states it

Carbon bisulphide a good disinfestant, though it must be kept away from heat and flame

is spoken of as "high-life." It is a colorless, watery liquid which evaporates quickly when exposed to air having a temperature not lower than 75 degrees Fahrenheit. The gas is explosively inflammable, even by hot steam pipes or the spark from an electric light switch, and therefore fire insurance companies place the same restrictions on its use in or near buildings as those imposed for the use of gasoline. The gas is also poisonous to human beings, though not nearly to the same extent as hydrocyanic gas.

The gas is heavier than air, and therefore first occupies the lower places. It is destructive to weevils and other pests that injure stored grains, and also to lice and mites, rats and other rodents. The impure, commercial grades obtainable at the lowest cost are used for fumigating purposes. The vapor and the chemically pure liquid are not at all injurious to fabrics, though impurities in the commercial liquid, carbon bisulphide, will stain fabrics. When it is desired to destroy pests in grains (page 476) these should not be heating at the time of application. A reasonably gas-tight receptacle or bin must be available.

A method of disinfesting grain

The liquid carbon bisulphide may be placed in a shallow dish and set on top of the grain, provided the latter is not too deep, or it may be poured directly onto the grain. If the grain is more than ordinarily closely packed, it may be necessary to force some of the liquid into the mass. Dry grains are not injured for seed purposes and no grain so treated is injurious for animal consumption after airing it.

2. *Hydrocyanic acid gas* is extremely poisonous to all forms of life as well as to the eggs of insects. (Page 342.) A very few inhalations of the gas

Hydrocyanic gas a deadly poison

are fatal to human life, and it is employed for this purpose in a few states in inflicting the death penalty on criminals in the so-called lethal gas chambers. It is not inflammable, nor destructive to fabrics, though it penetrates fabrics poorly. Its highly poisonous action makes it unsafe for use excepting under the direction of the trained expert. Usually the preparation used in calcium cyanide—in the presence of moisture, high humidity of air or in the ground of burrows, it forms hydrocyanic acid gas which is a deadly poison for man, animals, and insects.

3. *Sulphur dioxide* is much safer to use as a fumigant disinfestor than either hydrocyanic gas or carbon bisulphide. This gas is made by placing **Burning** flowers of sulphur or molded sulphur can-**sulphur is an** dles in iron containers and these in turn **established** are placed in tubs partly filled with water. **method of** In order to start the combustion of the sul-**disinfesting** phur easily some alcohol is poured over it and ignited. The resulting sulphur dioxide gas will destroy rats, flies, lice and mites, but is not positively effective against insect eggs. The room is to be kept sealed for from one to six hours. Though some forms of life are more susceptible than others to the action of sulphur dioxide gas, it is best to use an amount and a duration of exposure (four pounds of sulphur for each one thousand cubic feet of space for six hours) sufficient to destroy the most resistant. During World War I horses infested with mange mites were placed in sealed cells with their heads protruding. Sulphur dioxide gas was then passed into the cells so as to obtain a concentration of approximately five per cent by volume, and the exposure was continued for one hour. The mites on the protruding head of the animal were killed by local application of other agents.

4. *Kerosene emulsion* has been recommended to destroy mites and similar parasites in farm buildings. It may be applied to any of the farm animals **Kerosene** by means of a brush or spray pump with-**emulsion** out injury. It will rid the stock of lice. **sprayed on** Poultry lice are destroyed by dipping fowl **roosts con-** **trols mites** in it for one minute, and then the material

may be used to spray roosts and coops to rid them of lice and mites. Some of the mites have their abode in cracks and crevices, and leave these only during the time that a host becomes available for their nourishment, returning to their abode when their appetites are replenished.

Kerosene emulsion is an effective agent to destroy these parasites in their abode. It is made by boiling a mixture of one pound of hard soap shavings in one gallon of water until the soap is dissolved. Water must frequently be added to take the place of that lost by evaporation. Then move the solution to a safe distance from fire and slowly mix in four gallons of kerosene by continuous stirring. If properly made, it results in a thick creamy stock mixture—this is "kerosene emulsion." Dilute with ten parts of water before dipping poultry in it or before applying to animals or in buildings. It may be applied with a brush or spray pump. Chemical sprays or dusts—such as malathion are preferable.

5. *Pyrethrum flowers powders* (page 310) are the unexpanded flower heads of two species of the chrysanthemum. This is also known more commonly as Dalmatian, and Persian insect powder. Its color ranges from yellowish brown to yellowish green, the brown tinted powders being superior to those having a green tinge. Its active insecticide ingredient is a volatile oil which disappears as the powder ages. The active principles contained in the oil are pyrethrin I and II. The injunction therefore to use only the fresh powder or that kept in tightly closed containers is well founded. Under ordinary commercial conditions it is much too costly to use on animals as a delouser, but its price fluctuates and at times its use from this standpoint is permissible. It is effective against lice on cattle, sheep, horses and poultry, and ticks on sheep. It is not poisonous to livestock and therefore no danger attends

Persian insect powder an excellent delouser

its use. It may be used undiluted though for economical reasons it is best mixed with some inert substance.

The commonest mixture consists of one pound of pyrethrum and two pounds of white flour. The fur-

Methods of using Persian insect powder
ther addition of four ounces of powdered moth balls or naphthaline is also practiced, and in some instances, especially when blue lice are present, may enhance its value. One-half pound of the mixture is enough to give a large animal, such as a horse or cow, two treatments. It may be applied by means of a shaker, or small dust gun, though on the under parts of the body the application must be made by hand. The powder must be rubbed thoroughly into the hair, wool, or feathers. The second treatment may be applied fourteen days after the first. Used in the method described, it is a good disinfestant during cold weather, though there are better agents and methods for use during warm weather.

As an insecticide, and in measure as a repellent, for protection of dairy cows there is recommended a

Pyrethrum against stable flies on dairy cattle
preparation consisting of a mixture of one part of an emulsion concentrate containing one per cent of pyrethrins and 10 per cent of piperonyl butoxide (piperonyl butoxide is classed as a synergist or it is an agent that aids or cooperates with another) with nine parts of water. Most flies are killed or repelled if they attempt to feed during the first three days after treatment. Dairy cattle may be sprayed with a quart of the mixture every few days, (page 699) or many dairymen use pyrethrin sprays on the lactating cows—applied with a fogger.

6. *Allethrin* is the coined name for a synthetic organic insecticide. It was discovered in the Insecticide Division, Bureau of Entomology and Plant Quarantine. Chemically it is like the active principles in pyrethrum —one of the oldest and most useful natural plant in-

secticides. Like pyrethrum, allethrin exerts a rapid paralytic action on insects which is especially desirable in the control of disease carriers. It is commercially available. Allethrin finds its greatest use along the same lines as pyrethrum—for flies, mosquitoes, and household insects.

7. *Derris root* is derived from several species of plants known as derris, and particularly from the Derris

Derris root a highly lauded new dis-infestant elliptica. The Derris elliptica is the tropical fish poisoning plant; "an extract of the root is placed in a stream which causes the fish to rise to the surface, when they are speared or netted. Fish obtained in this manner have never caused ill effects in the people or dogs which have consumed them." Its active principle is a white crystalline material, "rotenone" which is present for an average of two per cent, but varies widely in different plants of the genus derris. The "devil's shoestring" contains as high as four per cent rotenone. A more reliable source of rotenone has been found in the South American cube root (Lonchocarpus nicou), which contains over seven per cent of rotenone. Probably the non-uniformity of rotenone content in derris root is responsible for the inconsistent results reported by field workers. It is considered to be a contact insecticide. In efforts to rid dogs of ticks, it has been recommended as a wash or dip. An ounce of soap and two to four ounces of derris powder (rotenone content four per cent) to a gallon of

Derris for ticks on dogs, and warbles on cattle water are used. Derris root in the form of an ointment or as a soapy wash containing the powdered derris has been found effective against ox warbles.

Ox warbles (page 706), "cattle grubs," may be controlled and practically eradicated if cattle herds are consistently treated for a three-year period, and no new infested cattle brought into the herd, or held in adjacent feed lots during March, April and May which is the heel fly period.

The most efficient methods of treating cattle infested with ox warbles are as follows:

Dust Methods:

1. One part derris or cubé powder containing 5 per cent rotenone, and one part tripoli earth, double ground.

2. One part derris or cubé powder containing 5 per cent rotenone, and one part wettable sulfur. (Wettable sulfur is a solution of calcium polysulphide and a solution of casein combined—it is sometimes called colloidal sulfur.)

3. One part derris or cubé powder containing 5 per cent rotenone, and two parts pyrophyllite.

Any one of the above three mixtures may be used, by pouring from one to three ounces of the powder over the back, from the shoulders to the hips and down about 12 inches on each side of the backbone. A quart can or jar with a tin lid, perforated by punching it full of holes with a 20-penny spike, can be used. The powder should be settled into the hair with the hand or a brush.

Spray Method:

7.5 pounds derris or cube (rotenone 5 per cent), and 100 gallons water.

A spraying machine which will develop 100 pounds or more pressure and which has an agitator to keep the rotenone in suspension can be used. About 75 feet of pressure hose, connected with about 6 feet of ½-inch gas pipe, having a hand valve where it connects to the hose and a nozzle which delivers a spray 6 inches in diameter when held 10 or 12 inches above the animal's back should be used. If the spray is too fine it fails to penetrate the hair and one too solid may waste solution.

The spray method is the most satisfactory for large herds where a machine is available, as it can be used for killing lice as well as ox warbles. For lice, two sprayings should be done 14 days apart.

Dip Method: (Fig. 189.)

10 pounds derris or cube (5 per cent rotenone), 2 ounces sodium lauryl sulfate and 100 gallons water.

The powder should be worked into a thick paste by adding small quantities of water in the vat and then the water is added to make 100 gallons. Let the suspension stand in the vat 2 hours before using. Hold cattle in the vat two minutes with their backs completely covered. Keep the dip agitated with a bucket by pouring and dipping. This method is not as popular as the dust or spray method.

Louse powder A louse powder control combination widely used in some states with favorable results is made of 20 pounds derris dust (5 per cent rotenone), 10 pounds pyrethrum flowers, 8 pounds powdered naphthalene, and 62 pounds talc or fine kaolin.

The powder is applied along the backs of cattle from the poll to the tailhead when the hair is dry. A second application fourteen days following the first kills lice that have hatched in the meantime. One pound will treat about ten head of cattle.

Powdered derris or cube rotenone (content five per cent rotenone) diluted with three parts of flour or calcium carbonate has been shown to be effective against fleas and lice of the dog, cats, and chickens. It has no appreciable action on the eggs of parasites and, therefore, fowl should be submitted to a second dipping in two weeks. One-fourth ounce of the powder in one gallon of water may be used for dipping lice-infested fowl. It is lethal to both biting and sucking lice.

For the destruction of so-called sheep ticks or ked by dipping in a rotenone solution the Agricultural Research Service, U. S. D. A. recommends as follows:

Dipping for sheep ticks "The formula for the dip is based on derris or cubé powder having a 5 per cent rotenone content. Shipments of the powder vary, however, from about 3 per cent to more than 6 per cent of rotenone. In preparing the dip it is necessary to know the rotenone content of the powder in order to have the proper strength of this material for the destruction of the ticks. A powder containing only 4 per cent rotenone, for instance, must be added on the basis of 6 ounces per 80 gallons of water, and one containing 6 per cent rotenone should be added on the basis of 6 ounces per 120 gallons of water."

"The derris or cubé powder works equally well in so-called soft and hard water, as well as in ditch water that carries small amounts of silt. However, soft water is preferable because it tends to wet the wool more easily than does hard water."

"Derris powder or cubé powder having a 5 per cent rotenone content was used in the proportion of six ounces of the powder to each one hundred gallons of water in the vat. Derris powder and cubé powder are marketed as light, finely ground powder that are difficult to wet. Therefore, it is suggested that the quantity of powder necessary to charge the vat be calculated. This amount of powder should then be placed in a wash tub, or other similar container; small amounts of water should be added gradually with constant stirring until a thin paste is formed. It is preferable to allow the paste to remain in the container over night, and pour it into the vat the next morning. Thoroughly stir the contents of the vat before beginning the dipping. It is not necessary to heat the water in the dipping vat, although some sheepmen prefer warm water for this purpose. Sheep should be held in the dip about one minute or until the fleece is thoroughly wet. The heads should be submerged twice for just an instant while in the vat so that all parts of the sheep become thoroughly wet. Sheep and lambs 'mother-up' well after dipping, which is not the case with some of the other dips used for the eradication of sheep ticks." (Consult page 710 about "Trolene" etc.)

"The best time to treat tick-infested sheep is within one or two months after shearing, and after all shear cuts have completely healed. This coincides with the time when there are fewer ticks on the sheep than at other seasons of the year, which has also proved advantageous in eradicating this parasite."

Best time to dip sheep

8. *Fluoride of soda* has been found to be an excellent disinfestant against biting lice but is not dependable against sucking lice. It usually remains on animals long enough to kill young lice that have hatched from eggs that were present at the time of application (page 723). The simplest method of treatment is the so-called "pinch method" in which a small amount of the powder taken between the thumb and finger is filtered into the feathers of the breast, back, fluff, thigh and wings. One pound is enough for one hundred fowls. Another method is to dissolve one ounce of fluoride of soda and one ounce of laundry soap in one gallon of water, adding one and one-half ounces of flowers of sulphur and dipping lice-infested fowls in it.

Fluoride of soda a favorite remedy to rid poultry of biting lice

Fluoride of soda has during recent years come into extensive use in the elimination of round worms in swine (page 673).

Also a new rat poison—known as "1080"—is chemically a flourine compound. It is the fluoracetate of soda—a dangerous poison (page 340).

If properly handled the fluoridation of human drinking water will benefit a community by considerable reduction in the incidence of decayed teeth (dental caries). Fluoride of soda is an active poison. It is a wise precaution to color this white chemical so as to distinguish it from flour and sugar. Its ingestion by humans demands the immediate attention of a physician.

Use in drinking water for humans

9. *Arsenical dips* and also such highly poisonous chemicals as fluosilicate of soda, and fluoracetate of

soda are very dangerous to use by attendants applying them and also to the animals treated.
Since the advent of D.D.T., benzene hexachloride, lindane, methoychlor, or malathion, these highly poisonous chemicals
have been entirely superseded.

**Highly
chemical
poisons
no longer
used**

10. *Commercial pine tar* in addition to being a repellent is also a disinfestant and is extensively used to
destroy and dislodge Spinose ear ticks
(page 716) in cattle. The tar alone is
somewhat irritant to the thin skin below
the ear and it is, therefore, diluted by mixing two parts of the tar with one part of
cottonseed oil to make a smooth mixture. It may be necessary to warm the mixture before use during cold
weather. As many as possible of the ticks are first mechanically removed by means of a piece of looped
rigid wire. With a blunt nozzled two-ounce metal dose-
syringe, about one-half ounce of the mixture is injected
deeply into the ear. It is a good plan to manipulate the
outside of the ear by means of the fingers so as to
spread the mixture into the deeper parts of it because
only those ticks will be killed that actually come in
contact with it. It is sometimes necessary to resort to
a second application of the mixture after a lapse of
thirty days. (More treatment on page 717.)

**Spinose ear
ticks in cattle
controlled by
means of
pine tar**

11. *Tobacco* and its active ingredient nicotine have
been favorite disinfestants for a long time. It is a contact poison. Super-fine tobacco dust containing not less
than one per cent of nicotine, though not much more
than this, may be used to destroy ox warbles (page
706). One pound of the very fine dust is enough to treat
from fifteen to twenty animals. It is best to apply the
dust carefully by means of a shaker can to each bump
detected on the animal by passing the hand over the
skin, and then work the material in with the tips of the
fingers or with a stiff bristled brush.

12. *Nicotine sulphate,* also sold under the trade

name "Black-leaf Forty," is in the form of a concentrated solution containing forty per cent nicotine. It is a highly poisonous agent, and even after its dilution, if this is not done in accordance with the permissible percentage, it has proven poisonous to animals.

13. *Benzene* (it is also incorrectly known as benzol) is a coal-tar product and must not be confused with the American *benzine* which is a petroleum distillate. *Benzene* is one of the best larvicides and is particularly deadly to the larvae of the screwworm fly. These are the so-called maggots that infest wounds on animals (pages 702-703), and may even cause the death of the latter by almost eating their way into the body of the host or into some vital organ. When the larvae are discovered in a wound, they should be killed. If they are mechanically removed from the wound, they should be killed to prevent further development. Those on and in the deep portions of the wound are best killed by placing on or in the wound a piece of cotton that has been saturated with benzene (gasoline is not a satisfactory substitute). The fumes of the benzene will stupefy the larvae in a few seconds, but it requires several minutes to kill them. If there is any pus or tissue debris in the wound, this must first be wiped away; otherwise the fumes will not reach the parasite. When the wound is a deep one, the benzene-saturated piece of cotton should be pressed into the deeper portion of the wound; a clean plug of cotton is used to close the wound, and oil of tar (must be from pine trees) smeared over the cotton plug. Examine the wound the next day, remove the dead larvae and daily thereafter apply oil of tar to the edges and in the wound to act as a repellant. It is very important to reduce bleeding to a minimum during the treatment, because blood invites fresh deposits of screwworm fly eggs.

Benzene, not benzine, is destructive to screwworm maggots

14. *Formula (or Smear) No. 62* (page 703). This preparation developed by the Federal Bureau of

A screw-
worm
specific
Entomology and Plant Quarantine is virtually a specific in screw-worm (page 703)
control. Its composition is as follows:

Diphenylamine (technical grade) 3½ parts by weight
Benzol (commercial) (Benzene) 3½ parts by weight
Turkey red oil (pH-10 or neutral) 1   part by weight
Lamp black_____ 2   parts by weight

"The diphenylamine is dissolved in the benzol
(benzene—not benzine) preferably by placing the two
substances together and allowing them to stand 12 or
24 hours. In no event should the dissolving of the
diphenylamine in benzol be attempted by heating over
an open flame. Benzol is highly flammable and should
be kept away from flames and lighted cigarettes or
cigars. If heat is used to hasten solution, the container
holding the benzol and diphenylamine may be placed
in a vessel of hot water, the benzol container being left
uncorked until the diphenylamine is dissolved."

"After the diphenylamine is dissolved the turkey
red oil is added and the mixture thoroughly shaken.
The lamp black is then stirred in gradually and the
mixing continued until the compound attains a smooth,
even texture of about the consistency of molasses. It
is then ready for use."

*"Prepare the remedy well away from open flames
and do not have lighted cigarettes or cigars around
during the process."*

"Benzol in the form in which it occurs in the smear,
is highly volatile and will evaporate quickly from the
smear if left in an open container. *It is therefore advisable that the smear be kept tightly covered in a cool
place when not in use.* It is also recommended that only
an amount necessary for a few days' use be removed at
a time from the larger supply container. Even when
animals are actually being treated the container should
be kept covered as much as possible. In case the smear,
through evaporation, becomes too thick for easy ap-

plication, an additional amount of benzol may be stirred in to bring it back to its original consistency."

"The remedy is best applied with a 1-inch paint brush." (Consult "Smear EI-335," page 303.)

Applying No. 62 to wounds
"In treating an animal infested with screwworms, the material is swabbed into the wound, care being taken that it is pushed well into all the pockets made by the maggots and painted around the wound where blood and wound exudate have made the surrounding tissue attractive to flies and susceptible to infestation or to fly blows."

"It is not necessary to remove the dead worms from the wound, but most of the larger dead worms may be picked or wiped out with the brush if desired. If the worms are removed the wound should be treated again with the smear before the animal is released."

"For protecting uninfested wounds, such as those caused by shear cuts, castrations, dehorning, and docking, it is sufficient to cover the raw tissues and surrounding area thoroughly with a coating of the smear. In treating castration wounds some of the material should be pushed slightly into the openings of both sides of the scrotum."

"This remedy kills screwworms quickly, and after its application large numbers of them soon drop out of the wound, carrying a considerable amount of the protective chemical with them. For this reason it is indicated to be a good practice to apply a second treatment from 24 to 48 hours after the first one to insure a proper coating of the wound surface. Thereafter, under average conditions, regular treatments twice each week should be given until the wound is healed. It is especially recommended that infested animals be kept in a hospital pasture when this schedule of treatment is followed. When flies are unusually active and abundant more frequent treatments may be necessary."

"This material has been applied to wounds on several hundred sheep, goats, and cattle, and no harmful effects have been observed."

(The preceding paragraphs in quotation marks are from mimeographed circular E-540 of the Bureau of Entomology and Plant Quarantine, U.S.D.A. by Melvin, Smith, Parish, and Barrett.)

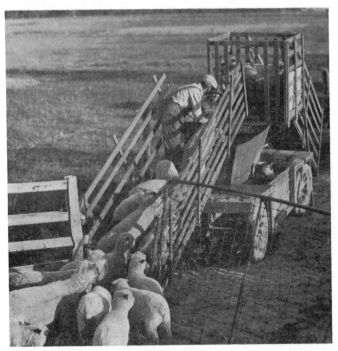

FIG. 65. A field dipping vat.

15. *Coal-tar dips* are extensively used and sold for farm use in ridding animals of lice and other parasites. They consist of a mixture of cresylic acid with soap. Cresylic acid covers those cresols and other phenols derived from coal tar, none of which boil below 365° F. nor above 482° F. When the material is diluted for use as a dip it should contain 0.5 per cent of cresylic acid.

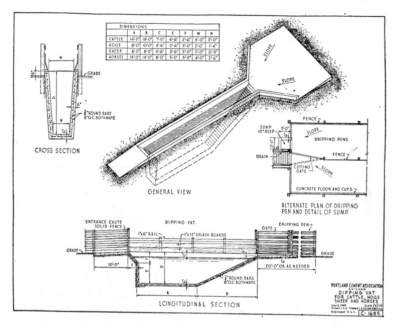

FIG. 66. A well planned dipping vat for animals of all sizes.

Coal-tar dips are useful against lice on cattle and horses

The manufacturer's directions for their use as given on the original container should be followed. Soft water or softened hard water must be used. These dips are much more effective against lice on cattle and horses than on hogs, because of the longer, more closely matted hair of the former animals which has a tendency to hold the dip, thus insuring a longer contact with the lice. Taken as a whole, the coal-tar dips do not compare favorably as liquid disinfestants with D.D.T., B.H.C., etc.

16. *Crude petroleum,* unprocessed or processed, formerly extensively used as a disinfestant has been almost entirely discontinued in favor of D.D.T., benzene hexachloride, lindane, etc. Even the old-fashioned hog oilers have fallen into discard.

17. *Lime and sulphur* dipping fluids are standard for the purpose of freeing animals, especially cattle and

sheep, from the mites that are responsible for scabies or mange, though these also are being displaced by the chemical agents.

Lime and sulphur dip intended for dipping sheep (Figs. 65 and 66) should contain eight pounds of unslaked lime and twenty-four pounds of flowers of sulphur to 100 gallons of water. For cattle and hogs it should contain twelve pounds of unslaked lime, otherwise the same as for sheep. The lime is to be placed in a mortar box and sufficient water added to slake the lime and form a sort of paste or putty. To this the finely sifted sulphur is added and the mixture thoroughly stirred. This is then placed in a boiler, thirty gallons of water added, and the mixture boiled for at least two hours with frequent stirring, occasionally adding fresh water to retain the original quantity. This is then placed in a cask or other receptacle and allowed to settle for several hours. When fully settled, the clear liquid is drawn off into the vat and sufficient water added to bring the total quantity up to 100 gallons. Instead of preparing the dip for smaller numbers of animals, it is quite convenient to purchase in a drug store the concentrated lime and sulphur spray of orchardists, and diluting this for animal use in accordance with the directions printed on the original container. Irrespective of the kind of lime and sulfur dip employed, the following general direction should be adhered to:

1. The temperature of the dipping vat should be constantly maintained at from 103 degrees F. to 105 degrees F.
2. Each animal should be held in the vat for two minutes, and completely immersed twice.
3. The dipping should be repeated in from ten to fourteen days to destroy the parasites that may have hatched out subsequently to the first dipping.

18. *Quaternary Ammonium Compound:* (pages 117, 279) has been used with apparent success on dogs as

a flea and lice insecticide; also for nits eight ounces of a ten per cent solution added to a gallon of water is the recommended strength. The diluted preparation,

A dog wash to combat fleas and lice

is used as a wash applied over the entire body. It is odorless and not sticky. One treatment is claimed to be sufficient, though if necessary it may be repeated three weeks later. This chemical is not effective against ticks. For ticks six ounces of a twenty per cent D.D.T. emulsion in a gallon of water is used. (Page 295.)

REPELLING EXTERNAL PARASITES

Repellents may be applied directly to the host. Usually these agents are obnoxious to parasitic pests so

Oily repellents on horses result in a loss of hair

that animals so treated are avoided by them. Some species of animals, horses in particular, are likely to suffer from a loss of hair when oily mixtures are used frequently and when rubbed deeply into the hair coat. Their value is limited, and their action transient.

An excellent fly repellent may be made by mixing one ounce of fresh pyrethrum (page 309) flowers

A good fly repellent

and one gallon of kerosene. This should be permitted to macerate or "soak" for six weeks. It is then to be strained through cotton flannel. Finally one ounce of cedar oil is added. It may be sprayed on animals, or lightly brushed over the hair, but its application must be repeated daily or sometimes oftener. (Also see page 310.)

Oil of tar (must be from pine trees) has considerable value as a repellent. The fly (oestrus ovis) respon-

A method of preventing "grubs in the head" in sheep

sible for the presence of its larva in the head cavities or sinuses in sheep, commonly designated "grubs in the head" (page 712), may be quite successfully repelled by the use of this agent. The usual procedure is to bore some holes having a diameter of two inches and approximately the same depth in a log. Salt is placed in the bottom of these holes and oil of tar smeared around the sides. In reaching for the salt, the sheep smear the nostrils with the oil of tar. The oil is obnoxious to the fly so that its eggs which later become larvae or grubs are not deposited in the sheep's nose.

(For information about the use by humans of insect repellents the reader is referred to U. S. Dept. of Agriculture, Bur. of Entomology and Plant Quarantine circular E 698 (Revised) entitled "Use of Insect Repellents and Toxicants" by Travis, Morton and Smith.)

CHAPTER XX

RATS AND SOME OTHER RODENTS, AND THEIR CONTROL

The attempt to exterminate (page 824), or at least to control, rats and other rodents from buildings and their surroundings appropriately falls in

Rodenticide and Raticide defined the field of disinfestation. The word rodenticide applies to all poisons that are lethal to rats, mice, squirrels, gophers, prairie dogs and other rodents; raticides are agents specifically intended for the poisoning of rats.

Rats eat or spoil an estimated 200 million bushels of farm grain annually at an estimated value of one-half billion dollars at least. A mature rat

Damage by rats may eat fifty pounds of grain and spoil or waste another one hundred to one hundred and fifty pounds annually. This means a loss of from $6.00 to $8.00 a year for each rat on the premises, simply from grain waste. In addition, rats kill baby chicks and even mature poultry, and gnaw into buildings, and start fires by damaging electric wiring.

Furthermore rats spread diseases to humans and animals, and from this standpoint alone

Disease spread by rats they should be exterminated. It is on this basis that action against them is discussed in this book.

The following are some of the diseases that may be transmitted by rats:

1. *Murine Typhus* (rat typhus, flea typhus). This disease is transmitted from rats to man by means of the rat flea, *Xenopsylla cheopis*. It is the carrier of the true cause, the Rickettsia prowazeki

Rats responsible for these diseases mooseri. Murine typhus is closely related to the louse-borne typhus of Europe and of the Rocky Mountain Spotted Fever though less fatal than either of these diseases. The general symptoms are weakness, headache, chills, fever and sometimes a skin eruption.

2. *Leptospirosis* (pages 535 and 826). (Weil's disease; infectious jaundice; Stuttgart disease of dogs). It is primarily a disease of dogs and rats with rats the chief offender in spreading the disease to man. It is due to a cork-screw shaped organism that the infected rats spread by means of their urine and thus to human and animal food. There are other means of spread but not for discussion here. The disease has been observed in man and in animals in all parts of the United States. One publication states that 40 per cent of the rats in San Francisco carry the infection, though without outward evidence of it. The symptoms in man are frequently alarming and appear quite suddenly. There are muscular pains, a coated tongue, kidney involvement, enlargement of the liver and spleen, and jaundice in about one-third of the cases. The condition ends in either recovery or death about the fifteenth day.

3. *Plague* a disease of man. One form of it—bubonic type (page 824)—is transmitted from rats and other rodents to humans by means of infected fleas. The infection is *Pasteurella pestis*. Epidemics of this disease have at times wiped out large segments of the human population. It is essentially a tropical disease; in colder climates the infection occurs in rodents such as rats, ground squirrels and prairie dogs, but it seems to be self-limiting. While murine (rat spread) plague plays a negligible role in the United States the infective agent has been demonstrated in rats and field rodents in the western half of the country. It requires eternal vigilance by health and sanitary control agencies to check on the possibility of the potential spread of the infection. Bubonic plague in man is characterized by swelling of regional lymph glands known as buboes, fever, depression, great prostration and death in more than fifty per cent of the cases. D.D.T. (page 291) in rat burrows kills the fleas

and thus assists in controlling the spread of "plague." Antibiotics (page 248) are effective in the treatment of infected humans.

4. *Tularemia* (Rabbit fever). Rats are of minor importance in the spread of this disease though they may harbor the infective agent. (See page 604.)

5. *Rabies* (canine madness) (page 544). Rats may spread the causative virus to man but seldom do so.

6. *Rat-bite Fever.* (Sodoku in Japan). This is primarily an infection of rats caused by the *Spirillum minus,* a flagellated organism. Apparently it causes them no inconvenience and is spread to man by rat bites. It is relatively common in man, but it is not contagious, and therefore it is limited to the bitten person. Children under one year of age are most frequently involved. In those bitten there is a rather severe local inflammatory reaction at the site of the bite with swelling of neighboring lymph glands. These symptoms are accompanied by severe intermittent attacks of fever. Mortality in humans is said to range from six to ten per cent.

Food Poisoning. Food soiled by rats is always potentially dangerous to the human or animal consuming it. Rat droppings and their urine have in them germs capable of setting up ill-health in man and beast. Food so contaminated is always a health hazard. Rat droppings if present are clearly visible though rat urine is not nearly so evident and may escape detection; it may even be disregarded by some human food handling agencies.

Many more human and domesticated animal diseases in all parts of the world may be traced entirely or in part to rats because of their close association with human activities. Fortunately most of these diseases are not present in America. Rat eradication would remove at least one factor in the fight on human diseases.

Three kinds of rats have been recognized in America. They are as follows:

Kinds of rats

Norway Rat (house rat, brown rat, wharf rat, sewer rat). This species has a total length of 16 inches—the tail being 7½ inches long—and weighs near 11 to 12 ounces, though very large individuals may weigh as much as 24 ounces. The fur is generally brown with scattered black hairs, and the under surface of the body a much lighter shade. The female averages eight to nine young in a litter, and has four or more of these each year. In many places the Norway rat, because of its boldness and large size, has driven out other kinds of rats.

Roof Rat (Alexandrine rat, gray rat) is smaller than the Norway rat. It weighs eight to nine ounces, is about 15 inches long from tip of the nose to the end of the tail which represents from 8½ to 10 inches of the total length. The fur on the back and sides is gray to gray-brown, and the under surface of the body is almost white. This rat breeds four or more times a year with an average of six young in each litter.

Black Rat resembles the roof rat in every way excepting color which is a solid black, or nearly so.

The house-mouse is another nuisance, having some rat characteristics. These small rodents frequently have their nests in cast-off clothing, bales of straw, or bales of other material. They climb readily and therefore enter all parts of buildings, though seldom do they burrow in the ground. They can pass through any opening one-half inch or more in diameter. During summer warmth they frequently leave buildings returning to shelter upon the arrival of cooler temperatures. The mothers average five to six young a year, and captive mice have produced as many as 100 young a year. Although a house-mouse begins to breed at 42 days of age, it seldom lives longer than a year.

House mouse and its habits

Rats and mice have in the front of the mouth two pairs of chisel-like teeth that grow out continuously

Rat and mouse characteristics

and are self-sharpening. These rodents have no tusks. The cheek or grinding teeth are small with rough grinding surfaces. The claws are sharp so as to assist in fighting and climbing. While the rat does not leave much odor perceptible to humans, the mouse leaves a strong unpleasant "mousy" odor.

Rats and mice have poor vision, though their senses of hearing, tasting and smell are very acute. They do not fear accustomed noises though the slightest strange noise will send them scurrying.

In human dwellings, especially tenement houses, and farm buildings rats and mice are frequently

Evidence of rats and mice

present though the residents are unaware of their presence. In fact, there may be the contention that these rodents are not present on the premises. Evidence of their presence is their tell-tale droppings, the sounds they make, paths and holes, gnawed places, smears from their greasy bodies around rafters and on their paths, and if there are comparatively large numbers on the premises they may occasionally be seen.

Efforts to control rats and mice

Efforts to control and exterminate these rodents from the vicinity of or in human and animal habitations take many different forms. No one of these efforts by itself is sufficient, though a combination of selected methods appropriate to a given situation can be made effective as evidenced in communities that have followed carefully laid plans for rat extermination.

Buildings rat proofed

Concrete, masonry or sheet metal walls cannot be penetrated and form effective barriers. Walls extending upwards from foundations at least two feet deep with a broad outward flange at the bottom are effective. Screens made or reinforced with hardware cloth (Fig. 67) having ¼ inch meshes over all openings, cement or metal around all openings (Fig. 68) where pipes or conduits

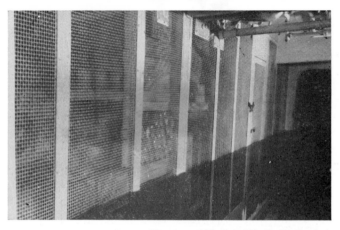

(Courtesy of U. S. Public Health Service)

FIG. 67. Example of wire mesh partitioning between store and passage way to exclude rats.

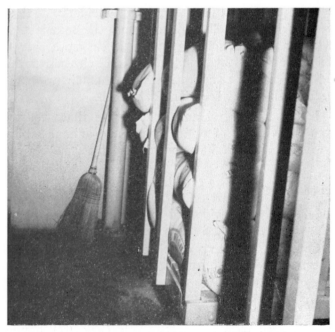

(Courtesy of U. S. Public Health Service)

FIG. 68. An approved method of storing flour, dry grain and sugar. Note collared pipes passing through concrete floor.

pass through the walls, and tight fitting doors also form effective barriers to the passage of these pests. However, even the best constructed buildings should have frequent inspection as these rodents will take advantage of every opportunity to gain admission. Open doors and windows at night are important avenues of admission. Feed bins in buildings should have protective metal coverings. Many other details of construction may be obtained from federal and state agencies, and from building contractors.

Insanitary surroundings always invite vermin (Fig. 69). Manure piles, decaying hay, straw and other feeds

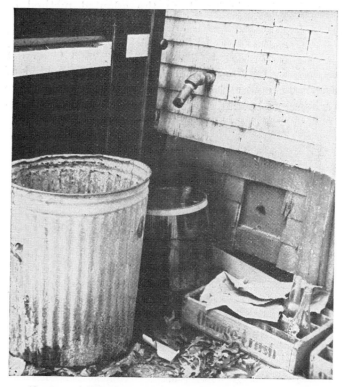

(Courtesy of Federal Security Agency, U. S. Public Health Service)

FIG. 69. An invitation to rats and flies. Poor garbage disposal facilities—worn-out, uncovered garbage can on ground, barrel containing water, and scattered trash.

Rubbish in and near buildings in close proximity to habitations, and baled feeds inside of buildings—unless the latter are rodent proof—are invitations to rats and mice. Such conditions provide shelter and are a source of food supply. Insofar as it is possible keep premises sanitary and free from rubbish of all sorts.

Placing straw, hay, fodder, and comparable feeds on platforms so that eradicating methods can reach the underneath spaces is to be recommended. In some instances sheet metal fencing thirty-six inches high and set six inches into the ground surrounding out-of-door stored feeds has been the adopted method of preventing rat and mice infestation. Small-**Storage of human and animal food** er amounts of grain such as chicken feed may be stored in garbage cans (Fig. 70) or similar receptacles. The same kind of receptacle, new and clean, as well as 2-10 gallon size crocks, glass bottles, and small covered cans is service-

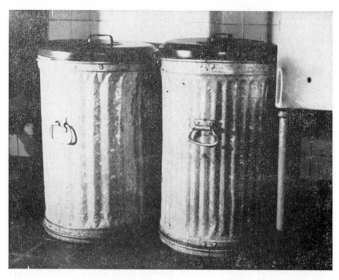

(Courtesy of Federal Security Agency, U. S. Public Health Service)

FIG. 70. Thorough cleansing of garbage cans is necessary to do away with roaches and other threats to food.

able and effective as preventive against rodent contamination. Table scraps thrown about promiscuously as feed for animals invite rats and mice, as well as serving as fly breeding places. If it is necessary as an economical procedure to feed farm animals on table refuse then the feeding places should be cleaned daily.

It is stated on good authority that odors of various substances are objectionable to rats. If at the same

Odors objectionable to rats

time such odors are not objectionable to human beings when placed in close proximity to food products then they may serve a useful purpose in protecting certain foods. Among the odorous substances used as rat deterrents are the wood-tar and coal-tar derivatives, creosote, carbolic acid, naphthalene, kerosene, and the oils of wintergreen and peppermint. Substances not likely to contaminate foods are commercial dry lime-and-sulphur mixture, powdered sulphur, lime, or lye and strong red pepper. The actual destruction of rats and mice that infest buildings and premises is along several lines each having some merit. However, some methods are dangerous to both human and animal life.

A good rat dog, such as a small terrier, can be trained to hunt rats though not molesting other forms of farm life. A dog of this kind under ordinary good surroundings will keep farm buildings practically free from rat infestation. Good cats are rare, and furthermore they are destructive to bird life. However, in warehouses cats can render very useful service. Ferrets

Destruction of rats by natural enemies

are not of great value except in the hands of trained personnel. Hawks and owls keep down rodent infestation though unfortunately some of these also prey on poultry and other farm animals. Bull-snakes in barns are said to be of some value in holding down the rodent population but their mere presence is so obnoxious to the average human that they are of little help.

Trapping is the preferred method of rodent con-

trol in offices and human dwellings because of the
easy removal of the caught animal thus
Trapping avoiding undesirable odors. Probably the
rats and wooden-based spring trap is most gen-
mice erally used, though the No. 0 steel trap,
as well as box traps are also employed. Rats are trap-
wise or rather they avoid new objects. It is sometimes a practice to set an unbaited, sprung trap near
the runways for several days so as to allay the rats'
suspicions. Then bait and set the trap. Ingenuity on
the part of the trapper overcomes many difficulties in
catching rats. Electronic traps are expensive though
no more effective than others.

The principal objection to rat poisons is that any
one of them may be accidentally consumed by animals
other than rats or mice, or even by humans
Rodent with fatal results. Possibly the only so-
poisons called rat poison that is not particularly
toxic is red squill, because all animals can vomit it
though the rat being physiologically unable to vomit
dies as a result of consuming it. "Warfarin" is practically non-poisonous, though if ingestion is repeated
day after day it is fatal. The Federal Insecticide,
Fungicide, and Rodenticide Act of June 25, 1947,
provides that rodent poisons intended for interstate
commerce must be so labelled as to indicate the nature
of the poison, the percentage of the poison ingredient,
and the proper antidote to use in case of accidental
poisoning.

The kind of bait to use is of as great importance
as the nature of the poison. A survey conducted in
regard to this matter seemed to indicate
Kind of that from the standpoint of gustatory
bait to use attractiveness to rats the preference in a
decreasing order is as follows: raw meat, raw fish,
rolled oats, whole wheat, corn meal, bread crumbs,
canned fish, canned meat, cooked cereals, cheese, meat
scrap, powdered milk, fish meal, fresh vegetables,
cooked vegetables, and fresh fruits. Meat and fish

baits, and wet baits should be changed daily because of spoilage.

Prebaiting If unpoisoned baits are used for several days it will allay the rats' suspicions. Then poison the bait and usually if the place is badly infested a large number of rats will be killed followed by decreasing numbers so that after the third day there are no more poisonings. In another two weeks, or as late as three months, if there is evidence of rats repeat the prebaiting and the baiting. As rats eat less and less of poisoned bait the amount of poison in the bait should be increased from day to day.

Placing and handling of bait and poison Baits and poison should be placed with a long-handled spoon—rats fear the odor of humans. The poisoned bait needs to be placed in burrows and near the rat runs on floors. It should never be placed on human food containers. Care must be exercised to keep these highly poisonous substances away from people —especially children, pets, and domesticated animals in general. Poisoned rats and mice and uneaten poisoned bait must be burned or buried at least two feet deep. Unless 90 per cent or more of the rat population is killed in a poisoning campaign, the remaining population will soon reestablish themselves because of high fecundity.

1. *"Warfarin"* (3-(alpha-acetonylbenzyl) — 4-hydrophcoumarin) (the Communicable Disease Center of the Federal Security Agency designates this preparation as "Compound 42") (one trade name is dethmor) is a chemical that consists basically of dicumarol—formerly known as dicoumarin—found in spoiled sweet clover (page 462) and now also synthetically made.

Origin and nature of "warfarin" It was developed at the University of Wisconsin by Prof. Karl P. Link and his associates. It is patented by the Wisconsin Alumni Research Foundation and the initials of this association form the first letters of the proprietary name of this rodenticide. It kills rodents by means of its anticoagulant effect on the blood, and in order to produce a fatal effect repeated ingestion of feed containing the chemical is required. Internal hemorrhage is produced in its victims. Warfarin blocks

How does "warfarin" act? the action of vitamin K, the substance present in green plants which is necessary for the animal to produce prothrombin, one of the essentials for blood clotting. When warfarin is consumed over a period of time, from four to ten days, hemorrhages occur first in the lungs and then in other internal organs, and the animal ingesting it bleeds to death. This bleeding is not painful to the animal so it goes right on consuming the chemical-treated food or water. "Warfarin" is marketed as a concentrate which consists of 0.5 per cent of the chemical and 99.5 per cent starch. In preparing bait the 0.5 per cent concentrate is mixed with corn meal, or a mixture of corn meal, ground wheat, oats and barley at the rate which gives the ratio of 1 to 1000 of the pure warfarin. In other words, 19 parts of

Ratio in mixing the poison freshly ground corn meal and one part of the 0.5 per cent warfarin concentrate are thoroughly mixed and placed in clean containers, the latter not over three inches high. Several bait stations should be set up on the premises.

In order to prevent other animals from reaching the bait, place an inverted orange crate over it with openings to admit rats, or place the bait under a board nailed in a length-wise leaning position to form a tunnel. Keep plenty of the bait available in the containers at all times because an abstinence for a few days permits recovery to take place. Otherwise, the animal weakens so much that it can only crawl to the bait and death results.

The weakness in the foregoing plan of rat or rodent poisoning is that there is usually so much other food available to the rats that most of the time, on farms at least, they are satiated and therefore they leave the bait alone. However, rats must *drink* as well as eat. A late product which is to be used in water consists of "warfarin" coated on grains of sand at the old ratio of 99.5 per cent sand to 0.5 per cent of the chemical which is packaged in one-third ounce packets, and when the content of this packet is mixed with a quart of water it will give the correct ratio of one part of warfarin in 20,000 parts of water. The solution is usually put in a quart jar which is then upended on a baby-chick fountain, and it is ready for use. The chemical-treated water should be safeguarded from other animals. The sand settles to the bottom, the "warfarin" is in the water. Reports of fatalities in other animals have not been authenticated, and since several or repeated ingestions are necessary to produce a fatal effect such reports are of doubtful accuracy.

A water soluble "warfarin"

2. *Red Squill.* This is an onion-like appearing bulb. It is marketed in both liquid form and as a reddish powder. In humans and in animals capable of the act its ingestion is followed by vomiting, and as a rat cannot or does not vomit, the poisonous quality of the red squill is absorbed killing the rat. This is the reason that red squill has earned the reputation of being a specific rat poison. Unfortunately all red squill bulbs do not have uniform poisonous qualities. For this reason campaigns in which it is the mainstay of the efforts sometimes fail.

Some poisons

Mix one and one-half ounces to form a paste with water, and incorporate this in fresh ground fish, or unseasoned hamburger steak. Or add an equal amount of squill to a pound of oatmeal, corn meal or bran and moisten to a mushy consistency with milk or water. Liquid red squill may be mixed with a dry bait such as stale bread.

Squill mixtures

3. *Barium carbonate* — precipitated form — is a

white, heavy, odorless and tasteless powder. The foregoing attributes make it of value. Its disadvantages are
that though it is not a violent poison, it is poisonous for
humans and for domesticated animals. It is comparatively inexpensive but it is rarely obtainable. The
barium carbonate at the rate of one part of it to five
parts of bait (see page 334) and moistened is the
formula. The finished bait and poison mixture should
be in a sufficiently fine state of division so that rats
cannot drag it from place to place. Barium carbonate
containers should be labelled "Poison."

4. *Arsenic*—also known as arsenic trioxide, arseni-
ous acid, and white arsenic—is a slow acting poison
though rated as highly toxic for all warm
Undesirable rat poisons blooded creatures. One part to twenty
parts of bait is generally used. Containers
must be labelled "Poison."

5. *Strychnine sulphate.* This is extremely poisonous
and has an intensely bitter taste, and because of its
taste must be disguised. Rats take it poorly. Due to
its rapid action poisoned rats and mice die in the walls
of buildings and decomposition odors are frequently
very noticeable. Its use on city dumps is quite general.
But burial of garbage and other refuse in deep trenches,
with frequent covering, is preferred as a sanitary
disposal method in city dumps and at military posts.

6. *Yellow phosphorus* is luminous in the dark. It
is the poison in many commercial rat and mouse poisons. It is sometimes said to be a fire hazard but this
may be disregarded when the phosphorus is finely
divided as it is in rat poisons. It is poisonous to humans
and animals, and a good deal of technical knowledge is
required to prepare it. Yellow phosphorus is not generally recommended.

7. *Thallium sulphate* is a powerful slow acting poison. Because it is without distinctive odor or state it is
readily mistaken for some harmless substances. It
may even be absorbed through the skin and thus exert

its toxic properties. It is not recommended for general use. It should always be clearly labelled "Poison." Experiments are in progress to combine tartar emetic with the thallium so that cats and dogs will vomit if accidentally poisoned.

8. *Antu Raticide* is so named after the first letter of the components as chemically expressed.

A new rat poison It is Alpha-Napthyl-Thiourea. It is a fine gray powder with little odor or taste. One pound of the powder is capable of killing 300,000 Norway rats. The medium lethal dose is from 3 to 4 milligrams for a kilogram of live rat weight; it is about as poisonous as strychnine. Originally it was said to be poisonous only for rats but later experience has demonstrated that dogs, cats, hogs, chickens, and horses are susceptible to its action if the dose is large enough, and provided the animal does not vomit it up. If the stomach has fatty substances in it the "Antu" is more quickly absorbed and is therefore more poisonous. In this connection it has been found that Norway rats are much more susceptible to the action of "Antu" than are the black and the roof rats (page 328). Mice are relatively unaffected by it. Humans are about as susceptible to its action as they are to red squill (page 337). For use against Norway rats (page 328) "Antu" adheres well when dusted from a sifter on cut moist pieces of apple, sweet potato, ground meat or fish, or chicken head. In general from two to three parts of Antu by weight are added to 100 parts by weight of bait. "Antu" kills by drowning the rat in its own fluids —oedema of the lungs. This means that the fluids of the body overflow into the lungs. If the first ingestion of "antu" by a rat is not fatal bait shyness develops and may persist for as long as four months. The "Grote thio-urea test" is used for the presence or determination of "antu" in ingesta or vomitus. (Consult page 166, No. 35, Vol. X, April 1949 American Journal of Veterinary Research.) The resort to the stomach pump is advisable if there is time. Sulphur containing compounds are said to be the best antidote.

9. *Sodium Fluoracetate* (page 315) (compound "1080"). This compound, universally known as "1080," is a fine, white, fluffy powder similar in appearance to flour, powdered sugar and baking powder. The substance is readily soluble in water, and therefore this chemical, otherwise stable, leaches during humid weather. Also, it decomposes if subjected to temperatures higher than 230°F. It has no distinctive odor or taste and therefore it should be colored—nigrosine dye will color it black. There are several reported fatalities in humans following accidental or unintentional absorption of this chemical. The following seem to be some facts in regard to "1080":

A highly dangerous poison

1. Although "1080" is not volatile, it is dangerous if inhaled by humans handling it unless a respirator is worn.

2. It may be absorbed through cuts and abrasions of the skin and is poisonous should it enter the body in this manner. Therefore, protective gloves should be worn.

3. The principal danger is from getting small amounts of "1080" in the mouth and then swallowing it. To keep the hands away from the mouth while handling this compound the person should not smoke or eat. When through handling it the person should wash the hands with soap and water, and rinse with clear water. The waste water should not be discarded on vegetation that is likely to be consumed by domesticated animals.

4. "1080" should never be used in human or animal dwellings as this will be a potential source of danger to life. It may be used on guarded dumps, military establishments, ships and large commercial houses where it can be under the supervision of reliable personnel.

5. Dogs and cats are likely to die if they consume carcasses of rodents that have been poisoned by "1080."

6. Poisoning of cattle by "1080" has been reported, (page 435, No. 867, Vol. CXIV, June 1949, Journal of the American Veterinary Medical Association.)

When the use of "1080" is resorted to as a raticide the following points are to be borne in mind:

1. Poisoned bait should be placed out of the way of human or domesticated animals' activity.

2. Poisoned water should be carried in shatter resistant receptacles, and the contents are to be dispensed by means of a syringe or gravity-feed tubing. Squat-type containers, in order to avoid being up-set, should be used to hold the poisoned water. One-half ounce of "1080" in a gallon of water is the strength recommended for poisoning rats.

3. Dry poisoned bait must be of a nature that will not permit rats to pick it up so as to carry it to other places. Grain baits are satisfactory, or anything of a finely ground or crumb-like nature. One ounce of "1080" added to twenty-eight pounds of bait is proper concentration.

4. All uneaten food baits should be collected and burned. The bodies of dead rats and mice remain highly poisonous for an indefinite period, and therefore they should be burned or deeply buried.

Field rodents such as squirrels and prairie dogs are even more susceptible to the action of "1080" than is the rat. The outstanding susceptibility of dogs to the action of this poison is generally known because when used on city dumps dogs have picked up the dead rats and they, in turn, have been poisoned.

Poisoning of other rodents and animals

In a research project it was determined that sheep were poisoned when they were given as little as from 0.25 to 0.50 milligrams of "1080" for each kilogram of live weight.

As there is considerable danger of accidental poisoning in man and domesticated animals following the use of this poison, especially if carelessly or unwisely used, and as several people and many pets have already died because of it, the recommendation to limit its sale to those trained in its handling is a sound one. Because of popular articles dealing with "1080" the impression has gained ground that it is an ideal rodenticide, and that it should receive general application. This impression is erroneous if at the same time there is no mention of the potential danger to man and his charges. Whenever and wherever "1080" is used warning cards should be conspicuously displayed.

Dangerous for man and domesticated animals

In man and animals death, following its ingestion, is the result of greatly weakened heart action. When first swallowed there are no symptoms, and later when symptoms develop the compound has been absorbed to an extent that treatment is usually not effective. There is no known antidote to counteract the effects of "1080." A physician should be consulted at the very earliest moment.

Death in man and animals

10. *Calcium-cyanide* (page 307) dust is a valuable rodenticide to be forced into rat burrows (Fig. 71) and into corn under storage, or in fact into any place harboring rats, except closed habitations. This dust on the slightest contact with moisture gives off the deadly hydrocyanic, or prussic, acid gas. There is little danger in the use of calcium-cyanide dust in corn or other edible products because the poisonous gas is soon dissipated; this depends in a measure on the free circulation of air and if the residue is non-poisonous. The dust should not be handled in closed buildings, nor

on windy days. A small inhalation of the gas may be followed by serious consequences.

An effective antidote against cyanide is a combination of sodium nitrite and sodium thiosulphate intravenously administered. It is the same treatment that veterinarians administer to cattle following cane, sorg-

An antidote for hydrocyanic acid gas hum, sudan grass, and Johnson grass poisoning (page 437). Packages containing this dust must be kept tightly closed when not in use, and out of the reach of irresponsible persons and livestock. As a rodenticide the

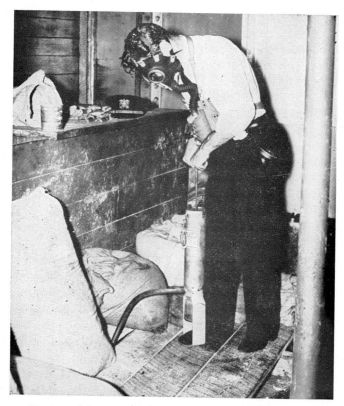

(Courtesy of Federal Security Agency, U. S. Public Health Service)

FIG. 71. Pumping calcium cyanide dust into inclosed harborage. (Note animal trap placed in run). U. S. Quarantine Station, Baltimore, Maryland.

dust is forced into burrows and stored animal feeds by means of dusting pumps designed for this purpose. Openings and exits of burrows should be tamped with soil so as to hold the gas in them as long as possible. Since the gas readily escapes from stored feeds its use under these circumstances is less effective.

11. *Fluosilicate of soda* spread on floors where mice and rats run gets on their feet, where because of its irritant action, it is licked off and thus reaches the rodent's mouth and stomach. If enough of the powder is ingested they die in three to six days. Though not highly poisonous care must be taken to keep it off food products. Usually it is placed close to a wall and then a board leaned over it—under this the rats and mice run.

12. *Carbon monoxide* gas from an automobile exhaust pipe forced into rat burrows, especially if the rats are under cement floors is a persistent and effective rodenticide.

13. *Rat "Virus"* recommended by some sources is not effective. The living organisms or bacteria in this virus belong to the food poisoning group (Salmonella) and may contaminate human food; therefore, the use of rat "virus" is discouraged. Neither has the virus proven to be effective as a rat controlling agent. Its sale is prohibited by law in some states.

Conservation Bulletin No. 8, Fish and Wildlife Service, U. S. Department of the Interior summarizes rat control as follows:

"The five essential steps in rat control, in order of importance, are as follows":

"1. Permanent rat control organizations should be provided for large cities and rural districts.

Essentials in rat control

"2. All shelter for rats should be eliminated and all garbage, trash, and other waste on which rats can feed should be promptly disposed of.

"3. All buildings should be made rat proof.

"4. The rats themselves should be destroyed by use of poisoned baits and traps. If it is desired to avoid the slight risk of rats dying in inaccessible places, traps should be used. Rat burrows and hiding places should be fumigated with poisonous gases.

"5. Natural enemies of the rat should be protected when they are not themselves destructive."

Unless mice are migrating in search of new home ranges, they usually travel less than 30 feet—some **Mice have** less than 10 feet. When disturbed, how- **a limited** ever, individuals may travel many times **range** these distances. Taken as a whole poison placements for mice should be fairly close, probably not more than 20 feet apart.

PART SIX

Non-Infectious, Sporadic Ailments

⚹⚹⚹⚹

CHAPTER XXI

GENERAL STATEMENTS AND SECONDARY AILMENTS

This includes those conditions that are not grouped, or, they are isolated. In human medicine it is stated that they are not epidemic, (the Greek **Sporadic ailments are not catching** origin of this latter word means "upon people"), and in animal medicine it is correct to state that sporadic diseases are not epizootic. (The word epizootic means literally "upon animals"). In further explanation, the understanding of sporadic diseases is that they affect only isolated animals here and there, and with no particular relationship in their occurrence. The usual statement that they are not "catching" is correct.

It is certain that many diseases of domesticated animals may be controlled by a rigid regard for the sanitary and other principles involved. Not infrequently an owner of livestock raises the objection that the care and attention to detail demanded in the correct handling of his charges is such as to make the recommended methods impractical. The answer to this is that nothing is impractical that makes the raising of livestock more profitable. If an owner feels that for reasons of his own he does not care to handle animals in this manner, or occasionally he may not have the

facilities, then he should be prepared to find that his
Poor venture is not going to bring him the
handling of maximum returns. The more he departs
livestock in the handling of his charges from ap-
entails proved methods of care, the more will
financial loss these charges suffer, and correspondingly
less will be his profits. These words should not lead one
to assume that all losses may be controlled by sanitation, since the millenium has not arrived, and there
are factors other than the matter of disease that influence the profitable production of livestock, but it is
generally agreed that disease stands at the head of the
list.

In the following pages it is intended to discuss the
nature of those ailments that frequently are observed
amongst America's herds and flocks, and in so far
as possible to suggest methods of prevention. The
cure of these ailments is properly not within the prov-
ince of this discussion; it belongs in the realm of the
practitioner of veterinary medicine. He alone has the
highly specialized training to intelligently handle
this involved question, and no better advice can be
given to the livestock owner than that he consult his
graduate veterinarian frequently.

The education of the modern livestock owner has
entirely eliminated belief in such fantastic ailments
Imaginary as "hollow horn," and "wolf-in-the-tail."
ailments Also, entirely disappeared is the formerly
extensively held superstitious belief in
the influence of the "signs of the Zodiac." In an entirely
different class there are the "secondary ailments."

These ailments are those that follow the introduction of some element not usually considered to be a
causative factor of, and usually not productive of
disease, though because of mass, force, or repetition it
ultimately results in an ailing condition. Frequently
there is no sharp line of demarcation between ailments
of this group and others of a sporadic nature.

1. *Loss of cud.* This is not a disease, as it is so frequently contended to be, but rather a symptom of disease. Neither must the words "loss of cud" (page 22) be interpreted too literally because there has been no loss, it is simply the failure of a physiological phenomenon to appear. The logical handling is to attempt to remove the true cause of the animal's ill health, and when this has been accomplished, the "lost" cud will be restored spontaneously.

"Loss of cud" a symptom of ill health

2. *"Proud-flesh."* Its appearance in a wound excites apprehension far greater than it warrants. It is really nothing more than perfectly normal tissue growing wildly or uncontrolled. Technically it is known as "exuberant granulations." The skin, by the pressure it exerts, prevents the deeper tissues from growing exuberantly. Therefore, when the skin is cut or incised, especially on those portions of the body such as in the "folds" of the legs where movement of the part prevents the edges of the skin from again joining each other, "proud-flesh" develops. (Fig. 53.) There may be so much of it that an affected leg becomes enormously enlarged, and the value of the animal is impaired. "Proud-flesh" is not of a cancerous or malignant nature. To those understanding the underlying causative principles which involve lack of skin pressure and the irritation resulting from movement, the proper method of prevention at once suggests itself, i.e., the application of artificial pressure by means of bandaging until healing has restored skin pressure and the avoidance of irritation by enforced rest. The ruination of many animals with greatly enlarged legs as sequelae of wire cuts or other forms of laceration may be prevented if the wounded parts are properly bandaged with judicious pressure, and the wound kept clean until healing is complete.

Proud-flesh may be guarded against

3. *Stomach balls.* Because of incomplete prelimi-

nary mastication and hasty swallowing of food, especially spiny or thorny, hard, dry roughages, cattle, sheep and goats frequently have these materials accumulate in the paunch as indigestible masses of varying volume. Russian thistle used as cattle roughage in the plains regions of the middle west during drought years are common causes of this trouble, if cut and cured too late in the season. Though they usually result in no apparent inconvenience to the animal, balls may at times be so voluminous (as big as a man's head) as to bring on unthriftiness because of impaired digestion. Prevention consists in withholding from animals roughages of the nature mentioned.

Stomach balls and hair balls occur in animals that eat indigestible forage, and those that swallow the hair of their coats when licking themselves

In the same general grouping there may be included the true hair-balls (page 23), wool-balls, and fur-balls of cattle, sheep and cats, respectively. Because of their cleansing habits these animals swallow these foreign substances which, cemented together by saliva, collect in the paunch, or in cats in the true stomach, in the form of matted balls. It is interesting to relate that the small hair-balls obtained from the stomach of a deer constitute the so-called mad-stone of former generations which when applied to the bitten portion of the body was empirically assumed to possess mysterious virtues in extracting from the wound the poison deposited there by a mad or rabid dog (page 544). There is no scientific basis for such an assumption, but the possessor of a "true mad-stone" was considered more than ordinarily fortunate in having a "charm" so "potent" in its action.

The mad-stone and its alleged properties

The hair-balls seldom cause trouble in ruminants, though they may be a source of indigestion in cats. Their formation is not entirely preventable because of the natural cleansing habits of affected animals.

Daily careful grooming (page 189) because it removes loose hair is helpful in this respect. In small animals the presence of hair-balls may be ascertained by an X-ray or fluoroscopic examination. Veterinarians accomplish their removal when necessary by surgical means.

4. *Stomach-dirt.* This is a common condition in horses and cattle occurring when these animals graze on loosely implanted vegetation such as the green wheat plant. It causes so-called "sand-colic." Unless there is a good root system, or when the ground is frozen, or when it has been well tramped down, the safest plan is to avoid pasturage of this nature. Death is a frequent sequel in horses, an autopsy revealing one to ten pounds of sand and soil in the stomach. Cattle become unthrifty, though they may be afforded relief by the performance of a rumenotomy.

Sand-colic and its cause

"Choke." Dry grains, including such feeds as beets, turnips and comparable material, do not always succeed in negotiating a passage from the mouth to the stomach. They become lodged in the oesophagus (page 17). Compelling animals, especially horses, to eat grains slowly (page 36) and reducing the size of roots fed to cattle will do much to prevent the trouble. The veterinarian has many surgical devices to correct the trouble, once it has taken place.

Preventing "choke" in animals

5. *"Crop-bound" fowl,* (impaction of the crop). In barnyard fowl the crop is that portion of the gullet that is a more or less distinct chamber, located at the entrance to the chest.

Occasionally coarse or stringy foods accumulate in the crop. At other times the bird over-indulges in the consumption of dry grains followed by water so that the grains swell. Also, the onward passage of foodstuffs in the crop may be hindered by a constriction in that portion of the gullet that is an immediate contin-

The cause of crop-bound in poultry

uation of the crop. Because of any or all of the foregoing conditions, and possibly others, the crop is subjected to repeated stretching and finally it becomes dilated to the extent that it no longer empties itself. The food in it sours and noxious gases are generated. If not relieved the affected bird dies.

The simplest method of handling is to introduce a small amount of olive oil into the crop by way of the mouth, then suspend the bird head downward and by careful manipulations of the distended crop by means of the fingers gradually empty the organ by forcing out the offending material through the mouth.

In very severe cases more heroic treatment must be applied. The feathers are plucked from the region directly over the crop, and the latter incised to a sufficient extent—not more than one inch long, preferably shorter—to permit of the gradual removal of the contents, then washing out the crop with clean warm water, and finally closing the wound by first sewing together the edges of the crop wound, followed by the skin wound, each to be closed by closely placed individual coarse stitches of silk or cotton thread. No food or water is to be afforded for twelve hours after the completion of the operation, and nothing but water and soft food for several days thereafter.

6. *Pendulous Crop:* Also known as "drop crop," "baggy crop," and water crop. This is not a secondary condition. It is described here because it bears a physical resemblance to the crop-bound condition. It is observed almost exclusively in turkeys.

A hereditary condition The tendency to develop this abnormality is generally admitted to be a hereditary factor. In some turkeys the crop has such weak walls that under the influence of a stimulus which has no effect on normal fowl, the crop promptly becomes "baggy" or pendulous. The stimuli responsible are increased fluid intake, excessively hot weather, eating coarse grasses, and other faulty diets. A crop that has once been dilated does not return to normal.

In fact because of an accumulation of stagnant sour food there soon are secondary developments such as ulcers and thickened crop walls. Final rupture of the crop is not uncommon. Since this condition is primarily a hereditary one birds affected in this manner or those that have a tendency in this direction should not be used for breeding purposes.

7. *Transportation Disease:* ("Staggers," "Railroad or Truck Sickness," Tetany, (page 501), "Stress," etc.) This condition—much rarer in sheep and horses—is most frequently observed in cattle, five years of age or older, that have been prepared for exhibition purposes for which transportation is involved. Hot, humid weather seems to be a factor.

Symptoms may appear during the later

Observed as staggering following unaccustomed transportation stages of a journey, and are most noticeable at the time of disembarkation. Mostly these are an unsteady gait, staggering, and finally, going down with inability to arise. Later, stupor sets in with general symptoms that usually are observed in cows affected with milk fever (page 509). Recovery generally occurs if, as the symptoms first appear, the animal is placed in a comfortable, shady place with all the drinking water it desires. It has been observed that cows that abort during an attack recover most frequently. It is a belief that if cows that have been on pasture are intended for transportation, they should be placed on dry feed for a few days before shipment. Thus an attack is less likely. Unnecessary excitement during the loading and unloading is to be avoided. Some veterinarians, because of the nature of the symptoms, are inclined to consider the condition a hypocalcemia—not confirmed—and medicinally treat it as such. This treatment must not be delayed. Since the animal's urine is in many instances not voided, catheterization of the bladder is advised.

8. *Awns in the lips, cheeks and tongue.* All herbivorous animals fed on roughage containing awns not in-

Injuries of the mouth from hard, rough forages frequently have the inner surfaces of the lips and other soft mouth-parts penetrated by these sharp, dried and hard vegetable barbs. If present in sufficient numbers they produce severe mechanical irritations which are sometimes followed by infections so as to interfere with eating. If discovered they should be carefully removed with a pair of tweezers, and the parts cleansed with a mild antiseptic wash.

9. *Thin Shelled Eggs:* This is largely a matter of heredity, and fowl having this genetic factor are most susceptible to a deficiency in the calcium and magnesium carbonates in the ration—the normal egg shell has approximately 94 per cent calcium carbonate, 1.4 per cent magnesium carbonate, and small amounts of phosphate and organic matter. Other causative factors are to a small degree responsible, such as high out-of-doors temperature, the beginning and the end of the egg laying period, pathological conditions in the oviduct, hormone treated eggs, Newcastle disease, infectious bronchitis, and advancing age, but heredity is the outstanding causative characteristic. The nutritional factors that must be given consideration are calcium, phosphorus, minute quantity of manganese, and Vitamin D-3—the latter from fish liver oils or irradiated cholesterol. However, if a hen has the thin-shelled hereditary taint, no matter what is the ration, the outcome is unsatisfactory. Culling is recommended for those not responding.

10. *Navel ailments.* This organ, technically known as the umbilicus, is a particularly vulnerable point of attack by disease producing factors from the moment of birth until the wound is **Navel ailments and infections are prolific sources of trouble in young animals** healed a few days later. During intrauterine existence, nourishment and oxygen by means of the blood as a carrier are transported through it from the mother, and some of the waste material is returned by this route.

Corresponding to the time of birth, or when the young creature enters upon an independent existence, the blood vessels, the "cord," constituting the main part of the navel are roughly severed, and thus opened and exposed to all the filth of its surroundings. In some animals the rupture takes place before the young creature has completed its passage through the birth canal so that the open stump of the cord is exposed to those infections that are present in the maternal genitals. Such a highly fatal condition as white scours (page 538) in calves may be contracted through the navel, and the even more serious blood poisoning of all newly born animals variously designated as "joint-evil," "navel-ill," and "joint-disease of sucklings" (page 537), has its origin through the navel. These diseases are relatively uncommon when the birth takes place in an open, sun-exposed place, away from animal habitations, and such diseases are most common under opposite conditions.

The mode and conditions of infection indicate the methods of prevention. If the young creature is to be born in an animal environment, this should be made sanitary. (Page 199.) Washing off the external genitals of the mother with soap and water, and douching the vagina with a warm one-half per cent water solution of carbolic acid shortly before the birth takes place is of value.

The greatest attention must be paid to the umbilicus itself (page 199). The attendant must be very careful to handle this organ only when his hands are clean. If the navel cord has not become severed, then as soon as pulsation in it has ceased it should be ligated about two to four inches from the body by passing around it a piece of string which has for some time previously been kept immersed in an antiseptic solution. By means of a clean knife or scissors, the "cord" may then be am-

The
prevention
of navel
infections

putated at some distance below the point of ligation. When the "cord" has become severed spontaneously, it is best not to ligate it, as this would simply imprison in it any existing infection. In either event attempts must be made to cause the stump of the "cord" to dry up as rapidly as possible. A dried "cord" stump is seldom a source of danger.

One good method is to paint the entire stump with tincture of iodine (page 276) as shortly as possible after it has become severed, and then hasten the drying by applying some good antiseptic dusting powder several times daily. A powder consisting of equal parts of alum, starch, wood charcoal, camphor and boric acid has been recommended. Another effective method is to dry the stump of the cord by immersing it in a two per cent solution of formalin (page 266). It is advisable when several births are expected, to have some of the formalin solution previously prepared and stored in a wide-mouthed bottle. This may be pressed against the navel region in such a manner as to completely immerse the stump of the "cord." Usually, as a result of any of the described methods the drying will be complete in twenty-four hours. These sanitary steps are surprisingly effective in the prevention of general diseases having the navel as their port of entry.

11. *Interdigital Pouch Obstruction in Sheep.* A careful examination of the space between the claws—in the anterior portion—will disclose a small opening about the size of a pin-head, or at this point it appears as if the skin is turned in. This is the outward opening of a bent tube or pouch extending in a backward and downward direction, though it soon changes to an upward direction, to end up between the first phalanges. The tube or pouch in mature sheep is approximately one inch long and one-fourth inch wide. The interior of the pouch is a gathering place for a colorless fatty substance which originates in sebacious glands in the vicinity of the pouch. It is important that the out-

side opening of the pouch shall not be obstructed in any manner so as to impede the normal discharge of the fatty contents of the pouch.

When sheep are kept on sandy soil, sand and other foreign material sometimes clog up the external orifice of the pouch. The result is that its fatty contents accumulate and frequently the pouch becomes tender to the touch and inflamed. Often the animal becomes lame and the region between and surrounding the claws is swollen. When these symptoms are observed the contents of the pouch—after a preliminary washing of the surrounding area with soap and warm water—are pressed out by hand. If there is evidence of infection a mild disinfection of the region is indicated. If several members of a band are affected, handling as advised for foot-rot (page 527) may be followed. If treatment is delayed too long infection may break into the neighboring joint cavity with serious results.

12. *"Rain-rot" in sheep.* Heavily fleeced sheep exposed to prolonged damp atmosphere and drizzling rains occasionally have enough moisture penetrate down to the skin where, because of inhibited evaporation, maceration results with loosening of the wool so that patches of it fall out. This trouble may bear a close resemblance to a somewhat similar phenomenon observed in mange (page 727). It is said that the older, less thrifty animals are most susceptible, possibly because of the reduced amount of the protective yolk in their fleece.

Loosening of the wool in sheep may be due to excessive moisture

Prevention consists in placing affected animals in drier surroundings before, or as shortly as possible after, the onset of early symptoms. Clipping the wool may be necessary when serious skin involvement is threatened.

13. *"Hardware disease"* (traumatic pericarditis). The condition so designated is observed most frequently

in cattle and other ruminants, quite often in swine and less so in other animals. It is essentially an accumulation in the digestive tract of foreign bodies such as nails, bolts, shipping-tag clips, pieces of baling wire and other hard substances. In ruminants these for-eign bodies are almost always present to some extent in the reticulum (page 23), and in swine, if present, in the true stomach. Many of these foreign bodies, as a result of partial solution or corrosion, be-come needle-sharp so that they penetrate the wall of the digestive compartment in which they are lodged, to travel in various directions leaving a train of infections in their wake. Abscess formations (pus pockets) are not uncommon in different parts of the body including the abdominal

Animals likely to consume hardware with their food. It frequently results in a serious heart ailment

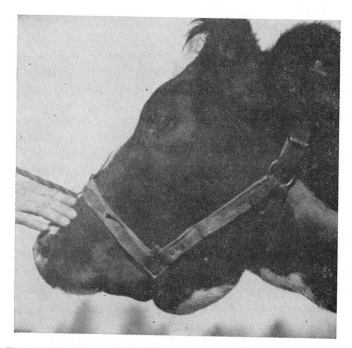

FIG. 72. Swelling under the jaw, and a prominent jugular vein in traumatic pericarditis ("hardware disease").

and chest walls. In cattle there is a very close anatomical relationship between the reticulum, which is
the stomach compartment in which the foreign body
is most frequently lodged, and the heart and its surrounding sac (page 23).

As a sequence of the normal stomach contractions,
it is very common for the sharp-pointed foreign body
to be forced in a forward direction so that its tip ultimately penetrates the heart sac (pericardium), or it
may actually enter it in its entirety (Fig. 72). Such a
chain of events is almost invariably followed by death.
This heart involvement is known as traumatic pericarditis. It is of very common occurrence in cattle—
especially those that are closely confined and fed, in
contradistinction to those that are pastured at some
distance from habitations.

The reactions in swine are seldom of the same nature as in cattle, being more in the nature of digestive
disturbances.

Prevention to a considerable extent is possible and
practical. On those farms and dairies where the ailment had previously resulted in several deaths yearly
from traumatic pericarditis, it has almost been obviated as a menace by precautions on the part of caretakers in avoiding the promiscuous scattering of nails,
baling wire, and shipping-tag clips in the vicinity of
cattle foods. In some instances the careful screening
of the finer foods has been an additional precautionary
preventive step.

Powerful magnets located at strategic places in
feed mixing establishments, shifting from wire to
twine for baling hay and bedding material,
Prevention   and awareness of the danger of hardware
in cattle feeds have all helped in reducing this hazard.

Veterinarians can successfully remove these foreign
bodies from the digestive tract by surgical means, and
operations on the heart sac have even been performed.
Unfortunately, however, in the early stages of "hard-

ware disease" when treatment will do the most good, the clinical symptoms are not so pronounced that a diagnosis is clear-cut. In a measure the comparatively early diagnosis has been helped by use of a "mine-detector" applied on the outside of the body over the region of the organs of digestion. Unfortunately a "mine-detector" gives no indication of the

Mine-detector use for diagnosis
nature of the metal object, its exact location, nor the lesions that may have been caused by the suspected presence of a metallic foreign body. The X-ray has also been used for early diagnosis (Figs. 73 and 74). This

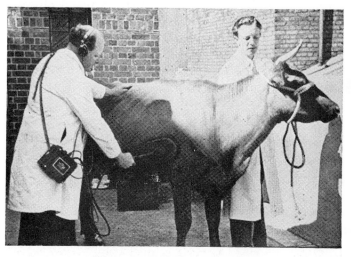

(Photo reproduced from Black's Veterinary Dictionary)

FIG. 73. Mine detector to aid in determining the presence of metal in stomach in hardware disease.

X-ray diagnosis
machine is expensive, and to apply it the animal must be taken to the machine which is frequently at some distance. The radiologic examination is not on a practical basis, and finally when the heart and its sac are affected, it is usually too late to expect beneficial results because of the hazardous nature of the operation.

A unique form of prevention and treatment has recently been introduced. It is a powerful magnet—the

A magnet in the rumen or paunch to attract metals

"reticular magnet"—which is administered orally by means of an ordinary instrument—every veterinarian has one or more—known as a "balling gun."

The "balling gun" is loaded with a "recticular magnet" so that the latter is passed through the animal's mouth and the gullet (oesophagus) into the rumen or paunch where it remains throughout the life of the cow. The magnet is so comparatively small, and so powerful, that it causes no noticeable inconvenience to the animal, although it continuously stops and retains foreign metal objects. It is said finally to lodge at the entrance to the reticulum. It has been used so little that its real merit has not been established. The few that have resorted to the use of the "reticular magnet" hint that it has been helpful in the control of indigestion, bloat, and, the "off-feed" condition. Prevention by guarding

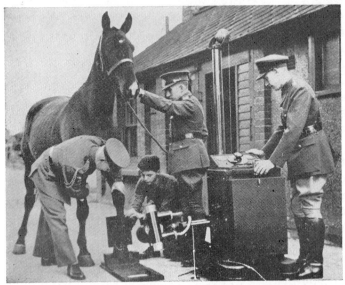

Fig. 74. X-ray as an aid in the diagnosis of lameness.

against the ingestion of metal objects is a better method.

14. *Acute Bloat*. This condition is common in cattle and sheep. It is the result of food fermentation with

Bloat is a frequent cause of death in several species of animals

the evolvement of large quantities of gas lodging in the rumen. So relatively enormous is the quantity of gas and so rapid its evolution that it distends the rumen to the point that the lungs and large blood vessels are compressed to the extent that death may result from suffocation in less than one hour. Sheep, because of a lesser chest cavity, succumb even more quickly than cattle. In horses death is due to rupture of the stomach rather than suffocation.

The foods usually responsible for acute bloat are the clovers, alfalfa, peas, beans, and other legumes, as well as grass, cabbage leaves, beet tops and others. When the foods named contain a relatively large amount of water, if they are wet as the result of frost, dew or rain, if they are wilted during the early stages of the curing process, or if they are undergoing heating, they are more than likely to be dangerous for use as foods. Soapy lather-forming materials (saponins) in alfalfa were recently shown to be one of the causes of bloat in cattle, sheep, and goats, and the discovery may be an important clue to one of the worst troubles of the farm and dairy.

When animals have been on a dry ration and are then suddenly changed to green feed so that they fill up on large quantities of the unaccustomed material, bloat may also ensue. Prevention consists in gradually changing from accustomed dry roughage to the succulent green foods. It is well before turning animals into unaccustomed green pasture to first give them a feed of their usual dry material. It is always hazardous to offer legume pasturage to animals if the vegetation is wet from dew, frost or rain. When offering cut green feeds it is best to mix them with some dry roughage.

Death from acute bloat is so quickly imminent that immediate steps must be taken if the animal's life is to be saved. Call the veterinarian and if his arrival is likely to be delayed beyond a few minutes, each affected animal should receive some medicinal agent at once to stop the fermentation. Cattle may be given two ounces of turpentine mixed in a quart of *raw* linseed oil; if the oil is not available, milk may be substituted for it. It is still one of the best, easily obtainable anti-ferments.

Thoroughly manipulating the rumen contents by slow boring movements with the closed fist in the animal's left flank will help to disseminate the anti-ferment through the frothing mass. Though this method of handling will not remove the gas that has already formed, it will control additional fermentation and is frequently the factor that saves the animal's life. Raising the animal's foreparts, or driving it up hill is a utilization of the gravitational pull to minimize pressure of the distended paunch against the lungs. Dashing cold water on the animal, or driving a band of sheep into a river when several are simultaneously bloated is said to stimulate contractions of the paunch, with at least partial relief as a result. The old practice of placing a stick crosswise in the animal's mouth, maintaining it there by a halterlike arrangement, favors tongue movements and the eructation of gas.

The administration of a highly polymerized methyl silicone injected directly into the paunch (rumen) increases the surface tension of the mass of ingesta in the rumen and thus prevents gas formation. The contention is that when gas forms the surface tension is decreased (Jour. Am. Vet. Med. Assoc., Vol. CXIV, No. 866, May 1949.)

Surface tension and bloat

The rather common practice of making an artificial opening or "sticking the animal" in the left side in the case of cattle, is to be encouraged only with considerable reservation due to the fact that a dangerous wound is created which seldom releases much of the imprisoned gas. This gas is in the form of millions of little gas bubbles intimately mixed with the ingesta, and therefore about the only result of the "sticking" is the emergence through the instrument of a small amount of a frothy material which does not in any sense of the term relieve the bloat. After the administration of the anti-fermenting medicine, it is best to await the arrival of the veterinarian so that he may exercise his professional judgment. This procedure usually resolves itself into removing gas and giving medicine by way of a stomach tube since the passage of a stomach tube creates no wound as does "sticking" or in more severe cases he may find it advisable to make a large opening into the animal's rumen, this being done under suitable anaesthesia and surgical asepsis, so as to remove the frothing ingesta handful by handful.

The prevention of acute bloat is currently receiving much research attention. Several preliminary reports have been issued.

Some of the results observed are as follows:

1. Michigan Agricultural Experiment Station has brought out that the incidence of pasture bloat was reduced by about two-thirds by feeding 100 milligrams of procaine penicillin per cow per day either with the grain or in salt on a free-choice basis. The value of this method of prevention seemed to decrease as the season advanced.

2. Based on a South African determination that a moist condition of rumen contents favors the escape of forming gas to an area above the ingesta rather than for it to remain as millions of bubbles mixed with the ingestia, the Kansas Agricultural Experiment Station decided to add a mucin-containing substance to the feed as this also seems to favor the escape of gas from froth-

ing rumen contents. Linseed meal is rich in mucin. In dry cattle two pounds of linseed meal daily in the feed reduced the incidence of bloat. In lactating cattle, on alfalfa pasture, two pounds of linseed meal per head in from two to four feedings prior to pasturing reduced the incidence of bloat, and those that did bloat recovered more quickly than the controls. An attempt is now being made to find a more economical source of mucin that may be incorporated in the feed.

3. At the Iowa Station, workers on the prevention of acute bloat reduced bloat very much by means of feeding water-dispersible lard oil mixed in the grain at the rate of 0.5 pound per day, or in drinking water—two per cent by weight; average daily consumption 0.65 pound. Soybean oil in the grain—0.5 pound a day—or sprayed on alfalfa ensilage also reduced bloat. They also report that penicillin daily in the feed lost its efficiency after a nine day trial.

4. In New Zealand (reported by Johns in the British Reviews and Annotations of April 1957) it is indicated that pasture spraying with antifoaming agents such as oil or tallow, (probably tallow oil R.R.D.) may be helpful. Also penicillin helped when only a small number of animals were involved.

Chronic bloat is an entirely different matter, and is not properly considered in these discussions. The causes of it, its nature, its correct diagnosis, and its treatment are so varied, that it belongs entirely in the realm of the veterinarian; death is never immediately imminent as a result of it. Tuberculosis is sometimes a factor especially when the bronchial lymph glands are tuberculous and press on the gullet to prevent gas belching.

15. *Sudden stoppage of milk flow.* There are many factors that influence milk secretion to a greater or less

The cause of a sudden cessation in the secretion of milk extent. Undoubtedly a certain balance of nervous impulses exercises considerable control over the secretion of milk. If this balance is disturbed there is likely to be a decreased milk flow, but this is seldom of more than a short duration. Sometimes the slightest influence will do this such as an unaccustomed milker, a change of surroundings, and heat periods because of nervous energy consumed that ordinarily is concerned in milk production. The drinking of unaccustomed ice-water may also stop the milk flow (page 114).

On the other hand, it is well recognized that if there is no absorption of food from the digestive tract as a result of disease, which usually means a disturbance of all physiological functions, the flow of milk must be greatly decreased, or possibly stopped entirely. When a milk-producing cow becomes ill, one of the first symptoms is always a decreased milk flow. There is plenty of clinical evidence to support the statement that the milk flow may be reduced before the cow shows visible outward evidence of being unwell.

In the very early spring months when vegetation is lush, dairy and other cattle that for several months have been carefully fed on dry and cured foods are frequently turned out to pasture. The ground is still cold and vegetation is drenched with dew or even frost. The winter-pampered animal fills its digestive tract with this unaccustomed, chilled food. The change is sudden and the shock is so great that, among other things, the delicate nervous balance that controls milk secretion is upset and when the animal returns to its quarters later in the day, there is no milk in the mammary gland. A few hours later on the animal usually "goes off feed" as well. In such instances, it always requires days of careful nursing to restore the animal to a near normal condition.

Prevention of all this trouble rests in observing care in changing animals to new and unaccustomed foods (page 37). It is always bad management, especially during the cold wet weather of early spring, to suddenly change winter-fed animals to pasture. The fact that animals that have been on winter range are not apparently deleteriously affected by being changed to spring pasture should not lead the unwary to assume that the "hothouse plants" in the form of many modern dairy cows may be likewise treated with impunity. Attention to careful feeding practices will control many dysfunctions of the mammary gland.

16. *Methods of drying up of the cow*. It **It is important to know how to stop the milk secretion** is desirable to dry up a cow at least a month before she again freshens. This gives nature an opportunity to prepare for the approaching birth. Furthermore, if the animal is milked continuously from one freshening period to the next, there is no opportunity for the secretion of colostrum. (This is the first milk after freshening having special composition and unusual properties.)

The question frequently raised is how best to dry up, without danger, the cow that has quite a heavy milk flow as the termination of pregnancy approaches. Three methods are in use, i.e.: (1) intermittent milking; (2) incomplete milking so as to gradually remove less and less; and (3) sudden cessation of milking. It is generally accepted that milk in the udder undergoing changes from the production to the drying up period is accompanied by an increase in numbers of germs. When the change has finally been made, the fluid in the udder more nearly compares to blood serum and white blood cells, and it suppresses germ growth. With intermittent and incomplete milking as methods of drying up the cow, there is maintained in her udder conditions favorable for germ growth. Sudden cessation of milking soon sets up enough intramammary pressure to control secretion and then the changed character of the fluid in the gland inhibits germ development.

To prevent undesirable conditions in the drying up of a cow, it is best to reduce the amount of food permitted the animal, and to stop milking her. If this method seems to cause too much swelling and distress in an occasional animal, then it may be necessary to decrease the intramammary pressure by withdrawing some of the milk. The grain ration may be completely withdrawn if advisable, and the cow taken out of the milking barn because the sound of others being milked and other common noises incidental to milking stimulates milk secretion in the cow that is undergoing the process of drying.

Ewes are usually dried up when the lambs are weaned at from three to five months of age when the older ones are marketed. If the ewe at this time has a large udder, or if there is still a good deal of milk secretion it is frequently advisable to partially milk her every three days until she goes dry.

Drying the ewe

17. *Teat Eversion.* When milking machine cups are pulled off the teats before the vacuum in them is entirely exhausted the lining of the teat has a tendency to become sucked out causing teat eversion. Prevention consists in shutting off the vacuum at the pail and inserting a finger between one of the inflations and the enclosed teat so as to permit air to enter. After a brief period of waiting all the inflations will loosen so as to destroy the vacuum, and the teat cups fall off.

How to guard against teat eversion

Pulling off teat cups before the vacuum is exhausted is painful to the cow, it results in hard milkers, and the everted mucous membrane of the teat is an open invitation to mastitis infection.

Many dairymen apply cloths wrung out of 130° F. water to the udder and remove a few strips of milk

Other
"vacuum"
injuries

from each teat so as to open the teat canal before applying the teat cups of the milking machine. If the udder is a healthy one the machine should remove all the milk within three to four minutes. Then the cups are to be carefully removed as described in the preceding paragraph. Permitting the vacuum to continue after all the milk is out of the udder will cause tissue changes in the teats. At first there is slight tenderness, followed by some difficulty in passage of the milk. If at this time the end of the teat is turned up to view, and the teat canal opened by pressure with the thumb and finger, it will be observed that instead of the normal pink smooth lining of the canal it will be reddened, hard and even scaly. At the outer opening the mucous membrane is frequently hardened and rough. This entire condition invites infection and possibly a ruined udder. Prevention consists in not applying the vacuum until the milk is ready to come down and carefully removing the vacuum or teat cups as soon as all the milk is out of the udder. Suction on an empty udder is to be avoided.

18. *Mechanical Teat Injuries.* Stabling cattle in stalls that are too small (page 127) results in frequent tread injuries to the teats. Barb-wire cuts may also in-

Small stalls
and
"spider"
teat

volve the end of the teat. Then when nature attempts to repair the injury it pays but slight attention to the mode of healing so that the milk sprays out or the animal is said to have a "spider" teat, or a low grade of infection produces "black spot." Prevention consists of having stalls of ample size. Prompt veterinary attention will prevent improper healing. Infections usually respond to local tincture of iodine applications.

19. *Fistula of the Teat.* Quite frequently barbed wire cuts involve the body of the teat so that the milk cistern is involved, and therefore milk flows out of

Milk from
the side of
the teat

the wound, provided the cow is in production. With a minimum amount of good care wound healing progresses satisfactorily up to the point that only a small opening remains and this latter refuses to heal, or a milk fistula has become established. During the milking process — sometimes between milkings — the milk escapes from the fistula. Healing is difficult to obtain so long as the teat is subjected to the manipulations of daily milking.

When not in production healing follows simple lines of surgical intervention such as scarifying the edges of the fistula, and if the fistula is a large one, holding the edges of the wound in apposition by suturing. The sutures must not penetrate the milk cistern or new "suture" fistulas will result. This is a job for the skilled veterinary surgeon. Prevention rests largely in the elimination of barbed wire fences from yards or corrals intended to serve for confining dairy cattle.

20. *Off-flavored Milk:* Well-informed dairymen know when dairy cows are on such green pasture as

Green feed
and off
flavors

wheat or rye plants that they will produce milk likely to have an objectionable bitter, or green food flavor. This condition is most likely to occur when the animals are first placed on green pasture. Also the consumption of various plants such as those named and described here-after along with some others, is at once reflected in the production of malodorous or bad tasting milk: (Figs. 75 to 84 inclusive.)

One of the symptoms of ketosis (page 505) is a decidedly "cowy" flavor of the milk. This symptom may be the only one in a mild attack of ketosis; therefore, apply the test (page 507) for ketosis.

It is not generally known that digestion disturbances and putrefactive processes in other parts of

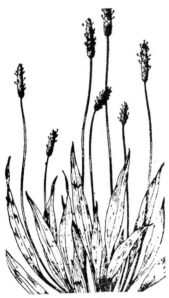

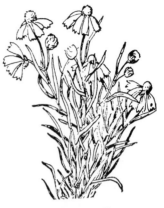

Bitterweed*

FIG. 76. Flowers are yellow. Plants usually about 20 inches high. Fibrous roots. The plant is poisonous to stock, causing sneezing. Not serious unless eaten in large amounts. Objectionable in h a y . Bitter, unmarketable milk is produced by cows that graze heavily on the weed.

To control bitterweed in badly infested fields, mow repeatedly before seed ripens in fall. Seedlings are smothered out somewhat if spring grazing is delayed until grass gets a good start.

Garlic or Wild Onion*

FIG. 75. Cows that eat garlic in pasture give milk with an onion taint—not poisonous, but enough to cause rejection of milk or cream at buying plants. To avoid taint, remove cows from infested pastures 5 or 6 hours before milking time. To get rid of garlic, plow late in fall and c u l t i v a t e thoroughly in spring. Follow with well-tilled row crops.

Upsets in digestion cause off flavors

the animal's body are occasionally reflected in the milk. Surrounding odors as of strong disinfectants are certain to taint the milk. There are occasionally bacteria in milking utensils that will impart a flavor to milk. Finally, especially in old cows and towards the end of the lactation period, there is the possibility that the milk may contain an excessive

*Descriptive material and illustrations courtesy Dr. Hess and Clark, Inc., Ashland. Ohio.

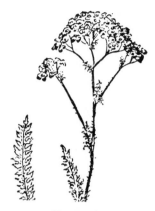

Yarrow*

Fig. 77. A perennial weed, c o m m o n in pastures and meadows. Plants may grow 3 feet high. Wh i t e flowers. Blooms J u n e to October. Leaves are more or less fuzzy. Fibrous roots. Plant has offensive odor. Damaging to dairy products when eaten in hay.

Many seeds are produced by each plant. Control consists largely of preventing seed production. Mow pastures or meadows when the plants are in early blossom stage (usually June). Not usually troublesome in cultivated fields.

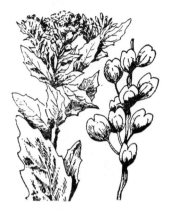

Stinkweed*

Fig. 78. Also called penny-cress and Frenchweed. Common in grain fields, waste places and pastures. Leaves have garlicky o d o r when b r u i s e d. White flowers. Blooms April to June. Seeds live for years in the soil.

In pastures and meadows, mow just before seed formation (May to August). Plants from seeds sprouting in fall should be killed by light cultivation; if left till spring, they have deeper roots and are harder to kill. Watch out for stinkweed as an impurity in clover or alfalfa seed.

amount of the enzyme lipase which is capable of splitting fats and thus producing a rancid flavor shortly after milk has been drawn.

Since heat destroys this enzyme it is suggested that immediately after drawing the milk it be heated to 150°

Testing for rancidity Fahrenheit and held there for thirty minutes. If the milk remains normal or does not become rancid after this heating it may be assumed that lipase is responsible for the rancidity. The other causes of "off-flavors" are preventable by avoiding in the feed, or surroundings sub-

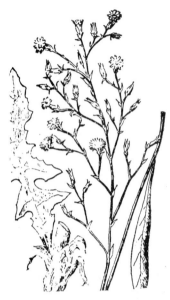

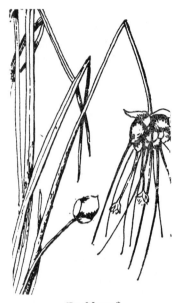

Wild Lettuce*

FIG. 79. This plant has abundant milky, bitter juice (like garden lettuce) which is capable of tainting milk. Plants have numerous yellow flowers about ½ inch across. There are spines on lower side of leaf midrib. To control, prevent seed production by cutting before blooming time in late spring or early summer. Plowing followed by corn or soybeans will get rid of this weed.

Buckhorn*

FIG. 80. Buckhorn belongs to the plantain family. Seed heads resemble those of timothy. Common in run-down pastures. Seeds of buckhorn are commonly present as an impurity in red clover and timothy. To get rid of buckhorn, plow infested fields and plant cultivated crops for two years. Small grain, followed by early plowing, will control buckhorn.

stances that are likely to taint the milk. The bitterish flavor of green pasture can be controlled by removing the cows from the green feed, to a dry lot or barn, for a few hours before they are to be milked. Early in the green pasture season it may be necessary to take the cows away from the green feed for three or four hours before milking, but after they are accustomed to the green material one or two hours is usually long enough to remove most of the off-flavor from the milk.

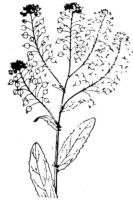

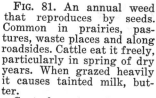

Peppergrass*

FIG. 81. An annual weed that reproduces by seeds. Common in prairies, pastures, waste places and along roadsides. Cattle eat it freely, particularly in spring of dry years. When grazed heavily it causes tainted milk, butter.

Control consists of mowing before seeds are ripe (May to October), and using farm seeds free from contamination. To avoid off-flavors in dairy products use supplementary pastures such as wheat, rye, etc. Remove cows from peppergrass pastures 5 or 6 hours before milking.

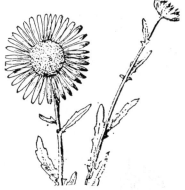

Oxeye Daisy*

FIG. 82. Common in meadows and pastures, where it is objectionable because of its ability to give milk a disagreeable taste. Plants also crowd out the grass. Reproduces by seeds, offsets and rhizomes. Flowers white with yellow centers, one at end of each stem.

To prevent spread of seed, mow pastures that are not g r a z e d . In meadows, cut flower stalks before they go to seed (June to August). When the weeds occur in plow land, rotation with a cultivated crop every 2 or 3 years will control them.

Digestion upsets and putrefactive processes are problems for the attending veterinarian, and bacterial contamination of milking utensils calls for the most careful cleansing with soap, or wetting agent (page 253), fine steel wool, scalding water, as well as direct exposure to the sun.

21. *Sweet Curdling:* This condition in milk may be responsible for the failure of the cream to rise. Usually the acid producing bacteria in milk dominate the bacterial situation from the time the milk is drawn, and they crowd out the rennin-producing bacteria which are nearly always present in small numbers. There are

Why cream fails to rise

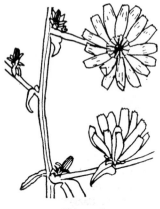

Chicory*

FIG. 83. Perennial, reproduces by seeds. Common in pasture, m e a d o w s , along roadsides—seldom in cultivated fields. Easily recognized by blue flowers along stems of the plant. Milky juice of plant is bitter, may taint milk. Chicory is a common adulterant in coffee, or substitute for coffee.

Destroy scattered plants by cutting below the crown. If troublesome over large areas, mow several times during the year to prevent ripening and distribution of seeds. Seeds ripen from July on.

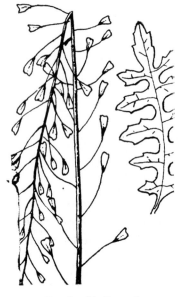

Shepherd's Purse*

FIG. 84. Found in poor pastures, cultivated fields, barnyards, etc. Flowers are small, white and occur mostly from February to June. Eaten by cows, c a u s e s tainted m i l k . Relished by chickens a n d causes olive color of egg yolks. To control in pastures, mow early in spring or pasture with sheep to prevent seed production. Improvement of poor pastures crowds this weed out.

several kinds of bacteria capable of producing rennin. When the acid producing bacteria have the upper hand the milk sours in due course; when as occasionally happens, however, the rennin producers gain the ascendency *sweet curdling* takes place and the cream does not rise. By way of explanation it may be brought out that rennin is a milk-curdling enzyme normally secreted by the cells of the true stomach (the so-called "fourth" in ruminants) to facilitate quick curdling in the process of milk digestion.

Some of the rennin producing bacteria are spore-producers (page 221) and are thus heat resistant; ordinary methods of sterilization do not destroy them. Furthermore heat sterilization of dairy utensils, if these rennin producers are present, frequently results in a thin film of coagulated milk proteins (known as "milk-stone") on the sides of the vessels, and this also serves to protect and harbor these heat resistant organisms.

Though *sweet curdling* bacteria are seldom in the udder, when only the milk of one cow raises no cream it is suggestive of udder contamination.

Some sweet curdling bacteria in the udder To test for udder infection sterilize a fruit jar, and separate lid, by keeping it in vigorously boiling water for fifteen minutes. When this has cooled enough so that it can be handled put lid in place so as to keep germs out of the jar. Take the cow some distance from the barn and wash her udder and teats with **A test for udder infection** a chlorine disinfectant (pages 257 to 258). Then carefully remove the lid from the jar and draw into it enough milk to half-fill it, and quickly replace the lid. Store the jar and its contents under the usual conditions. If this milk undergoes "sweet curdling" a veterinarian should be asked to apply udder disinfection to overcome the udder contamination. If, as is usually the trouble, the dairy utensils are the rennin-producing bacterial contaminants then the same scrupulous cleaning already advised for lipase in the milk (page 371) is recommended.

22. *Paralysis of the facial nerve.* In horses a very common ailment consists in bruising or permanent **Paralysis of the facial nerve is of frequent occurrence as a sequence of injury** functional destruction of the motor nerve (facial or seventh cranial) passing to the facial muscles that control the action of the lip and cheeks (Fig. 85). In its forward passage from the brain to the muscles of the face this nerve is located just beneath the skin, and it bends around

the border of the lower jaw at a point about two or three inches below the ear. In this vulnerable position it is frequently injured when the animal's head is caught in a door-way or stanchion with results that depend upon whether the injury involves one side only or both sides. In either event the prehensile power of the lips is interfered with, and in the more serious double-sided paralysis the prehension of food and liquids is impossible so that starvation may take place.

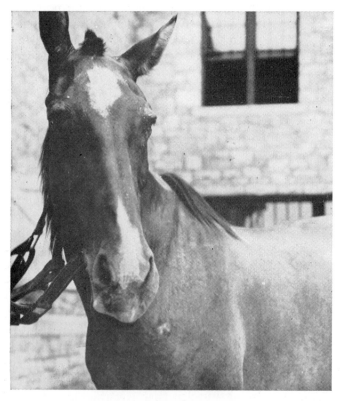

FIG. 85. Paralysis of the left facial nerve. Note the drooped half of the left upper lip.

Prevention consists in avoiding mechanical contrivances, including improperly controlled half-doors or occasionally entire doors, as well as any condition in which when standing or lying, the animal is likely to bruise the nerve in its most exposed location; this is especially important with animals when cast. When the nerve bruising has actually taken place professional aid should be secured at the earliest possible moment.

23. *Penis Sheath Obstruction* (page 192) (false navel rupture). In male hogs, the outward opening of the sheath of the penis is very narrow or small, and

Anatomy of sheath in boars and barrows just back of this exit the mucous membrane lining the sheath forms, above the tip of the penis, in a double pocket—anatomically named the "preputial diverticulum." Because of these anatomical structures the urine may not be properly voided, and collects in the preputial diverticulum to form a soft swelling filled with an accumulation of urine. Later there is inflammation and total inability to urinate. If not relieved, there may ensue uremic poisoning, rupture of the urinary bladder and death. In the early non-inflammatory stage the condition has the appearance of a navel rupture; hence, the name "false navel rupture." In the earlier stages a veterinarian can relieve the condition surgically.

24. *Feather plucking in poultry.* This vice is most frequently observed in those birds that are subjected to

Feather plucking is a common vice in poultry enforced idleness because of close confinement, and when a ration deficient in bulk is fed. Another possible factor is skin irritants in the form of lice and mites.

Prevention consists in so managing the flock that close contact of individual members is avoided; providing exercise that compels birds to scratch for feed in deep litter; providing a good ration including meat scrap, green feed, and oyster shell; and if necessary isolating offending members of the flock. Bulk in the form of wheat bran or beet pulp added to a concentrated dietary is a factor in preventing feather plucking as such feeds favor the retention of fluid in the lower gut which induces a feeling of satiety that inhibits the tendency to pluck feathers. With a file or nail clippers, three-sixteenths of an inch may be removed from the tip of the upper beak. If skin parasites are present, these must be removed.

25. *Cannibalism in chicks*. This vice usually starts in brooder chicks when they accidentally wound their toes with their beak when picking for food

Cannibalism of poultry is quite easily prevented

on the ground. The blood seems to incite the chick to continue pecking at its own toes, and frequently others attack the affected one. It is not uncommon for these cannibalistically incited chicks to attack other parts of the bodies of their victims, especially the vent, so that they may even cause partial disembowelment.

Prevention consists in isolating wounded birds. Keeping the flock busy by making them jump at suspended bones with particles of meat attached is a good device. Others report success by suspending cabbages or carrots for the fowl to peck at. Partially darkening the room in which the chicks are confined, or obscuring the red color of the blood by the use of transparent red paint on window panes, or by illumination through red electric bulbs are of value. Operating on the beak as described for feather plucking is helpful.

Oat hulls, oat mill feed, or whole oats added to the ration are believed to contain the cannibalism-preventing factor. The addition of an adequate amount of salt to the ration as a preventive, or the addition of plentiful salt to the ration for curative purposes has also been recommended. A tablespoonful of table salt to each gallon of drinking water for three mornings, with clean unsalted water in the afternoon frequently is helpful. Such conditions as "vent picking," "feather picking," and "pick outs" are all forms of cannibalism.

For cannibalism and associated vices
If the affected birds have been getting cracked or whole corn in the ration this should be discontinued and replaced with meat scraps two or three times daily for a few days, hand-fed if necessary. If this fails "debeak" as described on page 378.

26. *Prolapse of Cloaca* (prolapse of vagina). This condition observed only in laying hens is believed to be related, in some measure at least, to vent picking and cannibalism. Anatomically the cloaca in fowl is a tubular structure that terminates at the vent or anus. It is the passageway (1) for the terminal portion of the intestines, (2) for the urinary tubules from the kidneys, and (3) for the organs of generation—penis in the male and vagina in the female. The outstanding prolapsis symptom is that the cloaca appears outwardly at the vent in the form of a reddish, slightly bleeding, protrusion of tissue. In reality it is a turning inside out of part or all of the cloaca, and sometimes includes a portion of the anatomical structures that enter the cloaca.

A definite cause of the condition has not been determined; it has been ascribed to irritation of the cloaca by worms or by coccidia (page 735). Since the condition is commonest in pullets the straining of the first egg laying is also a possible causative factor. In older hens the "egg-bound" condition is thought to be a feature of the prolapse. Normally when an egg is laid the lining membrane of the cloaca is momentarily everted and when this is repeated daily the momentary protrusion may assume a more or less permanent nature which can be aggravated by the vent pecking (consult cannibalism) of other fowl. Some research workers (Wheeler and Hoffman, University of Georgia) have hinted at an association of the estrogen—a "heat" or estrus hormone (page 103)—blood level in laying pullets and hens.

Little can be done in the prevention of the trouble. Since "vent pecking" may be an aggravating factor, trap-nesting, which confines the bird until the normal eversion of the cloacal lining membrane subsides has been suggested as an aid in handling the problem where high producing fowl are affected. Unless the affected bird is a high producer, in which case isolation and trap-nesting are suggested, it is best to use the fowl for human food purposes.

27. *Turkey Mating Injury* (page 404). During the breeding season some males are so amorous that during the mating process they inflict more or less serious injury, with their talons, to the backs of **Male turkeys injure the females** the females to the extent that egg fertility is reduced, and the hen's general health is impaired because of the resulting secondary infections. If the hen is sufficiently valuable to warrant individual handling she may be kept away from the males for two or three weeks until the wounds heal. Badly torn skins need stitching. The application of tincture of iodine or Lugol's solution of iodine (page 276) is helpful, and flies should be discouraged by dusting the wound with a veterinary dusting powder of the kind quite generally used on large domesticated animals. When healing is complete it is best to return the hen to a breeding pen where there is an excess of females in proportion to males so that the hen will not be subjected to too frequent treading. It is quite customary in **Protecting the hen with a canvas "saddle"** the case of a valuable breeding hen to place over her back a canvas apron or saddle, made of reasonably heavy canvas. It has openings for the head and wings so that it is draped over all of the back region. Also about a week or ten days before the males are placed with the hens the talons of the males are blunted (page 404) by filing. Some turkey raisers amputate the end of each talon down to the sensitive tissues. If there is some slight bleeding following this operation

it is controlled by searing with a heated soldering iron. Futhermore, in the prevention of this trouble it is a good plan to separate the toms and the hens at about 20 weeks of age. The two sexes should be one-half mile apart because the toms will strut and fight with each other if the females are nearby. Some turkey raisers report good results, to control the fighting instinct by the use of diethylstilbestrol (pages 104 and 415).

28. *Increasing Egg Fertility.* Both male and female fowl may have the vent region so soiled with intestinal excreta, or the feathers so badly matted that there is not the proper contact for egg fertilization. In breeding fowl all accumulations should be removed from the vent region by washing with mild soap and tepid water, and by removing the fine feathers from this area.

Vent cleaning during mating

29. *Bumblefoot in fowls.* This is a wounding of the bottom of the foot so that pus-producing germs enter the deeper tissues of the part with resulting abscess (pus gathering) formation. The space between the toes then has a firm, prominent swelling (Fig. 86).

Bumble-foot in fowl is due to an infection and is preventable

Prevention consists in attempting to minimize injuries to the bottom of the foot. The edges of roosts should be rounded. The birds should not be required to jump down from roosts that are placed too high, onto hard rough cement floors. Roosts should be placed low, especially for the heavier breeds of poultry. If wounds of this region are detected because of symptoms of lameness, it is well to paint the part with tincture of iodine (page 276), and then confine the fowl for a time in a place without a roost. If abscess formation has actually taken place, the part must be lanced and treated antiseptically.

30. *"Pig-eating" sows* (cannibalism in sows). Sows on a deficient low protein ration frequently develop this

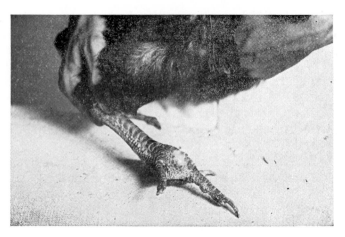

(Courtesy Dept. of Botany, Kansas State University)
FIG. 86. Bumblefoot.

vice. It is probably due to a desire for
phosphorus. Digester tankage has a high
protein content and contains as much as
15 per cent of phosphoric acid—if this is
placed before the sow she will frequently
take the tankage and forego the cannibalism. Smearing
the pigs with some bad tasting drug such as quinine
sulphate is a temporary control expedient. Veterinarians handle the extremely vicious sow by administering intravenously, subcutaneously, or for slower action
orally from 50 to 100 mg. of chlorpromazine hydrochloride—commercially thorazine hydrochloride—is the
tranquilizer used. It converts the sow into a docile
mother for a time but is not curative—rather depend
on phosphorus-containing tankage.

Sows that eat their offspring need protein

31. *Snake bites.* These are not usually deadly in
mature animals as their bulk protects them against the
comparatively small amount of venom
they receive though local swelling and
sloughing of tissue may take place. The
actual biting of the animal is seldom observed, the first intimation being swelling
of the head or less frequently of the limbs.

Snake bites are common though in the larger animals the termination is seldom fatal

Surgical treatment may be necessary at this late stage to assist in the removal of necrotic tissue, or to afford relief because of pressure by the swelling on neighboring organs such as the nose and windpipe. If the biting of one of the smaller animals by the snake is observed, or if it is diagnosed within a few hours after its occurrence the patient may be very much benefited by the administration of a specific serum known as "antivenin" procurable in most drug stores and from physicians and veterinarians in regions where poisonous snakes abound.

The Journal of Tropical Medicine and Hygiene, No. 2, Vol. 64, p. 46, Feb. 1961 reports favorable results in cobra poisoning, dogs from prednisolene succitate, and in humans following the injection of hydrocortisone.

32. *Electrocution Injuries*. Electrical discharges in the form of lightning—frequently transmitted to animals through non-grounded wire fencing, contact with

Electricity a danger to animals down-leads to wires from farm buildings, or fallen high tension wires may cause instant death, or severe burning. During a lightning storm cattle and other animals may gather under a single tree for protection from the elements and a single tree is much more dangerous than a grove of trees.

There are occasional livestock losses from contact with electrified fences used for stock control purposes. Such fences are commonly electrified from a six volt battery—such a battery is good for six months of continuous use and then must be replaced by a new battery. A dangerous procedure is to hook up the

A source of danger fence to a high voltage line without reducing the high voltage to six volts. There are on the market entirely safe convertible sets which contain an approved built-in one ampere fuse plug and which make it impossible to short circuit the 110 volts to the fence. Therefore when losses occur following contact with the fence it is usually because of improper connection with a high tension line, or because the one ampere fuse plug has been replaced with a stronger fuse, or a metal plug. Animals killed by electricity frequently show few evidences that can be clearly recognized and still this is of importance in order to be able to collect insurance. There may be only an irregular line of singed hair—frequently from the point of contact as in lightning from the tip of an ear down the side of the neck and down a leg into the ground. There may be a tuft of partially masticated grass in the mouth—death is so instantaneous. Foam may appear at the mouth and nostrils, and the blood is dark in appearance.

Basic prevention consists in having non-electrified fences grounded and electrified fences properly installed and operated. Instruct everyone on the farm how to disconnect the controller in case of an emergency, teach children not to play or tamper with an electric fence, and provide insulated gate grips for opening and closing gates. Do not depend on electric fences to restrain bulls, boars and other vicious animals, and keep the fence-line weeds mowed. If an owner has lightning livestock insurance he should at once notify the insurance adjuster, and a veterinarian for his professional diagnosis—without the latter, collection of insurance claims may be difficult.

Silo Poisoning (Silo Filler's Disease; Nitrogen Dioxide Poisoning). This is not an animal disease; it affects only humans engaged in filling or cleaning silos—usually it is corn silage. It is probably due to the reduction of nitrates in corn resulting in nitrogen dioxide—a heavy gas, yellow in color—that settles in the bottom of the silo. Sometimes the yellowish gas remains lodged in the chute, and this settles when laborers go into the silo to clean out old spoiled ensilage or to refill it. Animals have been poisoned by eating this discarded material.

A human disease

In humans a pneumonia, frequently followed by death, has been the result. Never enter a silo if a yellow gas is noticed, or if there is spoiled yellow ensilage. Always give the silo, and the chute, a good airing, especially at the bottom, before entering.

CHAPTER XXII

CONTROL, AND COSMETIC DEVICES, AND AILMENTS

Many species of animals are naturally endowed with defensive organs or parts that at times make them dangerous to others of the same group and to their attendants. Other animals, cattle, swine and sheep especially, need to be operated upon so that they may meet the requirements of domestication. These steps constitute control and cosmetic devices.

Cattle because of their size and strength need to be controlled by special methods of restraint. In the simpler procedures of control of cattle that are **Restraining** thoroughly domesticated, as the "family **cattle** cow," grasping the nostrils by means of the thumb and fingers is sufficient. In applying the same principle a metal nose clamp (bull leader, nose lead) may be used. For the domesticated, though always potentially dangerous, bull use a rigid staff or metal rod about six feet long snapped into the nose ring; it compels the animal to maintain a safe distance from his leader.

When cattle are to be branded, dehorned, spayed in the standing position, bled in the taking of blood samples, as well as during spraying, vaccinat**Special** ing and comparable procedures they must **methods of** ordinarily be confined in stocks, (Figs. 87 **restraint** and 88), a stanchion or "squeeze" (Fig. 89). For control during trimming of their feet it is desirable to have in the stanchion a sling so that the animal cannot assume recumbency. On large cattle ranches where numbers must receive treatment or attention some very ingenious devices in the form of alleys, corrals and gateways have been contrived. Many

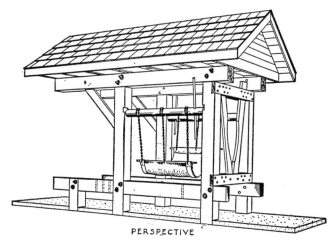

PERSPECTIVE

FIG. 87. Cattle stocks used in handling exhibition animals or valuable breeding stock where it is necessary to get the animal off its feet. The roof reduces deterioration from rain and sun.

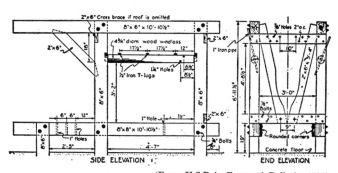

SIDE ELEVATION END ELEVATION

(From U.S.D.A. Farmers' Bulletin 1584)

FIG. 88. Details of the construction of the cattle stocks shown.

practicing veterinarians have stanchions that may be attached to their automobiles as "trailers."

There are times when it is most expedient or absolutely necessary to cast an animal for proper control.

Casting cattle
On ranches the young or smaller animals are cast by means of a lariat and a rider on a trained horse. Once down, the neck is twisted by pulling the animal's muzzle into an up-

ward direction; then another attendant seated behind
the animal pushes the undermost hind limb forward
with his foot just above the hock joint (Fig. 93) and
at the same time the uppermost hind limb is grasped
and pulled strongly backward. This is an ideal position
for the emasculation of either male or young females.

The casting of individual cattle of large size and
strength is sometimes necessary and for this the rope
Casting
individuals around the body is the standard method
(Fig. 90). The animal is tied, low down, to
a strong post or tree trunk. Then a
long rope—about one-half inch in diameter—is attached to the animal's head or around the neck, back-

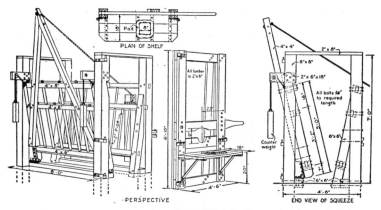

(From U.S.D.A. Farmers' Bulletin 1584)

FIG. 89. Cattle stanchion or squeeze with movable side. The
drawing in the center shows a detachable gate that is used
to stop the animal when it is to be branded and for holding
the head firm when dehorning. The padded hole for the nose
is shown at the top.

ward over the upper border of the neck and withers to
encircle the body just back of the fore-limbs, continued
backward along the region of the back up to the hip
bones, where the body is again encircled, and then
backward to a free end. At the points where the body
is encircled the rope must not be tied—simply a slip

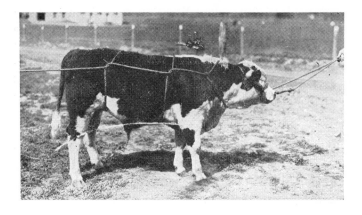

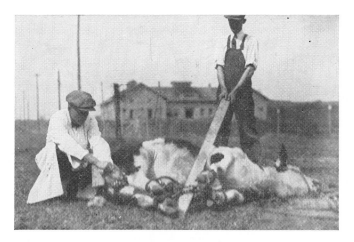

FIGS. 90 and 91. Half-hitch method of casting and confining cattle.

knot, so that when the free end is pulled upon the encircling rope will readily tighten around the two places of encirclement. A strong steady pull by one or two men will cause the strongest and most vigorous, and most recalcitrant animal to go down, so that its feet may be tied together and its head and neck twisted backward. When the feet are tied together a ten foot fence post of four inch diameter, may be laid cross wise over the body (Fig. 91) with one end under the tied feet and the other end held down by an attendant. This is known as the cattle-casting "half-hitch." The disadvantages of the half-hitch are (1) it compresses the heart and lungs thus affecting these organs especially in fat cattle; (2) it compresses the organs of digestion thus giving rise to bloat; (3) in male animals it frequently results in damage to the penis, and in dairy animals it exerts undue pressure on some of the mammary blood vessels.

Disadvantages of the "half-hitch"

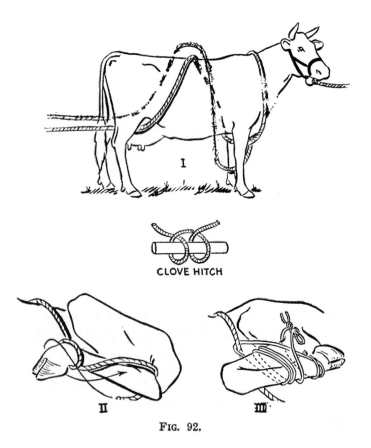

CLOVE HITCH

I

II   III

FIG. 92.

The objections against the "half-hitch" are overcome in an improved hitch (Fig. 92). Required are a strong halter, a bull lead and a 40 foot **An improved cattle-casting hitch** length of rope. Secure the animal by means of the halter. Place the rope over the withers and bring the ends down along the sides of the neck and backward between the forelegs to cross beneath the breast bone (sternum) ; continue the ends along the sides so that they cross over the region of the loins (dorso-lumbar area), and then downward and backward between the udder or scrotum and the inner surface of the hind limbs. The two ends should emerge a short distance above the points of the hocks. A strong pull on such a hitch will bring the animal to the ground. Separate lengths of rope may be used to confine the legs.

It is recognized that when deep chested animals such as cattle, sheep and goats are kept on their back or side (for a matter of minutes in the **Death as a result of back or side recumbency** case of sheep, longer in others) death from congestion of the lungs and closely related conditions — interstitial oedema, and alveolar hemorrhage—may occur. Bloat of the rumen is not a factor. Therefore, when

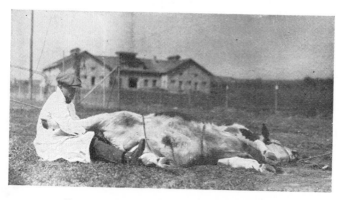

FIG. 93. Method of holding hind limbs.

these animals have been cast they must be released as soon as possible.

Lashing cattle against a board fence   Simply lashing a bovine against a strong board fence or gate is at times enough to obtain the desired degree of physical control over the animal.

In the quieting of cattle that, when in a corral, are difficult to approach, a solution of a tranquilizing agent is sometimes shot—by means of a special gun—into their muscles. This quiets the animals so that they may be approached.

Horses that are accustomed to being handled may, if necessary, be controlled by strongly grasping the upper lip (muzzle or "nose") with the

Twitching the horse's nose   fingers, or by using a mechanical device in the same manner. Usually this mechanical device is a piece of rope about twelve inches long and having a diameter of one-fourth inch passed through a hole in the end of a broom or axe handle and tied so as to leave a loop. This loop is placed around the animal's muzzle, and tightened by twisting the handle on its long axis.

It must be emphasized that to use such a twitch on a horse's muzzle for any purpose other than to obtain temporary control over the animal is inhumane. The horse's muzzle is probably its most sensitive organ —it is highly endowed with sensory nerves, and there-

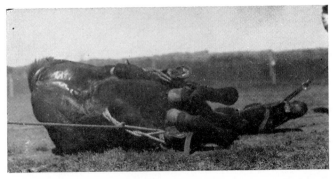

FIG. 94. A horse cast and tied for control in field surgical work.

fore a twitch applied unnecessarily, or for too long a time, for the objective of using it as a lead, or for the holder of the handle to rest a part of his weight on it is an abuse of power that no lover of the horse can

Casting a horse a major step condone. Sometimes a horse must be cast (Fig. 94) so as to have it under complete control but such a step is fraught with danger—broken bones and other injuries —and should therefore be attempted only by a trained experienced person.

Large hogs, especially boars, are very muscular, bulky and frequently dangerously vicious. There are

Boars snubbed to a post mechanical contrivances by means of which a piece of woven wire or light chain may be placed in the animal's mouth back of the tusks so as to encircle the region and the free end tied to a post. Sometimes a looped rope is used in the same manner. Confined in this way the hog will pull back to the limit of his power and during this time submit to many remedial or corrective steps. There are some occasions when the foregoing described method of control is only the preliminary step. Additional steps are to tie the four limbs together and then by pulling upward on the leg rope so as to keep the feet elevated from the ground, prevent the animal from getting on its knees.

Horses frequently attempt to tear surgical bandages off their limbs and other parts of the body by

How to prevent biting of wounds and "self sucking" means of their teeth, and cattle resort to "self-sucking" (page 415). Usually these practices may be inhibited by preventing the animal from backward bending of its neck. One method is to apply a "cradle" to the animal's neck. Such a device consists of ten or twelve rigid sticks, each eighteen inches to two feet in length, about three-fourths inch thick and one inch wide, laid parallel to each other—slightly divergent towards one end, properly spaced from each other, and held together by two straps of leather—one at the upper end and the other at the lower. When this is placed around the animal's neck it limits side movement of this member though it does not interfere with grazing or other necessary up and down motions.

Sometimes the desired degree of control can be obtained by placing a halter on the animal's head and **A simple device** a surcingle around the body just back of the fore limbs. Then attach one end of a rigid stick (broom handle) to the halter and the other end to the surcingle so that it will be either along the right or left side of the neck and shoulder. It should not pass between the fore limbs.

Ringing bulls and swine. Bulls are potentially killers. It is their inherited characteristics to perpetuate **The ringing of bulls is necessary to control them as they are usually very vicious** their control over their harem. This instinct of offense and defense is extended against all other living mammals including man, though not usually operative against the female of his own species. This natural aggressiveness frequently develops into actual viciousness, especially against man, because the latter is determined to maintain his control in general over the animal, thus resulting in frequent clashes, with man the usual winner.

The bull, however, does not forget his defeats. Close confinement, and the absence of free association with his females, together with the consciousness of his terrific brute strength make him a constant menace to those entrusted with his care and handling. The known vicious bull is usually watched but fatalities are common where an attendant is suddenly turned upon during a moment of unguardedness or possibly because of a misplaced trust in what he considers to be a comparatively gentle animal. No bull after having passed the age of calfhood is to be trusted in regard to the attitude he may assume towards humans. The latter's defensive forces must at all times be augmented by artificial devices. Furthermore, the bull must be made more susceptible to attack, and more amenable to handling by various agencies, of which the placing of a ring in the highly sensitive region of the nose to serve as a means of control is a preferred method (page 153).

The important point to remember is to place the ring through the septum just within the nostrils. If **The correct** it is placed higher it acts as a constantly **method of** painful agent which not only serves as an **inserting a** irritant, but which may even result in loss **ring in a** of condition because of the never-ending **bull** pain. Place it just within the nostrils, or in other words, just back of the muzzle. A rigid bull-leader or "staff" should be the control intermediary between the attendant and the ring in the animal, but leading should still be done by means of the usual halter or horn rope, because the staff and ring are purely control devices; the halter or horn rope is a leading device. To disregard the principle of each of these devices is to inflict unnecessary punishment upon the animal, and at times it may even result in lacerating the region by tearing the ring through the muzzle.

Neither should the ring be too large in relation to the size of the animal, as it then hangs too close to the mouth and interferes with grazing and eating.

Bulls that are free in a paddock or pasture may have a mask put over the face. Usually this is a strong **Restricting** halter with a metal shield securely **free bulls** fastened to it in such a manner that the eyes of the bull are covered; he can look neither sidewise, up or straight ahead, but he can look downward along his nose to the ground. It prevents sudden charges.

Ringing pigs through the rim of the snout is performed to keep these animals from harmful rooting— **How to ring** to inhibit lung worm (page 678) infesta- **a hog** tion for example—and it is quite effective. It is a harmless procedure so long as the rings are not placed too deeply. In the latter event, injury to the more deeply located tissues may cause so much discomfort that a minor unthriftiness results.

A more sound method of overcoming or preventing excessive rooting is to supply the hogs with a balanced ration including some protein (page 40)

A good protein ration obviates the necessity of ringing hogs in the form of tankage. It is recognized that excessive rooting is the animal's method of attempting to obtain protein in the form of grubs and other forms of subterranean life, and if this protein is supplied in some form in the regular ration, the animal's search for it will be discontinued.

Dehorning is practiced on cattle, sheep and goats. Unless the horns are desirable as a distinctive breed characteristic, their eruption and growth should be prevented, or their subsequent removal is to be advocated. When several horned animals are kept confined in a small space, they will inflict serious injuries upon each other.

Eruption of horns may be prevented if the necessary steps are taken during the first week after birth,

How to prevent horn growth or kids should be not more than three days of age. A small area about the size of a five cent piece is denuded of hair at the place where the horn usually makes its appearance. Brush the area as clean as possible with a stiff brush but use no water or other liquid. The solution used consists of drugs having the degree of purity listed in the United States Pharmacopeia and announced* as having the following formula: finely ground anhydrous antimony trichloride 28%, salicylic acid 7%, and flexible collodion 65%, all by weight. Applied to the horn button it is practically painless, non-toxic if used as recommended, not irritating to the udder of the dam, and very highly effective. It is applied to the horn button with a small brush. The

---

*This formula was developed and perfected by Dr. Hess and Clark, Ashland, Ohio, and is marketed by them under the trade name of "Pol."

calf is restrained until the solution has dried, this being hastened by blowing on it. The resulting film drops off in three or four weeks, without any evidence of scurs at a later period.

At a somewhat later period in the animal's growth when small horns have made their appearance, and **The removal** when they are no more than skin append- **of new horn** ages or they have not yet contracted a **growth is** union with the bones of the skull, they **described** may be surgically removed. At this period of their development the small horn when grasped is readily movable by shifting it and its surrounding skin.

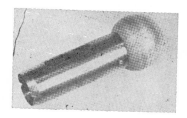

FIG. 95. Calf dehorner.

A humane method of surgical removal may be practiced under the influence of a previously injected local anaesthetic solution. Removal at this age does not involve the skull. In order to avoid infections, the wound should be kept clean. For this operation a dehorner having a full circle cutting edge (Fig. 95) is used on calves 2 to 6 months old.

When the horns have attained full growth, they are attached to the skull bones. As the animal ages, the **The relation** space or cavity in the horns becomes **between the** larger, and it is soon in direct anatomical **horn core** communication with a large cavity in the **and the** skull known as the frontal sinus; it, in **frontal sinus** turn, has a very small slitlike passageway to the nasal cavity or nose. All of these cavities and passageways are lined by a highly sensitive mucous membrane. The significance of this is that as a result of dehorning, the frontal sinus is opened, and unless protected, is exposed to germ contamination. As a result, a situation frequently ensues in which the animal suffers excruciating pain for days at a time, and there is a serious disturbance of the general health.

There are at least two mechanical devices for removal of the horns, i.e., the saw and the dehorning shear. Because of the toughness of the horn, the saw is the instrument of choice for dehorning the bull and older females. It should be a fine-toothed saw so as to reduce splintering of the tissues to a minimum. Furthermore, during the operation the animal's head is to be so inclined that none of the bone-dust and no dirt will fall into the frontal sinus. An electrically energized (Fig. 96) horn removing saw is on the market but it is noisy and frightens animals. It is not recommended.

Instruments and dehorning

The dehorning shears are preferred for the removal of horns wherever they may be successfully employed,

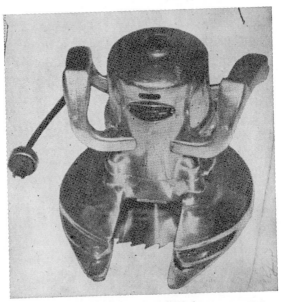

FIG. 96. Electrically energized horn remover.

which is on comparatively soft horn, on females, steers and very young entire males. The work may be more quickly performed than by other means, and there is no bone-dust to fall into the sinus.

In order to prevent the pain of removal and the possibility of subsequent sinus infections, the operation when practical, such as in the instance of the family cow or when only a few animals are to be operated upon, should be performed in as humane and clean a manner as possible. By means of the injection of a local anaesthetic solution over the sensory nerve supplying the part, or into the tissues surrounding it, the operation may be performed with practically no pain, and this is highly recommended. The graduate veterinarian is qualified to render this humane service to man's foster mother.

For some unexplainable reason, it has become a general custom to perform the dehorning operation **Sinus** without regard for the probability of seri- **infection** ous wound infection including that of the **following** frontal sinus, with the result that the after **dehorning** effects, especially in the more mature animals, are frequently quite serious. All of this may be prevented by being clean about the surgical steps and by applying to the wound an antiseptic dressing maintained in position by a bandage. All wound and sinus contamination may be avoided, insect infestation prevented, and bleeding controlled by resorting to good after treatment of the wound. EI-335 (page 303) is a good preparation to use, but keep it out of the sinus.

Horn weighting: There are no exact rules in regard to the "weighting" or training of the horns of show cattle. Quite often however because of show-ring demands horns have to be trained downward.

A good procedure in the case of 9- to 14-month-old calves is to use one-pound weights for each horn—for

Method of weighting older cattle use heavier weights. Leave the weights on for a week and then take them off so as to rest the animal. Further application of weights should be made at intervals until the desired downward curvature is obtained.

If the weights are too heavy or if left on too long the horns may develop a break and become unsightly. Unusual tenderness at or near the base of a horn will necessitate immediate removal of the weights.

Tail docking and castration of lambs. These operations are necessary to prevent soiling of the hind quarters, and to avoid the development of inferior meat on coarse ram-lambs.

The two operations are usually performed at the same time when the lambs are from seven days to two weeks of age. If the operations are delayed beyond this age there is more danger from bleeding, and because larger wounds are made there is more danger of infection.

The method of docking and castrating lambs The lambs are usually tightly grasped by all four limbs with their back resting against the body of an assistant. The greatest difficulty is experienced in cleansing the proposed site of the castration, because of its wool covering. This latter is also responsible for more than an ordinary amount of filth in the region. However, cleansing must be attempted, and should be reasonably well performed, including the use of some two percent water dilution of saponated cresol solution (page 263). Then the lower third of the scrotum is amputated with a clean knife, the testicles pulled down through the wound, and the cord divided about two inches above the testicle by means of scraping it with the edge of a dull knife; this method prevents bleeding. The wound is then to be douched with some of the clean antiseptic solution set aside for this purpose. *Caution!* Do not use the solution that has become impregnated with dirt during the preliminary washing of the scrotum.

The tail amputation or docking is then performed, preferably by means of the cherry-red heated iron docking pincers. The site of amputation is from two to three inches back of the tail's union with the body. In order to avoid burning the lamb, a device commonly used is a piece of board two inches thick through which a hole has been bored large enough to permit the tail being passed through; the board is held against the animal's buttocks and the amputation is then effected just back of the board by means of the hot pincers. The principal advantages in the use of the pincers are that if not used too rapidly, they sear the blood vessels shut so as to control bleeding, and at the same time they sterilize the wound.

During recent times a new instrument, the "Elastrator," has been introduced to American sheep raisers from New Zealand to be used for the castration and docking of lambs. By means of the "elastrator" specially designed elastic bands are applied to the neck of the bag (scrotum), and to the tail at the point it is desired to effect amputation. About two or three weeks later the scrotum and the contained testicles slough off with the wounds practically healed. During the fly season the tail is amputated by means of a knife, though leaving the elastic ring in position to slough off later with the distal stump of the tail. In view of the fact that tetanus is such a common sequel of the usually filthy areas in wooly animals it seems that this might be a complication here, i.e., the tetanus (page 542) germ localized in the raw wound, and its very potent toxin passing even the barriers interposed by the elastic rings. (Page 352 of the Nov. 1949 issue of the Journal of the American Veterinary Med. Assoc. reports tetanus losses following the use of the elastrator.) At any rate, watch lambs operated on by this device, and at the first sign

A new instrument for castrating and docking lambs

of tetanus use plenty of pure tincture of iodine on the recesses of the wounds. We can neither recommend nor condemn this instrument.

The Burdizzo emasculatome is the pincers used in the so-called bloodless castration of animals having a pendant scrotum such as bull calves and ram lambs. The jaws of the instrument must be placed on the cords of the testicles one at a time within the neck of the scrotum or bag. By this means the cord, which is the anatomical structure made up of the blood vessels and nerves and other structures to and from each testicle, is crushed in its natural location, and without creating an outside wound. The testicles shrink away if the operation has been performed by one skilled in the correct technique. If incorrectly performed a "stag" is the result.

Still another method of castrating and docking

For docking the Burdizzo instrument is clamped on the tail at the proposed site of amputation and all tissue-bone, muscle, and skin—is crushed. By means of a knife, while the jaws of the instrument are still in position, the amputation is effected just back of the point where the jaws of the instrument are applied; then the pincers are removed. In the few cases seen by us of docking performed in this manner the tail bone was so badly crushed that we would hesitate to designate this technique an approved surgical procedure. It may be classed with the blunt hatchet method, next described.

Some sheep herders amputate the tail by means of a dull-edged hatchet. If the hatchet is sharp there is likely to be a good deal of bleeding, though a dull blade crushes the vessels, and usually with only a minimum of bleeding. Unfortunately the dull-edged blade also crushes the bone and other tissues so that healing is delayed, and infection invited. The hatchet method of amputation, therefore, is not recommended.

Amputation may also be effected by means of a knife, though this is a slow method and not well adapted where many animals are to be operated upon. It necessitates encircling of the root of the tail with a piece of tape in order to control bleeding. This may be removed thirty minutes later. The skin of the tail is pushed forward as far as possible, then the amputation is effected through the joint. The skin then is permitted to slip back into its normal position so as to form a pad or covering for the stump.

An instrument for castration and docking intended for use when large numbers of animals are to be operated upon is the so-called "All-in-One" castrator.

In both the castration and docking operation, the important point is cleanliness, and occasionally the control of bleeding.

Failure to observe cleanliness is not infrequently followed by infection of the wound with the germ of tetanus or "lock-jaw" (page 542). The most pronounced symptom is rigidity or stiffness of all muscles. When it develops, the wounds must be freely opened to their deepest recesses, and pure tincture of iodine (page 276) applied. If the value of the animal warrants it, a veterinarian should be requested to administer the specific antiserum treatment.

Tetanus may be a sequel of filthy methods of operating on lambs

When excessive, from the docking wound, bleeding may be controlled by applying a tape around the root of the tail for thirty minutes. In the case of bleeding from the castrating wound, it may be best to try to locate the bleeding vessel and then tie a clean string around it. Failing to find the bleeding vessel, the next best step is to pack the wound cavity with some clean absorbent cotton which may be retained in position by a few stitches placed across the lips of the wound.

Amputation of the wattles or "dubbing" in fowls.
It is quite a common occurrence for fowls, males in
particular, to contract infections of the
Amputation
of the wattles wattles because of abraiding these organs
necessary to when they are dragged over the ground as
prevent the bird eats, and the germ of fowl cholera
infection also localizes there. The result of these infections is quite a severe swelling of the wattles referred to as "oedema of the wattles." The absorption
of germ toxins or poisons from the swollen organs induces a state of ill health accompanied by enough weakness so that the bird is not able to defend itself from
aggression by the more vigorous members of the flock.

Prevention is reasonably effective by keeping some
disinfectant such as permanganate of potash (pages
116 and 271) in the drinking water, so that whenever
the fowl takes a drink the wattles will be simultaneously suspended in the water and thus be subjected to
disinfection as frequently as the bird drinks.

A more effective and practical preventive frequently resorted to in those sections of the country
where intensive poultry husbandry is practiced, is to
amputate the wattles. The jaws of a pair of strong
compression forceps are made to encompass the wattles close to their attachment. By means of a pair of
curved scissors or a knife, closely following the under
surface of the jaws of the forceps, the wattles are cut
off. The raw edge of the wound is then brushed with
some tincture of chloride of iron in order to stop bleeding, after which the forceps are removed. If there is
any tendency to bleed afterwards, some more of the
tincture of chloride of iron may be applied, or some
powdered alum is almost equally effective. The fowl
recently operated upon is to be kept isolated until
healing is complete.

Claw and spur trimming (see page 380). The claws
of male birds occasionally severely injure the backs of

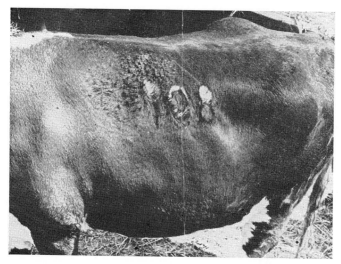

(Courtesy Lewis B. Jackson, Chm. Hide Co., Tanners' Council of America)

FIG. 97. Branding scar on a live animal. A valuable portion of the skin has been ruined for hide manufacture.

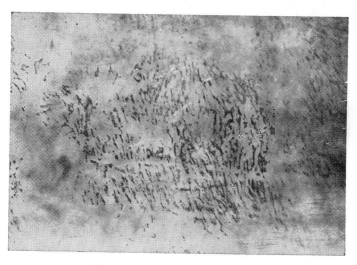

(Courtesy Dr. Fred O'Flaherty, University of Cincinnati)

FIG. 98. Bacterial hide damage from improper curing—unclean hide and salt.

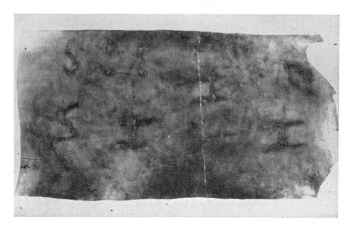

(Courtesy Lewis B. Jackson, Chm. Hide Co., Tanners' Council of America)
FIG. 99. Branding scars on a piece of tanned leather.

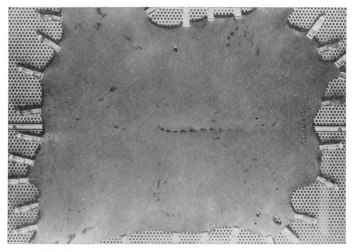

(Courtesy Dr. Fred O'Flaherty, University of Cincinnati)
FIG. 100. Hide damage by curry-comb markings.

Claw and spur trimming prevents injury to the back of the female the females. Spurs are potentially dangerous during fighting of cocks. Sharp pointed claws and spurs may be blunted by means of a file, or partially amputated with a tinner's shear, or any comparable cutting instrument. Caged birds such as canaries and parrots, because there is no wear on the claws, must be so trimmed.

Branding. When hot-iron branding is resorted to it should be applied to the less valuable parts of the hide **Place needed brands only on the jaw, neck or shoulder** such as the jaw, neck or shoulder. To brand in other places (Figs. 97, 98 and 99) reduces the value of the sole leather portion, and such a practice is estimated to cost American cattlemen several million dollars annually.

Sheep Branding: This is done for the purpose of establishing ownership, and paints are used during the breeding season. The ownership brand must be reasonably permanent, and at the same time it must be scour-

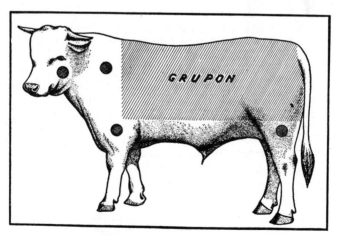

(Courtesy Lewis B. Jackson, Chm. Hide Co., Tanners' Council of America)

Fig. 101. No brand is to be placed on the "grupon." Preferred branding sites are indicated by circular markings.

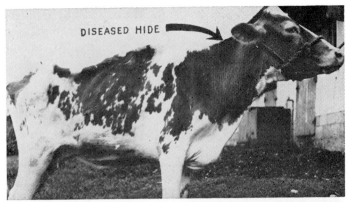

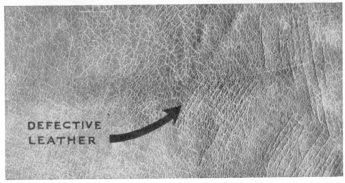

(Courtesy Dr. Fred O'Flaherty, University of Cincinnati)

FIG. 102. A defective hide from unhealthy cow.

A sheep branding formula   able from the standpoint of the wool processor. A formula for this purpose having the desirable characteristics (tentatively approved under the name "Development of Scourable Sheep-Branding Fluids" and issued June, 1950, by the Production and Marketing Administration, Livestock Branch of the U. S. D. A.) has the following composition:

Lanolin................................100 parts by weight

Carbon tetrachloride...........25 parts by volume

Pigment................................3 parts by weight

The pigments used during the research phase of the project were carbon black, chromic oxide green, ferric oxide yellow, ferric oxide red, and ultramarine blue. The black and the red colors were most satisfactory.

The scouring consisted of three 1-minute baths in 0.75 per cent soda (probably sal soda R. R. D.) 0.075 **Scouring fluids used** per cent soap at 130° F., and one 1-minute rinse at 110° F. Each bath was followed by passing the wool through a pair of squeeze rolls. All colors were found to be completely "scourable."

Hide injuries are also caused by deep currying (Fig. 100), parasites, skin diseases (Fig. 102), etc. Injuries and preventable skin diseases also constitute causes of skin injury. Cuts, deep scratches, mange (page 727), warble-fly (page 706), ringworm (page 567), bloody warts (page 428) all exact a toll from the hide.

Sexing Baby Chicks. The method most generally used in America was introduced by the Japanese who probably acquired it from the Chinese. It necessitates an examination of the vent or cloaca (page 24) of the day old chick. Because of the smallness of the vent at this age the difference between the two sexes is detectable only by those thoroughly familiar with the anatomy of the parts, and then only after a good deal of experience and practice. It is important to know how to apply the correct pressure on the abdominal region of the chick in order to expose the anatomical parts. The method consists in detecting the very minute male process, *which some pullets also have.* It appears as a small elevation about the size of the point of a pin on the floor of the median aspect of the urodeum, sometimes described as a white spot. The lining membrane of the cloaca of the chick is divided from the rear to the front by three folds; fold number one is the mucous membrane at the vent, fold number two is the beginning of the urodeum, and fold number three the coprodeum. The male process is located on the median ventral portion of fold number two. Important landmarks are enlarged folds situated on each side of the male process. These folds are usually identified before the male process can be located.

Location of the male process

Unfortunately no two processes in the same breed have the same appearance, and there are greater differences between breeds. *Many pullets show evidences of these processes.* The male process, "whether it is long or broad or both" is the characteristic of the male. Some processes are dark in color and others have the same color as the mucous lining of the cloaca. The chick is held up-ended so as to expose the vent. The fingers of the other hand expose fold number two, the urodeum. When there is any doubt further pressure so as to partially evert fold number two will cause all of this to disappear in the case of the *pullet.* The difference in size of processes is the distinguishing feature.

When a male and when a female

(Bulletin 307 entitled "Distinguishing Sex of Chicks at Hatching" has been issued by the Kansas Agricultural Experiment Station, Manhattan, Kans. It discusses sexing by various other methods.)

Sex Control in Chicks: There is a claim that if fertile hen's eggs are wetted, for a few seconds, before incubation, in a solution of a male hormone or a female hormone that the resulting hatch will be males and females respectively(the process is patented).

In regard to the above, research by an independent research worker, in general reports that: (1) Dipping of eggs in estrogen solutions is an effective means of penetration of the shell so that "embryonic sex differentiation is modified." (2) However, the testes at six months of age are small and there is delayed spermatogenesis. In females from eggs that were hormone treated, one oviduct, the left—the left is almost always the functioning one, the right rarely develops—was of insufficient size to receive the ovum resulting in abdominal cavity ovulation and therefore such females were frequently not layers of normal eggs. (See page 353).

Flight Control: There are several methods to control flight in both thoroughly domesticated fowl, and wild fowl held in confinement.

The simplest method is to shorten or clip the wing feathers. In wild fowl this usually means to start the clipping of the bird almost from the day that the wing feathers appear repeating the clipping **Clipping** every ten days or two weeks for as long **wing** a period as it is desired to keep the bird **feathers** in confinement. In birds intended for breeding or show sale there is objection to this method.

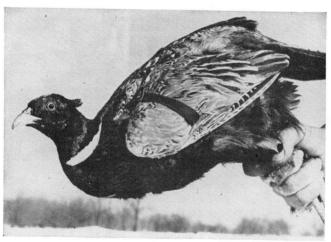

(Courtesy Joe Munroe—"Farm Quarterly")
Fig. 103. Brailing to control flight.

A second device (Fig. 103) much used to prevent flight of game birds that are temporarily held in captivity, to be released at an opportune time, **The use of** is to place a brail over one wing in such **a brail** a manner as to prevent the bird from extending its wing for flight at from ten to sixteen weeks of age, varying with different species. The brail is a Y-shaped leather thong with buckle.

The third method (Fig. 104) prevents flight though some of the birds operated upon may learn to fly well enough to escape from low type enclosures. It consists in the surgical division of a tendon so that the bird is not capable of extending the wing for flight. The ends of the severed tendon do not re-unite so flight is permanently impaired. Best results are obtained if the opera-

Division of a tendon

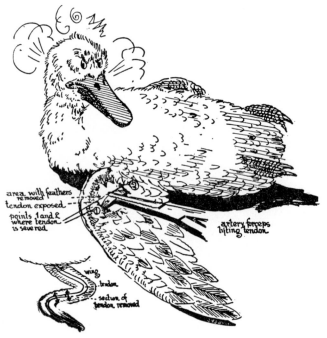

area with feathers removed
tendon exposed
points 1 and 2 where tendon is severed

artery forceps lifting tendon

wing
tendon
section of tendon removed

FIG. 104. Tendon division permanently destroys the ability to fly.

tion is performed with the surgical area under the influence of a local anesthetic.

The *wing-tip amputation* is highly recommended for permanent results. In it the wing tip external to the outer wing joint is removed, except for the small appendage on the leading edge. Feathers are removed

The wing-tip removal from the area, which is swabbed with grain alcohol (a 2 per cent procaine may be used for anesthesia). The skin is retracted medially as much as possible, and an incision made quickly in a circular motion down to the bone on all sides. The bone is cut with forceps, after which the skin and muscle tissue is permitted to return to position. The edges of the wound are drawn as closely together as possible and fixed by means of a mattress type suture to the underlying muscle tissue. The wound should be dusted with an antiseptic powder, and the bird released.

Even following this operation birds learn to fly in low circles so as to escape from predators. Wing feathers soon cover the incision so that it is almost impossible to detect the operation. In order to avoid needless mutilation this operation is best entrusted to the experienced veterinary surgeon. Sometimes there is bleeding so that ligation of blood vessels becomes necessary.

Caponizing: This is the emasculation of male fowl so that they lose the male characteristics. It is done to increase their weight and improve tenderness of the flesh for table purposes.

Surgically the removal of the cock's testicles is a major operation because of the intra-abdominal location of the testicles and their proximity to large blood vessels. To remove all of the testicular tissue and avoid **Surgical caponizing** injury to the near-by large blood vessel is a feat that can be successfully performed only by the experienced. Results are unsatisfactory if any remnants are left.

The testicles, usually about bean size though this varies in different breeds and at different seasons, are just below the anterior part of the kidneys. In fact, the right one is far enough forward to be in contact with the liver. The preferred age for the caponizing of cockerels is when they are from eight to ten weeks old. At this age Leghorns weigh about one pound and heavier breeds from one and one-half to one and three-fourths pounds. Feed and water are withheld from the fowl for 12 to 18 hours previous to the operation.

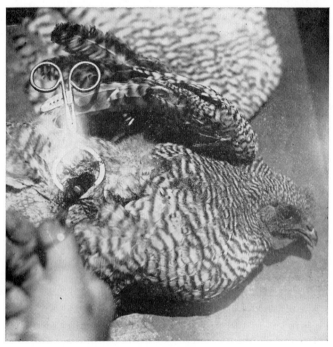

FIG. 105. In surgical caponizing the testicle is clearly visible through the center of the wound.

The testicles are reached through an incision between the two last ribs on the birds right side (Fig. 105). (For details of the operation the reader is referred to Bulletin No. 333 entitled "Capon Production in South Dakota" issued by Agricultural Experiment Station, South Dakota State College, Brookings, S. D., or Bulletin 315 entitled "Capon Production" issued by Agricultural Experiment Station, Kansas State University, Manhattan, Kansas.)

During recent years so-called *chemical caponizing* has been widely used. The chemical used is diethylstilbestrol; its shorter—though incorrect—name is stilbestrol (page 104). The chemical effect is to feminize the male. Usually the diethylstilbestrol which is a synthetic hormone—pellet, containing not

Feminizing by means of a hormone more than fifteen milligrams (this is maximum dosage permitted per bird by the U. S. Food and Drug Administration) is injected under the neck skin by means of a specially devised injector. The injection is not to be repeated. The maximum effects in male birds of any age are usually observed about six weeks after the implantation of the pellet. The time then is any time after male characteristics appear, or about six weeks before the marketing of broilers. The changes observed are loss of fighting instinct, paleness of the undeveloped comb and wattles, pale shanks and skin, and an increase in weight—the latter owing to the fact that the watery constituents of the muscle tissue are to an extent replaced by fat.

In older roosters with well developed sex characteristics the effects are the same as in broilers excepting that the already developed comb and wattles are not changed much from their usual male appearance. It is suggested that the heads be cut off before sale. The effects of an injection of diethylstilbestrol usually begin to disappear about eight to twelve weeks following the implantation of the pellet. This is the basis for the use of these pellets in controlling the fighting of young tom turkeys (page 380), though turkeys do not seem to fatten so much. All the available information indicates definitely that the meat of birds unsexed by means of diethylstilbestrol is not in any manner reflected in humans consuming the meat. Apparently diethylstilbestrol does not leave a trace of this hormone-like substance in the flesh of implanted or fed birds.

"Self-Sucking" of cows: (page 393). This is an established habit of the occasional dairy cow in which

she reaches backward with her mouth to grasp a teat and thus remove and ingest her own milk. The vice once established is frequently difficult to correct.

In attempting to control the vice the simplest methods should be used first. Rubbing into the teats, either in the form of an ointment with a vaseline base or as a powder, such comparatively harmless drugs as sulphate of quinine, barbadoes aloes, or cayenne pepper may cause the animal to desist after a few tastes of these bitter or hot agents.

Correction by the use of bad tasting drugs

The rigid stick alongside an animal's neck colloquially known as a jockey stick, or the application of a cradle (page 393) are effective means of inhibiting the practice in some cows.

By means of a jockey stick or cradle

There are on the market ingenious devices. One of them attached to the nostrils has a hinged metal plate which falls over the animal's mouth whenever the head is raised to the level of the udder. Other than causing some nose irritation it is a harmless and frequently effective contraption.

By mechanical means

Another type of mechanical contrivance also attached to the animal's nose has several sharp metal prongs which prick the udder when the animal attempts to grasp a teat. The disadvantage is that some cows turn the head back towards the udder so quickly that the prongs actually penetrate the udder so as to produce wounds that are very susceptible to infection.

A dangerous device

Some cows acquire the habit of sucking milk from their mates. A practical control device consist of two rather small linked bull rings. One of the two rings is placed in the nose as in the bull (page 394) and the second is an appendage of the ring in the animal's nose. It does not interfere with grazing if the rings are not too large, and it frequently controls the habit.

Such devices as tongue splitting and partial tongue amputation should never be performed unless all other less severe methods have failed in their objective and only upon the advice of and by the qualified veterinarian. These tongue operations are bound to cause the animal some future difficulty in the prehension of food, and if improperly performed may ruin an otherwise valuable beast.

Surgical steps

Entropion of lambs: (page 186). This is the condition when at the lamb's birth a lower eyelid is turned in so that the lashes irritate the eyeball; if not corrected it ultimately results in blindness of the involved eye.

Not hereditary but a decided tendency in this direction

When the condition is detected within an hour or two after birth it may usually be corrected if the attendant, several times in succession, will manually turn the offending eyelid in an outward direction. A small strip of Scotch adhesive tape, or even a "band-aid" attached to the outer surface of the lid and lower down to the region of the face will assist in holding the lid in its proper position.

If the condition is not treated immediately after birth the lid soon becomes fixed in its abnormal position, and then an operation by a veterinarian becomes necessary for correction.

CHAPTER XXIII

SOME SURGICAL AILMENTS

The few ailments described are placed in a surgical grouping because methods of handling them are usually instrumental in nature, and because they require the services of the technically trained veterinarian for their correction. Horses—racing and riding—are on the increase (1961) and therefore the following discussion about the teeth of these animals.

Dental ailments.
1. Failure of temporary incisors to be shed. (Page 9.)
2. Failure of temporary molars to be shed. (Page 10.)
3. Sharp points on grinding teeth. (Page 11.)
4. Remnant teeth or "wolf teeth." (Page 11.)
5. Infection and inflammation occur at the roots of the permanent molars (Fig. 106), especially the first three and at a time usually corresponding to their eruption, or about the time the temporary caps are being shed. The outstanding symptoms are cautious mastication and a hard facial swelling directly over the root of the tooth. Surgical removal is usually necessary.
6. Split-teeth, elongated teeth and decayed teeth, in fact, almost all sequences of root infections, are common conditions.

When a horse is unthrifty though supplied with an abundance of food, or if mastication is cautious as indicated by holding the head to one side when chewing or drinking, when partially masticated food is rejected from the mouth, when salivation is excessive, when many particles of whole corn or other grains are found in

418

the manure, or if there is a bad mouth-odor, diseased teeth are to be suspected as a possible cause of the trouble; correctional steps should at once be instituted.

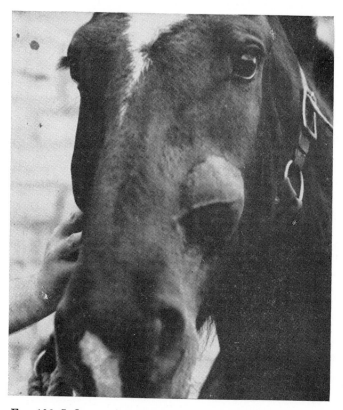

FIG. 106. Inflammation and infection at the root of a tooth.

7. Cattle are comparatively rarely affected with dental troubles (page 12) ; however, any of the suggestive symptoms in the horse should **Dental** also be considered suggestive in cattle. An **troubles rare** examination if positive will point to the **in cattle** proper method of handling and treatment.

Fluorosis (page 490) is a condition due to an excess of fluorine (page 83) usually in the drinking

The effect of fluorine on the teeth of cattle

water though also in some mineral mixtures. In humans mottling of the teeth and sometimes bone deformities are evidences of fluorosis. In animals mottling has no effect on the mastication of food, and because the life span of animals is so much shorter than in humans fluorine deposits on bones are virtually never observed clinically in animals, though the longer lived human may have bone deformities. Nevertheless the intelligent livestock owner will guard against an excess of fluorine in the water, minerals and feeds intended for his charges. Fluorosis is not a surgical condition; it is discussed here simply as a dental problem.

Sheep and goats have dental diseases as rarely as cattle.

Diseases of the teeth in dogs (page 12), especially the closely housed pets, are somewhat comparable to diseases of the human teeth. Caries or decay of the crown of a tooth is not uncommon, and may be treated by extraction, or sometimes burnishing and filling is practiced on these animals.

Dogs have dental ailments comparable to those in the human

A rather common ailment in house dogs, though also observed in horses and other domesticated animals, is an accumulation of tartar on the teeth usually at the point where the gums are in contact. If the tartar is not removed, infection will start its ravages in the gums followed by loosening and expulsion of the tooth. In house dogs it is an excellent plan to have the veterinarian scrape the teeth at least once a year to prevent excessive accumulation of tartar.

Castration of pigs and subsequent "bunch" formation. This operation is almost always performed as one of routine on the average farm by persons with no particular training in regard to surgical technique. The

Why
bunches
form fol-
lowing the
castration of
pigs, and
their pre-
vention

results are frequently disappointing, and still it is recognized that the value of the individual animal is so comparatively low that the employment of a trained and qualified person is seldom warranted.

Undoubtedly the commonest undesirable sequel of the improperly performed operation is the development of a "bunch," varying in size from a hazelnut to a man's head, in the scrotal region. Technically this is known as scirrhous cord. It is the result of filthy methods of operating, and of a faulty technique.

Prevention consists in being clean about the operation. The operator's hands and the operative area should be thoroughly washed with soap and warm water, to be followed by a rinsing with a two per cent dilution of saponated cresol solution (page 263). The instruments should be sterilized in boiling water.

There are three steps of importance to follow in performing the operation, i.e., to make a liberal incision over each testicle, to have the lower end of the incision well down between the hind limbs, and to divide the cord of the testicle about midway between the testicle and its point of entrance into the abdominal cavity.

If the incision is too small, it will heal on the outside before the inside of the wound has healed, with the result that any infection present in the deeper recesses of the wound is imprisoned. This favors "bunch" formation.

If the wound is not carried well down between the hind limbs there will result a "pocket" in which wound secretion will collect instead of being promptly evacuated. The accumulating material is an irritant and it favors "bunch" formation.

If the testicle is amputated from its cord at the point of union, it means that the long stump of the cord will be within reach of the infected outer portion of the wound where it is exposed to all sorts of irritation with the result that it will become inflamed; this favors "bunch" formation.

A careful regard for the sanitary and surgical steps outlined above will reward the owner of the animals with nicely developed barrows.

A very common practice in many rural communities of expectorating tobacco juice into the newly made castration wound is to be condemned as highly insanitary, and not likely to be followed by the best results.

Furthermore, a practice followed in both pigs and lambs of pulling out the testicles after their exposure is not in accordance with the best surgical principles, and though it is spectacular, it is not recommended.

Finally, when the operation is completed, and in season, the animal is to be turned into a clean, sun-exposed grass paddock. If the weather is unfavorable, a previously disinfected stall (page 215), well bedded with clean straw may be used for occupancy. Never permit animals recently operated upon to go into mud-wallows or dirty, dusty quarters; it is also best to keep them away from the dirt that is prevalent near the average barnyard habitation.

Actinomycosis or lumpy-jaw (page 801). This disease is observed in many species of domesticated animals, though with greatest frequency in cattle and swine. It results from the entrance into the hard or bone tissues of the ray-fungus *(Actinomyces bovis)*. These are widely distributed in nature on animal forage and surroundings. They enter the tissues through the wounds of recently erupted teeth or through injuries in the mouth from other causes, and through teat canals. It may even be inhaled into the lungs.

Actinomycosis occurs in various locations

It produces its characteristic symptoms wherever it locates. Thus in the region of the head in cattle it causes swelling of the bone of the jaw, (Fig. 107). In

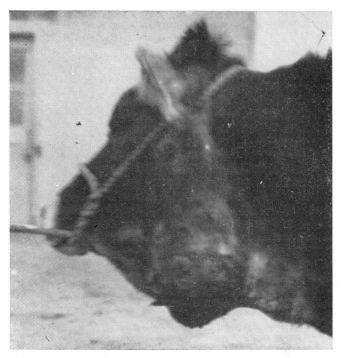

FIG. 107. Lumpy-jaw (Actinomycosis).

swine the usual site is in the mammary gland, the organism being acquired from contaminated ground as the teats drag over it (Fig. 109); in the male the testicles are not uncommonly invaded. Regardless of its place in the body the infection usually reaches the surface so that one or more outward openings or fistulae are established; avenues are thus created for the entrance of pus-producing germs or secondary invaders.

The handling of the condition is both surgical and medical. Surgical handling consists of lancing of the actinomycotic abscess so as to liberate the thick yellow pus contained therein. This pus should not be permitted to drain on the surroundings, but should be caught in an appropriate vessel. Otherwise, it will be a source of contaminating material for the later development

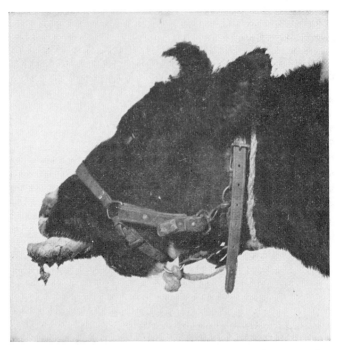

FIG. 108. Actinobacillosis of the tongue (wooden tongue).

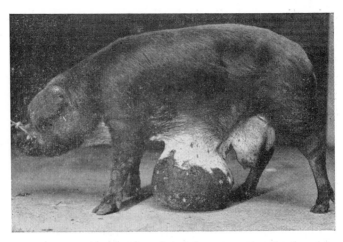

FIG. 109. Actinomycosis of the mammary gland.

of the disease in other animals. Medical treatment is used either to supplement the surgical treatment or alone when the ailment is in an inoperable region.

There is a disease of cattle, closely related clinically to actinomycosis, that is most frequently found in the

A disease resembling actinomycosis in the soft tissues
soft tissues of the jaw, and in the tongue —in the latter it is the so-called "wooden tongue." (Fig. 108.) This disease is *actinobacillosis* due to *Actinobacillus lignieresi.*

Both actinomycosis and actinobacillosis are iodine sensitive, though actinobacillosis is in addition very responsive to the sulfonamides such as sulfapyridine, sulfamethazine and sulfathiazole. These agents may well be used in addition to the conventional iodine. There is currently no form of vaccination.

Iodine in any of its various forms (page 276) is the most practical actinomyces destructive agent. In liquid form it may be packed into the wound on gauze saturated with it, or it may be administered by way of the mouth as iodide of potash. A particularly effective mode of administration is the intravenous injection of a single, sometimes a second, dose of iodide of soda (page 585). When animals are in the advanced stages of pregnancy there is an element of risk in the intravenous treatment. In swine, actinomycosis of the mammary gland is handled by complete surgical removal of all diseased tissue.

Fistulous Withers, and poll-evil in horses and mules. These are very common afflictions. The general nature

Fistula of the withers, and poll-evil are serious infections
of the two diseases is identical—they differ only in their location on the animal body. Both are more or less extensive invasions of the tissues of the regions mentioned, i.e., the withers, and the poll, with the germs of actinomycosis (page 422) (*Actinomyces bovis*) and brucellosis (page 578) *Brucella abortus* and various pus-producing germs. The exact reason for their predilection for the regions of the withers

and poll are not known, nor is there any certainty about predisposing causes though bruising is frequently accused.

The symptoms consist of a prominent swelling of the withers and poll. The swelling may be soft or firm, hot and painful, or without much inflammation at times. Usually it has broken open in one or more places with a discharge of pus and tissue debris.

Many unusual and sometimes harmful remedies have been employed for the attempted cure of these ailments. Some of the treatments in addition to being useless inflict torture upon the animal. In general, most of these so-called cures should be avoided. Fistulous withers and poll-evil are such complicated conditions that of all animal surgical ailments they are among the most difficult to bring to a successful termination. The underlying principles, in addition to recognized wound area preparation, that must be supplied are:

Establishment of good drainage so that wound secretions will flow away as rapidly as they form.

All diseased tissue must be removed from the wound, because as long as it is present, the outside wound will not heal.

The affected tissues must have a reasonably good blood supply or healing will be very slow and resistance to local infection will be very low.

A fistula of the withers in a horse is so situated anatomically that in some cases it is impossible to establish the drainage. These cases are incurable and no one can tell by an outward examination whether it is curable or not; in other words, it takes a complete, careful examination to determine the exact nature of the condition.

Fistula of the withers in the horse has in it a lot of dead neck ligament. So long as it is not completely removed surgically, the outside wound will not heal.

Sometimes this dead ligament is so deeply situated that it is almost impossible to get out.

The blood supply of the affected tissue in fistula is very poor, so that nature does not give very much assistance in this respect. Other factors to be considered are that in order to establish good drainage and to remove all diseased tissue may require such an extensive wound that it will blemish the animal badly, thus making it practically valueless even though the fistula may heal up satisfactorily.

Occasionally a fistula, because it is more or less superficial, will heal without very much treatment of any kind, but this is unusual. Many people believe in the use of different medicines to be injected into the fistula, but it is our experience that these have little if

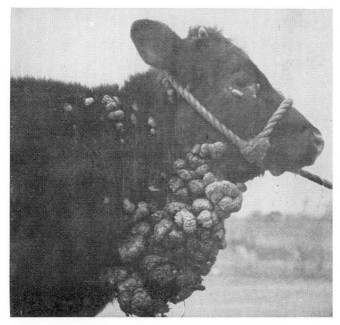

[Courtesy Dept. of Surgery and Medicine, School of Veterinary Medicine, Kansas State University]

FIG. 110. Bleeding warts contagious condition due to a virus.

any effect, and if healing follows their use, the chances are that healing would have taken place without the application of these remedies.

Taken as a whole, the question then resolves itself into the establishment of good drainage, surgical removal of dead tissue, and then trusting very largely to nature. If these principles can be established, all that remains to be done is to keep the outside of the wound clean. Furthermore, because of the highly technical character of all this work, a competent graduate veterinarian should be asked to do it.

Rupture or hernia in pigs. This is the passage of an abdominal organ, usually intestine, through a natural or artificial opening in the wall of the abdomen until it rests beneath the skin of the region. The natural openings most frequently involved are the navel in both males and females, and the inguinal passage ways for the cords of the testicles leading to the scrotum. Occasionally a pig receives an injury that tears the wall of the abdomen though it leaves the skin intact.

Research evidence indicates that the hernias through natural openings observed in many young pigs at ages varying from one day to one month are heritable (page 186), and that to a considerable extent their occurrence may be guarded against by the use of boars that are not ruptured or have never been ruptured. Furthermore, neither boar nor sow should be selected for breeding purposes if some of their litter mates were herniated. Such a program may not be entirely practical, nor does its rigid adoption insure all hernia-free offspring, but its adoption is advisable if the breeder is desirous of reducing the number of herniated pigs to a minimum.

Hernia in pigs inherited and its control

Bleeding "warts" on cattle; common warts of cattle (Fig. 110). These growths, technically *verruca vul-*

garis, are of common occurrence in cattle.

Bleeding warts of cattle are contagious. They spoil many other-wise good hides

It has been established that they are caused by a filterable virus. Their contagiousness is generally conceded and their inoculability is unquestioned because the appearance of one wart is usually followed by others so that several members of a herd may be affected.

Warts are commonest in young cattle, appearing on the sides of the head, neck and shoulders. Their size may vary from that of a pinhead to that of a man's head. When many of the larger warts are present, an animal becomes unthrifty.

Their principal economic importance rests in the injury they produce in the hide; tanners contend that holes appear in the tanned hide corresponding to the previous location of a wart. (Fig. 110.)

Because of the nature of the infection, prevention must rest largely in the isolation of affected animals until their recovery is assured. To disregard this is to leave open avenues for the spread of the condition.

The handling of the condition is both medical, and surgical, and possibly biological. The medical treatment is satisfactory only for the very small warts. The surgical treatment is to inject a local anaesthetic under each and then "cut it out;" simply "cutting off" the wart is of doubtful value. The biological treatment, the value of which has confirmatory clinical evidence, consists in using a formalin-killed wart vaccine. The services of a veterinarian will repay the owner in the handling of this condition.

Pasteurella mastitis in ewes; gangrenous mastitis in ewes; black garget; pink-bag; blue-bag in sheep (Fig. 111). This disease frequently affects several ewes in the same flock at lambing time. All the evidence points to an infection as the cause of the ailment —the germ *Pasteurella mastitidis* is the specific cause

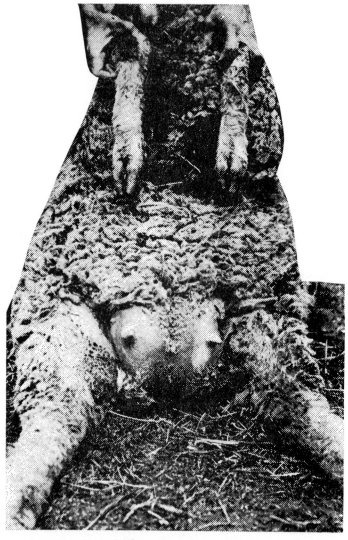

(Courtesy Montana Veterinary Research Laboratory)

FIG. 111. "Blue-bag" in a ewe.

Blue bag of ewes is a contagious condition. Its prevention is of the most importance though secondary germs usually invade the diseased udder as the ailment progresses. The discharge from the affected gland is highly infectious and ground contaminated by it is a source for the spread of the condition to other ewes. It may also be spread by the hands of the herder if it becomes necessary for him to handle these organs.

The condition develops as a hot, painful swelling of one side of the udder. Because of this the animal has a stiff straddling gait. Dullness, loss of appetite and general fever soon set in. Shortly afterwards dark bluish-violet colored spots appear on the affected portion of the udder; these soon coalesce so that all of the area is discolored. The discolored area becomes cold to the touch, and there is a dark reddish brown foul smelling secretion from it. Death is frequently the termination.

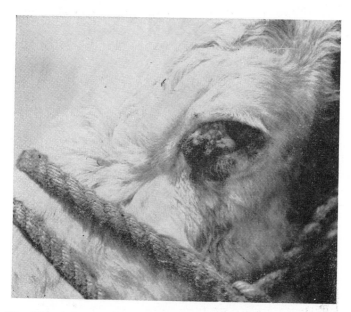

FIG. 112. A cancer destroying the eyeball. Surgery only offers relief.

Prevention consists in segregating an affected ewe as soon as the first symptoms are observed. Either disinfect the places contaminated, or if this is difficult due to the fact that the lambing pens cover a large space it may be simpler to move the ewes to a new place receiving no drainage from the infected yard.

In the "pink" stage of the disease, the intramuscular injection of 400,000 units of penicillin, and the oral administration of sulfamethazine, is helpful. In the later stages treatment calls for surgical amputation of the diseased portion of the gland. It is not uncommon for the remaining part of the udder to again become functionally active.

Cancer-eye: (Fig. 112.) This is a malignancy involving the eye-ball and immediately contiguous tissues. Hereford cattle are the ones most frequently affected. In some federally inspected abat-

Eye-lid pigmentation and cancer

toirs cancer eye was noted in 0.5 per cent of a total of 108,000 cattle slaughtered. Of this 0.5 per cent 95.3 per cent were

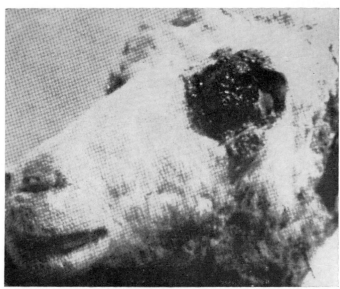

(Courtesy Journal of American Veterinary Medical Association)
FIG. 113. Cancer of lower eyelid in sheep.

Herefords, (Fig. 112) and 4.7 per cent other breeds. In sheep (Fig. 113) and swine the condition is rare. In addition to the unknown causes of cancer, the affliction in Herefords seems to bear some relationship to eye-lid pigmentation in that Herefords with red around the lids do not seem to be affected as often with cancer of the region as are Herefords lacking this pigmentation. Therefore, in the light of our present knowledge it is recommended that for breeding purposes there be selected those animals that are likely to transmit to their offspring the red pigmentation of the lids of both eyes. Bright sunlight is not so irritating to these lids.

When and if a cancer develops the veterinarian should at once be consulted before the tumor invades surrounding tissues too extensively. Surgically the veterinarian can remove the entire eye ball and then cause the lids to grow together so that there will be no hollow socket to invite insects, dust and other irritants. The animal will then present the appearance of never having had more than one eye.

Extra or Rudimentary Teats: (page 184). It is not uncommon for dairy cows to have more than the conventional number of four teats. The extra teats may be attached as small nipples to the regular teats, or there may be two undeveloped teats back of the regular ones. In some instances the extra teats are simply blind appendages with no excretory opening, and in others they have a connection with the secretory tissue of the mammary gland so that when the regular teat is manipulated during milking the extra teat will also discharge some milk. This makes a "messy" affair out of what should be a very sanitary procedure. Such cattle are discriminated against in the show ring.

Extra teats may discharge milk

Extra teats should be removed. This usually requires a surgical step which in some cases is only a minor operation. When the extra teat has connections with the secreting udder tissue it may be a hazardous step because of creating an avenue for a serious udder infection. All such operations should be approached with the same precautions as any other major surgical step, and preferably when the cow is not in production.

Leaking Teats: If this condition occurs only at milking time when the udder is full it is almost normal, especially if the cow is naturally an easy milker. The excitement occasioned by the approach of the regular milking period when a cow lets down her milk is too much for the circular muscle at the tip of the teat to stand. The sudden increase in intramammary pressure is responsible and this is not a pathological condition. However, there are cows that lose all or part of the milk at almost any time of the day or night. When these animals are at rest the pressure of the body on the udder causes a pool of milk to gather under them.

Some cows because of very weak sphincter muscles at the tips of the teats lose so much milk that the udder is practically empty as the regular milking period is approached. In the leaking condition described up to this point all four teats are usually involved. When only one teat is affected it is more frequently due to a previous injury of the teat or it may even be the sequel of an attempt to make an easy milker out of a hard milker. The cow that comes in to her milking time with an empty udder should be checked to determine whether she is actually a "leaker" in an aggravated form, whether she is addicted to "self-sucking" (page 415), or whether another cow in the herd has acquired the habit of using her mates as nurse cows.

Why do cows leak from the teats?

Sometimes simple remedies will control—not correct—the trouble. A wide rubber band applied to the teat—not so tight as to shut off all the circulation—will sometimes be sufficient. In other cases after each milking rub into the end of the teat a small amount of glycerite of tannic acid—this is an entirely harmless pharmaceutical which will draw the teat sphincter muscles more closely together. In most cases however, when the animal is dry the veterinarian's services will be needed for the injection of a very minute quantity of some irritant, by means of a very fine hypodermic needle, into the muscle surrounding the opening of the teat. Lugol's solution of iodine (page 276) has been used for this purpose. In very severe cases, as a last resort, then a small "melon sliced" piece of the sphincter muscle may be surgically removed, and the edges clipped together to promote quick healing. Because of the difficulty in estimating the exact amount of muscle to remove only the thoroughly qualified veterinarian should attempt it. Sometimes such cows are hard milkers when the teat heals.

Hard milkers: This annoying condition is exactly the opposite from those affected with "leaking teats" (page 434). Usually the sphincter muscle surrounding the teat opening—this is the lower end of **Cause of hard milking** the teat for an extent of three-fourths of an inch or less—is abnormally small either naturally or because of a previous teat injury. Various methods of handling are resorted to such as stretching the sphincter muscle by means of the spreading jaws of hemostats followed by the use of teat plugs for a few days to prevent contraction, up to radical surgical intervention which usually consists in four-way division of the sphincter muscle and the subsequent use of teat plugs until healing is complete. The services of a veterinarian are necessary.

Teat Stenosis or complete closure of the teat is usually due to an impermeability of the teat canal at some point along its course. If the teat fills **When no milk can be drawn from the teat** with milk which cannot be expressed then the canal at the end of the teat is impervious; on the other hand if milk does not enter the teat the obstruction is usually at the point of union of the teat to the udder.

In heifers a thin membrane frequently obstructs the teat high up. In older cows an early symptom of chronic mastitis (page 569) is frequently bean-shaped, or diffuse hardening (fibrosis) at the point of teat and udder junction. Thin membranous obstructions can quite readily be broken down; filrosis is much more serious and recoveries even after surgery are rare. Treatment in either condition should be prompt.

Warty Teats: Small warts, usually somewhat of an elongated shape show a predilection for being located on the teats of cows and the muzzle of horses. On the teats they are a source of annoyance at milking **How to re-** time. When the animal is not in produc- **move warts** tion the warts may be snipped off at the **from teats** level of the skin, and the resulting wounds painted with a drop of tincture of iodine (page 276). If this work is done when the animal is milked daily the necessary milking manipulations are very painful to the beast and also retard healing. Sometimes a milking tube must be used to draw the milk and this is hazardous because of the danger of introducing udder infection. Therefore, when in production a slower method is advised such as painting each wart three times weekly with a small amount of liquified glacial acetic acid.

Only the teat conditions that occur with the greatest frequency in the average dairy herd are described. **Teat** The teats and the udder are highly spe- **tampering** cialized organs, and they contain a fluid **dangerous** which is almost an ideal media for the growth of germs. When germs reach the deeper recess of the udder they are practically inaccessible. Therefore, any tampering with these organs is likely to be disastrous. The highly trained veterinarian should be consulted.

CHAPTER XXIV

PLANT, FOOD, AND CHEMICAL POISONINGS

There are many poisonous and potentially harmful plants and food substances. Only a few examples will be described. There are numerous bulletins, circulars, and textbooks in which may be found detailed statements about them. In general, animals are most likely to consume harmful vegetation when they are very hungry, and when the usual vegetation is scarce, as, for example, in seasons of drought and when pastures are overgrazed. In smaller pastures it is practical to eradicate all annual weeds including the poisonous ones by cutting them down before they go to seed; perennial plants may be dug up. Sometimes this type of vegetation may be smothered by heavy manuring or by planting other forms of vegetation capable of close, dense growth. Since some species of domesticated animals frequently are not so likely to be affected by certain harmful plants as are other species, a system of pasture rotation may sometimes be devised to control much of the trouble. Taken as a whole, in all areas excepting the large ranches, the control of food poisonings is largely a matter of careful eradication, and feeding substances of known wholesomeness.

Many poisonous plants

The control of many poisonous plants is one of general weed eradication

Prussic acid poisoning. Some plants extensively used as a roughage feed become *poisonous under certain conditions*, though ordinarily they are wholesome, and valuable animal foods. The roughages included in this grouping are cane, sorghum, Sudan grass, Johnson grass, and less frequently others. When one of the fodders named has been drought-stunted, frosted, developed a second growth, or when it has grown on heavily fertilized soil containing a large amount of nitrates, there is likely to be present in the plant a glucoside. This is known as dhurrin or it is parahydroxy-mandelo-nitrile—and an enzyme which when they unite or combine, form a deadly poison known as prussic acid or hydrocyanic acid. The combination of the two substances is most likely to result when the plant cells are burst due to freezing, crushing or bruising of the plant.

Of the domesticated animals cattle and sheep are most susceptible to the action of prussic or hydrocyanic acid as liberated from plants, and for **Cattle and** these animals the minimum lethal dose of **sheep most** HCN is close to 2.315 milligrams per kilo-**susceptible,** gram of body weight. Horses, swine, **and horses** rabbits, and guinea pigs are not nearly **and swine** so susceptible because as it is generally **are almost** held that the comparatively strong **entirely free** hydrochloric acid (page 18) in their **from this** stomachs combines with newly liberated **form of** prussic acid to form a much less poisonous **poisoning** substance. This theory is refuted by others who claim that the comparative immunity of horses, swine and other animals does not appear to be correlated with the normal stomach acidity of these animals. The fact remains, however, that horses and swine consume the prussic acid plants with impunity when under similar conditions cattle, sheep and other ruminants frequently succumb. It is also true that all animals exhibit a certain degree of tolerance to prussic acid and it is only when the prussic acid enters the blood stream, via the stomach, at a greater rate than the animal's tolerance for it that fatal poisoning results.

It has been quite well demonstrated that young plants less than two feet high of a dark green color are the richest in prussic acid and are therefore, the most dangerous to use for feed. The pale or yellowish green

Sudan grass less than two feet high is dangerous

plants are much safer. Plants grown on fields that are well fertilized with nitrogen fertilizers are more likely to contain a high prussic acid content, though when a phosphate fertilizer is also simultaneously applied, or when the soil is originally rich in phosphorus, the prussic acid content is much lower.

Plants that are drought-stunted are always more dangerous than others because their slower growth does not permit the prussic acid present in them to disappear, nor is there the normal amount of phosphorus to prevent the development of prussic acid.

Stunted plants are dangerous

Prussic acid-containing plants that are rich in this poisonous substance when made into ensilage or as quickly cured material, are likely to retain as much as 25 per cent of their poisonous qualities, unless there is a good deal of exposure of the plant in a slow curing process.

The question always arises, how to test a field of this roughage before animals are permitted to forage in them. This may be done by either a biological test or a chemical test, neither of which is one hundred per cent perfect.

The biological test is the more practical one of the two. It consists in testing a field suspected of harboring prussic-acid-containing plants by permitting one animal, usually the least valuable cow or steer, to graze in it for a period of ten days or two weeks. If there are no harmful results, it is reasonably safe to assume that the roughage of the tested field will be safe for consumption by other cattle.

There are many tests for prussic acid content

The chemical test is somewhat more technical in character and requires some equipment. Part I of the 11th and 12th Reports, page 495, of the Director of Veterinary Education and Research of the Union of South Africa states as follows:

"Picrate solution and papers, 5 gm. sodium carbonate and 0.5 gm. picric acid in 100 c.c. water. Wet ordinary filter paper with this, hang up to dry until only just 'perceptibly moist,' and cut into convenient strips, about 1 cm. by 4 cm. Papers should be made up fresh every week, as sensitiveness decreases with time. The solution keeps well for months in a stoppered bottle.

"Test.—Into a stout glass tube, about 1½ cm. by 7 cm. or other convenient vest-pocket size, push a few grammes of the moist shredded plant (or moist pulverized seed). Add two or three drops of chloroform to hasten autolysis, insert a slip of 'perceptibly moist' picrate paper at the top and cork tightly. Incubate in a vest-pocket, examining at intervals. Liberation of HCN is indicated by reddening of the yellow picrate paper—within a few minutes if the amount is large, after twenty-four hours if only traces are present. If the paper remains lemon-yellow it either means that a cyanogenetic glucoside is absent or that a hydrolytic enzyme is not intimately associated with it. In the latter case, chemical analysis may still show hydrocyanic acid, but with the majority of plants, analysis will not show much if the simple test fails. It may be added that the test is so delicate that cyanogenesis is revealed by a large number of common non-toxic edible plants, an easily comprehensible fact in view of the significance of cyanogen in normal plant anabolism."

Hungry animals of low vigor are more likely to succumb following the consumption of the prussic acid-containing plants because they consume larger amounts, and they lack the vitality to withstand its action. Animals that have consumed these poison-containing plants stagger, then fall to the ground, breathe rapidly and die in a few minutes from respiratory failure, the heart continuing to beat for sometime after the cessation of breathing. If the animal's life is to be saved, the poison must be prevented from forming by the combination of the enzyme and the glucoside (by themselves these two are harmless), or if the poison has actually formed and absorption into the blood stream has started, then a quick-acting antidote must be intro-

Symptoms of prussic acid poisoning

duced into the blood stream there to counteract its harmful results.

The first step to be taken in regard to the poisoned animal is to engage the services of a veterinarian so that he may inject into the blood stream any one of several chemical antidotes to neutralize the poison. In the meantime, while awaiting the arrival of the animal

Emergency treatment of prussic acid poisoning

physician, the owner or attendant should administer antidotes by way of the mouth. This can only be done before consciousness is lost, otherwise the medicine would simply be poured into the lungs with a fatal termination. The emergency antidotes may consist of a pint or a quart of molasses thinned with water to neutralize uncombined portions of the poison—the value of molasses as emergency treatment is debatable as some researchers commend it, while others were not able to demonstrate its protective action—or a better plan is to have ready during the season of the year when these plants are grazed, certain effective chemicals for neutralizing the poison before it has left the stomach to be absorbed into the blood stream.

These chemicals are dissolved in water to constitute two separate solutions, each kept separate, well corked, and in a dark place. Solution No. 1 is made by dissolving one ounce of carbonate of soda (washing soda) in one pint of soft water, and storing it in a long-necked quart capacity bottle. Solution No. 2 consists of one ounce of sulphate of iron (copperas), dissolved in one pint of soft water, and stored in a one-pint capacity bottle. When an animal is to be medicated, all of solution numbered two is to be added to solution numbered one, and the resulting combination measuring a quart constitutes one dose, which is to be administered as quickly and as carefully as the circumstances permit. The treatment outlined above is emergency handling and does not in any sense of the term supplant the intravenous medication by the veterinarian; in fact, the latter is far more effective and superior to any home treatment. The home treatment described is given because it is practical emergency handling and may be the means of saving some lives. The chemical antidote most frequently used is the intravenous injection of a solution of methylene blue which changes the oxyhemaglobin to methemoglobin which in turn forms a stable compound with the cyanide which is excreted as such. Others are sodium thiosulphate, sodium nitrate, and it has been found that sodium thiosulphate supplemented with sodium nitrite have a synergistic action so as to surpass the sum of their individual action so that the combination is $6\frac{1}{2}$ times as effective as methylene blue, and protected animals against 13 times the minimum lethal dose. The combination is given intravenously in divided amounts of the combination until recovery is effected.

Another question that arises is what to do with a growing crop of any of the roughages demonstrated to contain prussic acid. Horses and swine, also guinea pigs and rabbits presumably because of a higher degree of acidity in their stomachs (the acid destroying the enzyme necessary for the production of prussic acid) are not susceptible to this type of poisoning, and therefore these animals may be permitted to graze in the suspected fields. Others prefer to let the questionable roughage undergo a natural cure and then pasture it, as the prussic acid will practically have disappeared. Cutting the green roughage and shocking it for a slow cure is also a safe, approved practice. To summarize prevention bear in mind the following:

What use to make of prussic acid containing plants

1. Don't use too much nitrogen fertilizer, especially if the soil is deficient in phosphorus.

2. Don't pasture dangerous plants when they are young and dark green. Let them get at least eighteen inches tall before pasturing or cutting them for hay.

3. Don't pasture plants that have been stricken

by drouth while they were in the rapid-growing stage.

4. Don't pasture that new second growth that springs up after cutting or frosts.

5. Don't take chances with suspicious pastures. Try them out first on less valuable animals before turning in the entire herd.

6. Don't graze fields too closely. Such a practice increases the amount of that dangerous early growth that may be eaten by animals.

A system of crop management and growth will do much to prevent trouble. For example, in raising Sudan grass rapid growth is to be encouraged by either summer fallowing, or in regions of higher rain-fall the moisture must be conserved by every known expedient in order to have a continuous rapid growth of the plant. The plant should not be used for grazing until it is at least two feet tall, and for the making of nutritious hay free from danger it may be allowed to grow several feet in height. If two such pastures are provided the animals may be rotated from one to the other. Depending upon the region, whether south or north, there may

A method of crop management and growth to control prussic acid content in plants

be a spring planting, and a second one a month later. The first planting if on fertile soil with an adequate supply of moisture should be more than two feet tall in from six to eight weeks later. Then it may be grazed from four to six weeks and by that time the second planting should be tall enough for grazing so that the animals may be transferred to it. The plots should be comparatively small so that they will be grazed down rather quickly. If this grazing down takes too long there will be too much of the dangerous second-growth, though the small amount produced in the quick grazing process is usually not beyond the safe tolerance of the animal. This same general plan of pasture rotation may be followed, with modifications possibly, under various climatic conditions.

Cockle-bur poisoning. Cockle-bur (*Xanthium echinatum*) poisoning has been observed in hogs, sheep, cattle, and chickens. Hogs and sheep are equally susceptible so that the consumption of the very young plants approximately to the extent of one and one-half per cent of the animal's live weight is likely to prove fatal; one-half of this amount may result in the development of symptoms though with ultimate recovery. Cattle seem to require twice as much in proportion to their size, and chickens about six per cent of their live weight before serious results are observed. There is ample reason to believe that horses also are susceptible to the poisonous action of the cockle-bur though no cases are recorded—probably because these animals are more careful feeders. Daily sub-lethal doses of the plant are not harmful, or it is said that the poison is not cumulative, it being rapidly eliminated from the body.

Every spring there are numerous reported deaths among pigs, the owner being entirely at a loss regard-

Cockle-bur poisoning common in pigs

ing the cause of death. He will state that the animals have received no change of feed or care and, therefore, it is a mystery to him why several of them are found dead in the hog lot.

A careful inquiry into the handling of the hogs usually discloses that the day before the deaths occurred, the animals had been given access to a lot through which a small creek or other stream ran; that the water in the stream was very low; and that for several days the weather had been more than ordinarily springlike. This warm weather, combined with the necessary moisture requirements in the bed of the stream, resulted in a quick sprouting of the cockle-bur. When areas of this nature are examined they will be found to be literally covered with young tender cockle-burs that have just made their appearance through the ground. At this stage of its growth the young cockle-burs are appetizing and the pigs will eat almost any-thing of a green nature. So the stomachs of the dead animals are loaded with this cockle-bur.

Research work has demonstrated the fact that young cockle-burs are poisonous at the time that the first pair of leaves are partially developed or just after germination.

Pigs that have consumed the young cockle-burs in this stage may vomit, they are depressed, and before death, spasms may occur, though some animals die quietly. Death, when fatal doses have been consumed, takes place in from one and one-half to eight hours.

The obvious preventive measure is to keep pigs out of all lots in which cockle-burs are likely to make their appearance. After the plant has attained **Prevention** some growth, it is no longer relished by **of cockle-bur** pigs and apparently it also loses its poi-**poisoning** sonous properties.

Another preventive measure is to cut down the cockle-burs before the seeds have an opportunity to de-velop in the mature bur. In spite of the fact that the plant is an annual, this cutting down may have to be repeated for several years, for the simple reason that all of the seeds do not germinate the first year after they have fallen to the ground. Persistent cutting of the cockle-bur will eradicate it.

There is no specific remedy against cockle-bur poi-soning once the poison is absorbed. However, if the hogs are observed eating these plants they should at once be taken away from them and some fatty sub-stance should be given to them. If hogs can be induced to drink whole milk, this apparently contains enough butter fat to very largely control the poisonous action of the plant. Other fatty substances, such as unsalted lard, and linseed oil, possess properties which stop the poisonous action of the plant.

Futhermore, as soon as poisoning of the nature is suspected, a graduate veterinarian should be called, because he can administer remedies which will cause the hog to unload its stomach. If unloading of the stomach can be effected before the poison has been absorbed, it will of course control the entire trouble.

Oak-leaf poisoning. This is an ailment observed on the ranges of the southwestern United States, and it has also been reported from European countries. At least two species of oak have been incriminated, i.e., the *Quercus gambellii* and the *Quercus havardi*. The latter is also known as the shinnery oak. Cattle are affected,

Oak-leaf poisoning most frequently observed when other forms of vegetation are scarce and oak leaf consumed by them to the virtual exclusion of other forms of roughage will cause a serious disturbance in the digestive tract, manifested largely by constipation and loss of condition. Such other alleged symptom as bloody urine following the ingestion of an occasional mouthful of oak leaves is apparently not founded upon established facts.

When cattle are driven to the range in the early spring before grass makes its appearance, they eat quite a good deal of the early appearing young oak leaves. Less frequently they eat the older leaves later in the year.

The symptoms appear in from one to four weeks following the beginning of the oak leaf ration. The outstanding clinical symptoms are constipation with the passage of blood-stained, dark colored feces, and unthriftiness. From two to three per cent of the herd die, and some of the remaining ones are more or less permanently stunted.

Prevention of the appearance of ill effects consists in feeding a two-year-old steer at least three pounds of good hay or alfalfa daily. This means then that oak leaves alone are not a maintenance ration but when supplemented with a small amount of good hay they do not apparently produce a harmful condition. If hay is not available it is best to permit the animal to fill up daily on some other kind of roughage before being turned out to graze where oak brush leaves are the prevailing type of green vegetation.

"Acorn calves" are deformed at birth, they resemble so-called "bull-dog" calves. The latter is a
"Acorn calves" hereditary condition (page 182) so that they are dead at birth. On the other hand, "acorn calves" are born alive, and though unthrifty they can be raised to maturity. Usually the births take place between February and June, and mostly in the Sierra Nevada foothills where oak trees are abundant, and following a dry season when cows have been on a deficient ration for many months. The disease is never observed in irrigated valleys. The affected calves may have short heads, undershot jaws, the long bones of the limbs are noticeably short, walking is difficult so that the animal falls over backward or goes in circles; bloating is common. The California Agr. Exp. Sta. has definitely determined *that acorns are not the cause of the condition, and that it is not hereditary.* The real cause is a nutritional one, probably an avitaminosis, and most likely vitamin A, and possibly the B complex and D together with low protein in the ration of the dam. Good hay or other suitable roughage fed in abundance is essential as a preventive step, and breeding cows need concentrates. Actually the condition known as "acorn calves" should be discussed under the heading of deficiency diseases— it is handled here because of the wide-spread belief that it is related to the oak tree (see oak-leaf poisoning page 446).

Poisoning from seleniferous plants. Certain soils, especially shales are quite rich in an element known as selenium. It is more poisonous than arsenic. Some weeds, usually avoided by animals, always absorb a good deal of this element, while other plants normally not selenium feeders, become so if the soil and weather

Seleniferous plants cause losses at times

conditions are favorable, and if so-called "converter" plants have caused an excess of selenium to be drawn to the top layers of the soil. Under these conditions, ordinarily harmless, useful plants and their grains may absorb so much selenium as to become distinctly harmful to animals consuming this material. Thus wheat, corn, and barley have been incriminated as plants capable of being converted into selenium carriers. Sometimes the soil in a comparatively small area is rich in selenium, though by leaching, gravity, and by the droppings of animals that eat the vegetation, the small area may become considerably enlarged, and there are some soil areas in the western half of

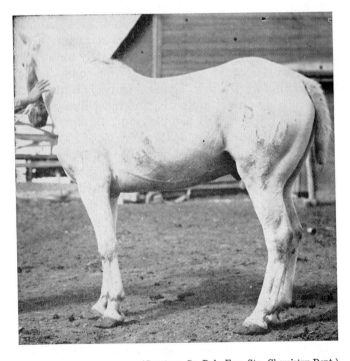

(Courtesy, So. Dak. Exp. Sta. Chemistry Dept.)

FIG. 114. Selenium poisoning. Note loss of mane and tail hairs.

the United States where large regions produce selenium-carrying plants.

"Alkali disease" a form of selenium poisoning   In the smaller areas the disease manifests itself in livestock as the "alkali disease" type of injury in which the animal is emaciated, with loss of hair, especially that of the mane and tail (Fig. 114) in horses, and deformed hoofs (Fig. 115) in both cattle and horses. In the larger areas the "blind stagger" type of disease is observed so that it is confused with loco disease. It has been claimed that an application of sulphur in some form to selenium soils will prevent plants from absorbing it, but careful research has demonstrated the erroneousness of this belief. Doubtless additional investigations now in progress in certain states will point the way to a control of this problem; in fact, it has

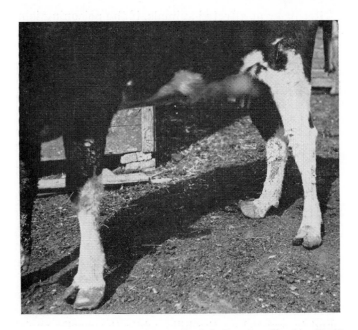

(Courtesy, So. Dak. Exp. Sta. Chemistry Dept.)

FIG. 115. Selenium poisoning. Note loss of tail hairs, and deformed claws.

Preventing selenium poisoning been demonstrated in experimental rats that the addition of five parts of arsenic (in the form of sodium arsenite) per million parts of water will prevent the symptoms of selenium poisoning when the ration consisted of eleven parts per million of seleniferous wheat. In the meantime, if selenium is suspected as a source of poisoning, the questionable plants or grains should be subjected to a careful chemical analysis, and if the presence of selenium is thus confirmed, the plants or grains containing it must be withheld as livestock foods.

Prevention consists in carefully guarding animals during periods of drought of sparse vegetation against grazing on areas normally avoided by them. Animals will eat selenium-bearing plants only when other vegetation is not available.

Recovery of affected animals, if the poisoning is not too far advanced, usually takes place if wholesome foods supplant the seleniferous material.

Loco-weed disease was formerly quite common in certain sections of the western U. S. *Loco-weed disease.* This condition has been generally observed in the semi-arid regions of the plains states and the Eastern Rocky Mountain region but since it has become better understood, and since much of its habitat is now under cultivation, the weeds are not so prevalent, and the disease is less common.

The weeds involved are the white loco or rattle weed(*Oxytropis lamberti*), the purple or woolly loco (*Astragalus mollissimus*) and the blue loco (*Astragalus diphysus*). In Texas the *Astragalus earlei,* and the *Astragalus wootoni* have been incriminated. Affected animals are horses, sheep and cattle.

The weeds grow from long roots that may extend two or three feet into the ground. The white loco is found in general on the hills, while the woolly variety occupies the depressions. These plants are legumes and apparently increase soil fertility.

Locoed animals act crazy. (The word "loco" is of Spanish origin and means crazy.) The outstanding

Symptoms symptoms are those of a nervous character including an involvement of eyesight and the sensorium. Affected animals are easily startled; they run into things and through barbed wire fences; at times they become very aggressive; and they seem to miscalculate distances or have a distorted vision as evidenced by their exaggerated efforts to pass over very minor obstacles. In the course of time they show evidence of malnutrition in a loss of weight and general weakness appears almost at the same time. Death is the final result if the animal is continued on an almost exclusively loco ration.

The loco eating habit seems to become established when because of droughts of more than the usual se-

Eating loco an acquired habit verity other vegetation is scarce. Before the loco eating habit is formed, animals pay but little attention to the weed, though once the taste is acquired they show a decided preference for it.

The actual poisonous principle or factor has not been well established. The chemical barium in the plant has been accused. Others contend that its action is largely the result of its exclusive use as an article of diet, or that it produces a nutritional disturbance. When other wholesome vegetation is available the grazing of the loco weed with it does not appear to be harmful.

Prevention consists in denying animals access to pastures and ranges where the weed is common until

Prevention of loco growth the latter have been dug out. By means of a spade the root may be cut off about two inches beneath the surface, resulting in death of the plant. There will be no new shoots from the root. The method must be followed up for a few years in order to destroy those plants that appear from seeds in the ground. These latter may remain dormant for several years.

Affected animals in an advanced stage of the disease are best destroyed as many of them fail to make a complete recovery. In the earlier stages of the disease and during less severe attacks medicinal treatment may be attempted accompanied by the administration of a good ration including alfalfa and grain, and laxatives in the form of linseed meal and bran.

Hepatic Cirrhosis, the "Walking Disease of Horses." "Walla Walla" (hard liver disease of swine and cattle). This disease has been observed in Nebraska and Washington as well as other parts of the world **An ailment** during the months of heavy growth of **due to** vegetation such as June and July. First **poisonous** there is yawning, then pushing of the head **plants** against fences and barns and a tendency to walk in circles and also straight lines apparently without any purpose so that wire fence entanglements or even walking over cliffs have been observed. Weakness finally sets in followed by death in most instances. Cattle are much less frequently affected with senecio poisoning.

Apparently the condition is due to the consumption of certain weeds especially the *Senecio* and the *Amsinckia intermedia* or the tarweed (Fig. 116) of the northwest which result in hardening and functional death of the liver, and distension and occasional rupture of the stomach, the latter probably because of the inability of this organ to free itself of large masses of indigestible vegetation. However, the seeds of the senecio are known to be toxic. The seeds are covered by a hard outer shell known as nutlets having a dark color and wrinkled. In screenings and **Seeds** grain mixtures the individual seed is dark **poisonous** colored, wrinkled, and about one-third the size of a grain of wheat. In one random sample there was one pound of tarweed seed in 450 pounds of mill screenings. The hogs consuming the screenings were unthrifty, and upon autopsy the liver was hard and

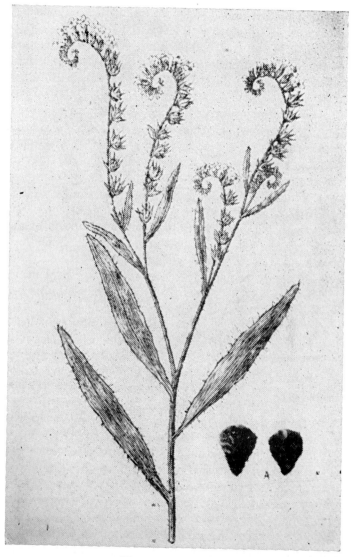

(Photo after Robbins et al. in Veterinary Medicine)

FIG. 116. Tarweed (*Amsinckia intermedia*) plant and seed.

small, and fluid in the peritoneal cavity. When the screenings were discontinued as a part of the ration no additional cases developed. (For the diagnosis of senecio poisoning in cattle the reader is referred to page 175 of the April 1953 number, Vol. XIV, No. 51, of the American Journal of Veterinary Research in an article entitled "The Bromsulfalein Liver Function Test and Biopsy of the Liver in the Diagnosis of Senecio Poisoning in Cattle" by Vardiman.)

In regions where this disease has been observed, prevention consists in keeping animals out of questionable pastures during June and July and removing the seeds of the tar-weed from the diet.

Crotalaria Poisoning: This plant is the *Crotalaria spectabilis,* a legume. Its common name in some sections is "rattle-box." In horses the consumption of another "rattle-box," the Crotalaria sagittalis, is claimed to cause "Missouri river bottom disease." It is a cover crop in many regions of the south and several of its species are non-poisonous. However, C. spectabilis has been demonstrated to be toxic for all species of livestock. In cattle (Florida) there sometimes is death within 24 hours, though most often it is **Crotalaria may result in quick death** the slower type of poisoning. The poisonous principle is the alkaloid monocrotaline $(C_{16}H_{23}O_6N)$. The green, wilted, frosted or dried plants are all equally poisonous. Sometimes death takes place several months after a sufficient quantity of the plant has been consumed though clinical symptoms are frequently not observed till the last week or two of life. On autopsy these animals have an enlarged, hardened liver (cirrhosis). In the more acute cases there are observed nervousness and excitability, stools somewhat bloody, and finally complete prostration and death. Keeping cattle away from *C. spectabilis,* or at least not including this species in the cover crop operations has been suggested. Most cattle do not take readily to this species but isolated animals will graze it if it is available. Curative treatment is of doubtful value because of the slow manifestation of symptoms.

Buckeye Poisoning: The young sprouts and nuts are poisonous to swine. The symptoms are incoordinated movement, paralysis, excessive salivation, dilated pupils and unconsciousness before death. There is no specific treatment—only symptomatic handling.

Black Henbane. (*Hyoscyamus niger*) is a plant about three feet high; it is an annual or biennial; flowers are dull yellow with purple veins **A very deadly plant** on short stalks, and the leaves of the plant are toothed, egg-shaped and wavy. The plant grows from the New England states to the Rocky Mountain region. Its alkaloids hyoscyamine and hyoscine are valuable in medicine as depressants. Poisoning in animals is indicated by loss of muscular power, stupor, and death from paralysis of the respiratory centers. Treatment is symptomatic.

Jimson Weed Poisoning: Also known as Jamestown weed and technically as *Datura strammonium* and *Datura tatula.* It is a malodorous plant refused by all animals excepting that swine eat the odor- **Animals do not like its odor** less seeds causing severe poisoning. The plant has funnel shaped white flowers and either a purplish or green stem. Its alkaloids or poisonous principles are comparable to those of henbane, and it also has the deadly nightshade alkaloid atropine. The symptoms of poisoning are very sudden and include pain, vomiting, dizziness convulsions and death. Treatment is usually to no avail because of the extreme rapidity of its development.

Nightshade Poisoning:—Botanically the *Solanum nigrum*—not to be confused with *Atropa belladonna* or "deadly night-shade" which is indigenous to Europe and Asia. The solanum is a member of the potato family. It has white flowers and black berries. The plant grows along the banks of brooks or in low-lying swales. In the middle west the plant occurs in patches

Occurs in wheat fields in the middle west

in wheat fields and as the crop is harvested with a "header" or "combine" the comparatively low night-shade is missed so that it forms a green oasis in various parts of the yellow ripened wheat plant stubble. Thus, it attracts livestock, especially swine, so that poisoning results. In this connection it is well to bring out that, in general, animals with a simple stomach (swine, dogs, horses, etc.) are more easily poisoned than those with multiple stomachs, or the compartments of ruminants. However, in the case of poisons not yet formed—such as prussic acid—the high acidity of the simple stomach is sometimes a protection in that it destroys one of the components before their union is effected. In animals ingesting freely of the solanum death takes place shortly thereafter. When smaller quantities are consumed there is usually vomiting in swine, some convulsions, and a greatly dilated pupil of the eye so that partial blindness is not uncommon. This pupil dilation is because of the active principle of the nightshade, and it is also in the poisoned animal's urine. A drop or two of this urine placed within the eyelid of a healthy animal will dilate the pupil. Prevention of this condition includes keeping animals out of infested wheat stubble fields, or before swine are admitted mowing the plant down. The veterinarian should be called at once so that he may hasten unloading of the animal's stomach through the use of quick acting emetics.

Animals with simple stomachs more susceptible

A test for this poison

Fern Poisoning: (Pteris aquilina). The bracken or brake fern is poisonous to horses and cattle. It is a perennial growing from one to four feet high. It has a scaly underground stem, and the leaves or fronds are three-parted or branched, which in turn are composed of many leaflets.

Description of the bracken fern

Cattle and horses will eat this fern in the late summer when green vegetation is scarce. Both cattle and
The effect on cattle horses show loss of appetite, great depression; bloody discharges from the mouth and nose are common, and in addition, cattle have intestinal bleeding. Death usually occurs in 12 to 72 hours.

Hay containing dry fern fronds should either have them removed or else the hay should not be offered as feed to horses and cattle. Hogs seem to suffer no ill effects from eating the roots. Cut the plant two or three times a year—June and August. Since the plant grows only in acid soil an application of lime to the roots will usually devitalize it or kill it.

Horsetail Poisoning (Equistum arvense). This perennial is poisonous to horses at all times of the year. Colts cultivate a liking for it. It grows in acid soil in waste leached hillsides and low depleted fields. Ap-
A year-round poisonous plant plications of lime to the soil will usually kill it. Sheep though not actually poisoned by it are nevertheless harmed following its consumption. The plant is five to twelve inches high with a yellow stalk; later this turns brown. Late in the spring the plant is bushy with a dozen or more pine needle-like branches at each joint. Remove the dried plant from hay and lime the soil to prevent plant growth. Poisoned horses become gaunt, and finally go down. Stimulants and physics, plus removing the animal from access to the plant, are beneficial in recovery.

"Water Bloom" poisoning (page 275). This disease of animals may follow the consumption of water badly contaminated with certain blue-green algae such as *Anabaena torulosa* and certain species of Microcystis—*Microcystis aeruginosa, Microcystis flos-equae,* and *Microcystis incerta* and some minor species. The
A water plant causes trouble algae may develop to such an extent that a body of water becomes covered with a thick layer resembling "thick pea soup."

It is the consensus that a very powerful poisonous substance is developed in connection with the concentration of the algae, as it exists in the water separated from the algae, though the nature of the poison has not been established; apparently the poison is not a very stable one because if the winds keep the algae near a certain shore long enough so that it decomposes to the extent that it is distinctly odorous it is no longer toxic. Cattle, sheep, horses, hogs, and fowl that consume lake water where the algae has piled up or concentrated because of hard or continuous winds from a certain direction may die. Death takes place very suddenly so that affected animals die on the margins of the lake. Prevention consists in fencing off the bodies of water that are covered with algae. Such bodies are particularly hazardous when prevailing winds have driven the algae shoreward to become greatly concentrated.

Halogeton poisoning: This plant (Fig. 117) is a relative of the Russian thistle and closely resembles it during the early stages of its growth, though in the later stages halogeton is more colored—reddish yellow—and the Russian thistle is more slender. It is not a native plant, it was first observed in Nevada about 1938; it has since spread to Utah, Oregon, California, Idaho, Wyoming and Montana. Early at-

The plant does not thrive under competition

tempts to eradicate the plant were not successful, and it is now believed that it will remain on the intermountain ranges as a permanent resident. In attempts to control it, reseeding of the ranges has been demonstrated to be helpful. Since the plant is sensitive to competition from vigorous stands of grass or perennial vegetation, it is a problem only in areas where the native vegetation has been depleted. The poisonous principle operative

Oxalic acid the poison

is oxalic acid, and this results in complete stupor an hour or two after the plant has been consumed in amounts of 1½ pounds of the dried plant for sheep, and 4 to 6 pounds for

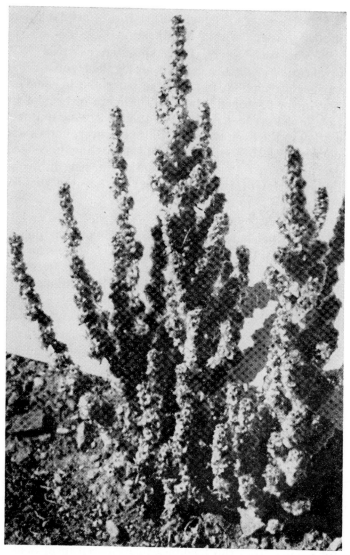

(Photo by U. S. Dept. of Agr., B. E. and P. I.)

Fig. 117. Halogeton, mature plant.

cattle. Death follows in 6 to 8 hours. The losses have been almost entirely in sheep, and sheep will not eat the plant if there is enough other forage available during the fall and winter months.

Potato poisoning: Green sprouted potatoes (*Solarium tuberosum L.*) contain an alkaloid, solanine, in various proportions in the green parts and to some extent in the "greened " tubers. There are records of injury to man from eating green tubers. Among animals, cattle are the commonest victims; however, horses and pigs have also died as a result of eating uncooked, green sprouted potatoes. Prevention consists in avoiding material of this nature as part of the diet of animals.

Trembles (page 830) *or milk sickness* (white snakeroot poisoning). This disease of cattle is due to the consumption of white snakeroot (*Eupatorium urticaefolium*). Ordinarily this weed is not consumed but in the late summer and fall when other vegetation is scarce it may be. "Tremetol" is the poisonous principle.

The white snakeroot is responsible for "trembles" in cattle

The symptoms are sluggishness, constipation, weakness, and loss of condition so that standing is difficult or impossible. The breathing is short, and the breath has a penetrating odor. Affected animals tremble, hence the common name "trembles." Probably its greatest importance rests in the fact that humans drinking the milk of affected animals also contract the disease, sometimes with fatal results.

Removing animals from pastures containing the white snakeroot, or grubbing out the latter causes the disease to disappear.

Cottonseed meal poisoning. The question of harmful results from the feeding of cottonseed meal is still somewhat of a debatable one. Research work in some of the Agricultural Experiment Stations (Arkansas and Louisiana) points to this valuable article of animal food as a possibly harmful one under certain conditions. Mature cattle, horses and sheep are seldom affected, though feeder calves and pigs are not nearly so immune to it. However, more and more research indicates that it is a deficiency condition rather than a poisoning (page 74).

The reported symptoms are those of impaired vision even to the extent of ulceration of the cornea, scurvy as manifested by unthriftiness, swelling of the limbs, a staggering gait, and nervousness. It has been reported to be responsible for some udder troubles, but careful experiments have demonstrated the erroneousness of this opinion.

Cottonseed is known to contain a poisonous principal known as gossypol which is contained in the germ portion of the seed. Therapeutists speak of this as a "cumulative" poison which means that it is not eliminated from the body as rapidly as it is taken in so that in the course of weeks or even after three or four

Poisoning from cotton-seed meal may be due to a poisonous principle or it may be caused by lack of vitamins months of feeding this material, so large an amount has accumulated in the body that it is outwardly manifested in symptoms of so-called cottonseed meal poisoning. In mature cattle as much as ten pounds daily have been fed in combination with suitable roughages and no harmful results were observed. In young animals it is best to limit the amount of cottonseed meal to one-half pound daily, gradually increasing this to one pound daily. Young swine and poultry seem to be relatively susceptible to the action of gossypol. It is entirely safe for swine and poultry if the germ portion of the seed is first removed—usually by a flotation process.

During recent years some evidence has developed indicating that some of the so-called cottonseed meal poisoning is in fact an avitaminosis—vitamin A is lacking, or in other words a deficiency disease (page

74). On the basis of this evidence it has been demonstrated that much of this trouble may be prevented by the simultaneous feeding of a forage rich in vitamins such as pea-green alfalfa.

At any rate when symptoms of so-called cottonseed meal poisoning appear the logical thing to do is to discontinue, temporarily at least, the feeding of cottonseed meal until all symptoms have disappeared, and then if necessary resume its feeding though in smaller daily amounts.

Sweet clover disease. Under certain conditions, consumption by cattle of the cured sweet clover plant is followed by harmful results manifested largely by a loss of clotting power of the blood (page 336). As a consequence the blood gathers in considerable volume in different localized parts of the body, especially beneath the skin, so as to form soft swellings of varying size (Fig. 118). Animals affected with this condition, though not having the swellings, do have non-clotting

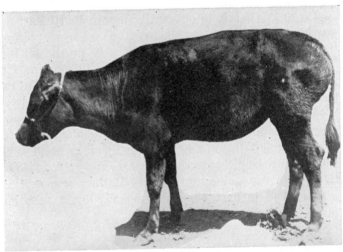

(Photo reproduced from Bul. No. 250, North Dakota Agricultural Exp. Sta.)

FIG. 118. Bodily swellings filled with bloody exudate as observed in so-called "Sweet Clover Disease."

Sweet clover disease is due to a chemical poison. It causes easy bleeding

blood, and therefore are likely to have a serious bleeding following injuries or surgical operations such as dehorning and castration. Conclusive evidence has now been presented that the disease is due to a chemical poison known as dicumarol—in human medicine it is a valuable anticoagulant—in the sweet clover. The chemical dicumarol is formed in the heating or spoiling process when the hay goes into the stack with too high a moisture content. The theory is that this chemical is responsible for the loss of clotting power in the blood. The rat-poison "Warfarin" (page 335) is related to dicumarol. This form of poisoning is observed, only when the sweet clover has been spoiled or damaged; clean bright hay is harmless, and the trouble is only rarely observed when the plant is pastured. The disease is one of young cattle—older ones are rarely affected. Sheep are only occasionally affected. In the prevention moldy pockets in the hay should most assuredly be discarded. A tobacco-like odor of the hay is an indication to discard it. Even the feeding of apparently clean bright sweet clover hay is hazardous.

Finally, the so-called "rabbit test" may be employed. It has been determined that rabbits are much more susceptible to the harmful qualities that the sweet clover plant harbors than are cattle. This fact is taken advantage of as a test when the sweet clover is fed as a regular ration of cattle. The test consists in maintaining a few rabbits in a pen and feeding them daily as their exclusive source of roughage on some sweet clover taken from the same part of the stack as that which is being fed to the cattle, and in addition a daily handful of whole oats. If there are harmful properties in the sweet clover, the rabbits will show the effects by the same symptoms as observed in poisoned cattle at least ten days before it is noticeable in the cattle. Prompt discontinuance of the sweet clover as a

A test to determine whether sweet clover is harmful

feed will prevent the development of the symptoms in the cattle.

If an animal is in an advanced stage of the disease it will usually make a very slow recovery providing the offending material is withdrawn from the ration. Curative treatment as applied by the veterinarian consists in the introduction of a relatively large volume of normal citrated blood into the blood stream of an affected animal. Vitamin K in amounts more than normally present in alfalfa may also be used.

Cornstalk Disease. The so-called cornstalk disease of the middle west results in the death of many cattle each fall and winter when this plant is used for forage. There is also a disease of horses occurring under apparently comparable conditions to the one in cattle; in horses, however, it is due to the consumption of moldy corn. The disease is unsolved, nothing being known about it other than the results observed in animals. Sometimes it causes sudden deaths the first time that animals are turned into the field, though it is not uncommon to find animals affected that have been in the same field for several days previously. Affected animals shiver, there are muscle contractions, frequent attempts at urination and finally they go down; death follows.

Cornstalk disease of cattle has not been entirely solved

The treatment by use of known agents has not been attended by even a fair degree of success. Veterinarians administer symptomatic treatment, and if this is started early during the attack, the animal's life may be saved, though the mortality rate is always very high. Though the disease has been under intensive investigation for years and many theories have been advanced as to its cause, none of these has been able to withstand the assaults of critical scientific research. It is only when the corn plant is permitted to undergo slow dissolution as it naturally occurs that it seems to cause the trouble, because when the plants of a previously dangerous field are cut and shocked or "sun-bleached," they soon lose their harmful properties.

With the present entire lack of a plausible explanation of the trouble, the best that can be done to prevent losses is to test the field first by turning into it for a ten-day period one of the less valuable animals, and if there are no harmful results, the remainder of the herd may be permitted, under constant surveillance, to graze in the field; immediate removal at the first sign of danger is highly important. Those fields known to contain dangerous plants need not be a total loss, as the plant may be utilized for animal feed by cutting and shocking it, then permitting it to "cure" in the shock for two or three weeks, after which it is reasonably safe to use.

Photosensitization in Cattle and Sheep: Literally this means sensitization to light. Usually it is characterized by inflammation of the skin in its white or lightly pigmented areas, and in severe cases by superficial death of the areas of the skin that are affected (Figs. 119 and 120). Jaundice is a frequent complication. The sensitization seems to be closely related to the ingestion of certain vegetation, such as buckwheat, St. John's Wort, alsike, crimson, white dutch and ladino clovers and others. Some plants are said to be

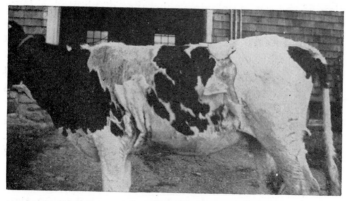

(Photo by Dr. J. R. Starkey, Goshen, N. Y.)

FIG. 119. Photosensitization dermatitis.

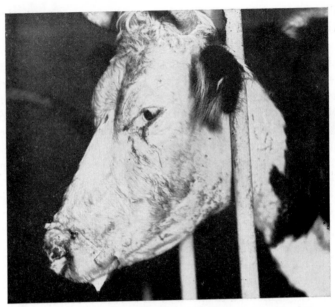

FIG. 120. Photosensitization dermatitis of the head region.

icterogenic or also as "hepatogenous photosensitivity" because in addition to their relationship to photosensitivity they cause degenerative changes in the liver and kidneys, usually with a fatal termination. It is ascribed to phylloerythrin which is a product of the degradation of the green coloring substance of plants—chlorophyll. Normally phylloerythrin is excreted in the bile with the feces.

When phylloerythrin accumulates in the liver it appears in the blood to sensitize to light the unpigmented areas of the skin, and as the liver is damaged jaundice also results. The "Geeldikkop" (Yellow Thick Head) of sheep in So. Africa, due to grazing on *Tribulus terrestris* is one of these diseases. When photosensitivity appears (see following statements about "Bighead" in sheep, "Dermatitis" and "Alsike Clover Sickness"), as a general preventive step to avoid overgrazing, mow down and remove or burn suspected vegetation, and transfer animals to other pastures or to the dry lot. For specific or symptomatic treatment consult the veterinarian.

Big-head in Sheep. This condition is also known as "swell-head in sheep," and "photosensitization," and in Europe as fagopyrismus. Photosensitization is an unusual phenomenon demanding increasing attention as a factor in animal diseased conditions. The nature of the processes in the plant and animal, and the relation of sunlight, plant and animal to each other in the production of disease is not yet clearly understood.

"Big-head" in sheep due to sensitization by a plant, and sunshine

Big-head appears suddenly about midsummer, affecting young, tender skinned lambs. In certain far western states the disease has been quite definitely ascribed to the consumption of certain weeds such as *tetradynia glabrata* (coal-oil brush; little leaf horse brush), and *Tetradynia canescens* or *Tetradynia canescens inermis* (spineless horse brush) without any mention of photo-dynamic properties in the plant, but in the midwestern states the same disease is common, and botanists contend that the far western weed does not grow east of the Rocky mountains. Other weeds that have been accused are ragwort, clover, smartweed and Sudan grass. In South Africa the *Tribulus terrestris* (puncture weed or Mexican sandbur) is incriminated. The general opinion is nevertheless frequently expressed by sheep owners that the animal does consume some plant which sensitizes it to the sun's rays with the production of the characteristic symptoms. Some support is offered this hypothesis by the fact that affected animals in the early stage of the disease almost always recover if they are carried or carted, not driven, to some cool, dark place.

It is to be emphasized that if the ailment is detected in an early stage the affected animal should be placed in the shade, *and all exercise avoided*. If the best results are to be obtained the patient must be carried or otherwise conveyed to the shaded place. The eyes should be cleared of gatherings by means of small pledgets of cotton squeezed out of some mild antiseptic, such as a two per cent water solution of boric acid (page 278), and the swollen head parts may be anointed with olive oil to prevent excessive cracking of the skin.

The prevention consists in keeping lambs in shaded places during bright sunlight, and permitting them to graze only during the night time especially if the pastures are weedy. Or it has been suggested to permit lambs to fill up on prairie hay before they are turned into weedy pastures and thus reduce the amount of weed grazing. It is especially recommended to follow these precautions when lambs have recently been received at a farm from some distant point.

Mold poisoning in general is frequently referred to in literature, but excepting in rare specific instances the importance of molds and smuts as sources of danger to animals consuming them is greatly overestimated. Certainly animals consume with impunity almost daily, "smutty" corn, or other cereals contaminated with stinking smut. Neither is it to be overlooked that many molds or smuts have a decided food value, though this information is not presented with the thought that these fungi should be used for this purpose.

Moldy foods are unwholesome, not desirable

Scabby oats infected with the fungus Giberella zeae —also corn and barley, are unpalatable but when eaten by livestock may be toxic. Toxins from this fungus fed experimentally produced vomiting and restlessness in swine. Researchers suggest that scabby oats might be fed to cattle (restricting the test to one animal) by including a known percentage in its regular grain ration and making observations for any bad effects.

Probably the best rule to remember with regard to moldy foods is that in the generally accepted sense of the term they are classed as unwholesome and therefore they are undesirable for animal consumption. Also, their possible dangerous character depends on the degree of moldiness. A good deal of judgment must be exercised by the feeder in this situation. Cattle are usually less susceptible to the possible harmful effects of moldy food than are horses. In offering it to cattle, the extremely moldy portions are best rejected, and the balance may be made safer by diluting it with clean, wholesome food, or by feeding it only occasionally, interspersing it with feedings of wholesome quality foods. If the material in question appears very undesirable following a physical examination, it may first be fed to a test animal for ten days or two weeks. Drying by direct sun exposure will also render moldy foods safer for animal consumption.

Forage poisoning. Food poisoning, ensilage poisoning, staggers, "cerebro-spinal-meningitis," and botulism (page 650) are terms that all refer to a group of diseases in which some agent, usually a harmful germ or mold, has been ingested by the animal with its food; mold poisoning (page 468), and moldy corn poisoning (page 470) may be included. Frozen or dwarfed rape can play havoc with cattle. Oat-hay poisoning (page 479) is another trouble maker. Whenever animals become ill following a change in the character of their feed, or if it is obtained from a different source, or if climatic and seasonal changes during its growth and storage are abnormal, and when various other factors are involved it is well to suspect the feed.

"Forage poisoning" is a general classification, and means that the animal is receiving something harmful with its food

It is not uncommon for ensilage to be fed regularly from a certain silo without any apparent harmful results, only to find that some portion of it in the deeper part of the silo has become the abode of the botulinus germ, *Clostridium botulinum* and its deadly toxin so that animals consuming this material die in from one to three days.

In almost all forms of this group of diseases spoken of collectively as "forage poisoning" there are nervous symptoms. Either the affected animal has a staggering gait, sleepy attitude, and dizziness or there is evidence of excitation as manifested by delirium, walking and running into fences and buildings, blindness, and pawing and kicking. Not infrequently there is more or less paralysis, the throat being first affected so that the swallowing of food and water is impossible. Attempted oral medication during this stage will result in the passage of the medicine into the lungs so that pneumonia will ensue.

The best assurance against this group of diseases is the feeding of wholesome materials (page 30). If there is reason to suspect the quality of food, or its contamination with extraneous harmful substances it is best to test it by feeding it to the least valuable animal of the same species as those for which the food is ultimately intended. The first step in the curative treatment is to withhold as animal food the suspected material; the second step is to call the veterinarian because the medical treatment of no two forms of the group of forage poisoning disease is identical.

Moldy Corn Poisoning in Horses. From the standpoint of observed symptoms this condition closely resembles "sleeping sickness" in horses, though it occurs during the late fall, winter and early spring while true sleeping sickness makes its appearance during the hotter months. Neither must moldy corn poisoning be confused with cornstalk disease in cattle (page 464) as the two conditions are seldom observed in the same field. Affected animals may have the sleeping form of the disease in which during a period extending from a few hours to several days after eating moldy corn there is gradually increasing sleepiness and finally complete unconsciousness, or the highly nervous type of the disease may be manifested. In this latter the animal may bite and kick, walk blindly into objects, have an unsteady gait, and frequently walk in circles. In either type which is at all advanced, death is the usual final outcome.

Horses succumb to prolonged consumption of moldy corn

Moldy corn poisoning has been produced experimentally by the feeding of moldy corn. During damp seasons it may occur when horses consume moldy corn as they are worked or pastured in corn fields.

The disease may be controlled by applying muzzles to horses as they are being worked in questionable fields. Moldy ear corn is not safe for graining horses. Shelled moldy corn may be made reasonably safe for **Prevention of moldy corn poisoning** animal consumption by placing it in a bucket of water and discarding the floating kernels. Upon the first evidences of this disease all corn should be removed from the ration, mangers and feed boxes scrubbed, and a ration of hay and oats substituted. Laxatives are recommended to hasten removal of unabsorbed molds from the intestines.

Botulism (pages 650 and 824) (Fig. 168). Sometimes conditions are favorable for the growth of germs **A food poisoning caused by a germ** in feed stuffs. An outstanding example of this is the *Clostridium botulinum*, an organism that elaborates a very powerful poison. It has been isolated from both human and animal food stuffs producing those fatal diseases known variously as meat poisoning, sausage poisoning, olive poisoning, forage poisoning, throat and tongue paralysis, and a host of others. It is one of the outstanding causes of the so-called limberneck (page 650) in poultry. Free exposure of animal food stuffs to circulating air and sunlight will do much to inhibit these harmful bacterial growths, or to destroy them once they have occurred.

Loin Disease of Cattle. This is an ailment, a food poisoning which in a measure is closely due to the same **Loin disease of cattle a germ disease** basic causes as rickets. Because of the low phosphorus content of soil and vegetation animals pastured in these regions acquire the bone chewing habit. Many of these bones are still in a "green" stage, or they have attached particles of decomposing, putrid flesh, which in turn harbors a poison or toxin producing germ—*Clostridium botulinum* (page 471). It is this flesh or germ poison that causes the bone chewing ranch cattle, eighteen months old or over, in certain areas in Texas to become weakened in the hind limbs so that they are unable to arise, and if enough of the poison has been consumed inability to control all otherwise voluntary muscles, together with other evidences of general illness.

Prevention consists in supplying with bone-meal, animals compelled to graze in low phosphorus territory so that the bone chewing habit, and the in-

Prevention of loin disease

cidental consumption of decomposing flesh particles will not become established.

Mildly affected animals usually recover from "loin disease" if they are deterred from bone chewing by being supplied with wholesome bone meal, and if laxatives are administered to hasten elimination of unabsorbed flesh poisons from the digestive tract. The handling of more severely affected animals is comparable, though recovery in these individuals is rare and may never be complete.

Ergotism. This is an ailment due to the consumption of ergot or rye smut, and other smuts replacing the grains of grasses. It grows on all plants

A smut of rye and other grasses causes serious trouble at times

included under the general name of grasses, especially rye. It has the appearance of blackened kernels (Fig. 121) resembling oats in size, though somewhat longer and more decidedly curved in its long direction. It is used in both human and animal medicine because it possesses the valuable properties of stimulating involuntary muscles to contraction, and it contracts the very small peripheral arterioles. It is this latter property that makes it harmful to animals, particularly cattle, hogs and poultry when it is eaten daily with the grain or forage, in that it contracts the small blood vessels in the extremities of the body so that their nutrition is interfered with and such parts die, or it is said they undergo dry gangrene. The tips of the ears, the end of the tail, the comb and wattles, and even the lower portions of the limbs may slough off because of this dry gangrene. (Figs. 122, 123 and 124.) Ergot has been accused of being responsible for premature births in cattle but when there are large numbers of these it is best to first eliminate Bang's abortion infection (page 578). Ergotism seems to be most common during the

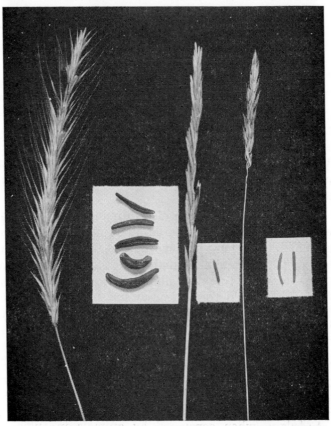

(Courtesy, Dept. of Botany, Kansas State University)

Fig. 121. Black kernels in the grain heads are ergot. Individual kernels are also shown. The larger ones illustrated are full size.

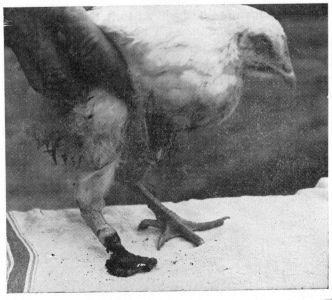

(Courtesy Department of Bacteriology, Kansas State University)
Fig. 122. Ergotism in a chicken.

colder months of the year, possibly because succulent fodder is not then so generally available; also, less water is consumed.

Prevention consists in discontinuing the use of the ergotized or smutty material. If it must be used for animal food it may be done quite safely by reducing the smut to a minimum, and at the same time permitting the animal to have a liberal allowance of succulent food either in the form of green material in season, or ensilage, and roots such as beets and turnips. A plentiful supply of water should be available at all times.

Vermin in food. This form of contaminated food stuffs occurs when they are badly infested with that type of life usually included under the designation of "bugs, insects, and worms." Many of these undoubtedly are harmful when consumed by animals in sufficient amount. Some of them excrete or have irritating subtances in the form of juices, and spines which

Vermin infested foods are not wholesome

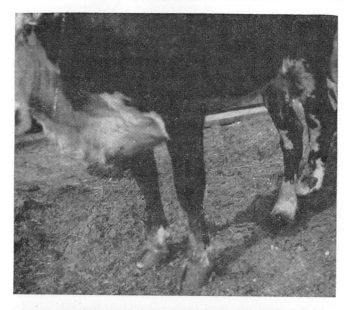

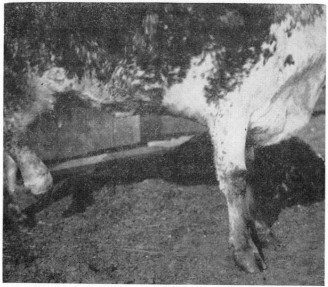

(Courtesy Dr. J. W. Lumb, Kansas State University)

FIGS. 123 and 124. Sloughing of the feet because of the prolonged consumption of ergotized grain and grasses.

doubtless injure the lining of the mouth and possibly the entire digestive tract. Furthermore, these forms of life in consuming the food stuffs leave the debris, and relatively enormous amounts of their excreta. If domesticated animals are offered as food this mixture of grain, grain husks, vermin life and vermin excreta, it does not constitute a very wholesome form of nourishment, and may be decidely harmful.

The entire problem may be controlled by so constructing grain bins as to make them vermin proof, or by frequent exposure to air and sunshine, and by subjecting the contaminated food to the action of mechanical blowers so as to remove the lighter particles and at the same time retaining the heavier, solid grains. Fumigation with a gaseous agent, especially carbon bisulphide (page 306) is valuable for the destruction of living forms.

Food poisoning in lambs. (Enterotoxemia (page 825) ; Overeating in Lambs; Food Intoxication; Indigestion; "Pulpy Kidney.") This is a form of food poisoning observed in lambs that are being fattened for market, and that are receiving more than a pound of grain per day, especially corn, peas, or barley. In an attempt to fatten range lambs so that they will be ready for market in ninety days the grain ration is pushed, and then this is complicated by the absorption of bacterial poisons *(Clostridium perfringens, type D)*. The fourth or true stomach and the intestines are inflamed, so that the poisonous products are more likely to be absorbed.

The overfeeding of lambs on grain may result in a form of food poisoning

The trouble almost always affects the fattest lambs. The early symptoms appear to be of a nervous character so that the head is directed backward; there is staggering, and finally recumbency, convulsions and death. Other nervous symptoms are running in circles, or pushing against a fence or barn. Occasionally the course of the disease is slower, with a loss of appetite and diarrhoea, inability to arise, and death at the end of several days.

Prevention is possible, but not always with financial gain. Lambs are fed to be in fat condition for the market in ninety days. If they are not fat they are not marketable, and if it takes more than ninety days the venture is not likely to be profitable.

All of the trouble in fat lambs on full feed may be stopped almost over night by withholding the grain ration. It has been suggested that grain concentrates be held to one pound for each lamb daily, and that this be supplemented with almost any fattening material other than corn, peas or barley. In the plains states where lamb feeding is not so intensively followed as in the mountain regions to the west, an excellent daily fattening ration practically the equal of corn and alfalfa consists of: milo grain, one pound; cottonseed meal, one-fourth pound; milo fodder, two pounds; and calcium carbonate or powdered limestone, one-fourth ounce. The Colorado Agricultural Experiment Station recommends feeding two per cent of flowers of sulphur in the ration of lambs to prevent enterotoxemia. A bacterin (Clostridium perfringens, type D) (—this is really a toxoid—) may be helpful in preventing the disease in lambs over two months of age, 10 days being required for the immunity to be developed. Bad results sometimes follow the use of the bacterin on newly shorn lambs. It is claimed, not substantiated, that vaccination of ewes at least a month before lambing will protect nursing lambs, or a serum may be used on the latter. Though the vaccines are very helpful the chief reliance in prevention is to be placed on careful feeding practices.

Other expedients that have some merit when lambs are turned into cornfields is to leave them there for a very short time only, or to place temporary fences across the field so that the lambs will have access to only a limited area at a time.

Experience also seems to demonstrate that it is advisable in order to aid in preventing digestive disturbances in lambs to feed whole grains in preference to ground grains. Sheep have a tendency to bolt the latter. Whole grains they masticate quite thoroughly.

The history of an outbreak of "food poisoning" (enterotoxemia) and the clinical symptoms manifested

Laboratory diagnostic aid

are usually sufficient on which to base a diagnosis. The disease has been at times confused with hemorrhagic septicaemia (page 547) and coccidiosis (page 733), as well as with plant and chemical poisonings. Laboratory diagnostic procedures are required to establish the exact nature of the ailment affecting the flock. In this case a tied-off section of the ileum (page 24) containing at least 30 cubic centimeters (about one ounce) of intestinal contents, as well as the usual tissues, should be sent under proper conditions to the laboratory.

Acute salt poisoning in animals. Two forms of salt poisoning are recognized, i.e., the one acute due to the

Acute salt poisoning is not of common occurrence

consumption of single large quantities of salt, and the other of a more chronic type (page 75) due to the daily or repeated ingestion of smaller amounts.

The acute type is observed in cattle after they consume four or five pounds of salt, in hogs after consuming about one-half pound, and in the dog after consuming a somewhat smaller amount. Chickens pick up pieces of rock salt instead of pebbles and are poisoned if enough is consumed. The excess of salt may be in food relished by the animal as when hogs receive salted kitchen waste, or brine from salted meats. A carefully controlled research project has shown that for pigs weighing 50 to 60 pounds a dose of four to eight ounces of salt—without free access to unlimited water—is frequently toxic.

Affected animals exhibit thirst, vomiting, pain, diarrhoea, muscular spasms, frequent urination, weak pulse and death.

An autopsy reveals congestion of the organs of digestion, and of the bladder, with occasional involvement of the brain and its coverings.

Prevention consists in withholding concentrated salt solutions from animals. Affected animals may have the stomach evacuated by means of a stomach pump, bland laxatives such as raw linseed and mineral oils administered, and large quantities of water given. (Consult pages 75 and 106.)

Oat Hay Poisoning (saltpeter poisoning; nitrate of potash poisoning.) Shortly previous to **1936** reports were made indicating that quite a large number of cattle had died after eating some cured oat hay. Carefully conducted experiments failed to disclose a toxic principle in the oat hay; the feeding of sufficient amounts of the oat hay resulted in the death of cattle but did not seem to be harmful to horses, sheep, rabbits and guinea pigs. Later results from another research source brought out that the toxic principle in the oat hay was soluble in water and resistant to destruction by heat; also that sheep could be poisoned though with more difficulty than cattle. Finally, after an interval of several years, it was determined that under certain growth conditions the oat plant contains a comparatively large amount of nitrate of potash (saltpeter) — concentrations of from 3.6 per cent to 4.91 per cent have been reported. In the outbreak in which the oat hay contained 4.91 per cent of nitrate of potash it had been grown in an old animal corral that had several years accumulation of manure in it. When nitrate of potash is consumed in sufficiently large amounts, by cattle in particular, it is in part changed from its chemical status of *nitrate* of potash (KNO_3) to the *nitrite* of potash (KNO_2) and the latter combines with the hemoglobin (red coloring, oxygen carrying blood constituent) of the blood so as to change

Cattle dead from eating oat hay

Saltpeter the real cause

it to methemoglobin which is incapable of releasing its oxygen to the tissues of the body or the animal dies of anoxemia which means "oxygen want."

There are recorded cases of well water contaminated by heavy manure seepage containing as much as 20.7 grams of nitrate of potash per gallon of water, and resulting in poisoning (methemoglobinemia) of cattle regularly consuming this water.

Prevention consists in not feeding to cattle cured oat hay grown on heavily manured soils. There may be other factors causing oat hay to take up large amounts of nitrate of potash but at this time they are unknown. Symptoms of oat hay poisoning in cattle include trembling, gasping for breath with bluish discoloration of the mucous membranes of the mouth and nose, frothing at the mouth, staggering gait, convulsions, sometimes charging attendants, and death, in untreated cases, in from two to ten hours. All the foregoing combined with oat hay consumption indicates need for the veterinarian in order that he may give intravenous injections of specific chemical antidotes—the same as for prussic acid poisoning (page 437). Even animals already unconscious may frequently be revived by this intravenous medication.

Nitrate Abortion: In some states there are comparatively large localized land areas of marsh—peat, a fuel, is harvested, and celery is grown on it—which also afford cattle grazing. There is a complaint that as many as seventy-five per cent of pregnant cows grazing on these areas have premature births or abortions. These cattle are brucellosis free. Conclusive research results are lacking, but preliminary reports (Univ. of Wis. Exp. Sta.) point strongly to the heavy nitrate content in much of the vegetation as the causative factor.

Marsh lands frequently have nitrates causing cattle abortion

"Soybean" poisoning, so-called is actually Trichlorethylene poisoning. Raw soybeans contain two sub-

stances that are harmful to young growing animals. One of these substances interferes with protein diges-

Harmful substances to be removed
tion—it is an antitrypsin factor. To re-move the harmful substance there are the so-called "expeller" process in which heat is used and much of the oil also is removed, and the "solvent" process by means of which almost all the fat is taken out. For the "solvent" process the relatively non-inflammable trichlorethylene was used. This chemical proved to be toxic, especially for cattle, less so for horses and sheep. In chickens, especially young and growing ones, extensive sub-cutaneous and intramuscular hemorrhages have been observed which are closely related to a ration of solvent extracted soybean oil meal—this meal is low in vitamin K (page 73) so that clotting time of blood is delayed. Supplemental alfalfa rations are helpful. In calves the elapsed time for death to take place varied from four weeks to over one year. The observed symptoms in

Symptoms in cattle
cattle are listlessness, depressed appetites, high temperatures and some times bloody discharges from the nostrils, and in the intestinal discharges. Post mortem examinations reveal extensive hemorrhages throughout the body, but par-ticularly in the body cavities. Pigs are quite resistant to soybean poisoning. As a result of the research work on this problem at several Experiment Stations the use of trichlorethylene in the processing of soybeans has been discontinued.

Chemical Poisoning. During recent years animal foods have frequently become the carriers of chemical

Chemical poisonings occur more frequently during re-cent years
poisons. The extensive campaigns against insect pests by the use of mashes contain-ing arsenic in some form, the use of chlo-rate of soda in the control of bindweed, the spraying of orchards with poisonous com-pounds, some of which is deposited on the vegetation below, are all factors in this form of food

poisoning. In order to be poisoned by any of these substances it is necessary that quite large amounts shall be consumed. This occurs only when an unnecessarily large amount of the poisonous agent is deposited in one concentrated area, or when hungry animals get a large amount of poison because they consume a full feed of vegetation previously treated with ordinarily safe quantities of poison. Care in the disposal of poisonous mashes and sprays, and in keeping animals out of pastures or lots so treated is an effective means of prevention. These are some of the chemicals that are most frequently responsible for these poisonings. The general use of powerful chemical insecticides (pages 291 to 297) is hazardous, and users of these agents should follow printed instructions on containers.

A wood preservative and lubricating oil ingredient the cause

Chlorinated Naphthaline Poisoning (hyperkeratosis; X-disease): This condition was designated as "X-disease" before its true cause was known (Fig. 125). It has now been determined that it is caused by a chlorinated naphthaline employed as a preservative of wood, and also in high compression lubricants. Manufacturers and processors have upon request discontinued the use of chlorinated naphthaline as wood preservatives and in lubricants. It seems that poisoning from this agent has almost disappeared.

Heavy death losses—59 per cent of those affected—are recorded, and therefore the disease is one of economic importance. Reports indicate that the disease is a more serious problem in some southern states than elsewhere, though it was formerly reported from many states. Young cattle appear to be more susceptible than the older ones, and the death rate is highest among them.

A disease of economic importance

There is a loss of condition, drooling, running at the nose and eyes, thickening of the skin and on the

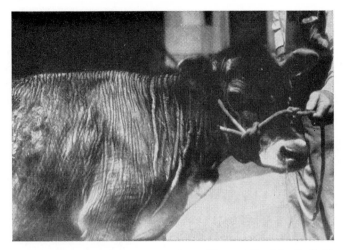

(Courtesy Dr. John D. Beck)

FIG. 125. X-disease.

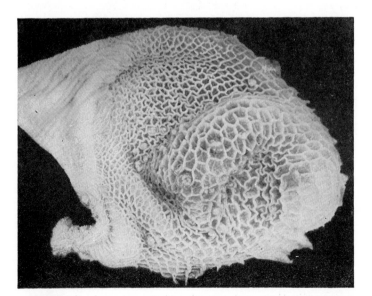

(Courtesy The New Zealand Veterinary Journal)

FIG. 126. Reticulum (honeycomb or second compartment of stomach) lining with raised necrotic ulcers in hyperkeratosis.

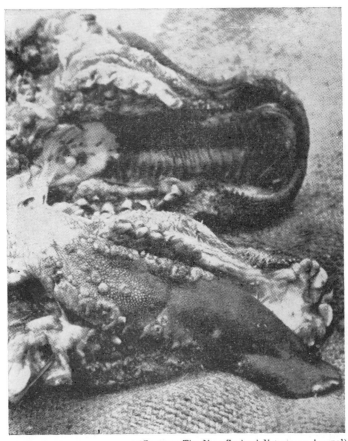

(Courtesy The New Zealand Veterinary Journal)

FIG. 127. Hyperkeratosis, mouth of calf, ulcerated.

Symptoms of X-disease
muzzle, and in the mouth. Diarrhoea may be a symptom but it is not constant in its appearance. The course of the disease varies from a few weeks to several months. The mouth thickenings on a post-mortem examination are frequently found to also extend into the gullet (oesophagus) and rumen (Figs. 126 and 127). Outwardly the most prominent symptom is thickening and hardening of the skin with loss of hair (Figs. 128 and 125) in the affected areas.

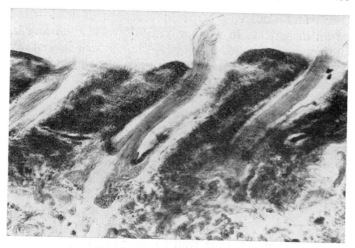

(Courtesy Dr. Fred O'Flaherty, University of Cincinnati)

FIG. 128. Microscopic section of the skin in chlorinated naphthalene poisoning (hyperkeratosis or X-disease) showing roots of hairs held fast by excess of keratin cells.

The naphthaline compound may cause trouble either by ingestion when present on contaminated feed, or by direct or indirect contact. The latter most frequently occurs when the compound has been used as a wood preservative.

In prevention it is essential to determine the source of contamination so that it may be removed. It is alleged that modern oils and greases do not now contain chlorinated naphthaline.

Mild cases usually recover when the foregoing has been accomplished. In more severe cases the outcome is questionable and therefore the prompt aid of the veterinarian should be sought.

Lead Poisoning: Lead is used commercially in various forms and all are poisonous. White lead (a basic lead carbonate) is the foundation of many paints; lead oxide (litharge in paint, and much used lead plasters and adhesive tape) ; red lead (this is lead tetroxide of paint) ; sugar of lead (lead acetate—used in the preparation of some pharmaceuticals such as Goulard's extract, and Goulard's cerate); arsenate of lead—used as an insecticide in the spraying of vegetation and in the manufacture of linoleum—the latter chewed by dogs when it forms the lining or flooring of their houses.

It is not at all uncommon for animals to lick the inside of paint receptacles, or recently painted buildings and fences. In times past it was quite common to transport drinking water for humans through lead pipes and thus lead was consumed; also the daily use of a paint brush in applying lead paint allowed enough lead to be massaged into the ungloved hand to cause "painter's colic" which is lead poisoning. It is well to bear in mind that lead is a cumulative poison—this means that small amounts of lead administered frequently will accumulate in the body to finally produce marked symptoms of poisoning. Vegetation in the vicinity of lead smelters may be the source of the lead. All poisonings mentioned in this paragraph usually are of the slowly developing or chronic form, though even from these sources—if the dose is large enough—acute poisoning may result. Affected animals are unthrifty, they have difficulty in breathing, colic is frequently noticed, and in some animals—especially in the horse and dog—a bluish line above the teeth on the gums is noted. This is the so-called "lead line." This chronic lead poisoning is very rare in animals as lead does not seem to be cumulative in animals as it is in man. One authority states in regard to the ingestion of lead compounds in cattle that "continued daily ingestion of lead in the very substantial dose of 8 mg. per kg. of body weight may be tolerated for months, and a level of 6 mg. per kg. of body weight per day may be tolerated for even three years."

Acute lead poisoning is commonest when animals consume vegetation in orchards after the trees have

Marginal notes:

Source of the lead that causes poisoning of livestock

Chronic lead poisoning rare in animals

Orchard grass and grasshopper poisons cause losses

been sprayed to control insect pests. Enough of the arsenate of lead spray is deposited on the underneath vegetation to cause the death of animals a few hours after its ingestion. In fact, hay produced from such sources may have enough of the poisonous lead on it to produce fatalities months after the spraying. Grasshopper poisons usually have arsenate of lead as the active ingredient, and there are plenty of recorded instances where cattle have had access to a pile of discarded bran grasshopper poison with the result that several died. However, in these conditions it undoubtedly is the arsenic component of the lead arsenate spray that is highly poisonous. Research indicates that acute lead poisoning is the result when lead oxide, lead carbonate and comparable compounds are ingested to the extent of from 0.2 to 0.4 gram per kilogram of body weight, and cattle more than four months of age require relatively larger amounts. Outstanding symptoms are slight temperature elevation, gradual loss of appetite and decreased water intake. It is even hinted that in pregnant ewes in an unthrifty condition abortion may take place.

Prevention consists in keeping animals away from recently painted structures; in fact, lead paints should have no place either for decorative or preservative purposes, nor should their containers be where animals can get to them. Grasshopper poisons, and other comparable insecticides, should be handled and disposed of with due regard for their dangerous qualities. Vegetation under trees sprayed with arsenate of lead is always dangerous. Veterinarians can save many animals that are acutely poisoned if the condition is not too far advanced. Chronic poisoning, once diagnosed, usually responds to withdrawal of the source of supply and the use of magnesium sulphate. Calcium versenate administered subcutaneously and intravenously is recommended. (Page 98, "Vet. Record" of Feb. 4, 1956.)

Arsenic poisoning: This is the condition when animals consume vegetation that has paris green or arsenite of soda applied to it, or when they drink some

Sources of arsenic

of the arsenical dip (page 315) in which they have just been submerged or which has drained from them. Occasionally arsenical poisoning follows the medicinal administration of an overdose of Fowler's solution of arsenic (Lig-Potassii Arsenitis) which has long been a favorite remedy with stablemen to "condition" their charges, and in the attempted cure of heaves in horses. Green paints have an arsenical base and may be causes of trouble. Some rat poisons have arsenic as their active agent and the promiscuous distribution of these is occasionally a source of poisoning of pets. The symptoms of arsenic poisoning are of a general character. Several deaths amongst livestock usually arouses suspicions of a poisonous agent, and more careful inquiry helps to confirm these. Trembling, staggering and

Symptoms of arsenic poisoning not characteristic

severe prostration occur. The animal indicates distress by groaning, restlessness and abdominal pain. In animals capable of the act such as sheep, cattle and swine, vomiting may take place; horses may retch. In chronic poisoning diarrhoea occurs as well as the odor of garlic from the breath. (Consult "Clinical Application of the Reinsch Test: A Rapid Preliminary Method for Identification of Arsenic" page 111, March 1950, number of "Veterinary Medicine" journal.) Treatment is usually without avail though to counteract unabsorbed arsenic in the digestive tract the freshly precipitated ferric hydrate is an old standby. This is usually prepared extemporaneously by mixing equal parts of ammonia water and tincture of chloride of iron; the resulting precipitate is squeezed out through cheese cloth and washed with water. Keeping animals from a source of supply, and due regard for the highly poisonous character of arsenic and its compounds will prevent losses.

World War II scientist developed a chemical now known as B.A.L., after the initials British Anti-Lewisite. Its discovery was the result of an effort to find an effective antidote against the dreaded war gas, Lewisite. B.A.L. was used in the form of an ointment because Lewisite affects the skin. Later the chemical was combined with peanut oil and benzyl benzoate for intramuscular injection. It is apparently an effective antidote for poisoning in humans from arsenic and mercury, and possibly gold and their compounds even after the poison has been absorbed from the digestive tract. It is explained that B. A. L. will draw the arsenic or the mercury from the tissues of the body and then combine with them, or the B. A. L. and the arsenic or mercury form a harmless combination. B. A. L.—it also is a poison—has not yet been used in veterinary medicine—it might have possibilities. One report states that in animals the intramuscular dose is one mg. per pound of body weight. From three to four injections are to be made the first two days and two injections the third day. Reports are so meager that extreme caution is advised in its use in animals. For details consult page 38, No. I, Vol. 40 of "Modern Veterinary Practice."

Mercury Poisoning: The medicinal preparations of mercury used in animal medicine are mercury bichloride (corrosive sublimate); mercurous chloride (mild chloride of mercury, calomel); mercurial ointment; and mercurial fungicides used on seed grains. Poisoning from these pharmaceuticals is rare in animals. The mercuric chloride is so quickly fatal that there is little chance to administer an effective antidote (page 275). The whites of eggs will combine with the unabsorbed mercury salt in the stomach to form an unabsorbed albuminate of mercury. B. A. L. (page 489) may be an effective antidote.

Deaths of swine have occurred as a sequence of the prolonged ingestion of seed oats, also seed corn, treated

Marginal note: An effective antidote for humans

with an organic mercurial fungicide. The reported symptoms throat paralysis, blindness, and a locomotor disturbance on post mortem examination brain and kidney lesions were found.

Copper Poisoning: (Blue vitriol, bluestone) (page 275). This occasionally produces poisoning in sheep because bluestone is a favorite and effec-

Sheep poisoned by copper tive remedy against stomach worms in sheep and to a less extent in cattle. It is a safe and effective remedy. However when mixed with salt so that every time an animal satisfies its craving for salt it also gets a dose of copper sulphate, poisoning may result. This then

Salt and copper injure sheep may produce chronic copper poisoning which in sheep is manifested by loss of appetite, jaundice and sometimes bloody urine. Its prevention consists in not forcing sheep or cattle to take copper sulphate with their daily salt ration.

Fluorine Poisoning (Fluorosis) (page 419). A high percentage of fluorine as an impurity in mineral mixtures, especially those having raw rock phosphate as one of the ingredients, may in rare cases result in softening of the teeth, and if the ingestion is continued there might be some softening and distor-

Fluorine poisoning rare in animals tion of bones. Mottling of the teeth, which is usually the first symptom, is of no particular significance in livestock, and seldom does an animal live long enough to get bone distortion. If the analysis of a mineral mixture indicates a high fluorine content good judgment will indicate not to feed it to animals. Animals need very minute quantities of fluorine which has been estimated to be 0.003 per cent for cattle, sheep and swine, and 0.015 for poultry on a total ration basis. Furthermore the upper limit of safety for cattle, sheep and swine is represented by 0.01 of fluorine in the dry matter of the total ration, and for chickens on the same basis it is in the neighborhood of 0.035 per cent. In

Florida a high level of 0.2 per cent of fluorine has been set as the maximum permissible content of this element in the phosphorus supplements offered for sale for feeding purposes.

Chlorate of Soda Poisoning: This chemical is extensively used as a herbicide especially in bindweed control programs. As used it is seldom a pure product. Stated otherwise it is a low grade commercial chemical having as impurities such compounds as calcium chloride, ammonium sulphate, and soda ash **A chemical** and others. When commercial chlorate of **used to kill** soda is used as a herbicide in an approved **weeds** degree of concentration in solution, and at the rate of approved application it may be considered non-toxic to livestock consuming sprayed vegetation. The approved strength for bindweed control is one pound of chlorate of soda dissolved in one gallon of water. An application of 200 gallons per acre in August, and a repeat of from 100 to 150 gallons per acre in September is the usual standard. In these strengths it has only very low toxicity for animals consuming sprayed vegetation. If too much is consumed, or if in too great concentration the animal appears distressed, bluish discoloration of the visible mucous membranes, convulsions, and possibly death will occur. Treatment is urgent and consists in intravenous methylene blue solution, and physiologic saline intravenously to hasten elimination of the chlorate iron.

2,4-D, 2,4,5-T. MCP Poisoning (2.4-dichlorophenoxyacetic acid, 2.4.5-trichlorophenoxyacetic acid and 4-chloro-o-toloxyacetic acid, their salts and esters). This group of herbicides, referred to as the plant hormones, constitutes by far the most widely used chemical means of controlling undesirable plants. As a group, these chemicals are practically non-toxic to experimental and farm animals. However, they do present indirect toxic hazards to livestock due to alteration of the plant itself rather than due to direct toxicity of the chemical. In laboratory animals the toxic dosage is 125 to 300 mg. per kg. of body weight.

Molybdenum Poisoning: Molybdenum is one element reported as being the cause of "teart" of cattle in England for more than a hundred years. The disease is a molybdenosis, characterized by anemia, diarrhoea, and loss of weight and milk production. It is due to the presence of molybdenum in the herbage of certain pastures. The California Agricultural Experiment Station has reported the presence of this poisoning in that state. The report indicates "that molybdenum is an essential micro-nutrient of plants, but when certain plants are grown in soils containing 1.5 to 3.0 parts per million they store up as much as 20 parts per million which is toxic to cattle." The Los Angeles County Livestock Department reports that animals in which a diagnosis of molybdenum poisoning had been made were placed on dry feed, and copper sulphate was administered at the rate of one gram per head per day; the cattle soon returned to normal.

Known for a hundred years in England

The disease in America

CHAPTER XXV

DEFICIENCY AILMENTS

Animals, much more frequently than humans, because of the comparatively narrow range of food varieties consumed by them, do not receive in their diets all those elements or compounds necessary for the normal functions of the body. As a result illness occurs. These ailments are collectively termed deficiency ailments. In some instances, "cottonseed meal poisoning" (page 460) is an example; the condition may, either because of its poisonous principle gossypol or as a lack of vitamins, be classed as a food poisoning or as a deficiency disease. Such hairline groupings may also be applied to other ailments.

Also there is a very close relationship between soil conditions and deficiency ailments in livestock. One of the principle functions of animals is to convert plants into animal tissue and necessarily if the soil is lacking in certain elements the plants grown on such soil will also be deficient and this, in turn, is reflected in animal ill health. In this connection it is well known that the vegetative part of a plant is more liable to nutritional variation than the seeds; therefore, the heavy roughage consuming animals are most likely to suffer from deficiency ailments. The use of natural manures, the growing of legumes, and possibly the use of fertilizers supplying calcium, phosphorus and potassium will overcome many of the deficiency ailments.

Soil conditions and deficiencies

Research agencies are still active in attempting to determine the best methods of curing roughages so as to maintain in them some of the unknown factors apparently more or less present during the growing

Other factors in deficiency conditions seasons. Young grass stimulates milk production beyond all other factors, but this same grass cured and used as a winter feed is lacking in this unusual lacteal stimulus.

Legumes harvested at a late stage of maturity do not have all the feed value of early young cuttings. Drought and other weather conditions during the growing season may prevent plants from taking up sufficient minerals for the maintenance of health in the consuming animals. When animals are fed for many generations on feeds produced year after year on the same farm, and no purchased feeds from other areas are used this may be reflected in a localized deficiency. Then there are the disturbances in metabolism in the animal economy that may be responsible for the most surprising upsets in animal welfare. (Consult Chapters IV and V).

Anemia in suckling pigs (page 86). In this condition the blood is deficient in red cells and the cells are low in hemoglobin content.

It is a condition affecting pigs, as well as calves and chicks occasionally that are continuously housed during the first few weeks of life. It is more frequently observed in spring than fall litters, **An ailment due to lack of soil contact, with subsequent iron and other mineral impoverished blood** because at the time of birth of the former the weather is frequently so inclement that there is no opportunity for soil contact by the little pigs. Later in the spring, or during the fall months the conditions for out-of-door life are more favorable. It seems that the appearance of the disease or its failure to develop is not influenced by sunlight exposure, or by a lack of green feed. The condition is apparently purely a nutritional disturbance caused by living conditions on cement, wood or other permanent flooring, and away from contact with soil which prevents the little animals from obtaining iron and copper, or iron alone, to replenish the depleted blood elements. All soil contains minute quantities of many chemical elements including the essential iron and copper. (Page 86).

The first symptoms usually observed are decreased vigor and unthriftiness. Even the slightest exertion causes fatigue and depression, and a short run may be followed by sudden death. An examination of the lining membrane of the mouth and adjoining regions discloses their markedly pale appearance.

The disease may be prevented by permitting the newly-born pigs to have access to soil from the first day following their birth. If the weather is **Prevention by** not favorable for out-of-door existence, **giving access** then some sod or even soil should be placed **to soil** in the pen so that the little pigs may have an opportunity to root in it, and incidentally to swallow some of it so as to obtain their quota of iron and copper. A more certain method of insuring this is to daily brush the nursing sow's udder with a solution made by dissolving a teaspoonful of copperas, (commercial sulphate of iron, this variety has minute quantities of copper in it as an impurity) in a quart of water. When the pigs are two or three weeks of age they usually begin to nibble at the sow's grain ration, and at this time the udder brushings may be discontinued, though the pigs still need iron. It is simpler to add it to the extent of one-tenth of one per cent to the

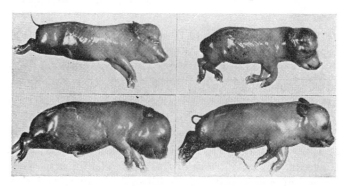

(Courtesy Dr. C. E. Aubel, Kansas State University)
FIG. 129. Hairlessness and big-neck due to iodine deficiency.

sow's grain ration so that the pigs may obtain it directly from this source. The small quantity contained in the food will not be harmful to the sow. When the pigs are eight weeks of age they are large enough— even during cold weather—to spend a part of their time out of doors to obtain the necessary soil contact.

Another method of handling is to thoroughly mix one pound of finely powdered iron sulphate, and one-fourth pound of copper sulphate. This

A practical method of getting iron and copper to pigs and sows

mixture is first mixed with a small amount of clean sand, and then with enough sand to bring the combination up to a total of 100 pounds. A little of the mixture is scattered over the floor of the pen holding the sow and her pigs. This is repeated each time the pen is cleaned. (Consult "Hemolytic Disease of Pigs," page 519.)

Shivering in Little Pigs (Hypoglycemia). Shivering, dullness and no desire to nurse are the first symptoms noticed in little pigs when they are

Shivering of newly born pigs

from 24 to 72 hours of age. The pigs when disturbed emit a weak squeal, the hair stands upright and they finally go into a coma.

Losses can be reduced by feeding the pregnant sow a liberal well-balanced grain ration. This will insure a good milk flow.

The little pigs should be closely watched during the first two or three days of life and if "shivering" develops they should be hand fed. Corn sirup diluted with an equal amount of warm water in doses of one or two teaspoonfuls every two hours is to be recommended. Call the veterinarian in order that he may administer glucose intraperitoneally—the response is much quicker than when oral medication is practiced. Later when there are signs of recovery a warmed mixture of two quarts of whole milk, the white of one egg, and three ounces of lime water is to be recommended. Do not over feed as this may result in scours. When four or five days old the pigs will usually be fed from a shallow pan.

Big-neck and hairlessness in pigs. (Fig. 129). In certain sections of the United States, especially the northwestern, and in some of the north central states, pigs at birth may be devoid of hair covering, or they may have "big" necks, or both. Research has demonstrated that the "big-neck" is due to an enlargement of the thyroid gland or it is goitre, and that both it and the hairlessness are the result of disturbed metabolism because of insufficient iodine intake (page 85) by the sow during the period of pregnancy. This same deficiency exists in the tissues of the young.

Diseases due to a lack of iodine

Prevention consists in seeing to it that the sow receives an adequate amount of iodine. When pigs are born "big-necked," or hairless, or both, it is prima facie evidence that the sows on that particular farm are not receiving the necessary amount of iodine—possibly because of a regional soil and water deficiency in this element. Making up this deficiency by feeding the sow iodine in the form of commercial iodized salt, or two grains of iodide of potash daily will prevent future trouble.

Prevention is simple

Nutritional blindness in cattle. In this condition the animals become blind, though it does not appear to be due to an infection as is so frequently the case. In this general grouping there must first be included the type of blindness usually associated with an excess of cottonseed meal (pages 74 and 460) in the ration, and without at the same time providing the animals with a balancing or compensatory ration. This particular type of blindness is sometimes referred to as cottonseed meal poisoning. It is usually the result of a lack of vitamin A (page 63) in the ration. Immaterial of the amount of cottonseed meal fed, if at the same time

This ailment is an avitaminosis

a part of the ration consists of a substance rich in vitamin A, such as a high quality of alfalfa, the blindness will not develop. In those animals in which this type of blindness has already made its appearance, the temporary or permanent withholding from the ration of the vitamin-A-deficient cottonseed meal, together with a liberal addition of vitamin-A-rich alfalfa will usually speedily overcome the blindness.

There is another type of nutritional blindness occurring in animals that are receiving some vitamin A in their ration at the time of appearance **The handling** of the blindness. Swelling of the legs is **of nutritional** frequently an additional symptom. There **blindness** are recorded instances where a portion of the ration consisted of yellow corn, which is vitamin-A-rich grain. The roughage fed at the same time was of the poorer quality, such as straw or corn fodder. This blindness has not been observed if a good quality of hay is fed with the yellow corn. Blindness of this type has associated with it an incurable degeneration or breaking down of the optic nerve, and therefore when the blindness is complete, it is also permanent. When the blindness is incomplete, or partial, it may be arrested in this stage by changing it to a wholesome vitamin-A-rich ration such as yellow corn and good quality hay. The theory has been advanced that it is not a vitamin-A-deficiency blindness, but rather a provitamin A shortage, and that the good hay supplies this.

Both of these somewhat identical types of blindness illustrate the importance of an adequate supply of vitamins in the rations of animals—without them there is potential danger. (Page 63.)

Starvation in Beef Cattle: Undoubtedly an insufficient quantity of total feed is the most frequent and, in general, the most serious nutritional deficiency affecting beef cattle—particularly those on the range. The available roughages often contain less than five per cent of protein (page 40). Less than eight per cent of total crude protein in the dry range forage is an absolute required minimum under the most favorable conditions—in this poorly digestible feed. At the same time phosphorus (page 83) is usually very low. These starved animals frequently turn to poisonous plants when under plentiful feed supply conditions they are avoided; thus, many die from poisoning. Others are so devitalized that they are ready prey for parasitism and because of a lack of resistance they contract and succumb to infections and contagious diseases. A plentiful supply of good nourishing feed is the answer to this problem.

Pregnancy disease in Ewes (page 39). Other names are lambing paralysis, old ewe disease, stercoremia, ketosis, and acidosis of pregnant ewes. As many as twenty-five per cent of the pregnant ewes may become affected, and ninety per cent of those in the more advanced stages of the disease die if treatment is delayed. If, therefore, the disease is diagnosed amongst

Pregnancy disease of ewes caused by a deficiency of carbohydrates in the ration a flock of ewes, it is well to ask a veterinarian to subject other ewes that are in advanced pregnancy to the so-called Ross test (page 507) by means of which the presence of ketones—these are the poisons responsible for the disease—in the urine may be determined. If found to be present curative and preventive treatment should at once be applied.

In almost every outbreak of this disease there are either two or three lambs in the uterus. The cause of the disease is believed to be largely the result of feeding a ration deficient in carbohydrates—this means sugars and starches. The disease is seldom or never observed in range ewes, and therefore the supposition that exercise is a preventive or, on the other hand, that a lack of sufficient exercise is a contributing cause. The symptoms most frequently observed are outstandingly of a nervous character. Some animals go down and are unable to arise, others push persistently with the head against some fixed object; gnashing of the teeth is quite common. When the animal is down it frequently makes trotting motions. On post mortem examination there are no outstanding changes in the carcass that are visible to the naked eye. The liver is frequently somewhat enlarged, the carcass has a good deal of fat, and there are two or three lambs in the uterus. Animals that contract the disease frequently die in less than a week after the first symptoms are noticed. Very little can be done in the way of curative treatment excepting during the earliest stages and at this time two ounces of molasses or brown sugar daily continued for several days is of value. Cortisone products seem to be helpful but are generally too expensive.

In the prevention of the disease the first important step is to see to it that during the last month of pregnancy, ewes take a reasonable amount of exercise daily. This is sometimes accomplished by compelling the animals to walk for some distance to the feed racks, then have the water tank placed in another direction and at some distance from the feed racks, so that the animal must exercise for feed and water. If the ewe will not take exercise otherwise, then she should be driven daily. Another most important preventive step consists in feeding a balanced ration which should contain a sufficient amount of *carbohydrates* (sugars and starches). Permitting the animal to partake of alfalfa at will, and in addition giving it about a pound of grain daily is satisfactory. The grain mixture may consist largely of cracked corn, and some ground oats and oil meal. Or, equal parts of bran, oil meal, oats and barley seem to be satisfactory. There are many other grain combinations that may be fed. In the absence of carbohydrates in the ration, a substitute consists in the addition of molasses—up to one-half pound daily—to the roughage.

The prevention of pregnancy disease

Since glycerine can enter into the carbohydrate cycle by being converted into glycogen and glucose, and since a feature of the disease is a disturbed carbohydrate metabolism, the administration of four ounces of it mixed with an equal volume of water has been found to be helpful in early cases.

During the early stages of the disease, a veterinarian should be asked to administer, subcutaneously or intravenously, a proper dose of "sugars" to supply the animal's immediate need. If the animal is constipated, this phase of the disease should be properly handled. In summing up the condition, then, the points to bear in mind are that pregnant ewes must have exercise, and they must receive carbohydrates in their ration in the form of grain, or, molasses may be given as a part of the ration.

After all is said and done, prevention is of the greatest importance, and the steps in prevention may be summarized as follows: (1) Ewes are bred on grass pasture—avoid rich succulent legumes; (2) during the fall months keep the ewes on good pasture—no grain is needed unless the roughage is not a good supplement; (3) at the beginning of the third month of the gestation period supplement with one-half pound of grain per ewe daily—this is gradually increased to one or one and one-half pounds daily during the last month of pregnancy; (4) compel the ewe to take daily limited exercise as described in a preceding paragraph.

Wheat "poisoning" (grass staggers, grass tetany, railroad sickness). The growing wheat plant is extensively grazed in the wheat growing sections of the nation. During the stage when it is grazed it is highly nutritious so that cattle on pasture of this nature gain up to $2\frac{1}{2}$ pounds daily. The wheat plant contains from 20 to 26 per cent of protein, and a high per cent of calcium, phosphorus and potassium, though sodium percentage is low. When cows in advanced pregnancy or early lactation have been on this pasture for 30 to

90 days—open heifers and steers are seldom affected—
the blood sugar level drops progressively from a normal of 50 to 60 mg. per 100 cc. of blood until it levels
off at about 50 mg. per 100 cc. The level is about one-
half that of non-ruminants. Hypoglycemia (low blood
sugar level) follows when the blood sugar

Blood changes in wheat "poisoning" falls below 20 to 30 mg. and it is accompanied by low calcium and magnesium
levels so that the former may be as low as
$3\frac{1}{2}$ mg. and the latter 2 to 3 mg. per
100 cc. of blood.

All of these blood changes are to be expected when
an animal has no feed other than the unjointed wheat
plant. Wheat plant is not grazed after it starts to joint
as this will prevent it from seeding. Therefore the normal magnesium-calcium ratio in cattle is about 1:35,
and in wheat poisoning it is about 1:14. In affected animals there are intermittent tonic contractions of the

Similar symptoms produced experimentally muscles accompanied by excitement so that
humans may be attacked. Later the animal
goes down, the third eyelid (membrana
nictitans) is protruded, the head is drawn
back, the heart beat is rapid and pounding, cyanosis (bluish discoloration of mucous membranes) sets in, the cell volume of the blood is frequently up from a normal of 30 per cent to as high as
45 per cent and abortion may take place. Almost all of
the symptoms mentioned may be produced experimentally in a normal cow by injecting intravenously
large amounts of chloride of potash. On good wheat
pasture a cow consumes as much as 10 ounces of nitrate of potash daily. Supplying the animals with the
proper minerals—ground limestone and salt mixed—
usually prevents the condition. If the disease has developed, it is usually promptly overcome in its early
stages by intravenous injections of a solution of calcium gluconate slowly injected to avoid heart block—in
rare cases to be supplemented by subcutaneous or in-

travenous administration of a solution of magnesium sulphate and normal saline.

Paralysis of the hind parts in swine. This disease is rickets occurring when the animals are fed largely on a cereal ration (page 80) and especially if there is a lack of vitamin D (page 71) (Figs. 14, 15 and 130)

Paralysis in pigs due to a lime deficiency and an avitaminosis
when insufficient direct sun exposure is provided, though the place of the latter may be taken by fish liver oils. It may involve the front limbs (Fig. 130). The incoordinated gait frequently observed in vitamin A deficiency (page 63) is of a

different nature. The disease is a lime (calcium) deficiency. The chief symptom is a loss of function of the limbs varying from a slight lameness to inability to walk. The rear part of the body usually goes down completely, though progression is still possible on the bent fore limbs. In advanced cases the joints may be enlarged. The appetite and general health are apparently unimpaired. In a few instances ketosis (page 505) is responsible if it occurs shortly after farrowing; these cases respond to the ketosis treatment.

Prevention consists in feeding a well-balanced ration including skimmed milk, protein in the form of tankage, and alfalfa in addition to the cereal grains. If the disease is not of long existence and not accompanied by prominent deformity recovery takes place by the addition of two per cent of finely ground limestone to the ration. Some swine feeders—depending largely upon cereals for their animal feed—feel that they have a preventive in a mixture of steamed bone meal and tankage in the ratio of nine parts of the former to one part of the latter kept before the animals so that they may partake of it at will. It is advisable to supplement this mineral allowance with daily small doses of fish liver oil, especially during gloomy seasons and low sun radiation. During the winter months sunlight has less than one-fifth the antirachitic value of summer sunlight.

A survey (1954) in New Zealand reported on page 157, No. 4, Vol. 3, Dec. of the New Zealand Veterinary Journal about "Posterior Paralysis in Pigs" indicates another situation in that region. It appears from the survey that pigs from a copper deficient region become paralyzed in the hind parts. Autopsies disclosed a low copper content in the liver and in some instances loss of nerve fiber sheaths (demyelination) in all areas of the spinal cord except the dorsal. Prevention of additional cases consisted in the use of copper sulphate in the diet.

In those cases in which a copper deficiency was not proven and in which no demyelination was present, recovery in an estimated 70 per cent followed the use of a fish-liver oil alone, or combined with either copper sulphate or yeast in the diet. Yeast was used for its high vitamin D content, and the fish-liver oil for its vitamin A.

Rickets in cattle. (Fig. 13) (page 72). This disease occurs in cattle but not with the same frequency as in swine, and it is most commonly a

Rickets in cattle a phosphorus deficiency phosphorus deficiency rather than a lime deficiency. The parathyroids (page 99) have been suggested—when affected with dysfunction—as a contributing cause.

Such symptoms as an appearance of general unthriftiness with or without bone deformities as bow legs or forward bending of the front legs are noticed. At times it is no more than a stiff stilted gait. During the earlier stages the animal may have a "depraved appetite" causing it to chew bones or other foreign substances, and in licking of barns, fences, and other wood-work give it the designation "licking disease." Foods rich in phosphorus such as wheat, barley, oats and cottonseed meal are recommended, to be supplemented by other sources of phosphorus, especially that contained in steamed bone meal. The bone meal requirement varies from one-half pound per week for growing calves, three-fourths pounds per week for

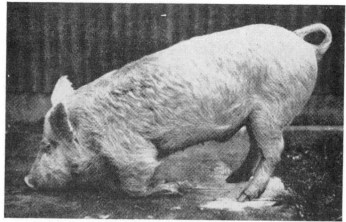

(Photo reproduced from Black's Veterinary Dictionary)
FIG. 130. Rickets following unbalanced ration.

growing stock over three hundred pounds in weight, and as much as two pounds or more per week for cows in full milk flow. Rations made up from several plant sources are more likely to contain the necessary elements than rations made up from one plant source. Vitamin D and sunshine—or fish-liver oils in place of the latter—also are needed (page 71).

It has become a custom to fortify commercial and home mixed calf feeds with vitamin D. In home mix-

Irradiated yeast in calf meal as a preventive of rickets

tures this is accomplished by adding one pound of irradiated yeast (this contains approximately four million units) to each ten pounds of calf meal. If clinical rickets is present additional vitamin D must be supplied—this may be in the form of ultraviolet light radiation.

False or Chronic Milk Fever, Acetonemia, or Ketosis in Cattle. (Consult Milk Fever, page 509.) This

An ailment due to a low intake of carbohydrate

disease closely parallels pregnancy disease in ewes with the exception that it is most frequently observed within the first six weeks after calving though it may occur at any time. It very seldom or never occurs in dry and non-pregnant cows, and steers and bulls. There is good foundation for the belief that the removal of sugars from the cow's blood as a result of pregnancy, the drain of heavy milk production, and possibly low intake of sugars and starches in a ration lacking adequate grain are all factors in producing the disease. Normally in cattle the blood sugar level is about 50 to 60 mgm. per 100 cc. (ml) of blood. In ketosis it may drop quickly to 20 to 30 mgm. per 100 cc., and associated with this is a rise in ketones from 1 to 5 mgm. in 100 cc. of blood to 20 to 80 mgm.; then clinical symptoms of ketosis become manifest. Pathologists sum up the situation by saying that in this disease there is a disturbed carbohydrate-fat metabolism in the liver, impaired kidney function, and functional damage to the central nervous system.

There are no characteristic symptoms in this ailment. General symptoms are observed such as loss of appetite, decreased milk flow—the milk frequently has a decidedly "cowy" flavor (page 369)—rapid loss of condition and constipation. Occasionally there are nervous developments so that affected animals run into fences and buildings, though more frequently there is listlessness and extreme docility. The back may be arched, and the gait wobbly or stilted. The temperature is seldom elevated.

A positive diagnosis can be made by the examination of the animal's urine by means of Ross' test (page 507). If the reaction is positive it indicates the presence of ketone bodies in the urine which is diagnostic of this ailment.

A test for "false milk fever"

In order to conduct Ross' test one gram of finely ground sodium nitro-prusside is thoroughly mixed with one hundred grams of ammonium sulfate. This mixture should be stored in an amber colored bottle in a dark place. The other reagent is stronger ammonia water (28%). To five cubic centimeters of urine in a test tube add one gram of the sodium nitro-prusside-ammonium sulfate mixture, and shake the tube until the solid material is completely dissolved. Then add two cubic centimeters of the stronger ammonia water and invert the tube a few times, after which it is set aside for observation. If the animal is affected with acetonemia the brown colored solution will soon change to a deep purple color.

Milk Test for Acetonemia or Ketosis: This is a test somewhat similar to the Ross urine test (page 506), though more readily applied. For making the test a nitroprusside mixture is used. It is made by grinding two grams of sodium nitroprusside in a mortar and intimately mixing with it 98 grams of ammonium sulphate. The procedure recommended for the milk

A new test for the detection of ketosis test is to add to 5 ml. (5 cubic centimeters) of whole milk 2.5 grams of the nitroprusside mixture. Mix well and add one ml. (one cubic centimeter) of concentrated ammonium hydroxide. A positive reaction is a pink or purple color which develops in about ten minutes. If the animal has been on formalin treatment the test reaction does not take place. No interference to the test is encountered from previous medication or treatment with turpentine, linseed oil, sulphonamides, iodine, strychnine, and sodium salicylate. Sour milk gives unreliable results. In acetonemia the concentration of ketones in the milk is about the same as in the blood—in the urine it may be 15 times that in the blood. Though there is no relationship of the reaction of the milk test and the severity of the clinical symptoms it is recognized that when the milk contains less than six mg. ketones in 100 ml. of milk the reaction in the milk test is only slightly positive.

Prevention of the disease is not always possible in the case of heavy milkers. The heavier feeding of

Prevention of "false milk fever" grains such as corn during the last month of pregnancy and the first six to eight weeks following calving is to be recommended. The addition to the grain ration of one quart of molasses per day is excellent.

Curative treatment also concerns itself with the administration subcutaneously or intravenously of comparatively large doses of chemically pure sugars, and the symptomatic handling of the patient. A diet rich in vitamin A (page 63) is very important; in fact, the attending veterinarian should be consulted as to the advisability of administering very large doses of this vitamin for at least three successive days.

The sugar used in the treatment is from 500 to 1000 mls. of 40 per cent glucose intravenously administered. The results are at once favorable but unfortunately most of the glucose is eliminated in the urine so that two hours later the animal is again distressed. There-

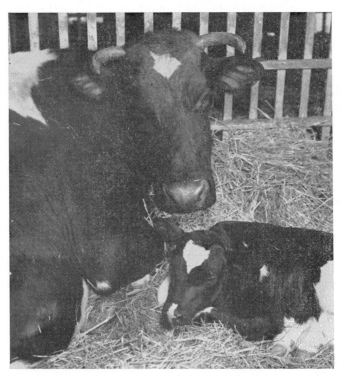

FIG. 131. Early stages of milk fever.

fore, veterinarians by means of a gravity apparatus continue the administration of the glucose so that the animal will receive from 150 to 200 mls. per hour until ketone levels in the urine drop materially. It is also desirable to give molasses.

Animals other than cattle, such as swine and goats may be affected according to early experimental evidence. Sheep have pregnancy disease which is ketosis (page 499).

Milk fever in cattle. (Consult "False Milk Fever," page 505). This disease, also known as parturient paresis, affects cows that have recently calved. In it there is a loss of calcium and inorganic phosphorus from the blood, and an increase in blood magnesium and blood sugar, this latter being the opposite from that in false milk fever or acetonemia (page 505).

The first symptoms are usually noticed in from twelve to seventy-two hours after calving, or they may be delayed for several weeks. The animal appears dull (Fig. 131), there is some muscular twitching, and inability to support weight especially on the hind limbs. When down, the head is turned back against the ribs,

Milk-fever is a disease closely associated with calving or if held forward the upper border of the back may have in it a peculiar kink. Complete unconsciousness usually sets in with the animal on its side, and paunch contents flowing out of the mouth. These contents are sometimes drawn into the lungs during breathing and then foreign body lung fever develops.

Untreated patients usually die in from a few hours to a few days. Properly treated patients usually recover, or in these the death rate is less than four per cent of those affected.

Prevention is reasonably effective; it is at least encouraging. It seems that animals having had one attack of this ailment are subject to its recurrence at subsequent calvings. In animals of this type it is a good plan for a period of ten days following calving to never

Prevention of milk fever

remove all of the milk. For the first few days milk partially every two hours; gradually increase the amount removed at a milking, and also the time between milkings so that at the end of the ten day period the milking approaches the normal. This entire procedure is comparable to the removal of the milk by a calf when nursing its dam.

The first successful curative treatment consisted in inflation of the udder with air. Apparently this method forces back into the blood stream some of the calcium which is quite abundantly present in the udder. This form of treatment in the hands of those not familiar with strict aseptic technique resulted in so many spoiled or ruined udders that it is not now generally practiced.

The early air treatment productive of unfavorable results

More recently the calcium deficiency of this disease has been rectified by the intravenous use of a solution of calcium boro-gluconate, supported in some instances by the subcutaneous injection of a sterile solution of magnesium sulphate, and other agents including dextrose.

Modern treatment and nursing

Good nursing practices in the form of placing the animal in a comfortable position so that it rests on its sternum or breast, fresh water, and mechanical removal of the urine are all helpful in preventing relapses and in hastening recovery. Never administer medicine by way of the mouth in the form of drenching as it is likely to get into the lungs with a resulting pneumonia.

Failure to respond to approved treatment may be ascribed to the fact that milk fever is occasionally complicated by other ailments such as poisoning from partially retained after-births, and other genital infections.

Sheep, goats, and swine are sometimes affected with a condition that closely parallels milk fever in cows. Sheep and goats respond favorably to the same treatment as cattle, and sows usually recover spontaneously following good nursing practices.

Crazy chick disease, nutritional encephalomalacia, epidemic tremors. This disease occurs suddenly at any age, usually between two and four weeks, or as late as eight weeks. They suddenly become very nervous and active, sit on their hocks and move backward by pushing with their feet, or they may wheel in circles, falling either forward, backward, or on the side. Trembling of the head and legs, with complete prostration is observed in advanced cases. The mortality rate is low and if not trampled to death, some will develop into broilers. Therefore, isolate.

"Crazy chick" disease prevented by the use of vitamin E

Prevention is comparatively simple by including in the ration some substances rich in vitamin E (page 72).

Black-tongue of Dogs (pellagra). This is a disease that also occurs in humans. It is due to a deficiency of the vitamin B compound known as nicotinic acid (page 70). Nourishing balanced food is the preventive. Curative treatment necessitates additional nicotinic acid.

Vitamin A Deficiency in Poultry: (Consult page 66).

Vitamin D Deficiency: (Consult page 71).

Perosis in Fowl: (Consult page 89).

Curled Toe Paralysis: (Ariboflavinosis) This condition is observed at times in chicks—especially males —about the third to the fourth week of brooding. The disease seems to affect the hocks (femorotibial articulation) so that the bird assumes a squatting position with the toes characteristically turned inward. On microscopic examination a morbid softening of some of the branches of the sciatic nerve is a lesion. The ailment is due to riboflavin—a vitamin B_2—de-

Curled toes due to riboflavin deficency

ficiency (page 69). In its early stage recovery is almost dramatic—in less than 24 hours—from individual dosing with about 10,000 micrograms of riboflavin.

Parakeratosis of Swine: a zinc deficiency. (Consult page 87.)

CHAPTER XXVI

MISCELLANEOUS SPORADIC AILMENTS

These are ailments, commonly observed, that do not lend themselves readily to any form of grouping. Most of them occur quite frequently, and veterinarians are well familiar with their treatment.

Azoturia, Monday disease, Holiday disease, Lumbago, Black water. These and other designations are used as terms to indicate quite a common horse disease. (Page 38.) It occurs most commonly in draft horses accustomed to daily exercise that are kept on full feed during a day of enforced idleness—hence the names Monday disease and Holiday disease. It is occasionally observed following accidental casting and the resulting struggling while the animal is stabled. When returned to work after the brief period of idleness the disease may develop.

An ailment observed in horses, accustomed to regular work, after a day of rest on full feed

The symptoms consist in profuse sweating, stiff gait, reluctance to move, and lameness in one or both hind limbs, or occasionally in the front. Finally the animal goes down in the affected limbs assuming a sitting dog position, to be followed by lying flat on its side. Severe struggling and sweating set in until exhaustion is complete.

The muscles of the affected limbs, especially those of the shoulders when the fore limbs are involved, are hard and board-like.

The characteristic symptom of the disease is the bright red or coffee-colored urine. As urination is usually scanty or suppressed it may be necessary to mechanically remove some of the urine to detect its abnormal color.

Prevention of this disease consists in either reducing the grain ration during days of enforced idleness, or exercising the animal during such days.

Prevention of azoturia Most horse owners prefer the latter mode of prevention as it leaves the animal in good condition for its work, though withholding the grain ration on days of idleness results in a lessened energy capacity when labor is resumed.

When the first symptoms of the disease make their appearance absolute rest is to be enforced for several hours, after which the animal may be permitted to slowly return to its abode. Recovery is the usual result following this method of handling. The continuance of muscular effort after the onset of the initial symptoms is almost certain to be ensued by a fatal termination. The services of a veterinarian should at once be engaged to insure the application of correct procedures for ultimate recovery. Heated clothes or blankets, hot water bottles, and comparable devices may be beneficially applied to the swollen and hardened muscles while awaiting the doctor.

White muscle disease; (Myopathy.) This ailment of lambs—calves and kids also—is not to be confused

An ailment of lambs characterized by stiffness and thought to be the result of improper feeding of the ewe with other conditions such as forms of food poisoning, brain diseases, tetanus (locked jaw), and others in which stiffness may also be observed as one of the symptoms. True stiff-lamb disease when it develops occurs in lambs at any age of one to eight weeks and when they are turned out to pasture—in calves any time from birth to four months of age, and especially after drought and short grass

season, rare after grass starts—or less rarely when they are still in the barn yard. A general contention is that it is a nutritional disease. On a postmortem examination the muscles of the affected parts—these are usually those of the hind limbs—are found to have

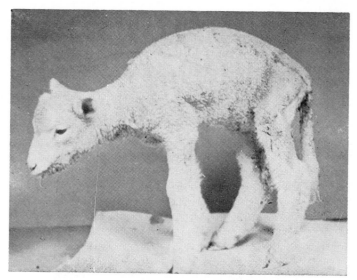

(Courtesy Dr. M. L. Gray, College of Veterinary Medicine, Michigan State University)

FIG. 132. Lamb affected with "White Muscle Disease" or "Stiff Lamb Disease."

whitish streaks in greater or less number and corresponding somewhat to the severity of the attack (Figs. 132, 133 and 134). Heart lesions in the form of round patches in size from pin point to 10 mm. in diameter are in the right ventricle.

The symptoms in the ailing lamb are disinclination to stand, with stiffness when compelled to move. As the disease progresses paralysis or total inability to use the limbs sets in. There is no fever and the appetite is not very much impaired, excepting during the stage before death, which is usual termination.

Though the cause is not definitely known —other than nutritional—it is quite a general belief that the severe exercise of gamboling in lambs may be an exciting cause. Since the condition is relatively rare after grass pasture becomes available—grass is rich in vitamin E—it points to a vitamin E deficiency (page 72). It is still a question whether the muscular changes

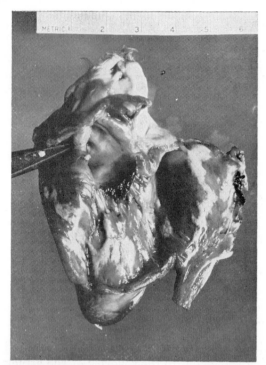

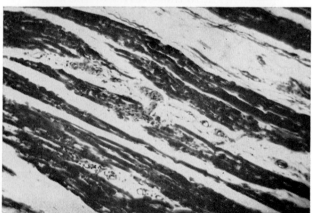

(Courtesy Dr. M. L. Gray, College of Veterinary Medicine, Michigan State University)

Figs. 133 and 134. Heart and skeletal muscles in White Muscle Disease.

observed in this disease are primary or secondary. Poor quality feed is predisposing, and in cows, a ration exclusively of second cutting alfalfa and red cull beans—this has a high calcium-phosphorus ratio—during pregnancy, resulted in myopathy in a large percentage of the calves.

Prevention consists in avoiding prolonged severe exercise during winter stabling and the pre-grass season. Ewes and cows should receive some bone-meal regularly before springtime pasture is available, and for creep-fed lambs and calves ground wheat should be in the grain ration. If wheat is not available the grain ration should be fortified with wheat germ oil because of its vitamin E content.

Severe exercise a predisposing factor

Wheat-germ oil in the treatment of early stages has not been successful because of its relatively low vitamin E content, therefore vitamin E either as its alpha-tocopherol fraction or the acetate is much more effective. In the early stages before extensive muscle changes have taken place alpha-tocopherol in an initial 500 mg. dose and from 100 to 300 mg. every other day until symptoms subside seems to be helpful. In calves the dose is doubled. Advanced cases do not respond to treatment because the muscle changes are not reversible.

In New Zealand when the pastures were top-dressed with superphosphate, magnesium, iron, cobalt and copper, and pregnant ewes grazed on these pastures, there were no cases of white muscle disease (page 214, Jour. Am. Vet. Med. Assoc., Mar. 1, 1958).

Deficiency of selenium in the ration is believed by some to be a contributing cause of white muscle disease. In addition to vitamin E in the ration of pregnant ewes, it was practically a preventive of the ailment when there was added 0.1 part per million of sodium selenite in the ration (p. 239, Mar. 1, 1959, Jour. Am. Vet. Med. Assoc.)

Icteric Foals (Jaundiced foals; hemolytic icterus in foals) : This disease was first observed affecting newly born foals in one of the great horse-breeding sections of the United States. It usually results in death of the foal once it is well established. An early preliminary examination of the dead animals failed to disclose any infection that might be held responsible. It appears that the foal seems normal at birth though in a day or two jaundice—as evidenced by a yellowish discoloration of the tissues—makes its appearance, and usually about the fourth day after birth the young creature dies.

Is there an incompatibility in the blood of the sire and dam?

An autopsy fails to disclose anything other than the yellowish discoloration of the tissues and organs of the body. The cause of the ailment is an incompatibility of the blood of the foal's sire and dam. In all cases of icteric foals the red blood corpuscles (erythrocytes) of the stallion were clumped together (agglutinated) by the blood serum of the mare when specimens of the two are mixed, and the red corpuscles of the foal reacted like those of its sire. Now when the blood of the mare is sensitized to certain types of red blood corpuscles by being bred to a stallion which transmits that type of corpuscle to its offspring the latter contracts the fatal icteric jaundice. The first milk of the dam (colostrum) contains the red corpuscle destroying antibodies of the mare, and when this colostrum is ingested by the foal it results in icteric jaundice. However, after a foal has reached the age of 36 to 48 hours it loses the ability to absorb antibodies from its digestive tract, and it is safe from this type of jaundice.

Blood reactions occur

Prevention of the ailment in foals consists in muzzling it immediately after its birth for a period of 48 hours. During this time it must be artificially fed. (Consult feeding orphan colts page 771.) The mare during this period must be hand milked every hour. At the end of the 48 hour period the foal may safely be permitted to nurse its dam.

Don't let colt have mare's milk for 48 hours after its birth

When the preventive steps have not been followed so that jaundice appears it is helpful to remove from 500 to 1000 ml. of the colt's blood, and immediately replace it with 1000 to 2000 ml. of compatible blood—in this connection it is necessary to remember that the foal is ill because it is carrying the red corpuscle destroying antibodies of its dam and therefore blood injected into the foal must be derived from a donor whose red blood corpuscles are compatible with those of the dam. When prenatal blood typing of the parents' blood indicates that the colt may develop the ailment in addition to withholding the colt from nursing its dam it is advisable as an additional preventive step to give the colt every four hours a 250 ml. blood transfusion from a compatible donor.

Hemolytic Disease of Newborn Pigs: This disease of newborn pigs is very similar to "hemolytic icterus" in foals (page 518), in that both of these ailments are the result of mating serologically incompatible parents.

Jaundice and anemia when the bloods of parents are not compatible

In these cases, the unborn pig inherits antigen from the sire which is passed to the dam so that in her body there is produced an antibody. An antigen is any substance such as toxins, toxoids, ferments, bacteria, viruses, etc., which when gaining access to the animal body causes the production of antibodies of a specific nature. For example, hog cholera virus forms an antibody that gives protection against hog cholera; blackleg vaccine has its antibody against blackleg, etc. Under certain conditions of placental—these are the membranes that envelop the unborn young—permeability of the antibody may pass into the body of the unborn young so as to cause its death, while it is still in the uterus. In other instances, the antibody concentrates in the colostrum—this is the milk of the dam, for at least a few days immediately after the birth of the young—so that the foetus is born normally and nurses normally. But during the first 60 hours of its extra uterine life the antibody it receives in the colostrum destroys its red blood cells with symptoms of profound anemia and varying degrees of icterus (jaundice), and causes its death. There is no known remedy against this condition other than to have normally born piglets from the moment they are dropped placed on the breasts of a foster mother, or fed artificially (consult page 773). The antibody in the sow is usually permanent.

Moon-blindness of horses, periodic or recurrent ophthalmia. This is an eye ailment affecting only horses. Formerly the recurrent nature of the disease led to the belief that the eyes of the horses were deleteriously affected by phases of the moon, hence the designation "moon-blindness," though the erroneousness of this theory is now universally conceded.

A mysterious periodic eye ailment frequently erroneously associated with the phase of the moon

The cause of the disease is not yet known although it has been demonstrated that riboflavin (page 69) deficiency is a factor in its development. It has been described as a heritable condition, and attempts have been made to incriminate various germs and viruses without success. In some European countries affected stallions are disqualified for public service as the fear exists that the disease may be transmitted to the offspring.

The first attack, usually affecting only one eye, sets in so suddenly that an injury is suspected though a careful examination fails to substantiate this. There is every evidence of pain in the eye, tears flow freely, the eyeball is discolored, and the lids are swollen. In a few days the symptoms disappear almost completely, but after a varying period up to three months a second more severe attack occurs, and as time passes there are succeeding attacks. Following each of these the clear portion of the eye gradually becomes more cloudy and the eyeball becomes shrunken until the eye function is permanently impaired. The second eye soon becomes involved in a comparable manner. There is no known method of prevention, nor is there a cure.

Heat stroke, sun stroke, heat exhaustion (page 107). Animals confined in humid non-ventilated quarters, or those compelled to labor during hot humid days, and heavily fleeced animals, or excessively fat ones are subject to this condition. In working animals not enough drinking water to compensate for the fluid lost by sweating is probably the principal cause. Also the excessive loss of salt (chloride of soda) during sweating soon reduces the requirements of the body for this chemical to a dangerously low point.

High temperatures, humidity, hard work, loss of salt, and low water intake are contributing factors in causing this condition

Prevention consists in letting working horses drink frequently and the addition of a smooth teaspoonful of table salt to each three gallons of drinking water is helpful. A veterinarian can treat affected animals by the intravenous use of a saline solution and heart stimulants.

"Gravel." (Water-belly of steers, urethral or urinary calculus). This is a condition which most frequently causes trouble in bulls, steers, rams, and wethers (Figs. 135 and 136). The gravel or stone develops in the kidneys or in the urinary bladder. Its cause is not understood though it is believed that a disturbed relation in the calcium, phosphorus, and magnesium intake is an important factor, and deficient vitamin A in the ration has been pointed to as another. The composition of the drinking water is of no significance. It seems that sheep fed beets and mangels are somewhat more frequently affected (Fig. 137). One research project (Swingle of

An accumulation of chemical substances in the urinary organs

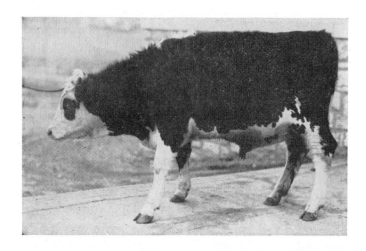

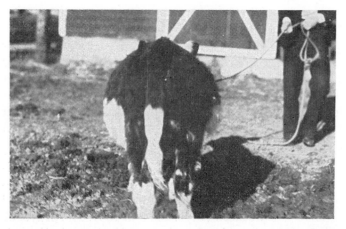

FIGS. 135 and 136. (Above) Swelling of the region of the sheath because of a "gravel" in the penis. (Below) Enlarged abdomen because of urine in it following rupture of the urinary bladder as a sequel of "gravel."

Montana Veterinary Research Laboratory) in 63 cases in range steers revealed protein and silica associated at times with calcium oxalate and magnesium.

In male sheep and cattle the excretory duct from the urinary bladder known as the urethra is of a very elongated funnel shape with a comparatively large opening at its origin from the bladder and a much smaller exit at the end of the penis. Also in these animals there is a distinct S curve in the penis. Because of the gradual decrease in size of the lumen of the urethra and its S-curved direction small gravel may readily enter it, though the forward passage is soon blocked with the result that urination is practically completely stopped. The affected animal shows evidence of pain by stamping of its hind feet and there is distinct pulsation of the urethra just beneath the anus and along the course of the sheath there may be swelling (Fig. 135). If not relieved the distended bladder finally ruptures and discharges the urine into the abdominal cavity so that this becomes enlarged (Fig. 136). The animal appears better for two or three days, then because of absorption of urine into the tissues death ensues from uremic poisoning.

If there are several animals affected on the same farm during succeeding years the animal food supply should be changed. A chemical analysis of the food

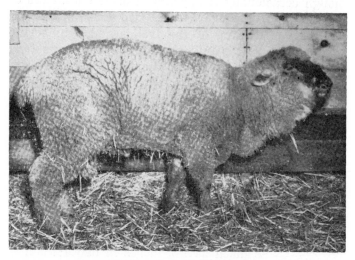

(Courtesy C. E. Lindley, Washington Agr. Exp. Sta.)

Fig. 137. Straining position of wether affected with "gravel" or urethral calculus.

as well as of the blood of affected animals should give valuable information for future guidance. The feeding of a ration rich in vitamin A (page 63) such as grass in season, and leafy alfalfa and yellow corn at other times may be helpful in relieving early stages of the ailment. In later well developed cases with complete obstruction of the urethra—before rupture of the bladder has taken place—a radical surgical operation may be performed to remove the gravel. Such animals may then be fattened or otherwise prepared for early slaughter. After the urinary bladder has ruptured the meat is urine tainted and no longer fit for human consumption.

A change of feed recommended as a method of prevention

"Gut Edema of Swine;" Enterotoxemia of Swine, ("Dropsy of the bowel.") This swine ailment, usually acute and fatal, has, during recent years only, been reported from various swine raising sections in the U. S., though recognized in England and Ireland since 1932.

Pigs up to 14 weeks of age are the usual victims though occasionally it appears in older ones. Loss of appetite and/or unsteady gait are early symptoms. Swelling of the eyelids and neighboring areas is an important diagnostic symptom. Later there may be diarrhoea, and complete inability to use the limbs. Death usually follows in most affected animals— sometimes in a few hours after the appearance of the first noticeable symptom.

Swollen eyelids an important symptom

The outstanding change observed during an autopsy is the presence of abnormally large amounts of fluid in the intercellular tissue spaces of the body—the so-called edema—as in the lower tissues of the body, the ears, eyelids, and especially along the greater curvature of the stomach to the extent of as much as 1½ inches in depth; fluid is also found in the mesentery supporting the colon—though not in the walls of the latter. In the

Fluid in many tissues

bodily cavities and in the heart sac there is more fluid. All this fluid gels on exposure to air.

The cause of the disease is not known—the most generally held opinion is that it is a bacterial toxemia due to the absorption of bacterial poisons. It is commonest after a change in management, feed or environment.

There is no known method of prevention other than good care, and no specific treatment—only symptomatic; this includes light feeding of a laxative nature such as linseed meal and bran. Antibiotics are not recommended at this time.

PART SEVEN

Infectious and Communicable Ailments of Farm Animals

✠✠✠✠

CHAPTER XXVII

INFECTIOUS OR NON-COMMUNICABLE AILMENTS

In this classification there are grouped those ailments that are due to germs, though within the usual meaning of the word they are not "catching" or communicable. These ailments are distinguished from the contagious ailments in that the latter are "catching" or communicable. The distinction is an important one because infectious diseases frequently affect only one animal of a herd or flock, though the contagious ones are much more widespread.

"Bull-nose" or "Sniffles" in Pigs (chronic rhinitis, necrotic rhinitis.) In this disease the necrosis germ (*Actinomyces necrophorus*), which is always present in manure and filthy surroundings as well as being a usually harmless inhabitant of the intestines in hogs, gains entrance to the tissues of the mouth and nose. This disease must not be confused with atrophic rhinitis (page 624). The mode of entry of the germ is through some small wound accidentally produced, or sometimes created by the removal of so-called black teeth in little pigs that during nursing

A germ
gains
entrance to
the soft
tissues of
the mouth
and nose

are believed to cause lacerations of the teats and udder of the sow. After the germ gains lodgement it destroys the tissues and causes swelling of them so that the little pig's face acquires a fancied resemblance to a bull's nose, and hence the name usually applied to the condition. The germ does not necessarily produce the facial distortion as the changes may be limited to small sores in the mouth and nose, and contiguous areas. The disease not infrequently becomes so serious as to result in very difficult noisy breathing and inability to nurse, so that unthriftiness and ultimately death is the final outcome.

Prevention consists in the raising of pigs in clean sanitary surroundings (pages 215 and 672) because "Bull-nose" is a filth-borne disease. Accidental wounds

Prevention is by sanitary methods in the region of the head in young pigs are difficult or impossible to guard against, though the injuries resulting from the "ringing" of very young pigs, and following the removal of black or other teeth may be controlled. If the teeth are so sharp as to cause laceration of the sow they should be dulled with a fine file.

During the early stages of the ailment, or when soreness is first observed treatment may be attempted by the application of pure tincture of iodine (page 276) to the wounds. As a home remedy ordinary vinegar for use as a wound wash has been recommended. Usually when noticed the disease is so advanced that it is more profitable to destroy the ailing creature.

Foot-rot or foot-foul in cattle. (*Infectious pododermatitis* (Fig. 138). This condition is due to infection with the germ of necrosis (*Actinomyces necrophorus*)

An ailment associated with insanitary corrals (page 531) which abounds in filthy places. When cattle are compelled to stand and walk daily in undrained insanitary lots the trouble is likely to ensue.

As a result of the wetness the skin between the claws and at the hoof head becomes macerated. This is soon followed by minute breaks in the skin because of walking on rough frozen ground or from sticks, stones and other material. Avenues for the entrance of the necrosis germ are thus created.

The first noticeable symptom is usually lameness. An examination of the foot may disclose little more than a painful redness in the skin between the claws or at the upper border of the hoof. In this early stage the progress of the disease may usually be stopped by thoroughly cleansing the part with soap and water, and then applying household vinegar (page 279) as an antiseptic, or painting the parts with pure tincture of iodine (page 276). The animal is to be kept on a clean dry floor until all evidence of the disease has disappeared.

Occasionally before its detection the malady has progressed to the point where the soft tissues of the foot are badly cracked, with a malodorous purulent discharge, and "proud flesh" (page 348) formation. The handling is the same as for the earlier stage though in addition daily antiseptic treatment, and bandaging, must be practiced.

In still more advanced cases—these are the badly neglected animals—the infection has passed into most of the tissues in the vicinity of the foot, frequently including the joint cavities. The entire lower portion of the limb is swollen, there are many pus discharging wounds, and the animal may exhibit symptoms of general poisoning from the absorption of the germs and their toxins. These animals can be satisfactorily treated only by the experienced graduate veterinarian. Not infrequently for the best results it becomes necessary to amputate the affected claw. Animals so operated upon soon walk as well as before on the remaining claw.

Not infrequently several members of a herd are simultaneously affected so that individual treatment is not practical. In these situations benefit may be de-

rived from compelling all animals of the herd to walk
(Fig. 139) through a one per cent water solution
of sulphate of copper (blue vitriol). The solution is
placed in a shallow container, to a depth of three
inches, and the latter set in a gateway between two
pastures or corrals. It may be necessary to repeat the
treatment a week later. The animals are also to be
moved to more sanitary surroundings.

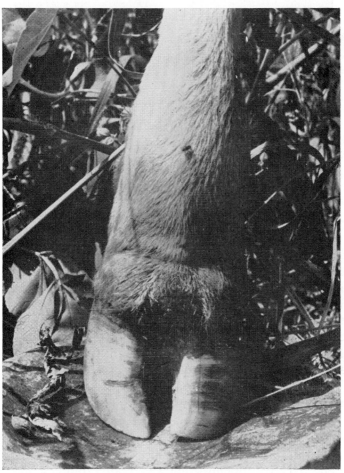

(Photo by County Agent Boberman, Seneca, Kansas)
FIG. 138. Foot-rot in cow.

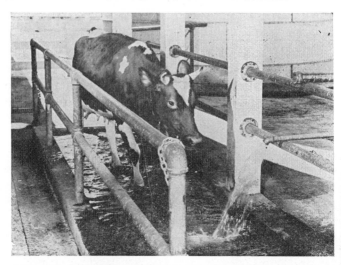

(Courtesy Bray's Island Plantation, Yennassee, S. Car.; photograph from National Cottonseed Products Association)

FIG. 139. Cow disinfecting feet.

Another generally resorted to form of control consists in placing in a shallow box at the doorway or gate a mixture of completely air-slaked lime and shavings in the proportion of one part of the former to five parts of the latter by volume, and compelling cattle to walk through this.

No form of treatment is satisfactory so long as the patient is not kept in a clean place during treatment, and repeated outbreaks may be expected if mud holes around door ways, water tanks, and other places (page 215), and general insanitary conditions in the corrals are permitted to persist.

Success in treatment depends upon clean surroundings

Since the advent of the "sulfa" drugs excellent results in the curative treatment—in addition to the sanitary steps—have been reported following intravenous medication with solutions of either sulfapyridine, sulfathiazole, or sulfamethazine. The best results were reported when the infection was treated in its incipiency, though many advanced chronic cases responded to this method of curative handling, but sanitation must still be practiced. The use of "sulfas" properly belongs in the field of the veterinarian.

Foot-rot in sheep is very similar to this condition in cattle. It is seldom possible to accord individual treatment to diseased members and therefore flock treatment is instituted by compelling the band to walk through the copper sulphate bath—the same as recommended under the heading "foot-rot" in cattle, and improving general sanitary surroundings by the removal of filth, and draining low places and mud holes near water tanks and other places. It is recommended that, in so far as this is possible, all necrotic tissue in the foot be completely removed, and then use the copper sulphate foot-bath. Changing the range to high dry land is very helpful, and there is no spread of the infection to the new range if it is dry. After 30 days on the high range the original range is again satisfactory—if it has been made sanitary for harboring sheep. (Consult page 355, "Interdigital Pouch Obstruction in Sheep.")

Infectious enteritis in pigs; necrotic enteritis; "necro" in pigs; swine dysentery; pig typhus; salmonellosis suis. This is one of the very serious infectious swine ailments occurring in the middle west. In some outbreaks it is contagious. Primarily the disease is due to a germ known as the *Salmonella suipestifer* though its principal lesions and symptoms are the effect of the necrosis germ. The two—*Salmonella suipestifer* (page 826)—also known as *Bacillus cholerae suis,* (page 826) and the *Actinomyces necrophorus* (page 527) (germ of necrosis)—always go hand-in-hand—the latter a secondary invader—in the production of this swine dysentery. Very frequently an outbreak may be traced to the recent introduction of new members into the herd. It is usually independently

[marginal note: A serious dysentery of swine believed to be one of a so-called group of filth borne ailments. A lack of vitamins is said to be a predisposing cause]

present on quite a large number of hog-raising farms. Young pigs up to four or five months of age are the chief sufferers. A lack of nicotinic acid—a vitamin B_2 fraction (page 69)—is said to be a predisposing cause.

In pigs dead of this disease the large intestines are found to have greatly thickened walls, and their lining is covered with a layer of necrotic, cheesy material which upon removal discloses reddish angry looking areas. These changes are so extensive that any one seeing them can readily understand why this stage of the disease is practically incurable, and why those whose lives are saved remain permanently "runty." The small intestines are usually free from the disease.

The outstanding symptom of the ailment is a bloody diarrhoea. When this appears within a week or two after new additions to a herd a diagnosis of swine dysentery may be considered to have been established. The animal's temperature at first high usually subsides as the diarrhoea sets in. Sometimes the disease becomes chronic in its character so that ailing pigs do not die though remaining permanently unthrifty. The death rate is highest in young pigs—forty to fifty per cent—, less so in feeder swine—ten to twenty per cent—, and even less in the mature animals that occasionally become infected—two to five per cent.

Sometimes the two diseases, hog cholera and swine dysentery, appear simultaneously in a herd creating a situation of unusual gravity. If in the attempted immunization against the cholera, use is made of both serum and virus— this is the older form of immunization, and the fully virulent form has been largely replaced by modified virus—there are likely to be many deaths from the "flare-up" that almost always ensues. Veterinarians have learned to limit their immunizing efforts to the use of anti-hog-cholera serum alone until a more favorable time arrives for the injection also of the virus. (Page 618.)

When hog cholera and "necro" appear simultaneously the situation is grave

The best method of prevention is not to introduce newly purchased swine into a herd until they have first
been held in quarantine for three weeks.
During this time care must be taken to
avoid the transfer of any existing infection from the quarantined group to others.
Many hog raisers are firm believers in alkalinizing the grain fed to their hogs to prevent this disease. Their procedure is to dissolve one pound of sodium hydroxide—usually this is Lewis' lye—in some water and then adding this to a barrelful (fifty gallons) of soaking grain. This material constitutes the sole daily grain ration permitted the herd. Keeping pigs at pasture away from farm buildings and animal habitations is a sound practice.

A method of prevention

Within recent time the claim has been advanced that a (page 283) nitrofuran, NF-180 at the rate of six pounds per ton of feed continued for 10 to 14 days at the beginning of the symptoms will control the condition.

In more advanced cases sulfaguanidine and the antibiotic streptomycin have been effective in the hands of veterinarians.

When the disease has established itself in a herd it is advisable to at once separate the apparently well animals from those visibly ill. The former should be placed in clean quarters that have not been occupied by swine for some time previously, and that receive no drainage or seepage from the lots occupied by the ailing swine. Disinfect (page 215) contaminated lots and hog houses with a 3% Saponated Cresol Solution.

Swine Plague: Hemorrhagic septicemia (page 547) of swine. It is pneumonia caused by the *Pasteurella suiseptica*—a hemorrhagic septicaemia organism. The same sanitary procedures are recommended as for hog cholera (page 616). This disease often complicates hog cholera, and it is difficult to draw a sharp line of demarcation between the two. When in doubt, treat as if it is cholera. The germ held responsible for this disease is harmlessly present in many swine, and only when the animal is unthrifty or devitalized does it become active. Therefore keeping swine healthy and vigorous and in sanitary surroundings is an important preventive step. Vaccination of healthy hogs with hemorrhagic septicaemia bacterin is frequently resorted to a few days before they are shipped as this latter is a devitalizing influence.

Calf Diphtheroid; calf diphtheria. This is a herd infection of housed, young, and half grown calves—it does not occur in animals on pasture. The name diphtheria as applied to this disease is misleading as it connotes a close relationship to true human diphtheria which is erroneous. It is in fact due to an entirely different germ from that responsible for human diphtheria, though symptomatically it bears a resemblance to it.

An ailment of calves resembling human diphtheria though it is not related

The disease is caused by the germ of necrosis—*Actinomyces necrophorus*—(see bull-nose, page 526, foot-rot, page 527, and infectious enteritis of pigs, page 531), which is widely distributed in nature. It gets on barnyard litter which is consumed by animals. Small scratches or other wounds permit the germ to enter the tissues of the throat. In the strict sense it is not contagious, though common in a herd.

Attention is usually called to the infection because of difficulty in eating, drinking, and breathing. An examination of the inside of the mouth and throat discloses the presence of yellowish crumbling masses and patches on the tissues. If these are removed, easily bleeding surfaces are exposed. The diseased patches are frequently deeply embedded. In the course of time other germs invade the diseased tissues, the affected animal becomes very thin, and usually dies because of the absorption of germ poisons.

Preventive steps to control the spread of diphtheroid consist in segregating afflicted animals. Dur-

Sanitation a preventive ing parturition cows should be in cleaned and disinfected maternity stalls (pages 199, 215), or during warm weather in the open, away from farm buildings.

The results of attempted curative treatment are not encouraging excepting in very mildly affected animals—others die. Sulphamethazine in doses of ¾ to 1½ grains per pound of body weight given by way of the mouth for each of two successive days is helpful in the early stages of mild cases. Careful mechanical removal of the false membranes by a veterinarian followed by disinfection of the denuded area may be tried.

Circling Disease: (*Listerellosis*) (page 829). This infectious disease has been observed in sheep, swine, cattle, goats, horses and man. In general it is an infection with the germ *Listerella monocytogenes* which has been recovered from the central nervous system—brain and spinal cord; therefore the usual symptoms are of a nervous character such as dullness, holding head to one side, sleepiness and drooping the ears. Sheep tend to move in circles. Swine show a tendency to drag the hind limbs. Death is a frequent termination especially in the young. In sheep the condition has been confused with pregnancy disease (page 499) though seasonal occurrence should distinguish it. Sanitation and prevention should follow general lines. Sheep have been successfully immunized with live organisms, but practical vaccination is lacking.

A brain disease; sheep circle

Leptospirosis of cattle: In man known as Weil's disease and leptospiral jaundice (pages 326 and 826). In cattle the disease is due to a cork-screw shaped organism known as a spirochete or specifically as *Leptospira pomoma* which occurs in the blood, urine, milk and other tissue in early stages of the disease. Usually in the early stages there are symptoms of general ill-health. Soon the milk and urine become blood-tinged, and the visible mucous membranes may appear yellowish especially in advanced cases.

Some cattle do not survive an acute attack though when recovery is to take place convalescence is very slow. An important point is that the apparently re-

Recovered animals are carriers for many weeks

covered animals continue to spread the infection to susceptible cattle by the latter inhaling spattered urine. Prevention consists in segregation of recovered animals for several months after apparent recovery. If newly purchased animals are obtained from a herd in which the disease has occurred then such animals should be kept isolated until an examination of specimens of blood and urine indicate that these tissues are negative for the specific spirochete. Treatment in the early stages by means of antibiotics (page 249) are said to be helpful.

A word of warning is not out of place in a textbook of this nature about the possibility of the contraction of

Urine of infected animals may contaminate human foods, etc.

leptospirosis (Weil's Disease or leptospiral jaundice) by humans since public health reports indicate that in the United States this disease in humans is on the increase. Sources of infection are in almost all instances through the contamination of food, swimming pools, etc., by the urine of such infected animals as cattle, swine, sheep, horses, goats, dogs, raccoons, and such rodents as rats and mice. Otherwise it seems to have been contracted from handling an infected pet, from contaminated moist soil, from the handling of infected tissues of recently slaughtered animals, from working in areas that are contaminated with urinary discharges, etc. Infection may take place through abraded skin or mucous membranes of the eyes, nose or mouth. However, the stomach secretions appear destructive to the organisms, and there are no records of human infection from the drinking of whole milk. Since more than half of the humans who contracted the disease were between the ages of 15 to 30 years it is assumed that occupational and environmental factors are important because infected animals and carriers are most frequently handled by persons in this age group:

Navel-ill; joint-ill; pyosepticemia of the newborn; omphalophlebitis. As at least one of the names of this disease indicates, it is an infection observed in the newborn. Foals, calves and lambs are the victims.

An infection gains entrance through the navel of foals. It results in a general poisoning

It usually makes its appearance in a recognizable form within the first week of independent life, though there are slowly developing cases that do not appear until up to six months of age.

The disease is frequently the result of infections contracted by the young creature from its dam before birth, and also through the navel immediately after birth.

The first noticeable symptom is weakness at birth, or listlessness shortly after birth. The temperature becomes elevated, there is at first slight lameness frequently giving rise to the impression that the young creature has been stepped on by its mother. Soon there is a hot painful swelling of one or more joints, suckling is no longer indulged in, and death is the outcome.

The modes of infection, i.e. from the dam and through the navel seem to indicate points of attack in the attempted prevention of the ailment. It is conceded that the dam that has given this infection to her offspring has developed resistance to it in her own blood or it is charged with antibodies, and if the newly born colt is given a subcutaneous dose of from four to eight ounces of its dam's blood, the colt's resistance will also be raised. Experience seems to demonstrate the soundness of this theory. (Page 771).

In order to control the afterbirth or post natal infections through the navel this organ should be subjected to thorough disinfection (page 353). One method is to immerse the navel cord up to the point where it joins the body in a solution made by mixing one

A method of disinfecting the navel

part of formalin (page 266), with twenty parts of water. The solution should be in a wide-mouth bottle so as to readily accommodate the navel when it is pressed against the navel region. This treatment usually results in drying up the navel within twenty four hours, otherwise another application is advisable. In the interval between applications, apply frequently— once every two hours is not too often—some good astringent antiseptic veterinary dusting powder (page 355). After the navel is thoroughly dried infection through it is not likely to take place.

In the prevention of this disease it is important that maternity stalls shall be thoroughly cleaned and disinfected (page 215) for the reception of the dam and her unborn young when she shows evidence of impending parturition, or better still, if the weather is not inclement, to have the birth take place in the open on a grassy plot some distance removed from dwellings and farm buildings.

Calf scours, white-scours, infectious diarrhoea. In addition to being undoubtedly infectious this disease of calves may appropriately be classified as contagious because the appearance of one case of it in a barn is soon followed by others.

A highly infectious diarrhoea in calves occurring within a few days after birth

The disease is the result of infections entering through the navel and the mouth, probably complicated by incorrect or injudicious feeding.

There are many types of dysentery affecting calves. It is, therefore, important to distinguish clinically between the comparatively harmless group and true white-scours, a feat that is sometimes impossible. In general, it is reasonably accurate to assume that a calf has white-scours if the symptoms appear within the first week after birth, and to consider those types that develop after this period as belonging to the group resulting from purely digestive causes and upsets.

The first symptoms are listlessness, loss of appetite, gaunt appearance, sunken eyes, temperature normal or elevated, and a thin white or yellowish diarrhoea. It is not uncommon to find undigested milk curds, streaks of mucus, and particles of blood in the intestinal evacuations. The hind parts are usually smeared with these discharges. Death is the outcome in most cases. Those that occasionally recover frequently remain more or less permanently unthrifty.

Prevention consists in having birth take place in the open during seasonable weather on a sun exposed plot at some distance from buildings. Otherwise a disinfected (page 215) maternity stall must be provided. All fluid matter is to be squeezed out of the navel cord (page 354) with clean hands, then apply a solution for about five minutes made by adding two teaspoonfuls of formalin to two ounces of water. Remove all adhering mucus from the nose and mouth of the calf. A closely woven muzzle should be placed on the calf during the first week, being removed only at the time of drinking. Milk vessels should be clean and scalded. If the attendant makes it a practice to insert his fingers into the calf's mouth to induce it to drink, he must first disinfect his fingers. One or two strips of the first milk is drawn off and thrown away, after which the calf is fed. For the first ten days of life, two drops of formalin (page 266) should be added to each quart of milk.

Prevention after the most rigid sanitary steps have been adopted

The milk supply of the calf should preferably be supplied from its own dam, and *it is important that its first few feeds be derived from its mother, either as colostrum or blood as serum* as these substances contain specific antibodies.

A method of feeding is helpful in affected animals

Prof. K. P. Link of the University of Wisconsin, the discoverer of warfarin (page 335), has developed an artificial colostrum which is marketed under the trade name "Kafmalak" (consult Milk Replacements page 50) by the Wisconsin Alumni Research Foundation, 209 So. LaSalle St., Chicago,

Link's colostrum formula

Illinois. The formula consists of 100 grams of dried blood serum from dairy or beef cattle, 25 grams of partially digested milk solids and 50 milligrams of vitamin K (page 73). This dried material is mixed with a quart of warmed milk or water and one-half of it given to the calf as shortly after birth as possible, and the remainder 12 hours later. This preparation is purely for preventive purposes—it is not curative.

Calves artificially fed (page 772) during the first day of their life should receive no more milk than 2% of their bodily weight; the addition of four tablespoonfuls of lime water is recommended. This may be increased ½% a day, so that at the end of ten days the calf will be receiving 7% of its bodily weight. Explained in other terms, this means that if a calf weighs 80 pounds at birth, it should receive not to exceed 1.6 pounds of milk the first day of its life. This may be increased by two-fifths of a pound daily. The additional administration of two teaspoonfuls of cod liver oil daily for the first two weeks of life is very helpful, especially in the winter.

As soon as a calf shows any symptoms of scouring, all milk is to be withheld from its diet, and in place of it, it is to receive barley water. This may be made by placing 3 quarts of cracked barley in a three-gallon bucket, then filling the latter with scalding hot water. When it has cooled, the calf may be fed on this barley water in the same proportions as recommended for milk in the preceding paragraph. As the diarrhoea is controlled, milk may gradually be substituted.

Scouring and coughing calves should be kept from the remainder of the herd and there should be a separate attendant for the sick animals. Such attendant should keep away from healthy calves, or he must wear "rubbers" while attending the sick calves. He must wash his hands in an antiseptic solution after handling sick calves.

The bodies of sick calves, especially the parts soiled with feces, must be cleansed with a mild antiseptic daily.

The barns sheltering both healthy and diseased calves should be thoroughly cleaned and disinfected at least once a week. The walls should be disinfected with a 3% water solution Saponated Cresol Solution, (page 263), and the floors brushed with lime.

Under no circumstances should young calves be permitted to come in contact with aborting cows. An **Other preventive steps** aborting cow is defined as having either given premature birth, or affected with retained afterbirth, or having a purulent vaginal discharge, or affected with garget. Any of the foregoing conditions, either singly or in combination, are highly suggestive of abortion disease.

A recent development in the control of calf scours consists in keeping these animals, during the season **A new sanitary device for the control of calf scours** that they are housed, on raised floors so as to provide drainage for liquid manure.

The first suggested floor of this nature was made of three-fourths inch mesh wire stretched over No. 9 woven wire fencing on a wood frame. Later the so-called "expanded sheet metal" was marketed. In still another development the floors in the pens are of wood—six-inch boards spaced with cracks a half to three-quarters inch wide. These are off the main floor about four inches. The sides of the individual pens are solid so that the calf cannot lick or nose other calves or cattle which might carry the infection of scours.

In those herds in which white-scours is prevalent, and if the value of the calves warrants, it is advisable to raise the calf's resistance immediately after birth by giving it an injection of calf dysentery serum or Prof. Link's artificial colostrum (page 540). Theoretically it is advanced that four to eight ounces of the dam's blood administered subcutaneously is of equal value to the much more expensive calf dysentery serum. The use of sulfaguanidine or sulfathalidine or the antibiotic (page 249) dihydrostreptomycin if begun early is valuable.

Tetanus or *"lockjaw"* (page 827). In this we find an example of a typical infectious disease, i.e., due to a well known specific infection and not in any sense contagious or "catching."

One of the grave commonly observed ailments of man and animals due to a wound infection

The disease is due to the bacillus of tetanus (*Clostridium tetani*) which lives indefinitely in soil, manure, the intestines, and similar places. Its distribution is world wide though most prevalent in the warmer climates. This germ must gain entrance to the animal's body through a wound or an abrasion. The wound may be so small that it heals outwardly, imprisoning the implanted germ. The latter does not leave the region of the wound to get into the blood stream as is so frequently the case with other germs, but remains localized though giving off a very powerful poison or toxin which it is said to be one hundred times as powerful as strychnine. It passes along the nerves to reach the spinal cord

The recognizable symptoms are shown as soon as the toxin establishes a contact with the spinal cord. This passage of the toxin from its place of elaboration in the wound to the spinal cord sometimes requires the elapse of quite a long period, and is an explanation for the delayed development of clinical symptoms; the wound heals frequently before the symptoms appear. In sheep castration and docking wounds invite the infection (pages 400 and 402).

Tetanus may affect horses (Fig. 141), cattle, swine (Fig. 140), sheep, goats and others. Its usual onset is in

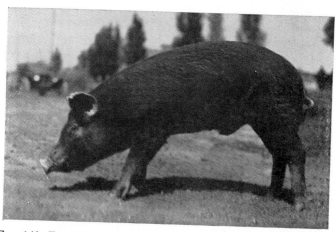

FIG. 140. Tetanus as a sequel of castration; note the generally stiff appearance.

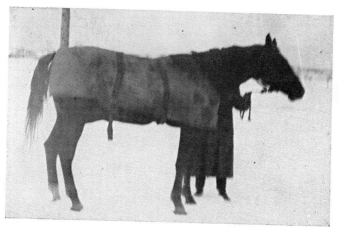

FIG. 141. Tetanus; note erect ears, and extended head and tail.

from a few days to several weeks after the infection takes place. The first noticeable symptom is stiffness which in twenty-four hours has become pronounced. Occasionally the stiffness affects certain groups of muscles more than others as in the so-called "lockjaw" in which the muscles of the jaw become set. The ears are stiffly upright, the tail is in a semi-rigidly extended position, and the eyes upon the least excitement are retracted into their sockets so that the third eyelid is protruded over the eye. Laymen speak of this latter symptom as the "hooks," or the "haws" (Fig. 141).

If the symptoms develop rapidly the termination of the disease is almost always a fatal one. If the symptoms develop more slowly or if the stiffness still permits the animal to eat and drink recovery is more frequent, probably somewhat more than fifty percent.

The termination of the disease is frequently a fatal one

Prevention of the disease consists in thorough cleansing of wounds as soon as they occur. Wounds with extensive laceration, and deep penetrating wounds are the most serious because their recesses afford hiding places for the germ. After all parts of a wound have been freely exposed full strength tincture of iodine (page 276) is to be applied daily until healing is well on its way. An injection of tetanus antitoxin will protect an animal for at least ten days. Tetanus toxoid will protect an animal for at least a year, and this method of immunization is resorted to as a routine measure in those countries or regions where tetanus is of frequent occurrence.

Prevention consists in thorough disinfection of all wounds as shortly as possible after their occurrence

Rabies, hydrophobia, "madness" (pages 327 and 829). This is an infectious disease due to a filterable virus. It is communicable by means of the bite so that saliva containing virus enters the wound. The disease occurs most frequently in dogs. Other domesticated animals usually contract the disease as the result of dog bites. Man is quite susceptible.

A disease that is more and more becoming a serious menace to human and animal welfare

The causative virus is in the nerve tissues of the brain and spinal cord, as well as in various secretions such as tears, milk, and saliva. A point of importance is that the virus has been found in the saliva at least five days before the infected animal has clinically recognizable symptoms of the disease. This means that the bite of a dog is always to be considered potentially dangerous, and the best procedure is to confine such a dog for daily observation; if no recognizable symptoms appear in the animal within a period of two weeks after it has inflicted the bite it is safe to assume that there was no rabies at the time of the bite. It is a serious error to at once destroy a biting dog because this also destroys the evidence the laboratorian needs to make a diagnosis. It is better to confine the dog until there is clear cut evidence on which to base a diagnosis.

There is no workable method of preventing this disease. It seems to be on the increase in America. Whenever the public becomes convinced of the increasing gravity of the situation in regard to rabies and will give eradication methods its support, the disease can be stamped out by methods comparable in a measure to those adopted by the federal forces in the handling of that highly contagious disease of cattle known as foot-and-mouth disease. This means the destruction of all stray and bitten dogs, and muzzling of others in the quarantined area.

No workable method of prevention

The method of vaccinating dogs against rabies as practiced at this time is of value, though no one contends that it is one hundred per cent efficient. Vaccination affords the best known protection that can be given an animal, but alone, and without additional quarantine measure, it will not eradicate rabies. Immunity in dogs following the use of living rabies virus—Flury strain—lasts at least two years. The virulence of the Flury strain has—in the making of the vaccine—been greatly reduced by serial passages through day old chicks. It is therefore

Vaccination is the best protection for the dog but it is not perfect

known as the "Avianized Flury vaccine." A single injection is given to immunize dogs.

Another vaccine is the phenol killed vaccine, also known as the Semple vaccine. It is the most frequently used human vaccine.

The latest in a human protection vaccine is a "duck embryo vaccine (DEV)," or a "chick embryo vaccine (CEV)," either for pre-exposure immunization.

A word about the disease in man. A bitten person should always at once consult a physician. If the bite

A person bitten by a supposedly rabid animal should have the attention of a physician

is in the region of the neck or head it is safest to at once commence treatment. *An anti-rabies hyperinimmune serum became available in 1954 for use within the first 72 hours after exposure,* and then followed by the usual anti-rabies vaccine. *This system is said to overcome the hazards of heavy doses of anti-rabies vaccine.* Do not wait for the establishment of the diagnosis in the dog, as the virus will travel rapidly to the comparatively nearby brain. A bite on the extremities of a person permits of confinement of the dog for the two weeks observation period, and if no symptoms develop in the dog during this time the wound need receive only routine care by a physician; if the dog does develop symptoms of the disease during the two weeks waiting period the person should then submit himself for treatments.

Whenever the symptoms of the disease are positively recognized in any species of animal it is best to destroy it as the condition is incurable. The head of the animal should be sent to a state laboratory for a confirmation of the clinical diagnosis by a microscopic examination of the brain. (Refer to "madstone," page 349.)

Mad Itch of Cattle (false rabies). This is a rather rare disease of an infectious character. It is re-

ported to have been observed in other lands in animals other than cattle. In America in the
In cattle rare outbreaks the affected cattle had al-
the disease ways mingled with swine; therefore, it is
occurs when with some justification the belief exists
associated that the causative virus of the disease is
with swine transmitted from the snouts of swine to
abraded areas on cattle. The outstanding symptom of
the disease is the intense itching so that the hair is
licked off or rubbed off against posts and buildings.

In one outbreak observed by the writer the itching
was so intense that recumbent cattle welcomed lacerations by swine. The swine were actually eating their
way into the living bovine. Death is the usual termination in 24 to 48 hours. During the last few hours of life
paralysis, bellowing, gnashing of the teeth, and convulsions may occur. Itching of the hind parts of the
body was controlled, for a short period only, by resorting to epidural anesthesia but when the effects of
the anesthetic wore off the itching reappeared. In the
light of our incomplete knowledge little can be done
to prevent the condition in cattle other than to take
all cattle away from swine, and away from lots, corrals or pastures in which the disease first makes its
appearance.

*Hemorrhagic septicemia, shipping fever of cattle,
stock-yards fever, stock-yards pneumonia, or lung
fever.* The name hemorrhagic septicemia
A frequently refers to a group of infectious diseases
diagnosed affecting cattle, sheep, swine, birds, and
disease of rabbits. In cattle it occurs most frequent-
animals ly after being shipped and it is, therefore,
commonly spoken of as "shipping fever"; as affected
animals have been in public stock-yards it is also designated "stock-yards fever," or "stock-yards pneumonia." In swine the common name is swine plague.
(Page 533.) It is undoubtedly an infectious disease as it

The causative germ a normal inhabitant of the respiratory tract

is due to a specific germ, (*Pasteurella*) and it is also in a measure "catching" or communicable so that it would not be incorrect to group it as contagious. The germ is found normally in the respiratory and digestive tracts of animals and in water, on soil and vegetation. The germ is very susceptible to the action of the mildest disinfectants. Usually it is a mild almost harmless organism though for reasons not understood it frequently and suddenly flares up. This may be due to changed conditions in its surroundings, or because of lowered resistance of its host such as occurs in cattle when they are subjected to the unaccustomed nervous strain and the rigors of being shipped to feed lots. This germ dies soon after its host dies, and, therefore, it is difficult to recover from the carcass excepting almost immediately after the animal's death.

The symptoms vary depending on the localization of the ailment

The symptoms of the disease vary depending upon the seat of localization of the germ, and in a measure on its virulence. Thus, there may be a lung form; a form with swellings in the regions of the throat, eyes, lower chest and others; a very acute form quickly causing death as from a severe blood poisoning. A brain form, and an intestinal form have also been noticed.

In the lung form the symptoms are those of lung fever with chilling, high temperature, difficult breathing, and coughing. In the intestinal form there may be bloody diarrhoea and colicky pains. When there are swellings in any one of different parts of the body an organ may be pressed upon so as to interfere with its function as difficult breathing when the throat is involved. In the acute form death is usually the result in less than twenty-four hours.

Prevention is difficult as there is no warning that an outbreak of the disease is threatened. In cattle

Prevention is difficult and necessitates special precautions

and sheep about to be shipped from the range to feed lots various animals are likely to have their resistance lowered because of the shipping and exposure from chilling in drafty conveyances. It is a good plan, therefore, to vaccinate them with a hemorrhagic septicemia bacterin at least ten days or two weeks before they leave the range or place of origin. The immunizing agent must have a species specificity. This time of vaccination is not an absolute preventive, though it offers a better chance of success than at any other time. Vaccination when an animal is in the early or more advanced stages of the disease is likely to result in disappointment. The use of anti-hemorrhagic septicemia serum is somewhat helpful in the curative treatment though good care and nursing must not be neglected.

At no time should the cattle be worried unnecessarily. Feeder cattle should be driven leisurely from the time of their removal from freight cars or trucks until they reach their destination, and then should have a plentiful supply of fresh water and limited feeding. In other words, they are to be brought gradually to a full fattening ration. It is important to protect them, until they are settled at least, from chilling rains and severe inclemencies of the weather. At the first sign of a "cold" or illness isolate the affected animal. The veterinarian can do much in the curative handling by means of sulfonamides and antibiotics, and therefore he should be called when the first symptoms appear.

An ailment affecting isolated groups of cattle and believed to be due to a virus

Malignant head catarrh, malignant catarrhal fever in cattle. This is an infectious disease observed amongst isolated groups of cattle, though seldom or never does it generally involve the cattle of a larger community or area. It is soundly assumed that the cause of the disease is a virus, presumably organisms so small that they are not visible by means of a powerful microscope. The virus has been demonstrated in the blood of infected cattle. It is not known how cattle contract the disease in nature.

The symptoms of the disease appear suddenly with virtually no premonitory signs. The appearance is that of a very sick animal with a high temperature, loss of appetite, extended head, involvement of the eyes, painful cough, and a thick discharge from the nostrils. As the disease progresses the animal walks with difficulty, finally goes down and dies. Secondary symptoms such as severe diarrhoea, or constipation may be present.

The mode of prevention of the disease is not known for the reason that the mode of infection is not understood. There is considerable evidence that the virus causing the disease is maintained by sheep, although the disease itself and its clinical symptoms do not occur in sheep. Therefore, if the disease appears in cattle on a farm, and if cattle and sheep are closely associated, it is a good plan to segregate these animals from each other immediately. In the light of our limited knowledge it is best to adopt the same sanitary measures as have already been described for other disease (page 215). However, many veterinarians that have had experience with this cattle disease are exceedingly pessimistic about its outcome; as soon as a clear-cut diagnosis is established in the first affected individuals the remainder of the herd is rushed off to market. Furthermore the condition seems to establish itself on certain farms for a term of years so that cattle raising, feeding, and breeding may need to be abandoned in that particular localized area. Possibly this may be explained in a better way by the fact that
Infection persists there is reasonably good evidence that the causative virus may persist in a recovered animal or host for several months. Recovered animals are apparently immune to the disease for a compara-

tively short time only—four to eight months, occasionally longer.

Curative treatment is likewise unsatisfactory though during the latter part of an outbreak the disease seems to become milder, and with appropriate nursing and treatment recoveries are more frequent. (Technical Bulletin 97, entitled "Malignant Catarrhal Fever," with full-color plates, may be obtained from Kans. Agricultural Experiment Station, Manhattan, Kansas.)

Mucosal Disease of Cattle: Although in a measure this is a local disease, it is rather wide-spread. It is characterized by ulceration of the mucous membranes of the body, though the absence of corneal lesions distinguishes it from malignant head catarrh. Its exact nature is at this time not understood, and the specific cause is unknown. Diseases of this nature can be handled by segregation of the well animals, and symptomatic treatment of the ailing.

Blackleg (page 825), *black quarter, symptomatic anthrax.* This is an infectious disease affecting cattle principally, though sheep and goats may contract it. It is due to a specific gas forming germ to which young cattle between the ages of six months and two years are most susceptible, though older animals may contract it. The germ—*Clostridium chauvei*—has a "seed" stage—bacteriologists say it is a spore forming germ (page 221)—which lives almost permanently in soil contaminated by it. The disease once prevalent in a community remains there as a permanent hazard to cattle raising. In this spore stage the germ may lie dormant for many years though suddenly becoming active when given the opportunity. The germ is usually taken into the animal's body with spore contaminated water or soil. The entrance of the germ through wounds to produce the disease is a possibility.

A widespread cattle ailment preventable by vaccination

Frequently the first noticeable symptom is lameness, which rapidly increases in severity until the animal goes down. Almost simultaneously the affected portion of the body—usually a hind quarter, the front shoulder, chest or back—becomes swollen. When the hand is passed lightly over these regions there is imparted a crackling sensation due to the presence of bubbles of gas beneath the skin. This is almost a characteristic symptom. Other general symptoms are high fever, loss of appetite, cessation of cud chewing, and extreme depression. Affected muscles if cut into are dark colored, with a frothy bloody fluid of a sweetish rancid-butter odor.

Many reports during recent years were evidence that the highly efficient blackleg vaccine did not seem to protect the vaccinated animal. Investigations disclosed that another disease—*malignant oedema* (page 825)—due to an entirely different germ—

A com-
plicating
disease

Clostridium septicum, also a gas former— was at the bottom of the trouble. Clinically it is impossible to distinguish between "blackleg" and "malignant oedema." Therefore, modern blackleg bacterins have, or should have, the power to simultaneously immunize against both blackleg and malignant oedema (also known as gas phlegmon). This has been accomplished by having in the blackleg bacterin equal numbers of both the killed *Clostridium chauvei* and the *Clostridium septicum*.

Prevention consists in the vaccination, with the double vaccine mentioned in the preceding paragraph, of all susceptible cattle between the ages of six months and two years. After the animal reaches two years of age a natural immunity gradually sets in. In regions where blackleg is prevalent vaccination must be practiced as a routine measure, otherwise a yearly loss of at least ten per cent of the calf crop may be expected. Vaccination with a correct dose of either blackleg bacterin, blackleg aggressin, or blackleg filtrate properly introduced under the skin is one of the most effective of all forms of immunization practiced against any disease. Disposal of carcasses should be in a sanitary manner (page 226), and opening of the carcass or incision of the swellings is to be cautioned against because of the grave danger of spreading the permanent spores over the premises.

In the very early stages of the disease before the animal goes down large subcutaneous doses of anti-blackleg serum seem to be helpful in aborting the attack—its use is recommended in very valuable animals. It is helpful only when blackleg is not complicated by malignant oedema.

Infectious anemia in horses; swamp fever; (page 760) *recurrent fever.* This is an infectious disease of the horse, mule and ass. Though the name "swamp fever" would seem to indicate a disease of the low lands it is observed with almost equal frequency on the higher areas away from swamps. It has a tendency to localize on certain farms though it is seldom observed in animals that are strictly stable fed and handled. The disease is widespread over certain areas west of the Mississippi and its delta, though less frequently in eastern United States. However, in 1947 there was a very serious outbreak in many of the large racing stables of eastern and northeastern United States. The financial loss resulting from this ran into millions of dollars.

An ailment that will require additional research to clarify all phases of it

The disease is due to a virus or ultra-microscopic germ which is in the blood of an infected animal. Animals that appear to have recovered from an acute attack of the disease still retain the virus in their blood, and such animals are, therefore, carriers of the disease. The virus is distributed from an infected animal through its urine, saliva and tears. The virus has also been isolated from the bodies of biting insects, and these are probably the most important—though not exclusive—means of transmission. Outside of the body the virus may remain alive for several weeks in contaminated straw and bedding as it resists drying, freezing, and putrefaction. The disease is contracted as a result of drinking and eating contaminated water and food, and by the bites of insects. It may be spread by means of a mechanical device such as a hypodermic needle.

The disease manifests itself in an irregular symptomatology. In an acute form death may take place in a few days. Others start with acuteness of symptoms which seem to abate so that the disease remains chronic for periods of months or even years though finally returning to the acute stage, and death. In the acute cases there is a sudden rise in temperature, extreme prostration, swellings in the lower parts of the body, jaundice with a reddish tinge, and frequently red spots on the mucous membranes of the eyes, nose, and in the female on that of the genitals. A pounding heart, easy exhaustion and sweating are noticed. In the slower type of the ailment the animal seems unwell without actually appearing sick enough to be withheld from work. There is loss of condition and occasional fever.

Prevention of the disease seems to rest on sanitary principles, and these should be practiced as a routine measure (pages 212 and 215). The promiscuous use of hypodermic needles (page 220) and other surgical instruments is a hazardous procedure especially in racing stables. The federal regulations now require that all antisera, made from horses, intended for interstate shipment must be heated from 58° to 59° centigrade for one hour which destroys the virus, thus removing these agents as possible avenues of spread. The disinfecting of premises (page 215), and the use of disinfectants—D.D.T. and others (page 291)—is of the greatest importance. One of the principal difficulties is the impossibility of positively diagnosing the disease excepting by removing some blood from a suspected case and injecting this into a known susceptible horse. If the disease de-

The application of sanitary steps is a sound preventive measure

velops in the latter a diagnosis is thus established, but under field conditions this is not practical, with the result that many mildly infected and "carrier" animals escape detection to continue as spreaders of the virus causing the malady.

In the present state of our knowledge a cure can not be effected. Sooner or later all infected animals die.

Sleeping sickness, equine encephalomyelitis (page 825). This infectious disease of horses has at times assumed alarming proportions in the United States. It is caused by a virus that has a predilection for the nervous tissues of the horse though minor natural outbreaks have also been observed in pigeons and pheasants. The causative virus has been recovered from several asymptomatic carrier birds so that these are also reservoirs. The disease is seasonal in character extending from early summer until frost makes its appearance in the fall. It has been demonstrated that during the colder months of the year the virus may be isolated from the body of the "assassin" bugs. (Figs. 142 and 143.)

Sleeping sickness assumed epizootic proportions during recent years

The virus is in the brain of an infected horse, and during the fever stage it is also in the blood; it disappears from all tissues a few hours after death. It is believed that the virus is transmitted from infected to susceptible animals by means of the bite of a mosquito (page 724) (*Aedes aegypti*). Other biting insects may be responsible for the transmission of the virus. In the United States there are several strains of virus. The eastern strain is the more virulent, and it has been known to occur only in outbreaks of the disease east of the Allegheny mountains—the western strain in all other sections.

Sometimes the symptoms of the disease are so mild that they pass unnoticed. Usually, however, nervous symptoms are pronounced. Affected animals may run

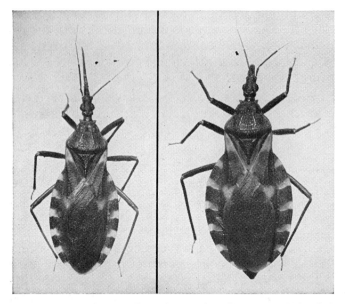

(Courtesy Dept. of Entomology, Kansas State University)

FIGS. 142 and 143. Male (left) and female (right) of Triatoma
sanguisuga (assassin bug) (Le Conte), reservoirs in nature
of the virus of horse "sleeping sickness."

into and over things, though this soon changes to
coma or the drowsy stage. When forced to walk the
animal circles endlessly in the same direction. Towards
the end standing straddled with head hanging low,
and eyes closed is observed. There is almost always
inability to swallow, because of paralysis of the throat.
Other muscles of the body may become paralyzed so
that the animal goes down, and death ensues. The
chances of recovery are better in those diseased animals that remain on their feet. It is estimated that
in 1948 twenty per cent of the horses infected with
the western strain of the virus died, and ninety per
cent of those infected with the eastern strain.

Prevention of the disease consists in the vaccination of all horses as soon as the disease makes its ap-

Annual vaccination a preventive

pearance in a community. If the disease has been present in a community during a previous year it is advisable to vaccinate all horses a subsequent year. Two subcutaneous injections of the embryonic-chick-tissue anti-encephalomyelitis vaccine must be administered with an interval of one week between the two. Solid immunity will be established in a minimum period of fifteen days after the injection of the second dose of the vaccine, and it will persist for at least six months. The vaccine must be handled very carefully especially in regard to exposure to warm or high temperatures. The injections should preferably be made on opposite sides of the neck and with a regard for the very strictest aseptic precautions or there may be undesirable sequelae. It is best to employ a veterinarian to apply the vaccine.

More recently the vaccine in one cubic centimeter doses is administered intradermally rather than sub-

A later method of vaccination

cutaneously, the interval between the two doses being one week. The immunity following this technic is as good as when the vaccine is administered subcutaneously, and unfavorable sequelae, such as serious swelling at the site of injection, do not seem to occur.

Preventive steps other than vaccination consist in the isolation of infected animals in screened enclos-

Other preventive steps

ures, or by applying to them insect repellents (pages 289 and 323). Horses not affected should also have repellents applied. Keeping horses stabled during seasons of insect prevalence, and where "sleeping sickness" is abroad is a good plan. Animals dead of the disease should be promptly and properly disposed of (page 226). Places and buildings that have been used by infected animals should be disinfected (page 215), preferably with formalin (page 266).

*Horses are not spreaders of equine encephalitis—
the infection stops in them or it is designated a "dead-
end" disease. Birds are principal reservoirs.*

Curative treatment is largely symptomatic and
best entrusted to a veterinarian. Combined with it
there should be good nursing, including some sort of a
device, such as a sling, to support the animal and to
maintain it on its feet.

Petechial Fever (purpura hemorrhagica; morbus
maculosus.) This disease of horses—in rare instances
cattle—is an anomaly in that the exact cause is unknown. Nearly always it is a secondary condition following lung fever, strangles, infections of the genitalia,
badly infected surgical and mechanical injuries, and
other conditions. It is a disease of the circulatory system; one of its earlier symptoms is bloody spots
(petechia) or actual bleeding in and from the nostrils
—hence the name "petechial fever."

Later symptoms include swelling of the head—the
so-called hippopotamus head—, limbs, under surface
of the body, sheath and other organs. The eyes may
be swelled shut so that vision is seriously
impaired. Swellings around the nose may
cause difficulty in breathing, and those
in the sheath difficulty in urination. The
temperature may be slightly elevated. The
appetite is usually quite good provided the
swellings do not interfere with mastication and swallowing. A very serious result of the bleeding is a great
decrease in the number of red blood cells so that weakness is an early symptom.

Bleeding and swellings the outstanding symptoms

Depending upon the severity of the attack and the
earliness with which treatment is instituted the death
rate may run as high as fifty per cent of affected animals. Veterinarians usually resort to frequent blood
transfusions, together with supportive and symptomatic handling. So long as the cause is not known it is
difficult to outline sanitary steps. The use of sulfona-

mides (page 280) in the handling of the primary disease—petechial fever usually being a secondary ailment—and keeping wounds as free as possible from germ contaminants is advised.

Blue-Tongue of Sheep: (Catarrhal Fever of Sheep.) This So. African sheep ailment was diagnosed during 1952-53 in California, Texas and Utah. The disease is due to different strains of blue-tongue virus, not spread by contact, though transmitted from infected to susceptible sheep through the medium of biting insects. One of these, a biting gnat *(Culicoides varupennis)* has been found to harbor the virus. About 30 percent of a flock may become affected and of these 90 per cent usually die. The disease is most prevalent during warm wet summers, and in those localities where it is observed it is safe for ranging between sunrise and sunset.

Safe in high places, and during daylight hours

Moving sheep during night hours to high ground is apparently a good preventive step. Cattle may contract the disease though they are much more resistant to the infection than sheep.

The symptoms appear in a few days following infection. The first symptom is a rise in temperature to as much as 107°F. followed in a few days by reddening of the lining of the mouth, and tenderness so that there is a disinclination to eat. The tissues of the mouth, including the tongue, swell and become bluish and purplish. Soon these parts become raw and bleeding, and the mouth area is frothy and even purulent so that there is an offensive odor. Foot lesions, nasal involvement and diarrhoea may all appear. Mild cases frequently recover though with loss of condition.

Prevention consists in dipping in repellent coal-tar preparations, and some of the more modern agents such as B.H.C., lindane, dieldrin, etc. (pages 300, 303, and 304) have been suggested. Keeping sheep and cattle away from low, moist pastures during the night hours in sheds or on high ground is advisable. In South

Africa "polyvalent" vaccines prepared from a number of anti-genetically dissimilar selected strains of blue-tongue virus grown on chick embryos are regarded as promising for immunization purposes. American firms are also making a preventive vaccine from local virus strains.

*Scrapie of Sheep:** This is a nervous disease of sheep and goats known for many years in France and England that has during recent years been observed in several flocks in California and the middle west. It is due to a virus though its mode of natural trans-
A disease of mature sheep mission is unknown. It is seldom observed in animals less than 18 months of age. The early symptoms are restlessness, grinding of the teeth, trembling of the ears, lips and limbs and excitement. Soon severe itching develops so that large areas of wool are scraped off. Finally the emaciation and weakness cause the animal to go down, coma sets in, and the termination is usually a fatal one; few recover.

Since the mode of transmission is unknown no effective preventive steps have been de-
Vaccines not effective veloped. As the disease is one of a very chronic nature it is doubtful if an effective vaccine can be found. In the United States if the disease is detected in a flock regulatory officials destroy the sheep and impose a strict quarantine on the premises.

Balano-Posthitis of Sheep: (Necrotic Venereal Disease; Sheath Rot; Pizzle Rot.) This ailment of sheep—wethers, rams, and ewes—is an infection with a virus and the necrosis germ—*Actinomyces necrophorous*) as a secondary invader. The disease is quite common in the U. S.

---

*Scrapie of Sheep, leaflet number 457, is for sale for five cents by the U.S. Superintendent of Documents, Washington 25, D. C.

Transmission is by the breeding contact. Symptoms are redness and ulceration of the sheath opening and the lips of the vulva. Many sheepmen call this stage "urine burn." If not controlled in this early stage by antiseptic washes the tip of the penis be-

Control the
disease early

comes swollen and ulcerated so that urination is difficult or impossible, and in this event the termination may be a fatal one. Prevention consists in stopping all breeding operations. Clipping of the wool around the sheath orifice, carefully removing scabs with mild soap and warm water, and the local application of a 5 per cent copper sulphate (page 275) solution or tincture of iodine (page 276) is helpful. In ewes the treatment is the same. Care must be taken that these irritant disinfectants are not injected into the sheath and vulva—their application is to be purely local.

Rabbit-Fever (page 828), (tularemia; deer-fly fever). It is not a livestock problem though there are reports of its occurrence in sheep. It has also been reported in the dog. It is of the gravest import to man as the causative germ—*Pasteurella*

Dangerous
to man

tularense—is very generally present in the blood of the cottontail rabbit but not in the domesticated species. It is also found in the jack rabbit, as well as in several other rodents, but without noticeable evidence of illness in these animals. Blood sucking ticks and flies on these rodents also carry the infection. Predator animals have infected mouths from their prey. In dressing wild rabbits for human food, or from bites derived from their ticks or other insects man contracts the ailment. Streams (small ones) and water holes may harbor the organism derived from infected water rats and beavers. Humans, it is reported, have contracted the disease from contact with such water.

Persons handling or dressing wild rabbits, to a less extent other rodents, should wear protective gloves (page 828). The meat after cooking is safe for human consumption. Infected persons usually start having severe general symptoms about three days after their contamination. More specific symptoms are soreness at the site of infection and painful swelling of the regional lymph nodes. Occasionally these symptoms are absent and then the disease is said to be "typhoidal." There may be ulceration of skin areas and glands, as well as eye involvement. In 1942 the death rate in man was computed at 6.9 per cent. One attack of the disease renders recovered persons permanently immune to future contamination. In humans the antibiotic "streptomycin" (page 248) is said to be a specific; penicillin is apparently without value. The use of a detoxified vaccine has been recommended for persons that do commercial dressing and handling of rabbit carcasses. It is of the greatest importance that a physician be consulted at the very first sign of the disease. (The name "tularemia" was attached to this disease following its detection in Tulare County, Calif.)

Symptoms in man

Psittacosis (page 828) (parrot fever). This virus disease of the parrot family may appropriately be considered communicable, though grouped here with the non-communicables. It is usually referred to by the names at the heading of this paragraph. Because other birds such as chickens, canaries, pigeons and others may also carry the psittacosis-like virus the disease is designated by some as *ornithosis*. The virus has been found in turkeys in all parts of the United States, and as a result poultry pickers and eviscerators have contracted a serious infection. Large turkey flock losses have also taken place. When the disease appears in humans employed in poultry processing plants there should be frequent observations for new cases. In the early stages treatment with tetracycline antibiotics is very effective. In humans the disease is undoubtedly contracted from parrots, some of which come from pet shops. It is an inapparent latent infection of parrots, canaries, pigeons and other birds.

Man in handling these birds may contract a pulmonary disorder characterized by high fever; this is the reason for its importance as it is a human disease factor. Man contracts the disease by inhaling parrot or bird dried **A danger to humans** excreta (droppings, urine, feathers) contaminated with the virus, occasionally through bite wounds, and from handling turkeys in slaughter plants. With the exception of the very mildest cases in man the lungs are always involved; "rose spots" may appear on the skin; the general symptoms may be very severe with occasional relapses. It must always be viewed with suspicion if two or three weeks after the acquisition of a parrot or parakeet a member of the family become afflicted with an atypical pneumonia. Canaries and finches are rarely affected.

Some states in which the sale of parrots, parakeets, canaries, finches and others is a comparatively important commercial venture have sanitary regulations—evidenced usually by leg banding of pet birds offered for sale. These include quarantine and laboratory tests before the birds may be released for sale. The laboratory test consists in using a percentage of the birds, at regular intervals, for autopsies; the spleens of these are tested by mouse inoculations. There are records of human patients infecting their nurses with psittacosis.

Q-Fever: (page 829). An infection due to a minute organism—a rickettsia—specifically *Coxiella burnetii* of cattle. It is an occupational disease of man.

It is a disease without recognizable symptoms and, on an autopsy, without lesions. In humans it may be confused with influenza.

Its principal importance is the transmission of the infection to humans—mostly through milk—though the infection is also in the urine, intestinal discharges,

tissue of the udder, neighboring lymph nodes, and in
the fluids and membranes incidental to
Cattle and calving. Cattle and sheep are simply in-
sheep are cidental hosts of the infection. Ticks har-
reservoirs of
the infection bor the infection and may also be a means
of spread.

In man it may be a mild illness of a week's duration
or a more severe attack of three weeks. There is fever,
headache, weakness, malaise and severe sweats. There
may be an atypical pneumonia. It may resemble brucellosis (page 578), typhoid fever, psittacosis (page
562) and atypical pneumonia.

In regions where the disease is present the milk
should be pasteurized. Ticks may be intermediate hosts
and should be controlled.

Chapter XXVIII

CONTAGIOUS OR COMMUNICABLE AILMENTS

Taken as a group these diseases are of far greater import than the sporadic or non-communicable ailments. In the United States immense financial loss has been occasioned by tuberculosis, hog-cholera, Bang's disease, foot-and-mouth disease, and a host of others. Enormous sums have been and are being expended in efforts to eradicate them so that at this time no country is as safe as America for the raising of livestock. Those diseases that have not been eradicated are so well under control that they are not of great concern to the large body of live stock producers.

An added feature of the greatest importance is that several of these diseases are communicable from animals to man. Human welfare is thus involved. (Page 823.)

The medical or curative treatment of the contagious disease is with a few exceptions not to be encouraged for the reasons that most of them do not respond favorably, and during the period of treatment the ailing patient is a reservoir of infection or menace to the animals of that region. It is much better to occasionally sacrifice an individual than to jeopardize the lives of all others.

Calf Pneumonia. This is an infectious lung fever of calves less than four months old, appearing on single farms. If sanitation is not practiced it may be a cause of extensive yearly losses. It frequently follows "white scours" (page 538).

Devitalizing factors make animals susceptible to this infection

Apparently the first case of the disease on a farm may be ascribed to lowered vitality induced by faulty sanitation and other factors. Chilling from faulty ventilation (page 154), and oxygen starvation—anoxia, (page 154) from inadequate ventilation, together with overcrowding, age susceptibility, the calves being usually less than two months of age and seldom over four months, debility from other ailments such as diarrhoea are all contributing factors in giving infections an opportunity to attack the lungs so as to set up pneumonia. Furthermore once the disease has become established in an animal domicile where other calves below four months of age are housed it frequently spreads to several of them. A virus that seems to be specific has been isolated.

The general symptoms such as dullness, poor appetite, rough coat and weakness are usually present. More important diagnostic symptoms are the rapid breathing, abnormal lung sounds such as hissing, bubbling and gurgling. Coughing is quite easily induced by tapping against the chest wall, or by compressing the chest between the hands.

Prevention consists in correcting those errors in housing and ventilation named as contributing causes in the production of the disease. As soon **Preventive** as there are symptoms of pneumonia in **steps are** an ailing calf of the susceptible age group, **of a** two weeks to four months, it should at **sanitary** once be placed by itself in a warm com- **nature** fortable enclosure in a separate building, with separate feeding and grooming utensils and with a separate attendant. This attendant must have no contact with the healthy age susceptible calves, and preferably he should remain away from other animal habitations. He should wash his hands in an antiseptic after taking care of the sick animal and before leaving the building in which it is housed. To avoid carrying the infection of the disease on his shoes he should wear rubbers or overshoes, and these are to be left in the building. The stall occupied by the ailing calf before its isolation should be cleaned and dis-

infected (page 215), and no calves of an age susceptible to calf pneumonia should be placed in it for the
remainder of that season. Every possible effort should
be made to prevent the spread of the infection from
the animal primarily infected. Vaccination with an
autogenous calf pneumonia bacterin as a routine measure on farms where this disease has made its appearance is not to be discouraged, though its helpfulness
is admittedly uncertain.

During the early stages of the disease curative
treatment offers some hope of a successful issue, but
during the later stages of the condition when the
changes in the lungs are extensive or severe complete
recovery to robust health is never to be expected, and
more frequently death is the outcome. The best curative
results during the early stages of the condition have
been obtained from the use of sulfamethazine (page
281). Recovered calves are immune.

Lamb Pneumonia: The sanitary prevention and the
curative handling of this condition are very similar
to that of calf pneumonia (page 565). In the clinical
handling there are reports of good results during the
early stages from the oral administration of sulfathiazole (page 281).

Ringworm (page 277) ; *barn itch; tinea tonsurans.*
This skin disease occurs most frequently in cattle,
though all other animals and man are sus-
A contagious ceptible to it. It is caused by a fungus
ailment which grows in the outer layers of the
due to a skin, and in and around the hairs. The
fungus fungus has seeds or spores and these live
for a long time in barns and elsewhere. The fungus
spreads from infected quarters or animals to non-
affected animals, and may also be transmitted by
curry combs, brushes, and by rubbing on contaminated
fence posts. The spores remain alive in dry protected
places for as long as eighteen months.

In affected cattle the disease appears especially in
the vicinity of eyes and ears, or the root of the tail,

though the sides of the neck also are frequent sites. (Fig. 144.) Rarely is the entire body covered. Affected areas have the appearance of grey asbestos-like patches gradually increasing in size. Hair usually disappears

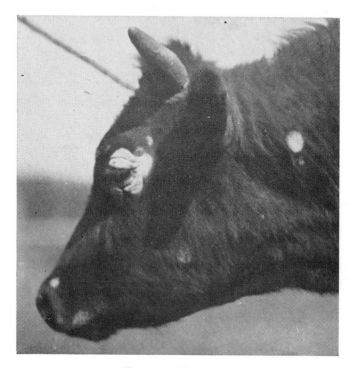

FIG. 144. Ringworm.

from the region, though short broken hairs are common at the margins of the patches. Mild itching is an almost invariable symptom in cattle, less so in other animals.

Prevention consists in disinfecting everything with which ringworm infected cattle have been in contact (page 215). The "Lime and Sulphur" (page 321) is effective when applied to inside of barns, pens, fence-posts late in the fall, followed in a week or two with white wash (page 256). The affected animals should be isolated until all evidence of the disease has vanished.

The handling of the ailment is quite simple as it responds well to mild treatment. It is well to remove all scabby material by stiff brushing, sand-papering, or by means of druggist's green soap (saponis viridis), and then apply tincture of iodine (page 276) every third day until the condition clears up.

Chronic mastitis; garget; caked bag. This is a disease of the cow's udder found much more frequently in dairy breeds and is due to an infection.
A very Apparently one germ, the *Streptococcus agalactiae,* is the causative factor in approximately ninety per cent of the cases. Other organisms are *Strep. dysgalactiae, Strep. uberis,* and in some cases *Strep. pyogenes;* when one of these organisms is the cause the response to treatment is less favorable. There also appear to be certain predisposing causes such as too much protein in the ration, chilling of the udder by lying on a cold stone or concrete floor, rough handling of the udder during milking or during nursing by a vigorous calf, too high vacuum in the milking machine—above fifteen pounds —and others.

(margin note) A very serious udder disease spread in various manners

The greatest source of the infection is the cow with a "caked" or gargety udder. It may be spread to healthy udders by the milker's hands, by milking machines, by contaminated bedding and surroundings, by milking tubes, and dilators. A very common reprehensible method of contaminating the surroundings is to discharge on the ground the milk from diseased or caked udders. Less potentially serious for other members of the herd, though more so for the individual involved, is not to remove the contents of a caked quarter; that is to take only the milk from sound quarters. Serious flare-ups follow this practice.

The symptoms of chronic mastitis develop very slowly, and when it does become sufficiently marked so

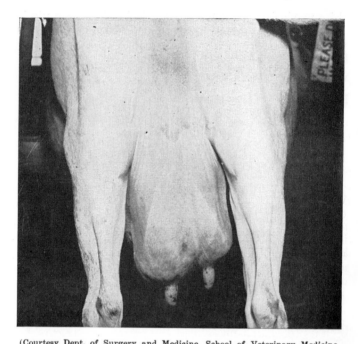

(Courtesy Dept. of Surgery and Medicine, School of Veterinary Medicine,
Kansas State University)

FIG. 145. Chronic mastitis; note swelling of left rear quarter.

as to be noticeable it usually is already in quite an advanced stage. In most cases the first noticeable symptom is the presence in the milk of small clots or flakes, no larger than a pinhead. The clots cannot escape attention when they become larger or stringy as the disease progresses. Towards the later stages the milk is frequently of a watery character. With these changes in the character of the milk the udder has developed in it areas of hardening or "caking." Not uncommonly the first indication of approaching "caking" is a small nodule or lump in the udder at the point where it is joined by the teat. Gradually this lump enlarges until the quarter is "caked" (Fig. 145). Other quarters soon become involved so that the entire udder may be uniformly "caked," or local areas are so affected.

The early diagnosis of chronic mastitis is a matter of considerable importance in order that the spread of the ailment to other members of the herd may be controlled. A positive diagnosis can be made from a bacteriological and microscopic examination of the milk, and this method is recommended when such facilities are available. Many dairymen depend upon the detection of the first small clots in the milk for a diagnosis, and for this purpose they either pass the first few strips of milk from each quarter through a piece of black cloth; the white clots if present are readily visible on the black cloth background. In another method, the first three or four strips of milk are passed through a very fine meshed sieve of one hundred meshes to the inch, so as to detect the minute clots. This latter test is called the strip-cup test.

Early diagnosis of great importance

Methods of diagnosis

For more complicated tests consult the following:
1. California Milk Test (C.M.T.), p. 199, March 1, 1957 Journal of the American Veterinary Med. Assoc.
2. The Christie-Atkins-Munch-Petersen test (Camp test), p. 133, Jan. 1952, The Cornell Veterinarian.

There are other technical and chemical tests that have value in the hands of the trained veterinarian under field conditions. Among these are the bromthymol-blue test, the Hotis test, the chlorine test, the catalase test, the rennet test, and others. Finally the physical examination of the suspected udder by an expert clinician may be a method of the greatest value in the attempts to establish a diagnosis.

The keeping qualities of milk are of importance in determining the presence of mastitis. It has been observed that milk from a healthy udder when stored in a tall glass cylindrical vessel will show a clean cut cream line even at the end of forty-eight hours, with the sides and bottom of the vessel free from sediment when it is inverted. On the other hand, in mastitis milk comparably stored, in a period of six hours, if warm, there is a layer of whey between the milk and the cream, and there is sediment in the container.

Methods of control (page 259) advocated by the United States Bureau of Animal Industry (now designated "Agricultural Research Service" or simply A.R.S.) are as follows:

Methods of control   Because of the nature of the disease and the manner in which it is transmitted, there appears to be a good possibility of controlling the spread of infection by adoption of a program of management and sanitation which should lead finally to elimination of mastitis from the herd. Such a program consists in detection of infected animals by a qualified veterinarian and the use of sanitary measures to be described later.

When each animal has been examined and the condition of the udder determined, those animals which are found to have marked cases of mastitis should be removed from the herd and slaughtered. Such animals are of little or no value and they are the chief source from which infection spreads. The remaining animals should then be divided into three groups, the healthy cows in one, those which are suspected of having the disease in another, and finally animals which have slight cases of mastitis in the third group. Although these last cows have mastitis, they may be retained because the trouble has not progressed to the point where the milk is unfit for use and milk production has not decreased to an unprofitable point.

Following this division, it is desirable that cows of each group be stabled together and assigned permanent stalls. In this way a permanent order of milking can be established and followed with little difficulty. In case it is impractical to stable the three groups separately, at least the healthy group should be kept separate from the other two. Since the disease is spread during milking, it follows that the healthy cows must be milked first each time, the ones suspected of having mastitis next, and those having the disease last. When first-calf heifers are added to the milking herd, they can be safely included in the healthy group unless definite evidence of the animals' being affected with mastitis at the time of calving is observed. When animals have freshened again after division of the herd, they should be put back in the same group, provided that they have not developed mastitis in the meantime. If they have become infected, they should be placed in the third group. If a milking animal (any animal which has had one or more calves) is obtained from another herd, it should be bought only after the udder has been examined, or subject to such examination after 60 to 90 days if an examination cannot be made at the time of purchase. Such an animal should be kept isolated during that time. If the animal is found to be healthy, it is placed in the first group; otherwise it is rejected. Any member of the healthy or suspected group which develops mastitis must be immediately placed with the diseased animals. Such an animal is usually easily recognized by the secretion of abnormal milk or changes in the udder.

Before milking all udders should be thoroughly cleaned. A practical method is to cut small hand towels **How to clean an udder before milking** in half and place them in a suitable chlorine (page 257) solution, a strength equivalent to from 150 to 400 parts of chlorine per million of water. All containers of chlorine solutions should be made of porcelain, enamel, glass, wood, or granite ware; never use tin, galvanized iron, or aluminum. Remove a towel from the solution, wring out the excess fluid and wipe the udder thoroughly, using a separate towel for each animal. This cleanses the skin and leaves it comparatively dry. After each milking the towels should be washed, boiled, and, if possible, dried in sun exposure. When a milking machine is used, the teat cups should be rinsed in a chlorine solution of the above strength before each cow is milked. If milking is done by hand, the milker should wash his hands in warm, soapy water or chlorine solution, and dry them before milking the next animal. After milking, the teats of each animal should be dipped in a similar chlorine solution to disinfect the ends of the teats and any milk which remains on them. Between milkings the machine must be thoroughly cleaned and disinfected. (See Farmers' Bulletin 1315.)

Inasmuch as any injuries to the udder cause it to be more easily attacked by mastitis bacteria, as much care as possible should be taken while the

Injuries to be avoided

animals are in the stable, to prevent such injuries. This may be done by providing properly constructed stalls which allow adequate space for each cow, stall partitions to prevent cows from treading on one another's teats, and a well-bedded, dry floor. The generous use of lime (page 255) in the stable keeps the floor dry.

If the foregoing procedure is strictly followed, there should be no further spread of the disease to the healthy animals. Also there should be a reduction in the severity of the disease in the affected group. However, it must be emphasized that successful operation of this disease-control measure depends entirely upon daily observance of all of the points mentioned. Finally, adequate veterinary supervision of the herd should be maintained at all times.

Treatment by intra-mammary injections of various agents are best applied when the animal is not in production. These treatments are not always successful, and in other than the hands of the trained veterinarian may be dangerous. Penicillin and other antibiotics are being experimented with as a treatment in mastitis. (Page 249.) However, when any of the antibiotics are injected into the udder, the milk should not be consumed by humans for a period of ten days following the latest injection because in people who are highly susceptible, serious reactions may occur.

(The following named publications—distributed free of charge—are recommended:

1. "Infectious Bovine Mastitis," Bulletin No. 255, issued by Storrs Agricultural Experiment Station, University of Connecticut, Storrs, Conn.
2. The De Laval Handbook of Milking, (pages 22 and 23) published by The De Laval Separator Company, 427 Randolph St., Chicago, Illinois.)

Cow-pox (page 828) ; *variola*. This is a contagious eruption appearing on the teats of cows. In other animals, and also in man there is a corresponding disease though with more general distribution of the eruption. There is a close biological relationship between the filterable virus responsible for the production of variola in all species. The first realization of the possibilities of artificial immunization against infectious and contagious diseases rests on Jenner's discovery that persons that had contracted the comparatively mild cow pox as a result of milking infected animals had thereby acquired a strong resistance against human smallpox.

An old disease that still is a source of trouble. It is related to human smallpox

The virus of variola has unusual resistance against natural destructive forces so that it may persist in barns for a long time. It spreads to susceptible cattle through contact with contaminated premises, or by direct contact with an infected animal, or by means of the milker's hands. After the disease has once made its appearance in a herd, and if no efforts are made to control it, there is quite a rapid spread of the malady.

The eruption in cattle is found almost exclusively on the teats—even the udder being remarkably free from it. Dairy cattle are mostly affected.

The outstanding symptom is the development of a series of sores on the teats. These may be in the form

Character-ized by sores on the teats

of pimples, water-like or pus filled blisters, and either raw or scab-covered crater like ulcers. The latter may vary in size from one-eighth to three-eighths of an inch in diameter. Frequently the sores have a metallic bluish lustre. Not infrequently several of these sores become confluent resulting in a raw, denuded, cracked or fissured, easily bleeding teat. If as occasionally happens a sore develops on the end of the teat it complicates very much the milking of the animal. The disease may continue for so long as the animal is being milked because of the repeated infection taking place as a consequence of the milking process.

The milker may develop the infection on his hands and forearms unless steps are taken to prevent this.

Prevention consists in segregation of the affected animal as soon as the first symptoms of the disease

Care must be taken to prevent its spread

are observed. The stables are to be disinfected (page 215). The segregated animal should have a separate attendant. The latter must disinfect his hands and arms with a reliable agent—carbolic acid is not effective against viruses—such as a two per cent water mixture of compound solution of cresol (page 263).

The handling of affected animals consists in the application of a disinfectant—Tincture of Iodine (page 276) is very good—to the sores as rapidly as they appear.

Swinepox: This condition is quite common. It is said to be really two diseases that resemble each other clinically; one of these is a true vaccinia or pox, and the other due also to a virus that is not related to vaccinia. The evidence is that the so-called swinepox observed in America is the one due to the unrelated vaccinia virus. Hogs only are affected; swinepox cannot be transmitted to other domesticated animals. Neither does this form of pox appear to spread amongst swine by contact —the hog louse (*Hematopinus adventicius*) (page 723) is a spreader; (Fig. 146) flies and other biting insects have

Spread by means of the hog louse

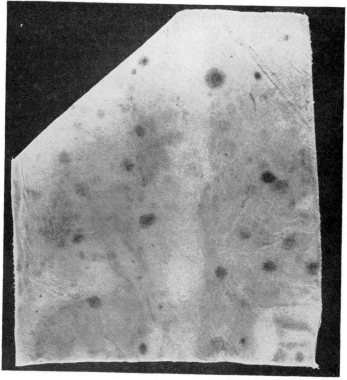

(Courtesy Dr. Fred O'Flaherty, University of Cincinnati)

FIG. 146. A piece of hog-hide taken from a pox infected animal.

also been accused. Affected hogs have the "pox" on the thin-skinned portions of the body, such as the belly, arm pits, inside surface of the hind limbs and part way up on the sides of the body. The disease disappears with the advent of cold weather.

Dipping swine in an approved **D.D.T.**, benzene hexachloride, or chlordane (pages 300, 297) solution is reported to be measurably effective in controlling the condition.

Sore Mouth of Sheep: Also known as contagious pustular dermatitis, and contagious ecthyma. It is a virus disease of young sheep. The virus is resistant to destruction by natural forces so that its presence in infected corrals is quite permanent, thus the young should be vaccinated. Older animals are usually immune. This virus causes the formation of sores and scabs on the outside of the lips. It makes

A disease of young sheep

the mouth region so sore that there is loss of condition, but in uncomplicated cases the death rate is very low as recovery usually takes place in approximately a month. In the southwest, however, screw worms or flesh-fly larvae (page 702), frequently change this low-mortality disease to one in which the death rate is high; in the northwest the germ of necrosis *(Actinomyces necrophorus)* (page 527) complicates the condition and raises the death rate. In lambs the disease may be prevented by vaccination with a contagious ecthyma vaccine. The vaccine is rubbed into the scarified skin of the inner thigh. Once recovered from a natural attack of the disease the animal is immune for several months to subsequent attacks. Non-immunized affected animals should be segregated, and the affected animals offered soft succulent feed. Antiseptic washes have not been found to be helpful.

Bang's disease of cattle; contagious abortion; brucellosis of cattle (page 824). This is a highly contagious disease of cattle. It is due to a

One of the most serious of animal infections. Humans also susceptible

specific germ—the *Brucella abortus* (page 425). A comparable disease in swine is due to *Brucella suis*, and in goats and man the *Brucella melitensis*. These suis and melitensis types are occasionally found in cattle, and the abortus and suis types in man. The observed symptoms in man are not at all similar to those occasioned in animals.

The Brucella abortus remains alive for several months in the uterus of the infected cow; for at least seven months in artificial media stored in a refrigerator; for approximately three months under moist manure—longer during the cold seasons—and for four to five hours only when exposed to the direct action of the sun's rays. Exact research indicates that the germ survived 749 days in milk and lake water at 40° F. below zero; at the some temperature it remained fully virulent in soil for more than 620 days, and in cow's urine for 218. On the other hand the germ, at 100° F., died in lake water in nine days. When not exposed to direct sunlight, that is when protected by manure piles and other debris, it survived for as long as two and one-half months; at 46° F. the survival period was six days in cow's urine, and 48 hours in unpasteurized milk. It is found in immense numbers in various organs of aborated or prematurely born calves, in the afterbirth, and in the fluids incidental to the premature birth. The germ though it may disappear from all other organs seems to be harbored indefinitely in the udder of infected cows. A cow once infected with Brucella abortus will remain permanently infected. The germ may enter the body through the genitals, through the digestive tract, the teats, and conjunctiva (the eye membrane).

When an abortion occurs in a pasture the tendency of many cattle is to lick the aborted young, or even the place where this has been deposited, thus a method of acquiring the disease. The virulence of the germ varies, so that it has been observed at times that the addition of an infected member to a herd of infected cattle, though the disease may be dormant in the latter, results in a sudden flare-up of the disease. The bull is not a spreader of the infection excepting when it is lodged in his testicles.

The symptoms of the disease are not always well defined. The outstanding clinical symptom—it may or may not be present—is the abortion or premature birth of the young. This may occur at any time during pregnancy. If the abortion occurs at an early stage the young creature may be so small that it is never found, and the owner's first intimation of the trouble is that a cow believed by him to be safely settled to service comes in heat again. During later stages of pregnancy quite a constant symptom is that the afterbirth is retained. In still other instances the virulence of the infection is so low or it was acquired during such a late stage of pregnancy that the calf is born at full term, and lives, though usually weak.

If at the time of the threatened abortion the pregnancy is quite well advanced there may be all the premonitory signs of a normal birth such as swelling of the udder, and sinking of the ligaments in the vicinity of the tail-head. It is quite common that animals having this infection, immaterial of whether the calf is or is not prematurely born, become barren so that they do not conceive readily or not at all. If the abortion or the full time birth has a leathery afterbirth it is considered to point to the presence of abortion infection. Because of the fact that a cow harbors abortion infection it does not necessarily follow that she will exhibit clinical symptoms of this. In reality she may outwardly appear perfectly normal, and her breeding record may be fairly satisfactory, but she is nevertheless a potential source of danger to other members of the herd. The situation in regard to the infected, though normal appearing cow is comparable to that of the human typhoid infection carrier who has the infection, and may spread it to other people, though himself not harmed by it.

Because of the difficulty of making a positive diagnosis based on clinical symptoms alone other methods are resorted to.

The first of these is the so-called "blood test" (page 758) which is an agglutination test on the blood serum

**A blood
test to
diagnose
the disease**

of the suspected animal; it is a laboratory test requiring the services of a trained person. This test is the most reliable and practical method of attempting to arrive at an accurate diagnosis, but because of its acknowledged limitations, and because there is lack of understanding by laymen it has at times been severely condemned. Though no definite figures are available it is safe to say that the "blood test" will detect more than ninety per cent of the infected animals in a herd, which is rather a high standard of efficiency. Virtually all of the failures are borderline cases that will respond more specifically when submitted to a subsequent retest. Also all premature births in a herd are not necessarily the result of an infection with *Brucella abortus* though the "blood test" will result in a positive reaction only when the suspected animal has this infection in her body. It is, therefore, not impossible for a cow to have a premature birth from any one of a number of causes other than *Brucella abortus* though receiving a clean bill of health when subjected to the test.

On the other hand, there is the animal that reacts to the "blood test" as a Brucella-infected cow though she always carries her calves to full term. This simply means that the cow in question is a carrier of the *Brucella abortus;* though herself with sufficient resistance, or because she is infected with an organism of low virulence able to resist giving clinical manifestations of it. In still other instances the actual contamination of a cow with Brucella abortus may have taken place such a short time previous to the application of the test that there has not been time for certain changes necessary for a reaction to the test to have developed in her blood. There are many other factors that influence this test which may be confusing to the uninitiated, but it must be repeated that it is a reasonably satisfactory, highly accurate, test for Brucella abortus infection, though not for other infections and conditions that may also have premature birth as one of the manifestations.

The "Ring Test,"—also known as the A.B.R. test after "Abortus Bang's Ring," for locating Bang's disease infection has received favorable consideration from scientists in this field.

A new milk test for Brucella infection (See page 360, No. 33, Vol. IX, Oct. 1948, American Journal of Veterinary Research; also page 1225, No. 9, Vol. 38, Sept. 1948, American Journal of Public Health.)

The test is based on the knowledge that the milk from a cow which contains "agglutinating substances" will show a positive color reaction when a few drops of a special antigen are added to a test-tube sample of milk. The antigen differs in general from that used in the older tube blood agglutination method in that it requires a larger quantity of bacterial cells.

The nature of the ring test The sample is incubated for an hour, and in the case of a reaction a blue color shows at the top of the fluid. It is well known that in infected milk Brucella organisms concentrate in the cream layer where they are as much as 50 to 100 times more numerous than in the underlying milk. However, the "Ring Test" may be used for skimmed milk or homogenized milk by adding two or three drops of negative cream to each milliliter of the product to be tested. Cream may be tested with a slight modification of the method. It appears that the chief value of the

Value of the ring test "Ring Test" lies in its ability to detect Brucella infection in a supposedly "clean" herd. The "clean" herd—demonstrated to be so by one of the standard blood tests, and because of calf vaccination—occasionally harbors a carrier that has failed to react, or new infection may be introduced at any time. If it becomes a routine practice to adopt the *Ring Test*, "carriers" and newly introduced infection may be detected at the very beginning, and disaster averted.

The vaginal mucus test is conducted by inserting a pledget of cotton or gauze into the vagina of the cow

Another accurate test

to be tested. It will soak up some of the vaginal secretion or contents—these are pressed out, and starting at 1-25 dilutions, they are submitted to the agglutination test. Since agglutinins are present in vaginal mucus before they are in the blood, it may appear positive on testing before a blood test indicates the infection.

The whey test is also being used to some extent. (Consult page 67, Feb. 1, 1958 issue of American Jour. of Veterinary Science—formerly North American Vet.).

The control of Bang's disease consists in the application of various measures either separately or col-

Method of control

lectively. If it is desired to maintain a clean herd or to establish one the "blood test" should be applied to all breeding animals. If there are positive reactions the test should be repeated once a month on all breeding animals in the herd, and after each test all the reactors must be removed from the herd, and the premises disinfected (page 215). After all diseased animals have been removed from the herd by monthly tests a period of six months may be permitted to elapse before the herd is again tested. When the freedom from infection in a herd has been definitely established retesting need be applied not oftener than once a year. However, "Ring Testing" (page 582) should be routine.

The premises must be cleaned and disinfected (page 215) after each reaction in a herd to the "blood test." No new members may be added to the herd unless the proposed addition fails to react to a blood retest after having been kept quarantined (page 212) for a period of sixty days. Care must be exercised that the *Brucella abortus* is not carried to the premises of the clean herd by visitors, wagon wheels and in other manners.

The method of control as described in this paragraph is essentially that followed by the United States Animal Research Service in its campaign against this disease.

Another method of attempted control is by means of protective vaccination against the disease. For no method of vaccination is it claimed that as a result of it infected animals will be freed of their infection or that they will be cured. At its very best vaccination can do no more than to protect a Brucella abortus free animal from the ravages of a subsequent infection. All methods of vaccination disregarding this fundamental principle of immunization have failed to produce favorable results. When mature animals are vaccinated they usually become permanent blood reactors so that in later testing it is difficult to distinguish between the blood reactor because of an active infection and a reactor because of vaccination. (Consult page 255, Volume 111, Jour. Am. Vet. Med. Assoc., and page 484, Volume 29, N. Am. Veterinarian about differentiating an "infection reactor" and a "vaccination reactor.")

The latest method of protective immunization is the so-called "calf vaccination." It concerns itself only with **Calfhood vaccination in the control of the ailment** calves between the ages of four to eight months. Mature cows should not be vaccinated until more information is available from research. Mature animals often fail to become blood-reacting negative following vaccination. The vaccine used is one made from a *Brucella abortus* strain of low virulence (United States Bureau of Animal Industry No. 19.) If properly applied it holds out hopes of protecting against Brucella abortus infection young females during their first, second, or possibly third conceptions. Many more observations must be made and much more research data collected before this method of vaccination may be unqualifiedly endorsed. "Calf vaccination" has at least one advantage over other previously attempted methods in that a calf so vaccinated does not become a permanent reactor to the blood test since she loses the vaccination-acquired sensitivity in less than eighteen months.

A third method of attempted control is to divide an infected herd into two groups. First the "blood test" (page 758) is applied and all animals reacting are kept in the second group. The two groups are kept separated with separate attendants. Calves from the infected group are removed from their dams shortly after their birth to form the nucleus of a clean herd.

Whenever an animal aborts immaterial of whether in a clean herd or in an infected herd it is necessary in order to prevent the spread of the disease to destroy by burning or deep burial, or by other sanitary methods of disposal all aborted calves and their membranes (page 226). The contaminated area must be disinfected (page 215) and the aborter segregated until there no longer is an abnormal discharge from her genitals.

Diseases and conditions other than Bang's disease in which abortions are observed   Though abortions, if they occur, are most frequently due to Bang's disease infection they are also sequelae of vibriosis (page 590), trichomoniasis, (page 749) injuries, drugs such as iodide of soda used in lumpy-jaw treatment, (page 425) high fevers, nutritional disturbances, hormonal imbalance, etc.

Occasionally an owner observes signs of an impending premature birth, and requests the veterinarian to prescribe something for administration to the cow to stop the abortion, but whenever an animal is so far advanced in parturition either as a result of *Brucella abortus*, or of natural processes so that she shows outward signs of it, there is no method of stopping the birth, in fact it would be

Undesirable to attempt to stop an impending birth

undesirable to stop it as the calf has at this stage become a foreign body in the uterus of the cow, and nature demands that it be expelled.

Bang's disease control is one of the major animal disease problems, probably also a human health problem as it is transmissible to humans (pages 589 and 824), confronting sanitarians. The losses it engenders annually are enormous, human health is jeopardized, and the American public is not one to complacently accept such a situation. Undoubtedly Bang's disease in the United States will go as tuberculosis of cattle, and other animal diseases, have already been controlled or eradicated. The control plan of the United States Bureau of Animal Industry, ably seconded by the livestock sanitary officials of many states, is beginning to make appreciable headway so that many states have now been declared as "accredited" or "modified certified free" areas. As this campaign has advanced, human infections have decreased correspondingly.

Brucellosis of Swine. This is a self-limiting infection of swine—due to the *Brucella suis,* an organism closely related to the germ that causes Brucellosis or Bang's abortion disease in cattle. It is not nearly so wide spread geographically as the cattle abortion. Outside the animal body its resistance to natural destructive influences is about the same as that of the cattle organism (page 578), so that under proper conditions it will remain alive for approximately three months. The infection in swine occurs because of contact with infected swine and surroundings. Cattle have been artificially infected with the swine strain (*Brucella suis*) of the Brucella infection; also kept in the same yards with *Brucella suis* infected swine they have acquired transitory blood changes, and during this period react to the agglutination blood test (page 758). As the question of the transmissibility of *Brucella suis* (the

An ailment of swine usually manifesting itself by premature births

swine strain) to cattle is frequently raised, especially
in regard to the following of cattle by infected swine,
it may be said that cattle may harbor the
The swine swine strain, it has been recovered from
ailment the milk of cattle, and artificially inocu-
may be lated cattle have aborted as a result of it
transmitted with the recovery of the *Brucella suis*
to cattle from the genitals, but under natural
conditions cattle seem to offer considerable resistance
to infection with the *Brucella suis* and seldom contract infectious abortion because of it. However, if
swine are known to carry the *Brucella suis* organism
it is safest to keep them away from cattle. As regards
the two strains, i.e., the cattle strain (*Brucella abortus*)
and the swine strain (*Brucella suis*) it appears that
the latter is the more virulent one.

The symptoms of *Brucella suis* infection are observed more frequently in the boar than in the female.
The outstanding clinical symptoms in the male are
swelling of the testicles, in some cases they are shrunk-
en, loss of sexual desire, and sometimes swollen joints.
In the female barrenness and abortion occur though
the latter is not nearly so frequently a symptom as in
brucellosis of cattle. Observations indicate that brucellosis of swine is a transitory condition, and that it
does not remain in the individual for longer than
five months.

Prevention consists in disinfection of the premises
(page 215), and suitable disposal of aborted material
(page 226). The male known to be infected should be
disposed of as he is a source of danger.
Preventive Females lose the infection in about five
measures months. Infected animals should therefore be kept segregated for at least five months
and then if they are negative to a blood test, returned
to the herd. The herd from which the infected female
was removed should be blood tested monthly until
there no longer are reactors.

Brucellosis of man (undulant fever) (page 824). Though brucellosis is primarily a disease of domesticated animals man is susceptible. In man the infection arises from animal sources, and rarely if ever from human cases. The *Brucella melitensis* (goat strain) is particularly virulent for man either as the result of drinking contaminated goat's milk or by laboratorians in their researches. It is known as Malta fever, or Mediterranean fever because of its prevalence in those regions. The American public is more concerned, because of their more general prevalence in animals, about the transmissibility to humans of the cattle strain (*Brucella abortus*), and the swine strain (*Brucella suis*). It has already been pointed out in the discussion about brucellosis of swine that cattle may become infected with the swine organism—*Brucella suis*. Human beings in certain sections of the United States, especially the midwestern and southern, contract the swine strain (*Brucella suis*) most frequently, and in other sections the cattle strain (*Brucella abortus*).

Man susceptible to what is primarily an animal ailment

Humans may then become infected with the *Brucella suis* (swine strain) as the result of consuming milk derived from cows that have contracted this most virulent of the Brucella group of organisms. Humans may also become infected with the cattle strain (*Brucella abortus*) from the drinking of contaminated cow's milk, but here the danger is not as great as it may seem to be because of the comparatively low virulence of this organism, and the additional fact that there are usually only few of them in the milk. There is no attempt here to minimize the danger to humans from the use of raw Brucella contaminated milk, and the practice of pasteurizing such milk, as well as removing from the milk line known infected cattle is to be encouraged, but this danger must not be unnecessarily magnified. Compared to the total number of raw milk drinking people there is an insignificant prevalence of brucellosis in humans; however, more knowledge of diagnostic procedures has resulted in a significant rise in the detection of brucellosis in humans. Many cities have ordinances prohibiting the sale or distribution of dairy products within their borders, unless derived from brucellosis-free animals.

Many reliable sources indicate that humans may be infected with the Brucella organisms through the skin, and it is not unlikely that many humans contract the disease in this manner. This explains the comparatively high incidence of the disease in bacteriologists that handle the germ in their laboratories; in veterinarians that frequently contact infected secretions from their patients; in packing house employees where infected animals are handled; and the higher percentage of cases in farm men than farm women— the former having the most frequent contact with animals.

It has also been demonstrated, though it is a point of minor importance, that Brucella infection may be transmitted by biting insects.

Undulant fever (brucellosis of man) in humans can be a very serious condition. The pasteurization of all milk (page 235) or the sale of milk derived from Bang's (Brucella) free herds are effective safeguards. Also the stamping out of cattle infections has been followed by decreased human infections.

The announcement that some of the antibiotics— terramycin and dihydrostreptomycin—are virtually specifics in the handling of Brucella abortus infection, which is the usual "undulant fever" of humans in the United States, was encouraging to sufferers from this malady but later reports indicate many relapses. Reports are that aureomycin is not effective against Brucella melitensis infection. This is the goat strain responsible for much of the undulant fever of humans in Mexico.

For detailed information about the symptoms, diagnosis and treatment of brucellosis in man consult a physician, or an appropriate text on human ailments.

Vibriosis in Cattle: An ailment caused by infection of the genitals of cows and ewes with the *Vibrio fetus*— not infectious for man, and resulting in sporadic or mild general outbreaks of premature births, retained afterbirths and delayed conceptions. It is a complicating factor in herds that are free from brucellosis though continuing to have abortions. Retained afterbirth is an almost constant sequela, though failure to settle to service is not so frequent. The mode of spread of this infection is unknown though believed to be similar to brucella infection. The isolation of the causative organism from birth fluids, the afterbirth or the fetus itself is evidence of the existence of the disease. An agglutination blood test with an antigen made from different strains of vibrio fetus is promising in that it indicates herd infection though not necessarily leading to detection of the disease in all of the infected animals in the herd.

Complicates the abortion problem in Bang's disease-free herds

The infection shows a decided tendency to limit itself in a few months because cattle are relatively resistant, and therefore the disposal because of the infection in an individual is not recommended. The general preventive steps consist in isolating aborting cows and ewes until all abnormal discharges from the genitals have ceased, and if there is retention of the afterbirth as well the animal should be given a four month period of sexual rest before rebreeding. During the rest period antibiotic injections into infected genitalia by means of an inseminating catheter are indicated.

Sheep (Ovine) Virus Abortion: Formerly a reportable form of abortion occurring in Europe and Great

**Common
in Europe
now also
in U. S.**
Britain, it is now so effectively controlled by vaccination that in these countries it is no longer reportable. The disease is clinically indistinguishable from vibrio abortion. A positive diagnosis which may be made at any time from three months before parturition up to nine months after it by the demonstration of complement-fixing and/or agglutinating antibodies. The disease is naturally transmitted by way of the mouth. Non-pregnant ewes are less susceptible than those pregnant, by aborted fluid at the time of lambing. After one abortion the ewe is permanently immune. Vaccination confers a solid immunity.

Anthrax (pages 109 and 823) ; *charbon*. This is a widespread communicable disease of all warm-blooded animals including man. Cattle and sheep appear to be most susceptible. Swine are also susceptible. Certain sections of the United States are known as anthrax districts (page 110) because of the repeated appearance there of this disease. The death rate is very high.

**A deadly
infection
of warm
blooded
animals**

Anthrax is caused by the *Bacillus Anthracis,* a spore forming organism (page 221). The seed or spore lives permanently in the soil, and is also in the intestinal discharges of infected animals. It may furthermore be in the bristles of shaving brushes (page 266), hides, wool (anthrax is frequently called wool-sorter's disease), roughage, bones and bone meal, and other inedible products. Animals contract the disease from grazing over infected pastures, through bites inflicted by insects, or it may occur following the common use of surgical needles and other puncturing instruments, and open wounds invite it.

**Its spore
lives
permanently
in
contaminated
soil**

The vegetative anthrax germ in an unopened carcass will die within 36 to 72 hours in the presence of anaerobic putrefactive germs. These are the germs in a carcass that cause putrefaction. But the spores of the anthrax germs (page 110) are much more resistant, and these spores contaminate the surroundings; however, in an unopened cattle carcass on the open range during hot summer weather the putrefactive changes will eliminate the danger of spore contamination of the soil within a period of three weeks. The foregoing statement is based on the assumption that the carcass is not opened by humans, rodents, buzzards or predators.

Symptomatically the disease manifests itself in from a few days to two weeks after the germ gets into the body—this is usually during the grazing season. In apoplectic anthrax in sheep, occasionally this is also observed in cattle, death may take place in a few minutes up to two or three hours. In these cases there is usually frothy blood from the natural bodily opening. Quick death is usually due to asphyxiation because the intense blood damage results in anoxia (page 154).

In a somewhat slower form of the disease, observed in both horses and cattle, there may be swellings of the lower part of the body with high fever, and blood tinged milk and feces. Hogs have throat swelling with the possibility of death from suffocation. Chickens may eat anthrax cadavers—as a result they die quickly.

In man the disease manifests itself as a local malignant pustule, or if the infection is inhaled into the lungs, as in woolsorter's disease, the **Symptoms in man** symptoms are similar to those observed in animals. Attempted curative treatment in man and animals is by the administration of large doses of anti-anthrax serum, aided by local treatment of infected wounds.

The control of the spread of the infection in animals consists in deep burial or burning of the carcass without removing the hide or in any manner opening the carcass. In order to discourage flies, predators, crows, buzzards and the like from spreading the infection, the carcass immediately after death is to be covered with kerosene or crude oil (page 321). Never feed carcasses—cooked or raw—of anthrax victims to other animals. Bloody manure, and bloody discharges from other parts of the body must be disposed of in a manner similar to that of the carcass, and contaminated areas must be disinfected—lye (page 253) in 5 per cent solution is one of the most effective agents, and fenced off so as to make them inaccessible to animals for several years to come. If it is necessary to send

How to prepare tissues for shipment to a diagnostic laboratory tissues to a laboratory for diagnostic purposes this must be most carefully done so as to avoid infection of the operator, and contamination of the surroundings. A good method is to tie two strings about an inch apart around an ear, then cut it off between the two strings, and sear the raw wounds with a blow-torch flame. The amputated ear is then to be shipped under refrigeration to the laboratory, and as expeditiously as possible because putrefactive processes in it will destroy the evidence of anthrax infection.

Another even better method is to thoroughly sterilize an empty tetanus antitoxin syringe and draw into it two milliliters of blood from the jugular vein of an animal that has just died. If taken too early or too late there may be no germs, but the blood of an anthrax subject has in it millions of anthrax germs immediately before and immediately after death. Wrap the entire syringe well and be careful to disinfect everything that has contaminated blood on it such as the needle puncture wound, the point of the needle or the body of the syringe. Enclose it in a mailing tube. The anthrax blood is such a dangerous product that only the trained laboratorian or veterinarian should do work of this kind.

Vaccination against this disease is of some value, though not entirely so. In general there are four

forms of immunizing agents: (1) the
Vaccination anti-anthrax serum used for curative pur-
of some poses (its protective power lasts for about
value ten days); (2) anthrax bacterin which
may safely and quite effectively be used for immunizing purposes in herds when there are no ailing animals, (it protects for a period of approximately one
year); (3) anthrax intradermal vaccine which protects for about one year. This product is highly recommended when animals are on grazing fields that may
be anthrax contaminated but in which there is no active anthrax. Its injection demands the services of the
veterinarian; (4) attenuated anthrax-spore vaccine
which should be used only in herds where the disease
has made its appearance, and when the occupied pastures are known to be contaminated. This vaccine is
simply greatly weakened or attenuated anthrax spores,
and under proper conditions might lose its attenuation
to become fully virulent so as to be a means of contaminating previously anthrax clean pastures. (It is the
most potent of the anthrax vaccines.) The methods
of immunizing animals are so fraught with potentially
dangerous complications that they should not be resorted to without professional veterinary advice. Anti-
anthrax serum made from horse blood is a harmless
product in itself, but when injected directly into the
blood stream of species other than the horse may result
in a very severe shock, even fatal.

A very important curative development within recent times is that such antibiotics as penicillin, terramycin, and tetracycline—for man as
An well as for animals—are credited with
anthrax many cures in that the germ in the blood
cure is inactivated. However, this treatment
must be applied early in the course of the disease or
the treatment will not repair the tissue damage occasioned by the disease. The use of anti-anthrax serum
at the same time is optional though in general in valu-

able animals its use is advisable. (For complete details of handling an outbreak of anthrax consult "Anthrax Control Program," published in the Bulletin of the Kansas Veterinary Medical Association of April, 1958, Vol. IX, No. 3. The plan was effective in controlling a serious outbreak that occurred in several contiguous mid-western states in 1957.) (For additional information consult "The Oklahoma-Kansas Anthrax Epizootic" on page 125, Feb. 1, 1959 of the Jour. of the Am. Vet. Med. Assoc.)

Tuberculosis (page 827). This is a chronic contagious disease of man and animals. Of the latter, cattle, hogs, and poultry are the commonly affected ones.

A contagious disease of man and animals Man, poultry, and the remaining group of commonly affected animals are each most easily infected by their own specific bacillus of tuberculosis (*Mycobacterium*

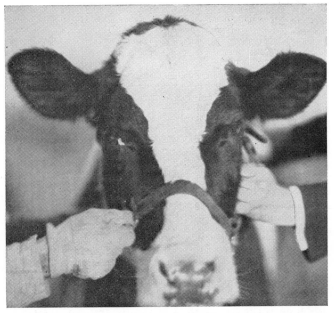

Fig. 147. An ophthalmic tuberculin reaction as indicated by the presence of pus in the animal's right eye.

tuberculosis). Thus the human, avian, and mammalian strains are recognized. There is, however, inter-communicability of the germ so that man may also contract the cattle infection; swine the cattle, human and avian (poultry) infection; cattle usually have only the cattle strain of infection, though they may be caused to contract a localized temporary infection following inoculation with the avian bacillus, and while so infected will react positively to a test with mammalian tuberculin.

The susceptibility of the various domesticated animals to the three strains of tuberculosis germs, i.e., the bovine or cattle strain, the avian or bird strain, and the human strain may be indicated as follows:

	Bovine	Avian	Human
Man	***	—	****
Cow	****	—	—
Horse	—	—	—
Sheep	—	—	—
Pig	****	**	±
Dog	*	—	*
Cat	*	—	*
Chicken	—	****	—

Key:
* **** — very susceptible, disease may be widespread.
* *** — quite susceptible, especially as children.
* ** — quite susceptible, but disease usually remains localized.
* * — slight, but occurs occasionally.
* ± — very rarely, if ever occurs.
* – — not susceptible, or at least occurs so rarely as to be of little or no practical importance.

Infection takes place by the consumption of tuberculosis-germ-contaminated liquid and solid food, and by breathing germ laden air. Thus calves **Modes of contracting the ailment** may get the disease by drinking milk from tuberculous cows—this milk may even have gone through processing in a creamery; hogs contract it by following infected cattle, and by eating on ground soiled by excreta of infected poultry, as well as by eating the carcasses of animals dead of this disease. Areas free from cattle tuberculosis still continued to have many tuberculous hogs until it was demonstrated that the hogs contracted the disease from poultry. All animals can acquire the disease by breathing tuberculosis-germ-laden air. Therefore, if cattle, swine or poultry, on farms where all three are present, have tuberculosis it is certain to be manifested in all of them. Freedom from the disease in one species of animals on a farm is necessary to eliminate it from all species on that farm. "Keep all chickens and hogs apart" or else the disease will occur in hogs.

The symptoms of tuberculosis in animals vary greatly, depending upon the infected organ or organs. If the disease is in the lungs there may be **Symptoms differ depending upon the center of localization of the infection** a cough; in the intestines, chronic diarrhoea; in the brain, nervous symptoms; in the udder, swellings; in the joints, and testicles, enlargement; and if the disease is of very long standing there is usually evidence of unthriftiness. Furthermore though none of the organs named may be visibly involved by a most careful examination including an autopsy, evidence of its presence in infected animals is in most instances found in the neighboring lymphatic glands.

A very important point is that infected animals may show no outward signs of the disease, many of them being pictures of perfect health. Herein is one of the greatest dangers in that the disease may make extensive inroads in a herd or flock without its presence being suspected until a "break" occurs so that the herd goes to pieces, as it were, or more serious when innocent children developed tuberculosis of the digestive tract or as a bone-deforming disease because of the drinking of tuberculosis-contaminated milk. One of the greatest accomplishments of the veterinary profession in America is the virtual eradication of bovine tuberculosis, with the incidental result that scrofula (tuberculosis of the glands of the neck), intestinal, and bone deforming tuberculosis of children have also disappeared.

A diagnosis of tuberculosis in infected animals may be established by the inoculation (page 759) method,
Methods of diagnosis and by a reaction to a tuberculin test. The inoculation method consists in the injection into both guinea-pigs and rabbits of some of the suspected tuberculous material so as to cause lesions of tuberculosis in these laboratory animals, followed by the recovery of the germ of tuberculosis from the lesions. From such a sequence of events there can be no question regarding the accuracy of the diagnosis.

A tuberculin test (page 598) necessitates the injection into the suspected animal of a diagnostic agent known as tuberculin. This agent is a solution of the products of the germ of tuberculosis—it contains neither living nor dead germs as they have all been removed, and therefore, the injection of this diagnostic material cannot cause tuberculosis.

Three different methods of tuberculin testing are recognized: (1) The ophthalmic tuberculin test (Fig.
The tuberculin tests 147) in which a small quantity of a concentrated tuberculin is placed within the previously sensitized lower eyelid of an animal to be tested. A reaction consists in the development and discharge of muco-purulent material from the instilled region within six hours. The ophthalmic method is seldom used as a routine test. (2) The subcutaneous tuberculin test, or "temperature test" consists in first determining the normal temperature curve of the animal to be tested, then injecting subcutaneously from two to four cubic centimeters of standardized tuberculin, and beginning eight hours thereafter the animal's temperature is again determined each hour until eighteen hours after the injec-

tion of the tuberculin. If the post-injection temperature curve is two degrees Fahrenheit higher than the pre-injection curve it is considered to be a reaction, and the animal is said to be tuberculous. So many hazards, dishonest methods, misinterpretations, and uncertainties complicated this test that it is no longer generally resorted to. (3) The intradermic tuberculin test or "tail test" is the almost universally used method of determining the presence of tuberculosis in animals. It consists in the injection into the skin of a drop or minim of concentrated tuberculin; it must be between the layers of the skin, not under it. The site of injection is the thin hairless skin of one of the two folds, caudal folds, beneath the root of the tail. Seventy-two hours later if the animal is infected a swelling will be manifested at the site of injection. The size of the swelling may vary from three sixteenths of an inch to almost two inches in diameter. This test is considered to be highly reliable, though because of faulty technic, faulty reading, and other known and unknown factors it may occasionally fail to meet the demands made of it. It is the official test of the United States Animal Disease Research.

The "Stormont test" is based on the fact that an intradermal tuberculin injection site—usually the side of the neck—becomes increasingly sensitive and therefore a second injection seven days after the first will result in a reaction when the first failed to disclose the infected animal. In skin tuberculosis the Stormont test is no more nor no less reliable than the single injection method.

More recently the "cervical tuberculin test" is sometimes used. It is based on the fact that certain skin areas—the skin of the neck or cervical region is one of these areas—are highly sensitive to tuberculin.

The control (page 827) of tuberculosis rests entirely upon the destruction of reservoirs of infection—the

The control of tuberculosis rests upon the destruction of the tuberculous animals   tuberculous animals. In the United States no other method is practiced if it is to receive official recognition. The periodic tuberculin testing of herds, and at least once in three years in herds believed to be clean, with no untested non-reacting additions, with the elimination and slaughter of all those reacting to the test is the approved method which has resulted in the reduction of the disease among cattle in the United States to less than two-tenths of one per cent, the so-called "modified accredited areas."

If an area has less than 2/10 per cent tuberculosis it may become a "modified accredited area" for a period of six years. If there is more than 2/10 per cent though less than ½ per cent it becomes "modified accredited area" for three years and then the area must be retested. In addition there are many individual herds that are entirely free from the disease, or they are fully "U. S. Accredited." General sanitation by cleaning premises (page 215) must follow the removal of diseased animals from the herd.

Vaccination not successful   Vaccination against tuberculosis of man and animals has been tried, and it appears to be in a measure successful in man, but in animals this has not been practical nor reliable. The adage, "once a reactor always tuberculous," is still trustworthy in the case of animals.

The use of meat derived from tuberculous animals for human consumption   A question frequently raised is in regard to the safety for human consumption of meat derived from animals that have been slaughtered because of a previous reaction to the tuberculin test. Many of these animals are condemned for food purposes and are converted into tankage, while others are condemned only in part; that is, the tissue or part of the body that is in the tuberculous region. Careful study by veterinary pathologists has demonstrated that at the time of slaughter the tuberculous lesion may be a purely localized one, and that it is not justifiable to condemn the remainder of the carcass, any more than when the housewife uses for family food a potato after she has pared away a black spot, or when she uses a bunch of grapes after discarding wilted ones.

Johne's disease; paratuberculosis; chronic bacterial dysentery. This is a chronic incurable contagious dis-

A false
tuberculosis
of cattle

ease of cattle. Other animals such as horses, sheep, and goats are susceptible though it is rarely observed in them. This disease is due to a specific germ, resembling that of tuberculosis, *Mycobacterium paratuberculosis*. This organism lodges in the intestinal lining, and leaves the animal's body only with the feces. It is much more resistant than the germ of tuberculosis to destructive influences, and, therefore, it presumably remains on a contaminated farm for a very long time to be a potential source of danger to the cattle kept there.

Symptoms of the disease seldom manifest themselves until several months after the germ gains en-

Symptoms
of Johne's
disease

trance to the tissues. The animal becomes thin, and it is affected with a persistent diarrhoea which usually so weakens it that death is the final outcome. Upon autopsy the lining membrane of sections of the small intestine is found to be thickened and thrown up in the form of folds and ridges.

There is a method of testing animals to determine whether Johne's disease is present. The diagnostic

A test
for Johne's
disease

agent most reliable is known as "johnin." It is prepared from the *Mycobacterium paratuberculosis* in a manner similar in general to the preparation of tuberculin from the germ of tuberculosis. It is not as reliable as tuberculin. In the test the normal temperature of the animal is determined, then a dose of johnin is injected into a vein, followed by the reading of hourly temperatures for twelve hours following the injection. A rise of one and one-half degrees if it persists for three hours or more is considered to be a positive reaction. Cattle having a preinjection temperature of higher than 103 degrees Fahrenheit are not tested until their temperature more nearly approaches the normal.

The control of Johne's disease is in general similar to that of tuberculosis, but where this has been at-

The control of Johne's disease has not been entirely encouraging tempted the results have not been entirely encouraging. The lack of a high degree of accuracy of johnin as a diagnostic agent; the absence of characteristic symptoms; the resistance of its specific germ to ordinary destructive measures and its consequent persistence on a farm; and the general lack of interest in the disease are all factors responsible for this situation. If the ailment ever becomes widespread its control will be more vigorously prosecuted. General sanitation is recommended (page 215).

There is no curative treatment though such an antibiotic as streptomycin is effective against the causative organism in the laboratory test-tube; but in the living animal it has not affected the course of the disease. The feeding of a dry ration may temporarily control the diarrhoea with an improvement during this time in the animal's general condition.

Pink-eye in cattle, infectious bovine keratitis; contagious ophthalmia in cattle; infectious conjunctivitis.

A common eye ailment of cattle This is a very common ailment of cattle. It is observed most frequently in range cattle during the hot summer months, though occasionally reports of its occurrence are received during the colder months of the year, especially when the ground is covered with snow. It is always more prevalent when cattle are on the

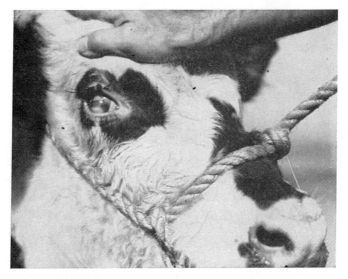

Fig. 148. Blindness caused by "pink-eye."

Most prevalent in animals subjected to bright summer light

range without opportunities for protection from intense light by shade-trees or other means.

Glaring light, insects, irritating vapors, and dust are usually held to be predisposing causes.

There is some proof that the actual cause of the disease is due to a germ or germs, though the evidence is not entirely convincing about this—the germ *Moraxella (Hemophilus) bovis* is an accused organism. At any rate infection by itself is not enough as cattle do not seem to contract this disease simply by contact of diseased and healthy animals if predisposing causes are not present.

The symptoms in the beginning of the attack are those observed in most painful eye ailments. There is profuse running of tears, partial or complete closure of the eyelids, and the eye itself is hot, painful and swollen. Soon the clear portion of the eye becomes discolored to a yellowish tint, and new blood vessels

develop at its periphery. In many instances this part
of the eye bulges and may even rupture with a protrusion of some of the iris from the wound. In other
cases ulcers develop on the eye. In almost all cases
the original disease in its later stages is complicated
by various pus producing germs so that the early
watery discharge becomes decidedly pus like. In the
earlier stages of the disease the animal's temperature
is elevated, the appetite is affected, and there appears
to be suffering. The final termination of the disease is
partial or complete blindness in the affected eye (Fig.
148.)

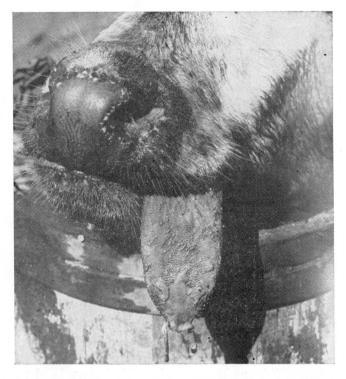

(Courtesy Press Service, Office of Information, U. S. Dept. of Agriculture)

FIG. 149. Blisters on cow's tongue in foot-and-mouth disease.
The blisters break, making it painful for the animal to eat.

Prevention consists in removing an ailing animal from the remainder of the herd as soon as the first symptoms manifest themselves. This step is recommended as the diseased animal is doubtless the greatest source of the infection. In so far as it is practical shade is to be provided, especially for all cattle of a herd in which the disease has made its appearance. Vaccination of non-affected animals is also practiced but uniformly beneficial results have not been obtained. The vaccine used is a bacterin containing the *Moraxella (Hemophilus) bovis* as the main organism.

The curative treatment as applied by a veterinarian varies depending upon the stage of the ailment and the severity of its manifestations. The owner's part of the handling is to provide a darkened sanitary place for occupancy by the patient, and to follow the principles of approved animal care.

Foot-and-mouth disease; epizootic aphtha, (Figs. 149, 150, 151, 152, 153, 154, 155 and 156.) (Pages 109 and 828.) This is a highly contagious disease of cloven-hoofed animals such as cattle, swine, sheep, goats, deer, and others. Horses do not contract the disease. Man is susceptible to a mild extent.

A plague of cloven-footed animals that has repeatedly made its appearance in the United States, and that has as frequently been stamped out

The disease is caused by a filtrable virus, a substance, presumably living organisms, so small as to be invisible through the most powerful microscope, and capable of passing through the finest filter. Three types of foot-and-mouth disease virus are recognized, A, O and C. The virus is in the blood, milk, and saliva during the fever stage of the disease, and in the blisters that occur during the ailment. It may be eliminated in the urine for as long as 246 days after inoculation, thus indicating that it may be carried in the blood for a much longer period than formerly known.

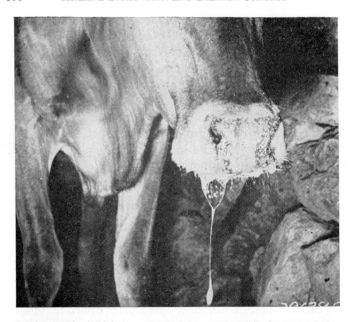

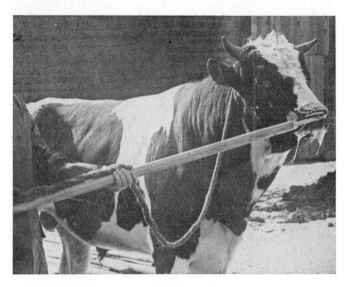

(Courtesy Press Service, Office of Information, U. S. Dept. of Agriculture)

FIGS. 150 and 151. Ropy saliva dropping from the mouth, in foot-and-mouth disease.

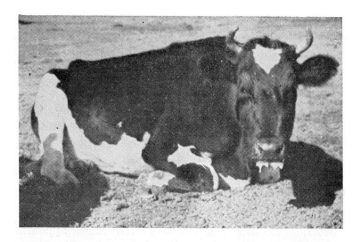

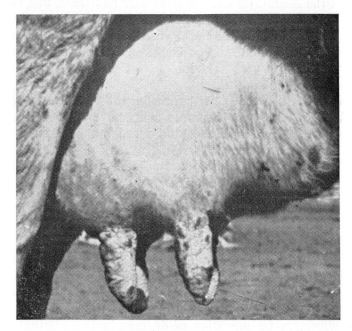

(Courtesy Press Service, Office of Information, U. S. Dept. of Agriculture)

FIGS. 152 and 153. (Upper) Sore feet that cause animals affected with foot-and-mouth disease to lie down much of the time. (Lower) Blisters and erosions on teats of cow affected with foot-and-mouth disease are accompanied by rapid drop in milk production.

The virus may be spread by contaminated litter, by such mechanical means as wheels of conveyances, by the feet of animals and man, by garbage, by vaccines, and in other direct and indirect way. Saliva from infected animals is a potent source of spread.

The disease is much more severe in some outbreaks than others; in sheep and swine it is usually mild. An attack of the disease confers an immunity which rapidly disappears after three months, so that at the expiration of eighteen months the animal is as susceptible as ever.

The symptoms of the disease consist largely of blisters, containing a straw-colored fluid, appearing in the mouth, on the muzzle, udder and teats, and between the claws of the feet. Most of the blisters are small, though on the upper surface of the tongue they may be from one to two inches in diameter. The blisters soon rupture leaving a raw, reddened, painful area. Because of these, eating becomes difficult, and there is slobbering with drooling of saliva. Because of the blisters on the feet lameness is a prominent symptom and affected animals are prone to assume recumbency. A slight fever is usually present at the beginning. The milk flow is reduced and loss of condition is quite marked.

In swine the blisters frequently are found only between the claws and on the under surface of the foot; rarely are they on the snout.

In man the disease may occur as the result of direct contact with animals having foot-and-mouth disease, or by the consumption of meat or Humans milk derived from them. In man there is also a sensation of dryness in the mouth folsusceptible lowed by the formation of small blisters. Occasionally the blisters also occur on the tips of the fingers especially at the base of the nails. Mild fever and vomiting are the general symptoms in man.

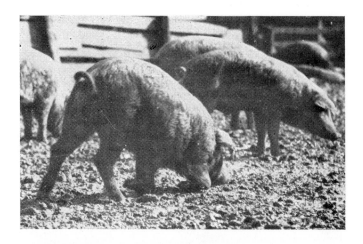

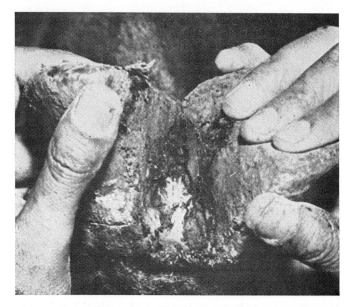

(Courtesy Press Service, Office of Information, U. S. Dept. of Agriculture)

FIGS. 154 and 155. (Upper) Foot-and-mouth disease in swine; the feet of affected hogs are so sore that they walk on their knees. (Lower) Eroded tissue between the claws.

The losses from foot-and-mouth disease are heavy in those countries where the disease is permanently established. The loss is due to decreased milk and meat production as recurrent and repeated attacks leave the animals in thin condition. The death rate in

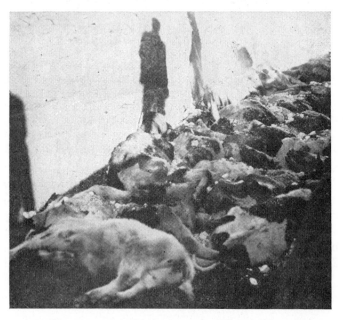

FIG. 156. Slaughtered animals covered with quicklime and in a trench for burial following exposure to foot-and-mouth disease infection.

an acute outbreak is not large, being not more than three per cent.

Control in the United States consists in the mandatory slaughter of all exposed and affected animals, and the sanitary disposal of the carcasses (Fig. 156). Quarantine measures by state and federal authorities are very stringent, but are warranted as indicated by the fact that the outbreaks in the United States have been prevented from getting a permanent foothold. In the Mexican outbreak in the middle forties, due to various factors, the results by this method were discouraging.

Scientists have announced the discovery of what they claim to be a safe, effective, immunizing agent that will actively protect against infection for approximately six to eight months. Its value remains to be established. It must be kept at temperatures ranging from 38 to 42° F. The use of vaccines is not approved in the United States as there is great danger that the disease would become widespread before vaccine immunization could become established. Curative treatment is not attempted in the United States.

For disinfection of premises Federal agencies use five pounds of hydrated or water slaked (not air slaked) lime (page 255), one pound of lye or caustic soda, both dissolved in ten gallons of hot water. Almost as efficient is a solution of two pounds of lye (page 253) in ten gallons of water. By means of a power sprayer the solution is freely applied. For blankets, ropes and finished surfaces use a four per cent solution of formaldehyde (page 266) or in a tightly sealed building resort to formaldehyde fumigation (page 269). Clothing worn by workers in the eradication program includes rubber coveralls and boots, and these are disinfected with two per cent lye solution, and carefully and immediately rinsing off contacted skin with water; otherwise burns develop. Cresol solutions are valueless for foot-and-mouth disinfection.

Hay in stacks that have become contaminated may be made safe by removing superficial layers for burning and spraying the remainder with a four per cent formaldehyde solution. Manure may be safely handled by spreading it in a thin layer over sun-exposed arable land.

Vesicular Stomatitis and *Vesicular Exanthema.* Both of these diseases are contagious and therefore routine sanitary steps must be used in their control. They are of the greatest importance because clinically they bear a very close resemblance to *foot-and-mouth disease,* but lack the highly volatile character of the foot-and-mouth virus. Therefore when domesticated animals become affected with a disease in which there are blisters and/or related symptoms it must be positively determined at once whether or not the condition is *foot-and-mouth disease.* The following are distinguishing features between *vesicular stomatitis, vesicular exanthema, and foot-and-mouth disease:*

Must be distinguished from foot-and-mouth disease

1. Foot-and-mouth disease affects only cloven footed animals.

2. Foot-and-mouth disease does not affect horses.

3. Vesicular stomatitis affects cattle, swine and horses. A significant point is that when cattle are injected intramuscularly with the suspected virus they will not develop symptoms if the virus is derived from a vesicular stomatitis patient. On the other hand, if the virus is derived from a foot-and-mouth disease patient the inoculated bovine will soon manifest clinical symptoms of foot-and-mouth disease.

4. Vesicular exanthema is almost exclusively a swine disease (swine may become infected with foot-and-mouth disease) though horses are slightly susceptible to it.

5. Horses are highly susceptible to vesicular stomatitis, slightly susceptible to vesicular exanthema, and apparently completely resistant to foot-and-mouth disease.

6. Guinea pigs, in the hands of laboratory technicians, may be infected with the viruses of foot-and-mouth disease, and vesicular stomatitis, but are resistant to the virus of vesicular exanthema.

The usual outstanding symptoms of vesicular exanthema are blisters on the mucous membrane of the

Clinical
symptoms of
vesicular ex-
anthema
snout and on neighboring skin. Sometimes vesicles (blisters) also occur just above the hoof and foot pads so that there is lameness. The blisters contain a clear straw-colored fluid. Refrigerated meat from an ante-mortem infected animal retains its contagious virus for at least two months and therefore the danger in feeding raw garbage containing pork scraps. Residual infection in pens persists for at least 72 hours. Affected hogs lose weight and their marketing is delayed for 30 to 60 days.

Federal regulations governing interstate shipment of infected or exposed hogs are (1) swine fed raw

Shipping
regulations
garbage can be moved only for slaughter and special heat processing and only if accompanied by a permit and certificate of a veterinarian stating that prior to shipment there were no revealed symptoms of vesicular exanthema; and (2) that all swine from a quarantined area must before moving for slaughter be accompanied by a certificate of a Federal veterinarian, or a federally approved veterinarian, stating that prior to shipment an examination failed to disclose evidence of the presence of this disease.

Prevention consists in avoiding the feeding of raw or uncooked garbage. Many states now have regulations requiring the cooking of garbage (page 48). The practice of cooking garbage also greatly reduces the infestation of swine muscle with parasite *trichinella spiralis,* and secondary infestation of humans following the eating of improperly cooked pork. (Page 681).

Disinfection in general is the same as for foot-and-mouth disease (page 611). Preventive vaccination is valueless.

In concluding this presentation of three animal diseases i.e., (1) *foot-and-mouth disease,* (2) *vesicular stomatitis,* and (3) *vesicular exanthema* only the first of the three named is of nationwide economic importance; and the last two of local significance. By the most careful and searching laboratory and clinical methods it is imperative for the welfare of the American livestock industry that an unquestioned diagnosis or refutation of the presence of foot-and-mouth disease be established. No animal disease diagnosis is of greater importance. Therefore, the veterinarian and the laboratorian should be brought into the picture at once to establish either a positive or negative diagnosis.

Glanders; farcy (pages 759 and 825). This is a contagious disease affecting horses and mules. It is communicable to man, though the condition has always been rare in the latter. The germ is the *Malleomyces mallei.* The disease has practically disappeared, since the advent of the automobile keeps the horse in quarantine on the farm. The diagnostic agent is mallein. Affected animals are to be destroyed, and the premises disinfected.

Strangles in horses; distemper in horses; colt distemper; infectious adenitis. This is a communicable disease of horses and mules, especially the younger ones, due to a germ (*Streptococcus equi*).

A disease most common in young horses and mules

The disease sets in with high fever, soon followed by an abundant discharge of pus from the nose. At the same time the glands under the jaw became hot and painful, and pus gathers there with final breaking open of the pus pocket.

Ordinarily when the disease has localized in the nose, and in the glands under the jaw recovery takes place following appropriate treatment.

Control of the spread of the ailment consists in placing affected ones, at the first appearance of the symptoms, in rigid quarantine (page 212).

Influenza in horses; shipping fever of horses; pinkeye of horses; horse "flu." This is a highly contagious disease of horses and mules. It makes its appearance wherever large numbers of horses are brought together as at shipping centers, in army camps, and in remount stations.

An ailment of horses that usually makes its appearance wherever large numbers of these animals are brought together

The disease is probably due to a virus though little is known about its nature.

The symptoms of the disease are not at all uniform. Always there is a high temperature and general evidences of ill-health. Most frequently the disease lodges in the upper respiratory tract so that there appears to be a bad cold with coughing and a discharge from the nose. If the eyelids become puffed out and swollen it is called "pink-eye."

Control of the disease in sales barns, camps, and other horse concentration places is almost impossible. For the average farm the best method of prevention is the placing in quarantine, for a period of one month, of newly purchased animals, especially if they have been through a public sale. The use of an anti-influenza serum, to be given to protect horses before they are to go through public sales, and also for curative purposes, seems to be of some value.

Virus pneumonia; influenza in swine; hog "flu." This is a highly contagious disease of swine presumably

A strange form of disease-spread and development

due to a combination of a filtrable virus, and a germ *(Hemophilus influenzae suis).* The germ can live indefinitely in the respiratory organs of swine. The virus is not persistent in swine, but it is harbored in the true lung worm larvae, as well as in the earth worm which is the temporary host of the lung worm. In the early fall and winter months many swine have in their bronchi and lungs the germ *(Hemophilus influenzae suis)* which is quite harmless; then the swine in rooting in the soil acquire the lung worm, and the virus in the latter cooperates with the germ already present in the lungs to produce "hog flu." Experimentally, the virus-carrying earthworms, when fed to hogs produce no disease, but if several intramuscular injections of the germ *Hemophilus suis* are made, many of the hogs develop typical swine influenza. It therefore appears that the germ is an excitant only.

From the standpoint of symptoms and pathology the disease is a broncho-pneumonia. It suddenly makes its appearance in a herd with several or all members affected. There is a high temperature, thumpy coughing, and a discharge from the eyes and nose. The animals are disinclined to get up to eat or drink. The death rate is very low, probably less than two per cent. Recovery in most cases occurs in a week or ten days. However, there is quite a loss of flesh during the attack and an animal may have recurrent attacks as an attack does not immunize against subsequent ones; thus the total loss may be quite large.

Very little, if any, thought has been given to the control of the disease by sanitary means, probably because it is of such short duration that segregation and quarantine are not warranted. Most swine raisers content themselves with a diagnosis by a veterinarian. To the uninitiated it is difficult to distinguish pneumonia from the early stages of hog cholera, but when this diagnosis has been established then apply the principles of good swine care such as an abundance of clean bedding in draft free, reasonably warm housing, and access to clean, and wholesome food.

The disease usually of short duration

Hog Cholera (pages 109 and 202). This is a highly contagious disease of swine—no other species contracts it. Before the discovery of a successful method of vaccination against it there were enormous annual losses. Since the advent of anti-hog-cholera serum these losses are much less. If vaccination were resorted to more generally, at least in an intelligent manner, all loss from this source can theoretically be eliminated.

A highly contagious disease of swine only

The cause of the disease is a filtrable virus. This may be disseminated from a diseased herd as it is con-

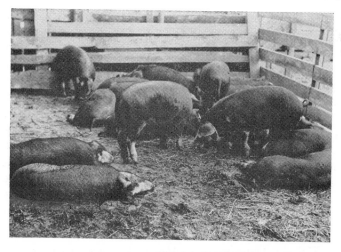

(Courtesy Associated Serum Producers)

FIG. 157. Cholera sick hogs pile up and bury themselves in the bedding.

Means of spread

tained in all the bodily discharges; the urine is an abundant source of it. Scraps of raw pork derived from cholera infected hogs contain the virus. This latter is a point of especial significance as it is a practice to rush to market the hogs of a herd in which the disease has made its appearance, and as many of these hogs—outwardly and inwardly still healthy appearing—have the virus in their bodies, it is spread far and wide when the pork is later distributed. Many outbreaks of hog cholera have been traced to the consumption of this tainted raw-pork garbage in which the virus may remain alive for at least eighty days.

The virus is said to remain alive for several months in hog wallows. It resists natural destructive influences for a long time, and under unusual conditions where it is afforded a measure of protection and not subjected to putrefactive changes, it may retain its vitality for months (page 202).

As in many other diseases the symptoms vary in different animals and herds. In the earlier part of an outbreak affected animals may die suddenly without showing recognizable symptoms. Later the disease is slower in its progress. There is loss of appetite, an elevated temperature up to 108 degrees Fahrenheit, sometimes there is chilling so that the animal buries in the bedding (Fig. 157), constipation alternating with diarrhoea, coughing, gumming of the eyelids with a sticky pus-like material, wabbling gait especially behind, and other general symptoms are noticed. In the more advanced cases there are reddish purple discolorations of the skin of the ears and the lower surface of the body. In only one other disease, that being swine erysipelas (page 620), do these skin discolorations appear.

Usually the history of the outbreak and the nature of the symptoms are so suggestive that it is not difficult to make a clinical diagnosis. In cases **A method** of doubt some of the filtered blood of the **of diagnosis** suspected animal may be injected into a **when** susceptible pig—if it is cholera the inocu-**in doubt** lated animal will come down with cholera in five to ten days.

In an outbreak of cholera in which no attempt is made to control the loss the death rate varies from 85 **Death** to 100 per cent. Those animals that do **rate very** not die usually go into a permanently un-**high** thrifty chronic stage of the disease so that they not only are worthless but they are also reservoirs of cholera infection. It is best to destroy them and to dispose of the carcass in a sanitary manner (page 228).

The disease is incurable. A highly effective pre-**The disease** ventive consists of vaccination with anti-**is preventable** hog cholera serum, frequently with the ad-**by a** dition of hog cholera virus. Properly used **highly** these agents will prevent cholera—improp-**efficient** erly used the virus is a potentially highly **form of** dangerous agent (pages 202 and 532). It **vaccination** may be a means of spreading the disease over a large area. Its use is rightly restricted to veterinarians, and other qualified persons. For some reason the thought has become prevalent that the vaccination of hogs is no more than the simple injection of the vaccine, but those persons that have observed the terrific losses that may result from the use of this material under improper conditions, or following a faulty technic are much more respectful in their attitude towards this problem. Many states now have regulations prohibiting the use of fully potent virus in the vaccination of swine.

Other vaccines such as "crystal violet vaccine" and B.T.V. (Boynton's Tissue Vaccine) have decided value as preventives though lacking "curative" properties and in general do not protect until two or three weeks following vaccination. They are less dangerous and also slower in their action and less permanently protective than anti-hog cholera serum and virus.

Still later vaccines have been produced to overcome some of the undesirable results occasionally following the use of living virus. In the new vaccines **A lately developed effective vaccine** (variously known commercially as "Rovas," "Swivax," "MLV," "Alocine," etc.) the virus is first passed through rabbits which so changes it that it no longer is capable of resulting in cholera in non-vaccinated hogs through establishing a life-long immunity against cholera as a vaccine. These newer vaccines cannot cause cholera, they cannot seed the premises and they confer lasting, three years or more, immunity. Since the immunity established by their sole use may be delayed for several days, it is always advisable at the time of the use to also administer a full dose of antiserum as this confers immediate, though temporary protection, during the few days that the attenuated virus is establishing permanent immunity.

Sanitation may be resorted to during and immediately after an outbreak to hold the disease in check,

Sanitary steps to hold the disease in check and to again make the premises safe for re-stocking. In no disease is the sanitary disposal of carcasses (page 226) and the cleaning and disinfection of the premises (page 215) of greater importance than following hog cholera. Carbolic acid is not an effective disinfectant against hog cholera (page 260), though lye (page 253) and Saponated Cresol Solution are (page 263).

The feeding of uncooked garbage, the indiscriminate use of hog cholera fully potent virus in vaccination, the failure to quarantine newly acquired hogs for at least two weeks, permitting visitors in the hog lots, failure to clean runs under buildings, the use of the same old straw stacks for nesting places, and other hazards, should be avoided in attempts to prevent the entrance of infection. If cholera occurs in a neighborhood, in addition to the preventive measures already mentioned, all hogs that have not been immunized, and that are within a radius of six miles of the infected animals should at once be protected by vaccination.

Swine erysipelas (page 827). This is a communicable disease caused by the erysipelas bacillus (*Erysipelothrix rhusiopathiae suis*). Man, pigeons, turkeys, lambs, rabbits, and mice may also contract the disease.

The germ has a wax-like covering which makes it resistant to many influences that ordinarily are destructive to germ life. It requires twelve days for direct sunlight to kill it; it lived for 170 days in pieces of bacon in pickle; in smoked hams it survived for more than three months; and in putrefying meat it was still alive at the end of four months. It is destroyed in ten to fifteen minutes by a one per cent lye (page 253) solution; by five per cent carbolic acid; by three per cent Saponated Cresol Solution (page 263). However, in barnyard litter and refuse the time required for its destruction is much longer.

A disease of swine— man also is susceptible— that is assuming greater importance

Because of this it may cause yearly outbreaks of the disease as new crops of pigs arrive.

The germ is found in all tissues and juices of the body in acute attacks of the disease, and in the chronic form it localizes in the tissue affected, such as the joints, heart, and skin. In healthy swine the germs may be lodged in the tonsils and in the intestines so that these animals are constant reservoirs of infection.

Healthy hogs usually contract the disease through the digestive tract by consuming contaminated food or water. Pork trimmings derived from infected hogs and fed in the form of uncooked garbage are an important source of the infection. The disease may also be communicated by means of direct contact through the skin.

Symptomatically at least three types of the disease are recognized: (1) Acute erysipelas; (2) subacute and chronic erysipelas; and (3) the urticarial type or "diamond skin disease."

The general symptoms of acute erysipelas are very similar to those of hog cholera such as high temperature, up to 108° Fahrenheit, loss of appetite, constipation or diarrhoea, burying in the bedding and reddish patches on the skin of the ears, lower surface of the body, and inner surface of the hind limbs. A characteristic alleged of these patches is that they blanch on pressure, a phenomenon not observed in hog cholera. From fifty to eighty per cent of the affected hogs die; those that recover may have no outward after-effects of the disease, or it may settle into the chronic form.

In the subacute and chronic erysipelas the causative germs usually localize in some organ such as the heart, gall bladder, tonsils or joints. Unthriftiness is a general symptom, with no other particularly noticeable signs, excepting when there is joint involvement. In this case, the joints are enlarged, and there is pain, and a stiff gait—this latter is arthritis.

"Diamond skin disease" (page 827) is the mildest type of erysipelas, and in the United States it is the most prevalent type. It may go unnoticed until the hog is scalded during butchering. In somewhat more severe form it is manifested by the appearance of raised roughly diamond shaped dark colored areas on the skin, which in two or three weeks slough off, or there may be the formation of large leather-like patches which gradually slough off. Occasionally large raw areas remain which become secondarily infected with pus germs. Usually animals affected with this severe form of "diamond skin disease" are unprofitable in the feed lot.

In cases of doubt about the diagnosis a laboratory agglutination test, or the inoculation of laboratory animals, pigeons and mice, may be resorted to (page 759).

A laboratory test may be necessary to establish the diagnosis If there is a possibility that a diagnosis will be delayed, and because of the close clinical resemblance of swine erysipelas to hog cholera, the latter being the much more common and serious disease, and provided the animals have not been previously immunized against cholera it is always wise to resort to the use of anti-hog-cholera serum and virus.

Sanitary steps used in the control of swine erysipelas are segregation and quarantine (page 212) of affected animals; disinfection of the premises (page 215) ; and keeping susceptible animals such as swine, turkeys, lambs, and others, off the lots and pastures previously occupied by swine erysipelas patients for at least a year. In those regions where the disease is or has been present it is an excellent procedure to resort to the use of anti-swine-erysipelas serum on hogs orig-

A method of protection by immunization inating from previously infected herds, hogs that have passed through community sales, and hogs that are affected with the acute type of the disease. This serum has a highly curative effect in the acute type of the disease, though it is of no apparent benefit in the chronic or urticarial forms.

On farms known to be infected the serum may be administered to each new litter of pigs, and then depending on the natural exposure to make the immunity permanent. The serum by itself immunizes treated animals for a period of eight to fifteen days. Though this is only a brief protection it is enough for curative purposes, and also to allow simultaneous natural infection to make the immunity permanent. The dose of the serum varies from five to thirty cubic centimeters depending upon the size of the hog, and larger doses are used for curative than purely immunizing purposes. It is best administered intravenously or intramuscularly; the subcutaneous route is less satisfactory.

A form of vaccination is the so-called culture-serum method. Its use at the time of this writing is permitted by federal and state authorities only in some states. It is effective.

Recently—about 1959—at least two new swine erysipelas immunizing agents have received U.S.D.A. approval for distribution or sale. They are "Eva" (Erysilpelas Vaccine Avirulent, Norden), and "Duragen, Lilly." When there is no erysipelas in a herd or drove either of these may be administered subcutaneously, at about six weeks of age, without the simultaneous use of anti-swine-erysipelas serum. Immunity is established in about 10 to 14 days. If the disease has already appeared, give both the serum and the vaccine at once—the serum for immediate, though temporary protection, and the vaccine for permanent immunity or at least to market age. Both products are veterinarian handled.

In humans this infection causes erysipeloid. Erysipeloid is not the same as human erysipelas.

Field reports seem to indicate that penicillin (page 249) in oil, in doses of 500,000 units, in addition to the

Penicillin in swine erysipelas

use of anti-swine-erysipelas serum, for pigs weighing 100 pounds or more is giving good results. The expense of the penicillin would warrant its use only in the case of valuable breeding animals.

Atrophic Rhinitis of swine: (Fig. 158) This disease was for many years believed to be "Bull-nose" (page 526).

The early symptoms are not characteristic. It starts with sneezing in one or two pigs in a litter. The affected ones remain runty, and by weaning time their facial bones show evidence of swelling, and there is a bloody discharge from the nose. No form of treatment has been found to be of value in reversing the changes in the bones. The specific cause of atrophic rhinitis has not been established up to this time. As the disease is spread by direct contact, sneezing pigs and sows should be segregated. All pigs having a deformity of the nasal region, or those showing clinical symptoms such as irritation of the

Due to an unknown infection

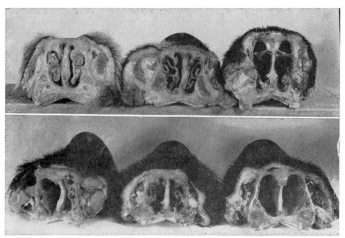

(Courtesy Dept. of Pathology, School of Veterinary Medicine,
Kansas State University)

FIG. 158. Atrophic Rhinitis in swine (cross sections of heads of six different hogs) showing progressive shrinking (atrophy) —from left to right and from above to below—of the turbinate bones in the nasal cavity.

nasal region, and an abnormal nasal discharge are capable of spreading the disease, as well as apparently healthy pigs from diseased litters.

Brood sows that were mature before an outbreak made its appearance in a herd are not infection carriers, and if adequate isolation can be maintained it does not seem to be necessary to dispose of brood sows that show no clinical evidence of the disease, especially if they are not raised on infected premises. However, the really safest procedure is to send the sow and her entire litter to a packing plant where federal inspection is maintained. Then the premises should be disinfected with a hot lye solution (page 253). In some states atrophic rhinitis is a reportable disease, and infected herds and premises are quarantined.

Contagious Pleuro-Pneumonia of Cattle: This filterable virus disease is not now present in the United States. It was stamped out several years ago.

It sets in slowly with cough and fever, and later the fever heightens, there is evidence of broncho-pneumonia, loss of appetite, difficult breathing, and muco-purulent discharge from the nostrils that may become bloody. The cough is painful. The mortality rate varies from 30 to 50 per cent—recovered animals remain unthrifty. The disease is of a contagious nature. Man is not susceptible. Control consists in slaughtering affected animals and vaccination of the non-affected. Disinfection of the premises must also be done. The carcass is best disposed of by burning or deep burial. In some countries, since the disease is not one of humans, the meat of mildly affected cases is used for human food.

One of the animal "national defense" diseases

Rinderpest of Cattle: This is a highly contagious disease of cattle prevalent in parts of the Orient,

A "Defense Against Animal Diseases" entity

though not in the United States. It is caused by a virus that in infected animals is present in the blood and various tissue fluids, and in the urine and intestinal evacuations during all stages of the disease.

The symptoms are general at first. There is diarrhoea. Later the reddened mucous membranes of the mouth and nose are covered with brownish crusts that leave bleeding areas when removed. Stupor is sometimes a symptom. Typical cases last four to eight days, and in a herd because of new cases for five to six weeks. The mortality rate varies from 90 to 95 per cent.

Symtomatically the disease bears some resemblance to "virus diarrhoea of cattle," to "malignant head catarrh" (page 549), and to the so-called "mucosal disease (rhina-tracheitis) of cattle" (page 551). Serological tests in early outbreaks are recommended in order to distinguish between these diseases.

Serums and vaccines, many of them effective, are used in those countries in which the disease is native. If it should appear in the Americas, the slaughter method of stamping it out—similar to the method used in foot-and-mouth disease (page 610) would doubtless be followed, with the exception that still healthy animals in a herd might be passed for human food. The carcasses of diseased animals reek with the causative virus. The virus is relatively less invasive for sheep and goats.

PART EIGHT

Some Infectious and Communicable Ailments of Barnyard Fowl

✦✦✦✦

GENERAL SANITARY MEASURES FOR THE CONTROL OF POULTRY AILMENTS, AND A DESCRIPTION OF SOME OF THE AILMENTS

It is very important in the prevention of diseases of poultry that there be a thorough understanding of the general principles of sanitation. To a considerable extent these have already been explained with statements about permanganate of potash (page 116) and iodine in the drinking water (page 117); ventilation (pages 154 and 159); poultry houses (page 133); droppings boards, roosts, and nests (page 141); sanitary runway (page 144); summer range shelters (page 144); graveled yard (page 174); manure disposal (pages 163 and 170); protection from parasites (page 144); destroying diseased birds (page 231); disposal of carcasses (page 229); incubator fumigation (page 269). In addition to the foregoing the information that follows is of importance.

A thorough understanding of basic sanitary principles essential to the control of poultry ailments

The houses and runs are best placed on soil of a light sandy type that slopes somewhat to the south. Such soil drains well, air permeates it, and the sun dries it, all factors that are not conducive to germ growth.

The right soil important

Shade is desirable for protection from a hot sun, but shade must not be of a type to shut off most air currents and sunshine, because dampness will be the result, and a continuously damp area is not a sanitary area.

Limited
shade
desirable

The small portable brooder house has many advantages over the large permanent one. The greatest dangers in the latter are the difficulty in keeping it sanitary, and the danger of keeping large numbers of chicks in close contact during the most disease susceptible period of their lives. Its chief advantage is that the routine care of the chicks is somewhat less when they are all together. The advantages of the small portable brooder house are that it may readily be moved to clean ground; it is easy to clean; and an outbreak of disease may be limited to a single small unit.

Small
portable
brooder
houses
are
recommended

A screening of hardware cloth or poultry netting of one inch mesh should be placed between roosts and droppings boards to keep the birds from picking at the droppings. The netting may be placed on frames that may be easily removed for cleaning purposes.

Poultry
netting
to keep
birds
away
from
droppings
boards

Feeding should preferably be done out of hoppers. The practice of compelling fowl to scratch for grain is not sanitary, and they do not need the exercise. The hoppers should be high enough to prevent the dirt scratched up from getting into them, and a one inch strip of wood or metal turned in along the top edge of the hopper will prevent the fowl from billing the feed out onto the ground. Wet mashes and liquid feeds soon attract flies, and as these are intermediate tapeworm hosts, the wet and liquid feeds should be in special pans in limited amounts so that they will be quickly eaten that the containers may be cleaned.

Wet foods
should
be kept
cleaned up

Feed from mills and feed stores should be refused if it is not in new clean bags. Used bags that have been on other poultry farms are important sources of spreading infections. Sometimes in order to avoid this disease menace it is preferable for the poultry owner to furnish his own bags as feed containers.

Danger in the promiscuous use of feed bags

In order to prevent fowl from picking in the wet area, surrounding most drinking vessels, these should be surrounded by platforms made of hardware cloth stretched over a frame. (Fig. 160.) All hardware cloth or chicken netting in frames should be cleaned frequently because the small amount of adherent intestinal evacuation is a favorite site of growth for parasites and their eggs.

Sanitary drinking arrangements

Constant Flow Chicken Waterers (Fig. 159) constitute a valuable addition to the poultry yard or house equipment.

If there is enough acreage to permit frequent changing of the range of young fowl this is desirable. A four year system of crop rotation may be practiced in which a legume crop such as clover or alfalfa may be used every fourth year as range for young fowl. It is recommended that the brooder house or range shelter be surrounded by a portable fence large enough to provide green material for one week. Then the fence and shelter are moved in an uphill direction so as to provide new range. This process is repeated weekly. At the end of the year the area is planted to crops for three successive years. During this time the soil will undergo self purification (page 246). If the acreage is not large enough to permit of this four year change it is desirable to adopt graveling or building permanent concrete runways (page 174).

A frequent change of range desirable

If old fowl are retained the young ones should not be permitted to mingle with them unless the former

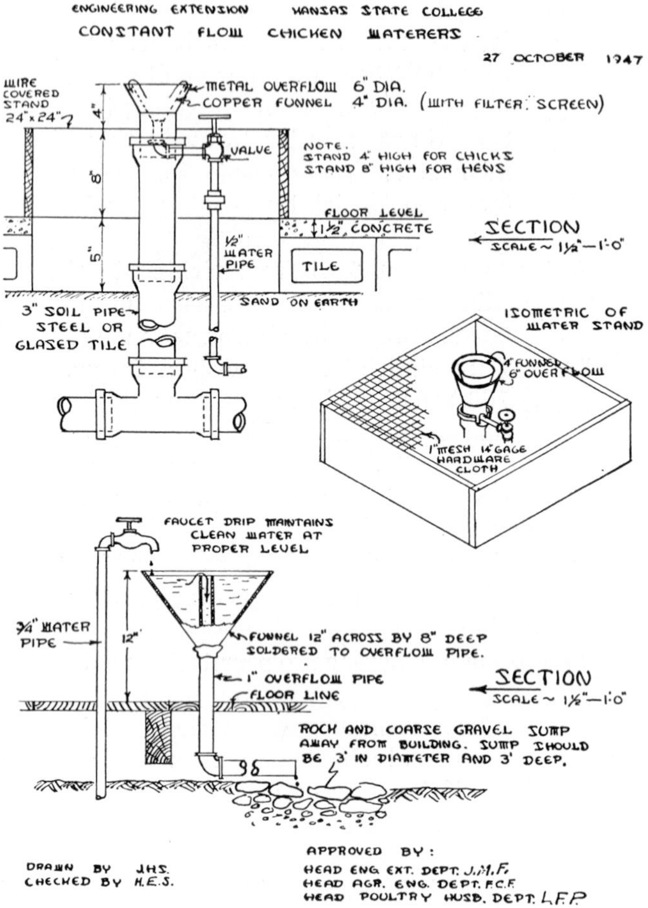

(Courtesy Engineering Extension, Kansas State University)

FIG. 159. A sanitary constant-flow chicken waterer.

Remove old disease-carriers before young susceptible stock is added to old flocks

have been thoroughly culled to remove chronic disease carriers. Research seems to indicate that it is desirable to retain old breeding hens, using as sires the sons of these hens, because of the immunity that has been developed in them as a result of exposure to various infections while they were aging. Breeding experiments indi-

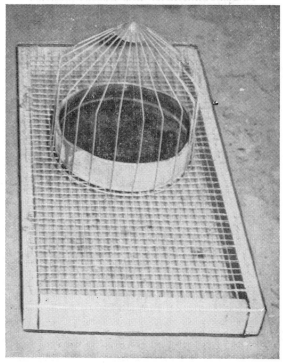

(Courtesy Dept. of Poultry Husbandry, South Dakota State College)

FIG. 160. A practical sanitary watering device for poultry. The pan rests on a hardware cloth platform, and the superstructure prevents fecal contamination of the water.

cate for example that the losses from range paralysis (page 640) may be decreased from year to year by breeding from those fowl that have shown natural resistance when the disease appeared in a flock; also chicks hatched from pullorum (page 651) resistant parents will be resistant, and those from susceptible parents will be susceptible.

When pullets are brought in from the range all those that are not vigorous and normally developed should be culled out and sold, because these are always the first to become diseased, after which they become a menace to the flock.

Newly acquired fowl and those returning from

shows shoulds be kept in quarantine for at least three
weeks. During this period it is an addi-
Keep tional good precautionary test to place in
newly quarantine with them a few fowl from the
acquired flock for the purpose of detecting carriers
birds in of disease. Some sanitarians are even rec-
quarantine ommending that birds that have been used
for display purposes at exhibits, fairs or expositions
must not be returned to the farm. Most poultrymen
prefer to adopt the quarantine method advised at the
beginning of this paragraph. Visitors in the houses
and on the range should be discouraged.

Tuberculosis of chickens. This contagious disease
in chickens is due to the avian (bird) strain of the
bacillus of tuberculosis (*Mycobacterium*
A wide *avium*). (Page 595.)
spread
disease The disease is worldwide in its distri-
of poultry bution. In the United States it seems to
be most prevalent in the north central
states—probably because it is the area of greatest poultry concentration. Fifty to sixty per cent of the flocks
in this area are probably tuberculous. In the United
States as a whole it is estimated to be between five and
six per cent of all poultry. The disease becomes more
prevalent in flocks as the ages of the members increase,
though generalization of the disease does occur in
young birds. In spite of these facts this serious situation is viewed with complacency by most flock owners.

The gravity of the matter is increased by
Poultry the apparent ease of transmission of the
tuberculosis disease to swine with the result that in
transmissible 1938 one out of every eleven hogs slaugh-
to swine tered under federal inspection was retained because of tuberculosis. A reasonable assumption for this is that swine contract the disease from
fowl, and not from cattle because there is less than
one-half of one per cent of tuberculosis in the cattle
herds of the country. Tuberculosis in fowl is, there-

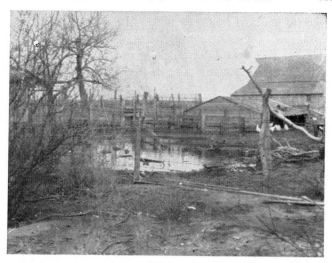

(Courtesy Dr. J. W. Lumb, Kansas State University)
Fig. 161. Tuberculosis was rampant in the poultry flock kept in these insanitary and disease-breeding surroundings.

fore, also an economic burden on the swine producing industry.

May occasion a reaction in contaminated cattle There is also evidence that cattle may react to the bovine tuberculosis test when they are free from bovine tuberculosis though temporarily infected with the avian organism. In order, therefore, to avoid loss from the condemnation of these cattle it would seem best to keep tuberculosis out of poultry flocks.

The source of infection in flocks is most frequently insanitary surroundings (Fig. 161) where fowl have been kept for many years previously. It may also be **The disease in poultry not transmitted through the egg** introduced by newly acquired birds that originated in a tuberculous flock. It is not introduced by newly hatched chicks, because there is no convincing evidence that the disease is transmitted through the egg to the chick immaterial of the origin of the egg, and even though the germ has been found in it.

The clinical symptoms of the disease are never characteristic, and in the earlier stages they are practically absent. In the later stages there **Symptoms uncertain** are lassitude, unthrifty appearance (Fig. 162), decreased egg production, and loss of weight. Diarrhoea is sometimes observed; the temperature is not elevated; and the appetite may remain good.

The best means of determining the presence or absence of tuberculosis in the individual suspected fowl is to kill it, and perform an autopsy. The **The best means of diagnosis is by an autopsy** lesions (Fig. 163) consist of numerous yellowish gray or flesh colored nodules in one or several organs such as the liver, spleen, intestines, lungs, trachea (wind-pipe), bone-marrow, and others. In all of these lesions the germ may be found; it has also been demonstrated in the blood.

The best means of ascertaining flock infection is to apply the tuberculin (page 759) test. In this test,

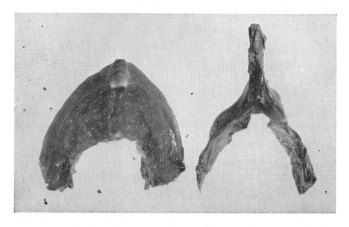

(Courtesy Department of Bacteriology, Kansas State University)

FIG. 162. Tuberculosis; (left) the breast muscles of a healthy bird, and (right) those from a case of chronic tuberculosis.

avian tuberculin is used. One drop of it is
A tuberculin injected into the skin of one wattle, the
test for other being left normal so that it may be
flock
diagnosis used for comparative purposes. If the injection is made too deeply no results will
be obtained, and if too superficially the skin is likely
to rupture. A reading is made forty-eight hours later.
A positive reaction consists in a doughy swelling of
the injected wattle. In the hands of the experienced
careful operator the test is a reasonably satisfactory
one—those not so qualified obtain indifferent, unreliable results.

No entirely satisfactory method of control of avian
tuberculosis has as yet been developed. It cannot be
based on the tuberculin test as this may
Control not detect all infected fowl, and if a single
not
entirely tuberculous bird remains in the flock it
satisfactory soon spreads to others. Furthermore, tu-
berculosis-clean flocks must be kept off
ranges that have been occupied by tuberculous birds,
because the avian tuberculosis bacilli may remain
alive and be virulent in soil for many years, and such
areas remain potentially dangerous for a long time.

It has been suggested that all fowl be disposed of at
the end of the first laying season, but it still remains
to be demonstrated that this will result in the stamping
out of tuberculosis, though it undoubtedly will reduce
very much the incidence of the infection in the flock.

The best approved method, though not 100 per cent
effective, is: (1) to abandon old equipment, and to
start on new soil. If this cannot be done
The best the premises should be plowed or spaded
approved
clean-up and it and the equipment should be cleaned
plan and disinfected (page 215). Three per cent
Saponated Cresol Solution (page 263);
or ten per cent formalin (page 266) are effective disinfectants. Fresh quicklime (page 255) is also of value
if scattered over moistened surfaces. (2) Applying
the tuberculin test with the disposal of the reactors.

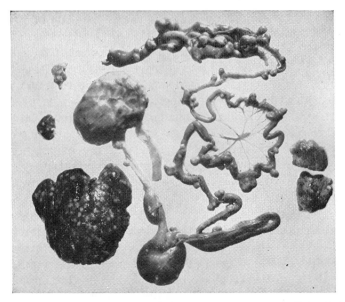

(Courtesy Department of Bacteriology, Kansas State University)
FIG. 163. Changes in the liver, spleen and other abdominal organs of a chicken due to tuberculosis.

Repeat the test every six months until the disease in the flock has been reduced to a low minimum. Also disinfect the equipment, houses and ranges that have been used by reacting fowl. (3) Remove all fowl over two years of age. (4) Do not introduce new fowl, other than chicks, to the flock unless they have originated from tuberculosis-free flocks. (5) The presence of pigeons, mice and rats should be held at the lowest possible minimum. (6) Maintain the premises and ranges in a sanitary condition.

If the principles outlined in the preceding paragraph are carefully followed they will be reflected in a healthier flock not only because of the comparative freedom from tuberculosis, but from other diseases as well. Also if swine are raised on the same farm there will be less tuberculosis among them.

There is of course no cure for tuberculosis. Vaccination has been considered and tried as a preventive but it is not now in a stage of development so that it may be given serious consideration for this purpose.

Laryngotracheitis; infectious tracheitis; fowl "flu." This is a highly contagious disease of the respiratory tract affecting chickens of any age and oc-

A highly contagious disease of the preliminary respiratory organs affecting chickens of all ages

casionally pheasants. The disease is due to a specific virus, an infectious agent so extremely minute as to be invisible by means of the most powerful microscope, found only in the respiratory tract, and which enters the body by way of the respiratory tract. Administration of the virus by way of the mouth, subcutaneously or intramuscularly does not result in the production of the ailment, though intravenous administration is occasionally followed by its appearance.

Apparently a bird that has recovered from laryngotracheitis remains a carrier of the virus for at least

Recovered birds are carriers

two years and it is therefore the source of the infection for future outbreaks. The virus in tracheal exudate is inactivated in one minute by five per cent carbolic acid (page 260); in one-half minute by three per cent Saponated Cresol Solution (page 263), and in the same length of time by a one per cent solution of lye (page 253). The mortality may range from five to sixty per cent.

The symptoms of the disease vary; in fact some fowl may have such a light attack as to escape notice.

Symptoms are those of difficult breathing

In general the disease spreads rapidly through a flock. Usually the first noticeable symptom is "watery" eyes. In mild outbreaks during the warmer months little else than "wheezy" breathing may be observed. In more severe outbreaks these symptoms are exaggerated. The breathing becomes very difficult; the head is extended; there is coughing with a bloody mucoid discharge; the mouth may be held open; there may be rattling and gurgling sounds; cheese-like masses are common in the head cavities and within the eyelids. A post-mortem examination in this disease discloses blood or bloody mucus in the trachea (windpipe), or it may be a cheesy plug, or a croupous exudate. The presence of mucus only in the trachea is of no diagnostic importance. In fatal cases death results from suffocation.

Control of this disease rests on sanitary methods, and, on vaccination. The former is seldom entirely satisfactory, and the latter is accomplished by means of a fully virulent virus which in the hands of the non-trained may set up centers of infection.

The sanitary means are: (1) disposal (pages 226 and 229) of all fowl that have laryngotracheitis, and those that have recovered from it; (2) cleaning and disinfecting all poultry houses, brooders, incubators,

Sanitary steps are not entirely satisfactory   utensils, shoes and clothing of attendants that have been contaminated (page 215), and leaving houses and range vacant for at least two months; (3) using new

stock should be from the poultryman's own hatching, or that obtained from flocks in which there has been no laryngotracheitis; and (4) careful management to avoid subsequent introduction of infection.

Vaccination is highly successful in so far as immunization is concerned, but in view of the fact that a

Vaccination is successful, though dangerous in the hands of those that are technically untrained   fully potent living virus of a readily diffusable nature is employed as the vaccine there are hazards in its use. The glycerinated virus, fully active, is brushed into the mucous membrane of the upper wall (bursa of Fabricius) of the cloaca (page 24) or vent. If properly done this cannot produce the disease as it has already been explained in a preceding paragraph that infection can take place only through the

respiratory tract. Birds over six weeks of age may be

vaccinated, preferably during the summer months. The simultaneous vaccination against fowl pox (page 643) may be practiced, but as there is an age limit for the latter—three months for the lighter breeds, four months for the heavier—the birds should not exceed this age limit in combined vaccination. A "take," which is necessary following laryngotracheitis vaccination, is evidenced in five days by swelling, redness, some slight pain and exudation in the cloacal mucous membrane.

Because of the potential dangers connected with vaccination it is recommended that it be applied either in: (1) an emergency where the disease suddenly appears in a flock; (2) in those flocks where the disease appears annually; (3) in those flocks where known "carrier" males are to be introduced; and (4) in newly established flocks in known infected colony.

The indiscriminate use of the vaccine is certain to be followed by dire results, and therefore the sound recommendation that its application be limited to the trained veterinarian.

Infectious Bronchitis (Gasping disease).

A respiratory disease in chicks less than three weeks of age This respiratory disease is observed mostly in chicks from two days to three weeks of age. Range aged chickens have only slight symptoms and light mortality. Mature laying hens may be without outward symptoms though egg production is seriously impaired, and the eggs laid are of poor quality. It is due to a filterable virus, and is acquired as a result of pen contact. Chicks that recover from this disease are still susceptible to infectious laryngotracheitis. As birds grow older they show increasing resistance to this disease; at eighteen months of age they are entirely nonsusceptible.

The symptoms are those of gasping, suffocation, and general unthriftiness, appearing usually about a week after hatching. The mortality rate varies from 10% to 90%.

The disease can be positively distinguished from infectious laryngotracheitis only by an immunological

Difficult to distinguish between respiratory ailments

test which consists in vaccinating a recovered bird with the laryngotracheitis vaccine. If there is the usual reaction on the fifth day to this vaccination then the disease cannot have been laryngotracheitis, though presumably is infectious bronchitis. From the standpoint of postmortem changes a bird affected with infectious bronchitis never has blood or a plug in the larynx as is observed in laryngotracheitis. In other words infectious bronchitis is primarily a disease of the lower wind-pipe or bronchi, and laryngotracheitis of the upper wind-pipe or larynx.

Because of the low value of the individual fowl, and because infectious bronchitis is of no danger to man

No form of immunizing in areas that are free from this disease

or other mammals, not much attention is being given to the development of a vaccine. However, in those areas where the commercial egg production industry is a paramount one, and where this disease is enzootic, it has become customary to infect artificially, by exposure, about one per cent of the flock at two to four months of age. The entire flock is thus exposed so that susceptibles contract the disease— non-susceptibles are not affected. Since immunity after one attack confers permanent protection, and the mortality rate is low, the egg production is not to any practical extent affected. *However, this form must not at any time be resorted to in areas where the disease is unknown or where it is not enzootic,* as it would simply be a means of introducing the disease to that area. (Consult spray immunization, under "Newcastle disease.")

Fowl paralysis; range paralysis; neurolymphomatosis gallinarum; leucosis; lymphomatosis. This is a widespread disease of chickens the nature and cause of which is not fully understood.

The disease has been ascribed to a virus, to heredity, to parasitism, to nutritional disturbances, and to
various well known germs.

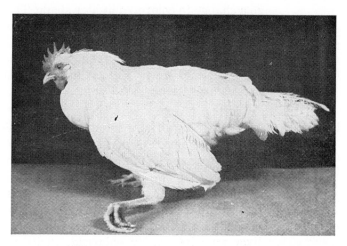

(Courtesy Department of Bacteriology, Kansas State University)

Fig. 164. Range paralysis—a typical field case.

The disease sometimes affects only birds of a certain group; those purchased from a single source; those
from certain parents; members of one breed only may
be affected though another breed is kept in the same
environment and under identical conditions.

An ailment
of chickens
characterized
by inability
to control
the action
of the legs
and wings

The symptoms of the disease usually do
not manifest themselves until the bird is
several months of age, possibly because it
is a slowly developing ailment. Authorities
are not agreed that they are all evidence of
the same disease.

The group of symptoms most generally observed
consist in a partial or complete inability to control or
use the legs and wings (Fig. 164) so that the affected
bird lies on the ground. Jerking and twitching, and
shrinking of the muscles of the affected parts are

common. The nerve trunk of the affected region is enlarged. (Fig. 165.) (This is "neural lymphomatosis.")

In another group of symptoms the disease, if it is the same, settles in the eyes so that these organs undergo a change in color to a lighter shade. This is "ocular lymphomatosis"; poultrymen refer to it as "white eye" or "gray eye." These affected eyes may bulge, and the pupil is either widely dilated or contracted to a comparatively small point.

Sometimes the ailment settles in the eyes

In the third group of symptoms there are tumor-like masses involving any of the internal organs, as well as the muscles and skin. The masses may be so large as to practically obliterate the organ to which they are attached. Some of the tumors are of a firm consistency, while others are mushy. Upon incision they are of a yellowish color. The liver may be greatly enlarged. Birds affected in this manner have a pale comb and wattles; are sluggish; lose weight in spite of a good appetite; finally they cannot stand, and death takes place after a rather prolonged illness. This is "visceral lymphomatosis." A rare form of the disease is that in which the

Occasionally there are large tumor-like masses involving various organs

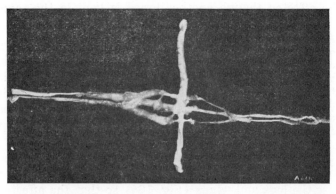

(Courtesy Department of Bacteriology, Kansas State University)

FIG. 165. Range paralysis lesion. Note the diseased and enlarged left nerve as compared with the normal right nerve.

bones of the shanks are thickened, hot, hard, and insensitive. (This is "osteopetrotic lymphomatosis.")

All of the groups of symptoms described may be present in one bird, or only a single group may be noticed.

Control of the disease must depend upon general sanitary measures until there is more specific information about the nature of the disease and **Until more information is available sanitary measures offer the best means of control** its mode of transmission. Prompt removal of affected birds and their disposal (pages 226 and 229); cleaning and disinfection of poultry houses and incubators; hatching eggs to be derived from a source known to be free from this disease; and establishing flocks from parents that through a long period of selection have demonstrated a resistance to the disease, are approved present day methods.

There is no known cure for the disease.

Fowl pox (page 828); *chicken pox; sore-head; contagious epithelioma; avian "diphtheria."* This is a **A highly contagious disease of poultry— not communicable to mammals** highly contagious disease of chickens, turkeys and other species of birds, though mammals, including cattle and others, are not susceptible to the avian (poultry) disease.

It is due to a virus which may get into the tissues through small wounds; through mosquito bites; it may be picked up with feed and water. The virus may be carried to neighboring farms on sacks and crates, and in various other ways.

There are two different types of the disease usually referred to as: (1) the skin form, (2) the diphtheritic or mouth and throat form.

In the skin form the disease localizes in the skin of the head region. (Figs. 166 and 167.) There are small, raised grayish blister-like spots which soon dry

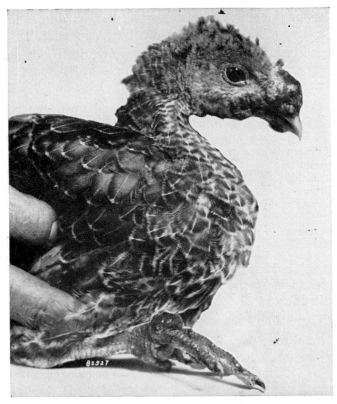

(Courtesy Dept. of Bacteriology, Kansas State University)

FIG. 166. Fowl-pox in the turkey. All poults of this flock seemed to be affected; old birds were not affected.

up to form brownish scabs and wart-like eruptions. Occasionally the skin of the legs, under the wings, and around the vent are also affected. In three or four weeks the scabs fall off leaving a dull appearing healed area. In the skin form there may be no general symptoms, though listlessness, and decreased egg production are sometimes observed.

The diphtheritic, or mouth and throat form of the disease is characterized by the formation of raised yellow canker sores or membranes on the tongue, mouth, throat, and windpipe. Occasionally an eye may

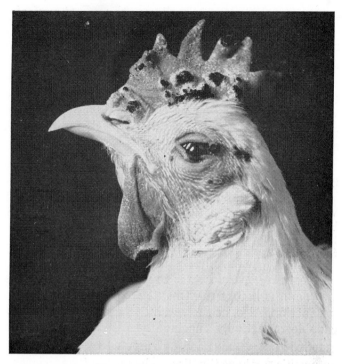

(Courtesy Dept. of Bacteriology, Kansas State University)

FIG. 167. Fowl-pox—this bird is a representative of a typical outbreak in a flock.

be destroyed as the disease extends to it. Difficult breathing is a marked symptom because of the mechanical obstruction in the mouth and windpipe. Difficulty in eating is due to the same cause, and this may result in rapid loss of weight and death. Both forms of the disease may be present in the same bird.

There is no statistical information to indicate the death loss from fowl-pox, though it is not believed to be large. The greatest loss is the result of unthrifty general condition, and suspended egg production. One attack of the disease creates long time resistance to subsequent infection.

Recovered birds are immune to future attacks

Control measures should be prompt.

As soon as evidence of the disease appears the affected bird should be killed and disposed of in a sanitary manner (pages 226 and 229), and the premises and poultry houses are to be cleaned and disinfected.

Vaccination in the United States is practiced by means of either a fowl-pox virus, or a pigeon-pox virus, the former causing a more severe and sometimes serious reaction though also resulting in a more solid immunity.

Pigeon-pox vaccine is frequently used in laying flocks, though it confers only a temporary immunity— usually about three months duration. In **Vaccinate before the third and fourth months** order to minimize untoward results it is best to vaccinate the lighter breeds before they are three months of age, and the heavier breeds before their fourth month of life, or a general rule is to vaccinate pullets at least two months before they may be expected to come into production. Also, as the vaccine is a potent living virus capable of actually causing the disease, it is recommended that vaccination be resorted to only in flocks on premises where the disease has made its appearance previously. Bad results are likely to ensue if the vaccinated bird is not in good physical condition.

There are two modes of vaccination, i.e. either by the "stick" method, or the feather follicle method. **Methods of vaccination** In the former a few feathers are plucked usually from the upper part of the leg. Then the tip of a guarded knife blade with a small amount of the vaccine adherent to it is pricked into the skin to a depth of one-eighth of an inch.

In the feather follicle method from six to eight feathers are plucked from the upper portion of the leg. Then by means of a small stiff bristled brush, or swab, the vaccine is applied into the follicles.

It is important that the birds be guarded against

unfavorable conditions for at least three weeks after vaccination. Eight to ten days following the vaccination several of the birds are to be examined to determine if there are "takes" at the site of vaccination as evidenced by swelling and scab formation. Under ordinary conditions if there are less than 80 per cent of "takes" it is advisable to revaccinate those that do not show a "take," though it must be remembered that absence of a "take" may indicate a pre-existing immunity.

Because of the great danger of disseminating the disease with the living potent vaccine, and the many

Danger in improper vaccination

factors that must be considered in the vaccination process, as well as to ensure the best results a qualified veterinarian should be engaged to do the work. All utensils and instruments, as well as empty vaccine bottles, should be sterilized or destroyed immediately after their use. If any of the vaccine is accidentally spilled steps must at once be taken to control spread from this source.

Fowl cholera. This is a contagious disease of chickens, turkeys, pigeons, ducks, geese and many wild

A very virulent disease of barnyard fowl

fowl. Of all birds, geese seem to be the most susceptible so that in them it usually assumes a very virulent form.

The disease is due to a germ known as the *Pasteurella avicida,* which is a member of the hemorrhagic septicemia (page 547) group of organisms; but there does not seem to be a species intercommunicability of the disease though rabbits succumb to fowl cholera inoculation. The germ probably enters the body through the respiratory tract when it produces the disease, because artificial production of it is successful by this route, though almost impossible to cause it by administering the germ through the digestive tract. The germ is readily destroyed by ordinary disinfectants. In the soil it may live for as long as three months. The disease may be introduced by means of cholera sick fowl, wild flying birds, pigeons, insects, and on the clothing of human beings.

The disease is so sudden in its appearance that the first indication of its presence may be the finding

The ailment appears very suddenly
of dead fowl, especially fat ones, under the roost. Though this evidence should not be considered conclusive sudden death is suggestive of cholera. In this acute type of the disease the comb and wattles are dark, almost purplish, in color. If life persists for a few days the droppings become pale colored with a mixture of mucus and blood though earlier in the disease greenish diarrhoea is a symptom. There is of course extreme prostration. In the slower or chronic type of the disease the bird becomes gradually emaciated; the comb and wattles become pale; frequently the disease settles in a joint so that lameness develops. Death may be delayed for several weeks.

The control of the disease rests in the application of sanitary principles. A sound management practice includes the separation of fowl of different ages because mature recovered ones may be carriers of the infection and by contact spread the disease to younger susceptible ones. As the germ may live and even propagate itself in the soil for a long time, it is essential in the control of the disease to change the

Sanitation offers most for the control of the ailment
runs. The poultry houses must be thoroughly disinfected (page 215). Dead fowl, and those sick with the disease should be burned (page 228). The killing of sick birds is best done by breaking the neck— at least no open bleeding wound should be made as that would be a means of disseminating the infection. (Fig. 205.) The feed hoppers and drinking vessels must be placed so that their contents will not be contaminated with the droppings. Birds to be

added to a flock should be held in quarantine for two or three weeks. The presence of wild flying birds should be kept at a minimum.

Vaccination has been tried and though it may not be condemned as being entirely valueless, still any successful immunization ascribed to it is very rare, so that taken as a whole it must be classed as of very low, doubtful value.

Sodium sulfamethazine or sulfaquinoxaline—the latter preferred by man (page 281)—administered either in solution in the drinking water or the mash is reported to control the immediate mortality in acute fowl cholera. A two-day treatment, then skip treatment for four days, followed by two more days of treatment. Since this treatment does not immunize or protect the fowl from the fowl cholera germ which is quite persistent in the soil of poultry yards and surroundings it is quite customary to commercially dispose of the entire flock before another outbreak occurs.

Fowl typhoid. This is a disease of all adult domesticated fowl though water-fowl do not appear to contact it so readily. It is caused by a germ known as the *Shigella gallinarum* which is quickly destroyed by direct sunlight, and disinfectants, though when buried in the soil it may survive for some time. It is in the droppings of affected fowl, and outwardly recovered fowl remain carriers.

All barnyard fowl with the exception of water-fowl are susceptible

The disease is geographically widespread. Up until comparatively recent times it was frequently mistaken for fowl cholera, which it resembles clinically. The comb and wattles are usually pale, and there is a greenish diarrhoea. In chronic cases life may persist for several weeks, and during this time, with the exception of listlessness, there may be no outward manifestations of the condition. A positive diagnosis may be made only by means of a laboratory examination.

Control of the disease consists in the application of the sanitary methods (page 215). As the in-

Sanitary measures most successful in the attempts at control

fection may persist in the soil for some time it is advisable to provide new yards that receive no seepage or drainage from the contaminated yards. As it is frequently impossible to detect "carriers" of the disease it is best to subject the entire flock to a blood agglutination test (page 758). In fact, the typhoid infected fowl will react positively to the agglutination test for *pullorum disease* (page 651) ; in other words when the pullorum test is applied there will be positive reactions by both the pullorum and typhoid infected fowl—provided both diseases are present in the flock. Destruction and sanitary disposal of infected fowl are important. Preventive vaccination with an autogenous bacterin—injected at two or preferably three different periods is claimed to be helpful by some, but most authorities express doubt in regard to its value.

Botulism (pages 471 and 824) ; *limberneck; food poisoning.* The cause of this disease is a very power-

A form of food poisoning in poultry

ful poison elaborated by a germ, *Clostridium botulinum.* The germ is readily destroyed, but it forms spores which are the seeds of germs and the spores are very resistant to destruction. Some spores resist boiling for as long as three and one-half hours. The germ is in the soil; in human foods that do not have air or oxygen exposure such as canned or tightly bottled material; in closely packed ensilage; in decomposing animal carcasses, and other places. Fly maggots feeding on carcasses may contain enough of the poison to kill fowl that eat the maggots. Poorly drained areas are favorite resting places of the spores, and when conditions are favorable the germ, which elaborates the poison, is developed.

The first noticeable symptoms are difficulty in walking and drooping of the wings. In severe cases there

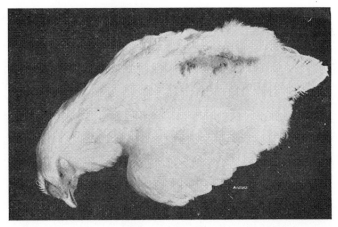

(Courtesy Dept. of Bacteriology, Kansas State University)

FIG. 168. Botulism (limber-neck). Note the paralysis of the neck and wings.

Early symptoms of paralysis observed
is inability to stand. Different groups of muscles become paralyzed especially those of the neck—therefore the name limber-neck—and throat so that there is inability to swallow. (Fig. 168.) The feathers may become loosened in chickens, though rarely in turkeys.

Prevention by withholding contaminated foods
Control of the condition consists in locating the contaminated food stuff, and destroying it so that no additional birds will contract the ailment. Low places that serve as harbors for the spores should be drained. Dead and decomposing animals should be burned.

If the unaffected birds of the flock in which the disease has made its appearance are of sufficient value to warrant the expense of using botulinus antitoxin, types A and C, this should be used as it confers a reasonably strong though temporary protection.

Pullorum disease; bacillary white diarrhoea; B. W. D. This is a highly fatal disease of baby chicks—

two week old or younger. Less frequently other fowl are infected—turkeys are quite commonly infected.

A highly fatal diarrhoea of young chicks

The causative germ is the bacterium *Salmonella pullorum* (page 826). It is found in all of the internal organs of the affected chick, and also in the ovaries of mature hens. (Fig. 169.) The eggs from infected hens carry the germ so that the little chick is infected when hatched.

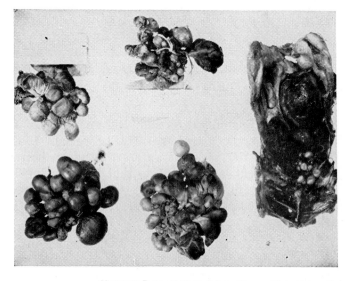

(Courtesy Dept. of Bacteriology, Kansas State University)

FIG. 169. Ovarian infection showing miscellaneous ovaries from birds affected with pullorum disease.

Most of the infected chicks die, but occasionally there are recoveries, and these recovered fowls perpetuate the infection to be passed on to the next hatching. Chicks born free of the disease also contract it from the diseased ones by contact, either while still in the incubator or later.

The symptoms in chicks consist outstandingly of a whitish, pasty diarrhoea, which is smeared around the vent. They are droopy and appear cold. There is little inclination to move; a painful chirp is common and the eyes are closed. Most of the affected chicks die within a week after hatching. (Fig. 170.)

Mature infected hens usually exhibit no clinical symptoms. On a post-mortem examination of the ovaries the attached ova (egg yolks) are visibly shrunken, misshappen, and discolored to a greenish lead-like tint.

The disease may be positively diagnosed by the isolation of the causative germ from the internal organs of a dead chick. Reasonably accurate evidence for diagnostic purposes may also be obtained from the lesions in the body of the dead chick. A high mortality rate in chicks because of a disease in which diarrhoea is an outstanding symptom is always very suggestive of this ailment.

The usual method of diagnosis is by means of the agglutination blood test (page 758) applied to the mature birds of the flock, and the subsequent removal of all reacting ones, because these are the most important sources of the infection. The test should be applied semi-annually, or if infection is detected in a flock a re-test should be resorted to every four to six weeks until reactors no longer appear. (Fig. 171.)

Mature birds are the source of the ailment, and the blood test should be used for its detection

The control of the disease rests in the removal from a flock of all fowl reacting to a blood test. (Fig. 172.) Eggs intended for hatching purposes, baby chicks and new breeding stock must be obtained from sources known to be free from pullorum disease infection. Sanitary conditions must be maintained in poultry houses, brooders and yards (page 215). Fumigation of incubators (page 269) is strongly advocated. Carcasses of dead birds should be carefully destroyed (pages 226 and 229).

Control rests in sanitation

There is no known form of immunization.

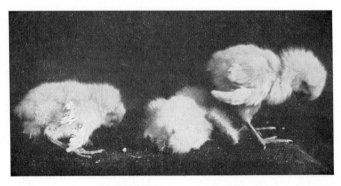

(Courtesy Dept. of Bacteriology, Kansas State University)
FIG. 170. Chicks artificially infected with pullorum disease.

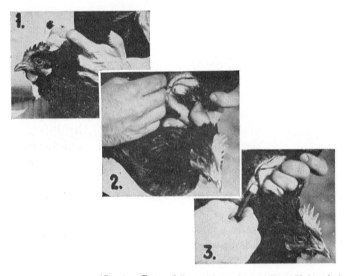

(Courtesy Dept. of Bacteriology, Kansas State University)

FIG. 171. Bleeding for pullorum testing purposes. (1) Method of holding bird preparatory to bleeding. (2) Vein exposed to be punctured for bleeding. (3) Withdrawing blood.

Because of the immense possibilities for widespread dissemination of this disease through the large traffic in baby chicks the federal government has formulated a "National Poultry Improvement Plan" which has for its goal the establishment of pullorum

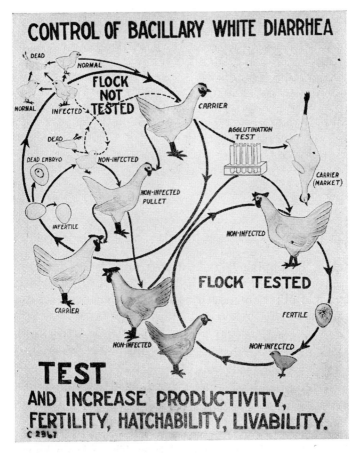

FIG. 172. Chart showing cycle of infection in pullorum disease of chickens.

control programs in every state, and to have every member of the industry participate in it. It consists in having all breeding birds blood tested under official supervision. Pullorum testing of turkeys had increased so that during July, August and September, 1953, there was an increase of 38 per cent over the same months a year previous.

Newcastle disease. (Fig. 173.) This contagious disease of fowl long prevalent in the Dutch East Indies,

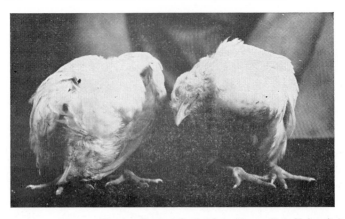

(Courtesy Dept. of Bacteriology, Kansas State University)

FIG. 173. Newcastle disease. Note the general paralytic condition.

India, Philippine Islands, Korea and Ceylon has now been recognized in the United States. It affects chickens and other fowl such as turkeys, ducks, geese, and guineas.

Symptoms consist of fever, loss of appetite, stoppage of egg production, foul smelling watery diarrhoea, a prolonged breathing act with head and neck outstretched, beak half-opened, and coughing and sneezing. There may be paralysis of the wings and legs. The death rate is high in foreign lands, though in America the disease has—up to the time of this writing at least—been of a mild type. There is no known cure.

The virus causing this disease enters by way of the mouth. Close contact is believed necessary. The droppings, infected premises and equipment **A serious** such as crates aid in spreading the disease. **threat to** The virus of Newcastle disease is in- **the fowl** activated in three minutes or less by the **industry in** following: Saponated Cresol Solution, **the U. S.** 1%, (page 263); bichloride of mercury, 1 to 1000, (page 276); sodium hydroxide, 2%, (page 253); and formalin, 10% (page 266).

After a positive laboratory diagnosis has established the presence of the disease, all infected fowl, including pigeons on the infected premises should be slaughtered. Feed bags or other equipment should not be permitted to leave the premises. Eggs should be dipped in a 2% solution of sodium hydroxide (page 253) for one minute.

Some of the older hens may have passed through an unobserved attack during the chick stage, or as a result of successful immunization. Such hens are usually solidly immune.

Hens that are solidly immune will pass on this immunity to the chicks hatched from their eggs through one egg laying period—the chicks are passively immune until about three weeks of age and at this age the immunity received from the hen wanes or has disappeared entirely, and the chicks must be vaccinated. No form of vaccination is effective during the three weeks that the chicks have the mother's immunity.

Until recently, all vaccines have been potentially dangerous, because being living virus material, there always existed the possibility that they could set up new centers of infection.

During the 1958 sessions of the Am. Veterinary Medical Assoc., the Bur. of Agr. Res., U.S.D.A., reported a new safe vaccine for the protection of fowl against Newcastle disease. **A new safe vaccine** The new vaccine made from the so-called G.B. Texas strain of the Newcastle virus—this is highly potent—is inactivated insofar as its disease producing power is concerned, by chemical means (beta propiolactone). This, however, does not affect its immunizing power—it is not capable of spreading the disease. Used at 14 days of age it protects chicks during the broiler growing period, and revaccination at approximately 12 weeks of age gives protection up to 32 weeks of age. Since it cannot spread the disease, if used consistently, it may ultimately result in the eradication of an infection.

Spray Vaccination for Infectious Bronchitis and Newcastle Disease: There are now available from veterinarians Aerosol Sprayers containing properly diluted preparations of embryo avianized B_1 strain of the Newcastle Disease virus and in combination with it a similarly treated Infectious Bronchitis virus. Sprayed over chicks, preferably at three days of age—it makes no appreciable difference if there is a parental immunity—it will protect the chicks until broiler age, or a second spraying at 20 weeks of age will protect to the breeding or production age. Spraying may be done while the chicks are in the brooder—fans shut off—or older birds while on the roost in the poultry house. There is usually a mild reaction for 4 or 5 days after the spraying though the mortality rate is less than two per cent.

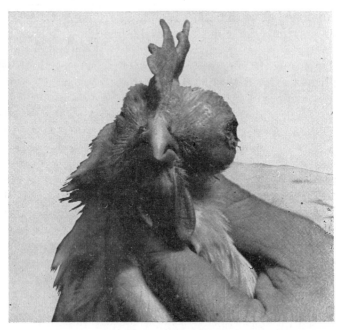

(Courtesy Dept. of Bacteriology, Kansas State University)
FIG. 174. Roup. This type of head swelling is the result of infection and not due to a lack of vitamins.

Infectious Coryza (Cold; Roup) (Fig. 174.) This is an infectious disease—the germ *Hemophilus gallinarum* is generally accepted as the cause of the "roup complex" (a combination of various symptoms). Since most "colds" are, to an extent at least, communicable

Handle as if contagious

it would not be incorrect on the foregoing basis to classify coryza as a contagious disease. From the standpoint of sanitation, the condition should be handled as if it is a truly contagious malady.

In this condition the eyelids may be glued together, there is a nasal discharge and this infection frequently involves the sinuses (head cavities) so that these become filled with a cheesy material and as a result the head in the vicinity of the eye becomes swollen; also as a sequence of these conditions there is mechanical obstruction to the passage of air so that the breathing is noisy. Affected birds usually weaken rapidly so that death takes place in a week or two.

In its clinical symptoms coryza resembles some other respiratory and nutritional diseases—laryngo-

A differential diagnosis important

tracheitis (page 637); infectious bronchitis (page 639); the mouth and throat form of fowl pox (page 644); Newcastle disease (page 655); A avitaminosis (pages 40 and 66); and others. Therefore, as some of the mentioned ailments are highly contagious a mistaken diagnosis could readily result disastrously to the flock. A veterinary diagnosis based on isolation of the specific germ is advised.

Prevention consists in destroying ailing birds—the value of the individual bird is so low that it is an

Destroy ailing fowl

error to jeopardize the health of the flock by maintaining in it a spreader of infection. If the fowl is an unusually valuable one it may be isolated—placed in quarantine (page 212), and treatment attempted by keeping the air passages cleared and by the use of sulfathiazole (page 281) in the mash.

In order to control the development of additional infection after the ailing ones have been removed, the drinking water of the healthy flock should be chlorinated (page 116), or permanganate of potash (page 116), or iodine (pages 117 and 276) added. Certainly running water, if it is available, is better to prevent the spread of contagious diseases than any medication of the water. Scalding drinking and feeding vessels once or twice daily is also an excellent practice.

Ulcerative Cloacitis: (Vent gleet). This is a condition characterized by an infection of the vent and cloaca (page 24). No specific germ has been isolated, and therefore it is usually ascribed to miscellaneous germs. By some it is listed as a venereal disease though there is no exact information on which to base this conclusion.

The vent and neighboring parts are irritated and inflamed and therefore there is straining Symptoms with the passage of small watery stools of "vent and mucus. Scabs and other forms of corgleet" ruptions soil the ailing area. The affected fowl as well as others in the flock peck at the sore vent so that ulceration sets in.

Prevention consists in isolating the affected fowl so that with appropriate handling including cleansing, mild disinfection, and the use of non-irritating dusting powders and ointments healing may be encouraged. Male birds should also be taken away from the flock so as to prevent the spread of the infectious material.

Fowl Plague: (Fowl pest; bird plague). This serious fowl disease affects chickens, turkeys and perhaps other barnyard fowl, though pigeons are generally considered to be resistant. It is due to a virus not present in the United States. It has however, at times gained a foot-hold, and only vigorous action by the U. S. Veterinary forces has on such occa-

Vigilance by sanitary authorities has kept this disease out of the United States

sions stamped it out in its incipiency. It it ever succeeds in firmly establishing itself the loss to the poultry industry could conceivably be proportionately as heavy as an outbreak of *foot-and-mouth disease* (page 605) would be to the cattle industry. Clinically the disease is easily confused with fowl typhoid (page 649); laryngotracheitis (page 637); and acute fowl cholera (page 647). Flocks in which the symptoms in general correspond to either or all of the diseases named, and when a clear-cut diagnosis cannot be established, should at once be placed in strictest quarantine. Notify the official Livestock Sanitary Authority at once.

One of the "Animal Defense" ailments

The disease is spread by direct contact and indirectly by feed bags, visitors, predatory animals, etc. The mortality rate is nearly 100 per cent. No vaccine that has been field tested is available, though as a last resort in widespread outbreaks the vaccination method of control may be tried. Usual control measures in isolated outbreaks is by quarantine, and by disinfection with a hot two per cent lye (page 253) solution or one of the approved cresylic acid (page 263) disinfectants. Fowl, from flocks in which the disease has appeared, that are still in apparent good health, may be used for human food since humans are not susceptible to this ailment.

Favus (page 661) (*White Comb*): This is caused by a mold that settles on the comb and wattles, and in severe cases may involve many parts of the body. The

A spreading disease

disease may spread rapidly to other members of the flock. Clinically it is characterized by the presence of white powdery material—sometimes also scabs—on the affected comb, wattles, and skin. On the latter the feathers become dry, brittle and break off or fall out leaving a depression in place of the feather.

Brushing affected parts to remove the powdery material and scabs and then painting the parts with tincture of iodine (page 276) will usually control the trouble in individual fowl. Affected birds should be kept isolated until the lesions are healed. If the disease persists in repeated outbreaks it becomes necessary to clean and disinfect poultry houses and runs (page 285).

Infectious Synovitis: This disease of poultry, very recently reported, seems to be due to a virus-like agent that produces erosions of joint surfaces. It appears to be spread by contact, after an incubation period of about 24 days. Chlortetracycline (aureomycin) in the feed in mixtures of one gram to the ton of feed for day old chicks for a period of 15 days, and up to as much as 1000 grams per ton for mature fowl, gave some encouraging results in the treatment.

Parasites and Disease

✄✄✄✄

PART NINE

SOME LARGER (MACROSCOPIC) ENDOPARASITES

Intensive animal husbandry necessitating confinement in crowded areas; repeated annual use of these areas, increased traffic in domesticated animals—often from widely separated regions, disturbance of normal relationships between intermediate and definitive hosts and parasites, and numerous other factors have resulted in widespread parasitism of all domesticated animals. Only a very few of the more important of these conditions may be presented in the following pages. Endoparasite: All of the parasites—down to and including "gizzard worms" are classed as endoparasitic as they live within the body of the host.

Liver rot; fasciolasis. This is a disease of sheep, cattle, particularly calves, and swine. It is uncommon

A livestock disease caused by a leaf-shaped parasite. It is found in swampy places

in horses and man. It occurs most frequently in low marshy areas along the Atlantic, Pacific and Gulf of Mexico coasts.

The disease is due to the common liver fluke, (*Fasciola hepatica*) a leaf shaped parasite approximately one inch long and somewhat less than one-half inch wide. The eggs of this parasite pass out of the body of the host, and after hatching enter the body of a snail where there is additional development. Emerging from the snail they get on blades of grass to be consumed by the final hosts to ultimately lodge in the liver, where they remain alive for from three to five years.

The symptoms do not usually manifest themselves until the fall of the year though infestation may have taken place several months earlier. Fre-

The parasite destroys the liver tissue, and unthriftiness ensues

quently during the earlier stages of infestation the host fattens, presumably because of stimulation of the liver by the parasite. Soon because of the destruction of liver tissue there is loss of flesh, the blood is altered, and its serum settles in the lower portions of the body so that there appear soft swellings under the jaw—the so-called "bottle jaw"—and along the belly. The symptoms mentioned are not sufficiently characteristic on which to base a diagnosis. Where the disease is suspected a post-mortem examination should be performed, and the bile ducts of the liver slit open. If present it is not usually difficult to detect the dark leaf-like slow moving fluke.

Prevention consists in keeping sheep and cattle away from low marshy places. Salt water marshes are

Prevention

not harbors of the liver fluke or its intermediate host the snail. The addition of one part of copper sulphate to approximately one million parts of swamp water is sufficient to destroy the snails in the water, and as the fluke cannot develop unless it is afforded the opportunity to pass a part of its existence in the snail this results in the death of the fluke. This amount should change the color of the water to a very light blue tint. Water so treated is not harmful to other animals or vegetation. Drainage of ponds, or fencing them off is helpful.

When larger areas are to be treated for snail destruction, use 33 pounds of powdered copper sulphate (page 275) dissolved completely in 400 gallons of water. A power spray maintaining 400 pounds nozzle pressure, with an agitator, should be used to spray the surface water and 10 feet of adjacent ditch banks. Unfortunately snail eggs are not affected so that a second spraying a month later is necessary.

If a diagnosis has been established, and if the infestation is not too severe, curative treatment may be attempted, under the guidance of the veterinarian, because all the drugs have harmful as well as beneficial qualities. Cattle have responded favorably to medication with a mixture of ten grams of hexachlorethane (C_2Cl_6, a colorless crystalline compound having a camphor-like odor) and 1.75 grams extract of kamala for each 70 pounds of live weight. For mature sheep dry pressed boluses (large pills) containing either 30 grams of pure hexachlorethane alone, or a mixture of 30 grams of pure hexachlorethane and 7.5 grams of bentonite (a hydrated aluminum silicate) gave good responses. However, it cannot be too strongly emphasized that prevention by keeping animals away from marshes, and destroying snails is the most important. When sheep and cattle reach the stage where treatment is necessary the liver fluke has already done immense tissue damage.

Tapeworm infestation (page 829). These parasites may occur in both herbivorous (vegetation eaters) and carnivorous (meat eaters) animals. Among the larger domesticated animals sheep are most frequently infested. In cattle and sheep it is usually the *Moniezia expansa* occurring in the small intestines, varying up to seven yards in length and about ½ inch wide. In sheep—sometimes in cattle— the "fringed tape worm" *Thysanosoma actinoides* is in the bile and pancreatic ducts, and in the small intestines. The segments are short and conspicuously fringed behind. During the month of August in some northern states there are

Prevention of tapeworm infestation in meat eaters is on a rational basis

occasionally heavy losses. Lambs infested with tape worms move short distances with short stiff steps, probably due to muscular fatigue, then collapse. Older sheep manifest a severe diarrhoea, loss of condition, weakness, and in instances high mortality.

All tapeworms regardless of the final host require an intermediate host for their development. For ex-

Intermediate hosts necessary for tape worm development

ample, in the case of herbivorous animals —cattle and sheep—there are certain grass mites; for fowl, ground beetles and flies are the intermediate hosts; and the dog and man acquire their tapeworm following the consumption of the "bladder" or cystic stage of the tapeworm in infested raw meat.

The adult tapeworm consists of a head, and body composed of several united flat segments so as to give a chain like appearance. The very minute eggs of the tapeworm pass out with the intestinal contents of the final host to be picked up by a suitable intermediate host—of a different species than the host of the adult

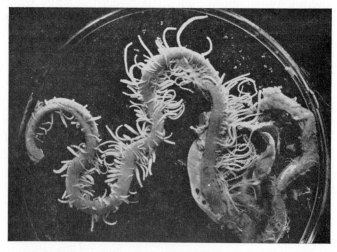

(Ackert, Zoology Department, Kansas Agricultural Experiment Station)
FIG. 175. Heavy tapeworm infestation of chicken.

tapeworm. In this intermediate host a larval stage occurs which is in the muscles. The larva consists of a tapeworm head and neck in a spherical or elliptical membranous bag of varying size filled with a clear fluid. This is the bladder-worm stage. The bladder-worm infested muscle is eaten by the final host to again develop in the intestines of the latter into the adult tapeworm.

In the case of cattle and sheep the best recommendation that can be made at this time is the avoidance of short pasture and thus control the ingestion of the intermediate grass mites. The prevention of the bladder-worm or larval stage of the tapeworm consists largely in keeping carnivorous animals— especially the dog—free from its adult tapeworm. In the dog prevention of infestation with its adult tapeworm consists in preventing this animal from eating uncooked meat, especially the offal and discarded parts of slaughtered animals, as well as carcasses of those that have died because of a disease.

Prevention of tape worm infestation

There are quite a good many remedies that are used to expel tapeworms from domesticated animals. They are not perfect in their action though in some species there is a degree of success—falling far short in others. The remedies vary for the different species and they are frequently dangerously poisonous for the host, so that the dosage must be carefully determined in order not to destroy the host as well as the parasite.

Lead arsenate of a commercial grade (98 per cent active ingredient) in a dose varying from one-half to one gram in weight, placed in a gelatin capsule, and administered by means of a balling gun to five months old lambs resulted in the removal of all the *Moniezia expansa;* however, there was a weight loss of from three to ten pounds per lamb. The smaller dose did not eliminate all the tapes—the larger did, and the latter occasioned the greater weight loss. The dose for calves is the same as for lambs, and for mature cattle it is doubled (2 grams).

In regard to the "fringed tapeworm" (*Thysanosoma actinoides*) those that are in the small intestine can be removed by the same agents as those effective in the infestation with *Moniezia expansa*, but this does not eliminate those lodged in the bile and pancreatic ducts. For the removal of these latter an involved chemical compound bis (5 chlor-2-hydroxyphenol) methane sold commercially as teniatol, teniathane, etc. has given encouraging results. For dogs a frequently used agent is arecoline hydrochloride administered hypodermically. Oleoresin of male fern, kamala, areca nut, and copper sulphate are some of the others.

Some very careful research workers in this field are exceedingly doubtful about the high efficacy of all of these remedies; their contention is—it appears well founded—the temporary starvation of the host, and also the mentioned remedies, will result in the expulsion of all of the tapeworm with the exception of the head or scolex, and that in a few days this will regenerate a whole new tapeworm. The failure of drugs in removing the head or scolex indicates the valuelessness of the remedy.

Tapeworms in fowl (*Raillietina cesticillus*): Several species of tapeworms are capable of infesting barnyard fowl. If present they are usually found in the first half of the intestinal tract. (Fig. 175.) Their size varies from those that are barely visible to the naked eye to those as much as ten inches in length.

The symptoms are most generally observed in young birds, but the symptoms are not characteristic.

A diagnosis based on the passage of segments
There is an appearance of unthriftiness. (Fig. 176.) The discharge of occasional tapeworm segments with the intestinal discharges is of value in establishing a diagnosis.

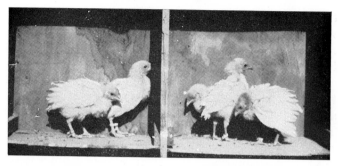

(Courtesy Department of Bacteriology, Kansas State University)

FIG. 176. Normal chicks on the left; tapeworm-infested chicks on the right.

Prevention is in a measure possible as the life history of most of the poultry tapeworms is well known.

Poultry acquire tapeworms by eating intermediate hosts such as flies, beetles, snails and others

In general the life history is similar to that of the tapeworm in other animals. The intermediate hosts consist of beetles —a single beetle after devouring a few tapeworm segments will develop several hundred larvae that are infective to fowl —house flies, stable flies, ants, snails, and others. The intermediate host consumes the tapeworm egg-infested droppings. The larval stage is in the intermediate hosts, and the latter are in turn consumed by the fowl so that the adult parasite develops in them.

Prevention of tapeworms in poultry, then, consists in frequently gathering up the droppings (pages 141 and 171) and disposing of them so that they will not be accessible to the intermediate hosts, and furthermore, in so far as practical, removing trash which frequently serves as hiding places for intermediate hosts. If food attracts flies it is best to offer it to fowl in such amounts so that it will be quickly eaten, after which hoppers are to be cleaned out. These methods though by no means perfect will hold tapeworm infestation in poultry to a minimum.

Curative treatment is very unsatisfactory because

the head of the tapeworm is so deeply embedded in the wall of the intestine. The contention of research workers is that starving chickens for 20 hours will cause them to lose all of the tapeworm segments (strobilae) except the head (scolex.) Due to the fact that most tapeworm remedies are recommended to be given after a preliminary starvation of the bird the remedy receives the credit while it is really the result of the starvation. Drugs used include kamala, turpentine and olive oil, arecoline hydrobromide, copper sulphate, and iodine preparations. Lead arsenate in a dose of 300 milligrams per fowl, after withholding feed for 18 hours before treatment and for four hours following treatment, will remove many tapes though toxic to some as evidenced by continued loss of weight. It is well to again explain that most of these drugs in order to destroy the parasite must be given in such large doses and in such concentration that they are frequently a source of danger to the host unless there has been careful discrimination in considering all the facttors involved. It is best to resort to curative treatment late in the fall months when insects have largely disappeared.

Ascarids (page 829) ; *Ascaris suis; round worms in pigs.* This parasite is extensively present wherever swine are raised. The loss occasioned by **This parasite is present wherever swine are raised** it is a relatively enormous one—at times it makes the raising of swine decidedly unprofitable. (Figs. 177 and 178.)

The mature worm is large, thick and round, of a yellowish or pinkish color. The male is from six to ten inches long, and the female may be up to twelve inches in length; they are about one-fourth inch in diameter.

The adult worms inhabit the small intestines of the hog. An enormous number of eggs are laid daily. These are passed out with the intestinal discharges of the host. These eggs are extremely resistant to the

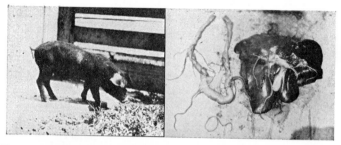

FIGS. 177 and 178. (Left) A hog infested with roundworms. (Right) Worms in a section of intestines and in the liver.

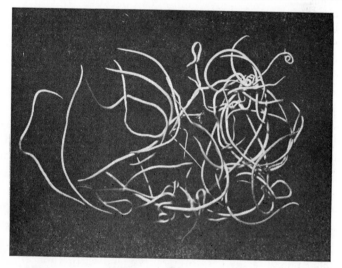

(Ackert, Dept. of Zoology, Kansas Agricultural Experiment Station)

FIG. 179. Large roundworms of the fowl; normal size.

usual destructive influences. In the egg a small larva develops which remains there until the egg is swallowed by a pig, then it emerges from its shell, bores through the wall of the intestine, and gets into the blood stream by means of which, after a brief sojourn in the liver, it is carried to the lungs. Here it escapes from the lungs into the wind-pipe, is coughed into the mouth to be swallowed so as to lodge in the intestines, where it develops into the sexually mature worm, thus completing its life cycle.

The symptoms are due to the mechanical damage inflicted by the parasite in its passage through the various tissues, and also by a poisoning process. The extent of the damage depends upon the numbers of parasites. Thus during its sojourn in the lungs there may simply be coughing, which the owner usually ascribes to dusty quarters, or there may be such inflammatory and destructive processes as to cause death of the host. The liver and kidneys may show extensive changes because of inroads made by larva. The adult worms in the intestines are harmful by their mechanical obstruction of the lumen of the intestines and bile duct; they often get into the latter. (Fig. 178.) Because of all these changes in various organs there are in infested swine varying degrees of unthriftiness. It is estimated that one-fourth of all the pigs farrowed die from the effects of these worms, and those that do not die are so unthrifty and so susceptible to bacteria infection that they are unprofitable.

When the parasite finally lodges in the intestines it has already inflicted much damage

Prevention consists in a swine raising practice known as the McLean County Sanitation System. It was first developed by veterinarians of U. S. Bureau of Animal Industry in McLean county, Illinois— hence the name. It consists in the following general steps: (1) Cleaning and scalding the farrowing houses with a strong lye solution using one pound of lye to thirty gallons of water. The lye dissolves the dirt, and the scalding hot water destroys the worm eggs. (2) Three or four days before farrowing, brush the sow as clean as possible to mechanically remove adherent worm eggs from her body and wash the udders with soap and warm water. Then place the sow in the cleaned farrowing house. (3) The sow and her pigs are kept in the farrowing pens for ten days. During this time the pens and houses are freed from intestinal discharges daily to

The McLean County system of prevention also controls other filth borne diseases of swine

minimize danger to the pigs through contact with the worm eggs discharged by the sow; however, there is no great danger of contamination from this source. (4) At the end of ten days the sow and her pigs are carted, not driven, as they would likely pick up worm eggs during this step to their permanent pasture. This latter must not have been used by other pigs within the last year. Until they are four months of age the pigs must have no contact with old hog lots or enclosures. Feed and water must be given them in the clean pasture. After they reach the age of four months there will be considerable resistance to round worm infestation, and at this time if it is found desirable to do so they may be returned to the old lots.

The McLean County Sanitation System not only controls round worm infestation in hogs, but many other forms of parasitism, as well as most filth borne diseases such as infectious enteritis, bull-nose and others. The "System" if carefully followed is one of the greatest benefits ever offered to the swine industry.

Effective worm treatment in swine is still in the research stage. In order to meet requirements, a rem-
Effective medication not always satisfactory edy should be (1) non-poisonous for the host; (2) easy to administer; (3) low cost; and (4) effective not only as a preventive but also as an expeller. In the case of *Ascaris suis* (round worms) the remedy should prevent the migration of the larvae through the liver and lungs—it is in this migration that the host's health suffers most.

Worm removal treatment consists in the use of such remedy as oil of chenopodium. More recently commercial phenothiazine (page 689) has been recommended as an unusually effective round worm remedy. Fluoride of soda (page 315), one part in 90 parts by weight of *dry* grain feed, fed for one day as the regular grain ration is also recommended. Fluoride of

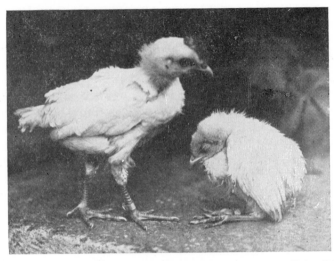

(Courtesy Department of Bacteriology, Kansas State University)

FIG. 180. Two chicks of the same age. The one on the left is normal; the one on the right is infested with roundworms.

soda (page 315) is a deadly poison and must be kept out of the reach of children and household pets and should be conspicuously labeled as "poison." It should not be given to pigs showing digestive disturbances, to sows in late pregnancy or to lactating sows. Under no circumstances may it be given in garbage, slops, milk, wet feed, in capsules, or as a drench. No form of curative treatment can equal the prevention of infestation. Where infestation is so bad that "curative" treatment must be resorted to, it indicates that most of the damage—by the passage of the larvae through the lungs and liver—has been already irreparably done.

One of the later remedies is *piperazine* (diethylene-diamine) marketed under the trade name of "Par-vex," (Upjohn). Fed at the rate of 0.26 gram per pound of body weight—in its administration it was mixed with one-fourth of the daily grain ration after 18 hours of fasting. Treatment was repeated 54 days later, and a third treatment was administered after a similar interval. After the second treatment the egg count was reduced to nearly zero, and remained thus for 21 days, indicating at least that this method of handling had effectively removed the adult *Ascaris suis* worms. It is not toxic in approved doses.

Hygromycin B (Lilly) is another of the agents under intense research at this time. It is an antibiotic which occurs in the fermentation products of a mold (Streptomyces hygroscopicus) found in the woods near Indianapolis, Indiana. In the feed it stimulates growth and reduces worm-egg production. It is quite effective in the removal of several of the intestinal parasites of swine such as whipworms, possibly red stomach worms, and to an extent the round-worms. Lung worms also were measurably reduced. There is a premix (Lilly) known as "hygromix." It has 12,000,000 units of hygromycin B in each five pounds of the "premix," and five pounds of the "premix" is added to each ton of basal ration. Largely as a preventive of infestation it was used in the ration of pigs for a period of two months. Another report indicates curative value in that a weak and emaciated pig, with no appetite, was given by way of the mouth 0.06 grams of hygromycin for six days. Shortly after diarrhoea ceased, appetite returned, and the pig started to gain weight. On autopsy the egg count was zero.

Unfortunately, in another research project a final report on five pigs on the level of the recommended dosage of hygromycin stated that it did not prevent the migratory phase of ascarids. This is the stage in which round worm larvae pass through the liver and lungs. Therefore, the greatest damage is done to the animal's tissues during this stage, and the animal's health may be permanently impaired.

The Thorn-Headed Worm: (*Macracanthorhynchus hirudinaceous; Echinorhynchus gigas*). This parasite of swine outwardly and in general resembles the "round worm" (page 670) in size and general appearance though they are not true "roundworms" since they have no intestine; in this respect they are like tapeworms. Their outstanding anatomical characteristic is that they have a spiny proboscis, or snout, by means of which they attach themselves firmly to the lining of the small intestine of the hog. Occasionally they migrate from place to place in the small intestine. As a result of this migration a small nodule or swelling remains as evidence of their former attachment.

Infected swine pass out the eggs with the intestinal evacuations; (Fig. 182) these in turn are swallowed by the larvae of June bugs which are also called May beetles, as well as comparable insects that serve as intermediate hosts. It is in their bodies that the eggs of the thorn-headed worm hatch, and in a very brief time the worm larvae penetrate the intestine of the larval beetle where they remain for approximately two weeks. They then migrate into the body cavity of the immature beetle, and as sausage-shaped affairs they are large enough to be visible to the naked eye. Finally after a period of 7-12 weeks they reach the infective stage that extends into the body of the adult beetle.

Life cycle of the thorn-headed worm

Swine rooting in manure or straw piles, or in low lying places find the beetle grubs, probably also the adult beetle, and consume them. The digestive juices of the hog liberate the small thorn-headed worm which migrates to the small intestine of its final host or hog where it attaches itself, grows, mates, and starts to lay eggs; thus, the cycle is completed.

Undoubtedly if present in sufficient numbers this parasite contributes to the general unthriftiness of the host, and there are recorded cases of intestinal perforations so that peritoneal infections and death from peritonitis could ensue. Intestinal injury produced in the hog does render the intestines unfit for use as sausage casings.

The usual worm remedies have no effect in the elimination of this parasite; it is too firmly attached.

In sections of the country in which it is most prevalent—the warmer climates, not the west coast—preventive measures consist of feeding swine and adequate protein ration because they root less on such a diet, ringing (page 394) and keeping the hogs away from places such as manure piles, decaying straw, vegetation accumulations, and low ground. June bug larvae abound in such environment.

Kidney Worm: (Stephanurus dentatus). This parasite appears to cause economic losses only in swine of the southern states. It discolors the kidney fat and even penetrates the kidney and injures muscles. This worm is mottled, thick—1/20 to 1/10 inch, and from one to two inches long. The eggs reach the urinary bladder of the host and are voided with the urine. Under proper temperature and moisture conditions the very minute macroscopic larvae emerge in a few days and after additional skin sheddings they are infective for any swine consuming them with the vegetation. Under conditions of warmth and moisture the larvae survive for several weeks. Direct sunlight, drying and freezing are unfavorable influences. There is evidence that the minute larvae under the influence of the warmth of the resting hog will penetrate the skin of the latter to reach kidney location. Regardless of their **Damage of the larvae of the kidney worm** mode of entry into the hog's body they get into the blood stream and pass through the various organs—liver and lungs in particular—damage all of these until they reach the kidney fat. They perforate the covering of the kidney so that their eggs may again be passed out with the urine. Those wandering worms that do not reach the urinary outlet lodge in muscle tissue and in other organs. Since these worms have no opportunity to reach the bladder, they cannot perpetuate their kind. The complete life cycle requires about six months.

A urinalysis usually discloses the presence of pus cells. Affected animals are unthrifty. Paralysis of the

Kidney worm symptoms

hind limbs is unusual and as it is observed in such a variety of swine diseases it is not at all characteristic. Internally the liver suffers considerable damage. Depending on the numbers of kidney worms that pass through it, it will show the tracks of the worms and more or less hardening. As a result many livers are rejected for human food purposes. Also, the loin muscles in the vicinity of the kidneys must frequently be trimmed out and thrown away; in fact, if there is much pus present the entire carcass is unfit for human food.

Prevention of kidney worms

There is no curative treatment for the elimination of the kidney worm. Prevention rests on destruction of the small larvae by direct sunlight, dryness and low temperatures, and in so far as it is possible keeping pigs away from the urine of sows and other older swine. To effect these conditions remove all litter and rubbish, drain low or swampy places, permit the sows to be with their nursing pigs only at the time of nursing by sending the sows to the pigs in high dry pig lots. The pigs are not to have access to the sow's feed lot. Wean the pigs as soon as possible so that they may be placed in a high dry pasture that has had no swine in it for at least a six months period.

Whipworms of Swine (Trichuris suis): This worm is about one and one-third to two inches long and located in the cecum and colon of swine. It is usually of minor importance. Treatment for removal is not effective and prevention rests on the McLean County System of Swine Sanitation (page 672). Also consult piperazine and hygromycin B (page 675).

Lungworms (Metastrongylus elongatus) (page 766). These are fine threadlike worms of a white or brownish color found in the air passages of the lungs in swine (other animals such as sheep and cattle also have lungworms. In cattle it is the *Dictyocaulus viva-*

parous, and in sheep the *Dictyocaulis filaria.*) The males are from one-half to one inch long, and the females from one to two inches.

The eggs of the lungworms are voided with the intestinal discharges of infested swine (Fig. 181). After hatching the larva is swallowed by an earthworm, where it undergoes partial development.

Lungworms of hogs are acquired following the eating of infested earthworms

The lungworm of sheep and cattle does not pass through an intermediate host such as the earthworm. Sheep and cattle get it from wet swampy pastures. Infestation of the pig results from the swallowing of the earthworm which it usually acquires during "rooting" in places where earthworms abound such as near manure piles, under trash and in most places. The evidence is that lungworm larvae have been found in the bodies of mature earthworms collected from a farm that had had no swine on it for at least four years, and that could not have become contaminated from neighboring hog lots. The lots had not been plowed during the four-year period. The lungworm larvae—after the earthworm has been ingested and the larvae thus released—penetrate the wall of the intestine, get into the lymph stream, are temporarily arrested in the mesenteric lymph glands, then pass on to the right side of the heart, and from here to the lungs, where they reach their full growth and maturity in about four to eight weeks after infestation has taken place.

Symptoms are not usually marked excepting when the infestation is severe in which instance coughing and even pneumonia may be observed. The symptoms mentioned differ in no respect from those produced by the larvae of the large roundworm of swine. (Page 670.)

Prevention of the infestation is not entirely satisfactory. It consists in keeping hogs away from those

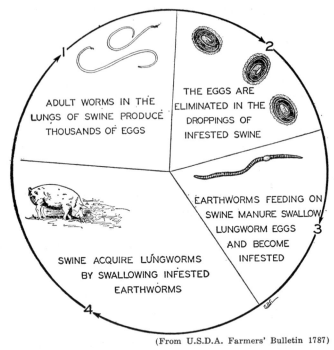

1   ADULT WORMS IN THE LUNGS OF SWINE PRODUCE THOUSANDS OF EGGS

2   THE EGGS ARE ELIMINATED IN THE DROPPINGS OF INFESTED SWINE

3   EARTHWORMS FEEDING ON SWINE MANURE SWALLOW LUNGWORM EGGS AND BECOME INFESTED

4   SWINE ACQUIRE LUNGWORMS BY SWALLOWING INFESTED EARTHWORMS

(From U.S.D.A. Farmers' Bulletin 1787)

FIG. 181. Illustrating the life cycle of the swine lung-worm.

Prevention not entirely satisfactory. In general it consists in keeping hogs from areas where earthworms abound

areas where earthworms are likely to abound. Removal of manure piles, trash, and low places—the earth beneath these is a favorite site for earthworms—is helpful. Feeding hogs on a balanced diet including tankage has a tendency to limit the animals' rooting proclivities to a minimum. If otherwise not controllable "ringing" the snout is effective to stop rooting. (Page 395.) The McLean County System of Swine Sanitation (page 672) is also recommended as a control measure. Furthermore frequent plowing of hog lots seems to reduce the numbers of earthworms and that is helpful. Cattle and sheep must be kept out of swampy infested pastures. Since older cattle and sheep are more resistant to lung worms, it is recomended that if it is not possible to keep all cattle and sheep out of infested pastures, by pasture rotation, only the older animals should be grazed in infested areas.

Curative treatment is not satisfactory as no drug is known that will reach the parasites in the lungs. Injections of medicines into the windpipe so as to establish a direct contact with the worms lodged there is an unsafe procedure, and is therefore not recommended. Good feed and care will permit the development of many mildly infested hogs so that they will be suitable for slaughter. The pork of these animals, if they are otherwise in good health, is perfectly fit for human consumption.

A drug that now has the approval of the U.S.D.A. for the treatment of lung-worm infested cattle is known scientifically as *cyanacethydrazide*. It has had extensive trials in both Great Britain and the United States and is commercially available to veterinarians in the United States under the trade name *dictycide*.

The trichina worm; Trichinella spiralis (page 829). This is one of the smallest round worms, the female being one-eighth to one-sixth inch long, and the male only half that size. It is rarely observed in tropical parts of the world. It is a parasite of meat eating animals, and it occurs naturally in polar bears and arctic foxes. It also occurs in man and pigs being of the most importance in these. It is much commoner in hogs fed on garbage than in those not receiving such material in the ration.

The adult male and female are in the intestinal tract of infested animals where mating occurs about a week after which the male dies. The females penetrate into the lining of the intestines, and produce their young or larvae in large numbers. The female lives for about twelve weeks.

The real damage is done by the larvae, which pass from the wall of the intestine into the lymph stream, then into the blood stream, and finally reach the muscle cells into which they pass. Here they grow until about 1/25 of an inch long. It then rolls into a characteristic spiral shape, and becomes surrounded by a capsule. In this environment it may live for years, or until the raw or insufficiently cooked muscle tissue is eaten by man or other species of meat eaters, usually the hog. It thus regains the intestines to start another life cycle.

The importance of trichina infestation in animals rests largely on the possibility that man will contract the condition if he consumes the raw or insufficiently heated pork. Pork products originating in a slaughter house or packing plant where federal meat inspection is maintained are so handled (page 245) that there is no danger from this source. This service is in all plants that are engaged in interstate or foreign traffic. When hogs, especially those that have been garbage fed are slaughtered on the farm or in the smaller packing houses without adequate meat inspection, and if such pork is eaten without thorough cooking, as sometimes happens with sausage, then there is the possibility of contracting the trichina infestation. Destruction (page 47) of trichina in pork may be effected by exposure to a temperature of $-18°$ C. for three days, or by a single rapid cooling to $-35°$ C. Research in 1954 indicated that exposure of pork to gamma radiation, using radioactive cobalt, sterilized contained trichinae so that their thousands of larvae could not spread through the bodies of those consuming the pork. If the radioactive cobalt could be made available cheaply enough from waste fission products of atomic piles gamma irradiation of pork products in abattoirs might become commercially practical.

The trichina worm is of importance because of the possibility of its transmission to man through the eating of insufficiently cooked pork

The symptoms in man vary depending upon the

number of parasites present. There is fever; digestive disturbance, swelling of infested muscles, with severe muscular pains including the breathing muscles. Death may result. The symptoms seldom set in until about ten to fourteen days following infestation. A specific skin test may be applied to aid in the diagnosis in man. This test is not practical in animals.

Prevention of the infestation in swine is important in order to remove a potential danger to man

Man must be certain that pork products are well cooked before eating

when he consumes the pork. Garbage fed hogs are most frequently infested. No practical method of controlling this phase of the trouble has been devised though cooking of the garbage is done in some countries and it is effective in reducing the infestation in swine and thus in man. Later statistics indicate that there has been a reduction of trichinosis in man as a result of the required cooking of garbage as swine food—this practice has been made compulsory in many states, primarily as a step in the control of vesicular exanthema of swine. Preventing swine from gaining access to raw pork offal is helpful as a method of prevention. Rats, frequently accused, are not important spreaders of this parasite, but from a sanitary standpoint they should be destroyed. Man should convince himself that the pork products he consumes have been well cooked.

Nodular Worm (Oesophagostoma columbianum) Disease of Sheep: This disease—also known as "pimply gut" or "knotty gut"—is so named because some of the little worms instead of escaping from the intestine become lodged in the walls of this organ producing small pea-sized swellings or nodules. Not infrequently the lining of the intestines is studded with hundreds of these nodules. Not only does this interfere with the nutrition of the animal, but it also ruins the gut for the future manufacture of that important human surgeon's suturing material know as "catgut" of which sheep intestine is the principle source. In 1947 at federally inspected slaughter houses, out of a total of 11,-165,026 sheep slaughtered, 6.36% of the carcasses were tanked and 710,358 casings were tanked because of nodular disease. Sheep get this parasite from eating contaminated vegetation, and in about 35 days the worm completes its cycle to lay more eggs which are passed out with the manure. Infested sheep fail to gain, and if badly affected they lose weight, the dung becomes soft or even changes to diarrhoea and straining, and the wool becomes dry, yellow and irregular.

There is no known remedy that will reach the encysted worms in the wall of the intestine, but phenothiazine (page 689) will remove the worms that are free in the intestine, and **A very serious worm disease of sheep** this will help that much, and is also effective against stomach worms and bankrupt worms (Haemonchus contortus). The dose is one ounce for mature sheep and one-half ounce for lambs. In northern climates the breeding stock should be treated for nodular worm infestation in the early winter after it is taken off pasture, and in the spring before being returned to the pasture. The lambs kept for breeding stock should be treated the following winter and spring. Phenothiazine (page 689) which is a water insoluble powder may be given in the required dosage mixed with some molasses and water by means of a syringe, or in capsules. In ground feed mixed with some molasses and water it is a satisfactory method of administration for ewes in advanced pregnancy.

In northern climates even moderate freezing will destroy the larvae or young worms. Therefore in the spring in these climates pastures are free from the parasite. This leaves old infested sheep as the sole source of contamination of the lambs. In general it is desirable to practice pasture rotation (page 220). During the period of rest the pasture may be used for other animals but not cattle and goats. Changing

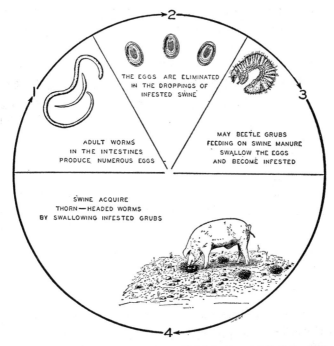

THE EGGS ARE ELIMINATED
IN THE DROPPINGS OF
INFESTED SWINE

ADULT WORMS
IN THE INTESTINES
PRODUCE NUMEROUS EGGS

MAY BEETLE GRUBS
FEEDING ON SWINE MANURE
SWALLOW THE EGGS
AND BECOME INFESTED

SWINE ACQUIRE
THORN—HEADED WORMS
BY SWALLOWING INFESTED GRUBS

(From U.S.D.A. Farmers' Bulletin 1787)

FIG. 182. Life cycle of thorn-headed worms of swine.

pasture every two months or oftener in the summer is best. Sheep pens should be cleaned before the lambing season.

Twisted stomach-worm of sheep; haemonchus contortus; bankrupt worms; twisted wire worms; "barbar" pole worms. This is a very common **A very common parasite of sheep** parasite of sheep. The male is from one half to almost one inch in length, and the female from three-fourths to one and one-fourth inches. They are a little thicker than an ordinary pin.

The eggs of these worms are passed out with the intestinal discharges of infested sheep. Depending upon warmth and moisture the eggs hatch in a few hours up to several days, or even weeks. The little larva is very resistant to most external influences, though direct sunlight seems to be destructive to them. This latter is usually protected against by seeking the shade of grasses. This small larva jells on grass and is thus swallowed by grazing sheep to lodge in the fourth stomach. A month later they are producing eggs to further contaminate pastures grazed by the sheep.

In the fourth stomach the worms attach themselves to the lining membrane. They frequently shift their position so that for each parasite there are usually several small wounds, each of which has been productive of some bleeding. The total loss of blood by the sheep is quite large.

Infested sheep have pale mucous membranes; sometimes there is a soft swelling under the jaws; the general appearance is that of unthrifti-

The effects of stomach-worm infestation ness; diarrhoea is frequently observed. On a post-mortem examination the muscles are pale, and the reddish parasite may be found either free in the stomach contents or attached to the lining membranes.

Prevention is not entirely satisfactory. In order to be effective it is necessary for young sheep to be kept away from vegetation that has been contaminated with the manure of older sheep, and in the warmer months of the year the animals must be changed to new pasture every two weeks. Pastures

Horses and swine may graze on sheep pastures remain contaminated for at least a year. This means that the pasture may be used for sheep, cattle or goats only two weeks out of the year, though horses and swine may be grazed there continuously. On most farms there is not enough land for such a program.

The next best plan is to provide separate pastures for the young and older animals; for the former

use upland pasture, with the lowlands for
Separate the older animals. In a measure the up-
pastures lands are washed free from parasites by
for dashing rains. Furthermore young sheep
young, and are more susceptible than the older ani-
old sheep mals. Also the parasites are more injurious to young growing animals. Frequent plowing is
helpful in the control of the degree of contamination
of a pasture. This entire sanitary method must in many
instances be supplemented by some form of elimina-
tive treatment. The copper sulphate treatment is the
one most generally used, and it is very efficient.

Copper sulphate, (page 275) for which the common
name is bluestone or blue vitriol is dissolved in water
as follows: Take one pound of finely powdered copper
sulphate and dissolve it in $9\frac{1}{2}$ gallons of warm water.
Use only clear blue crystals of the copper sulphate,
rejecting all white patches or crusts.

The dosage of the copper sulphate solution is as
follows:

Lambs 4 to 12 months old............2 to 4 ounces

Yearling sheep and above............3 to 5 ounces

Wormy sheep, during a period extending from the
first of May to the first of October, should be treated
once every month. During the cooler months of the
year, once every two or three months is sufficient.

In the use of the copper sulphate solution the animals should be deprived of feed for 12 to 20 hours
before they are dosed, and they should receive no water
on the day they are dosed, either before or after the
dosing.

An efficient method of administering the copper
sulphate solution consists in using an ordinary funnel
to which is attached a piece of rubber tubing three or
four feet long, and at the end of the rubber tubing
a piece of brass or iron tubing 4 to 6 inches long and
of proper diameter. The metal tube is placed in the

animal's mouth between the back teeth, and the animal is kept standing on all four feet, the head is very slightly elevated so that the solution will flow backward, and the dose of medicine is poured into the funnel. If at any time the animal appears to be strangled or coughs, the head should be lowered at once. A good rule to follow is to give the medicine slowly and never to elevate the sheep's nose higher than the level of its eyes at the time the medicine is given.

One part of phenothiazine (page 689) in twelve parts of coarse salt kept before lambs at all times, after first giving the copper sulfate treatment, or after a full dose of phenothiazine is a good treatment.

Ostertagia, Trichostrongylus, and *Nematodirus* of sheep are usually and in general spoken of as "stomach worms" or "intestinal worms." To the average untrained observer they bear a close resemblance to the true "stomach worm" (*Haemonchus contortus*). All of the foregoing named sheep worms or nematodes may be controlled by the use of phenothiazine (page 689). A mixture of one part of phenothiazine by weight and nine parts of salt is the proportion. If ewes get 1.5 grams of phenothiazine per day and the lambs one half of this amount, it will reduce worm numbers to a minimum in ewes, and will prevent clinical nematode (round worm) parasitism in the lambs.

A parasiticide for several sheep worms

This means that if the phenothiazine-salt treatment is offered throughout the year, and if at the time of shearing in the spring additional individual treatment is given, no extra handling of the sheep is necessary. For individual treatment lambs may be given one-half ounce, and mature sheep one ounce of phenothiazine. If in addition, sanitation and pasture rotation (page 220) are practiced, the seriousness of the parasite problem in sheep can be controlled. Sometimes lambs do not consume enough of the phenothiazine-salt mixture for maximum results; therefore, if any lambs show clinical evidence such as unthriftiness, diarrhoea, pale mucous membranes, or pouching (edema) under the jaw, they should be subjected to individual treatment.

Phenothiazine a complex chemical compound was presented to the American livestock industry in 1938 by the scientists of the Bureau of Animal Industry of the United States Department of Agriculture. It is said to be the "nearest ideal" worm medicine ever developed. In sheep and goats it is effective against stomach worms in general including bankrupt or twisted stomach worms, nodular worms that are in the lumen of the intestines—not encysted; the dose is ½ ounce for lambs and one ounce for adults.

Phenothiazine and its properties

In cattle it is effective for the control of nodular worms, stomach worms, hookworms, whipworms, and several roundworms known as Cooperia. One part in ten parts of salt may be kept before cattle. Individually mature cattle may be given at the rate of 2/3 ounce for each 100 pounds of live weight but not more than two ounces in a single dose; calves may be given from ⅔ ounce up to 1⅓ ounces. It may be given to cattle in dry feed or ensilage, as a drench, or in bolus or pellet form.

For hogs it is given for the removal of ascarids (page 670) and nodular worms; one-fourth pound of phenothiazine in the feed for thirty-five 30-pound pigs, for twenty-five 40-pounds pigs, for twenty 50-pound pigs, or for ten 100-pound shoats. Avoid overdosing of pigs as those under three months of age may have an undesirable reaction which normally wears off in a day or two.

For the control of cecal worms (page 695) in poultry the dose is one pound for 500 to 1000 fowl in a dry mash. The smaller dose is for the light weight fowl; the heavier breeds get the larger dose.

Individual treatment of horses infested with strongyles (palisade worms) should be left entirely in the hands of the veterinarian; in fact, before any treatment is attempted in any of the domesticated animals the veterinarian must necessarily be consulted in order to establish a correct diagnosis. This drug possesses no favorable anthelmintic action, for use in cats, dogs, and foxes.

Phenothiazine in sufficiently large doses frequently colors the urine red, especially in sheep; while this condition is without significance it will stain the wool of sheep in bedded stalls or corrals. Phenothiazine is a pale greenish yellow to dark greenish gray powder, granules or flakes. It is tasteless and has a slight characteristic odor. Exposed to air it darkens and this is best prevented by covering and storing in light-impermeable containers. It is insoluble in water but by means of wetting agents or molasses it may be held in temporary suspension in watery fluids (shake before using) or in more permanent suspension in emulsions.

Ascarids; round worms (page 829) *of poultry.* This worm *(Ascaridia galli)* in chickens is from one and one-half to four inches in length. (Fig. 179.) Its life history (Fig. 183) is in general the same as that of the round worm infesting swine.

Symptoms are much more commonly observed in young birds, because it is believed that as the birds age there are developed in them "growth inhibiting factors which react against the development of the worms." The usually observed symptoms are not at all characteristic as they are simply those of unthriftiness, its degree depending upon the extent of the infestation. (Fig. 180.) In the younger birds there is retarded growth, and in older ones reduced egg production.

Round worms of poultry are commonest in the younger members of a flock

Prevention is by far the most important method of handling the situation. In view of the fact that the

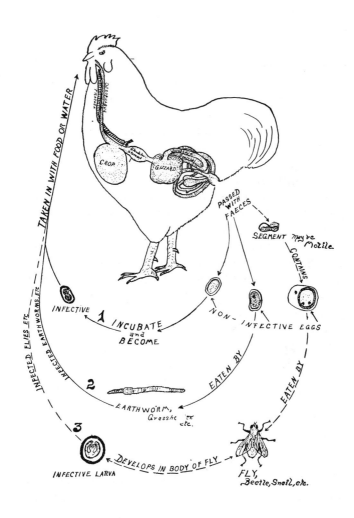

1 and 2 Roundworms

3 Tapeworms

(From Bulletin No. 473, Missouri Agricultural Experiment Station)

FIG. 183. A complex cycle of the poultry roundworm. Some poultry roundworms require no intermediate host.

A method of prevention eggs are in the droppings of infested birds, and that the eggs undergo their early embryonation best in moist surroundings—the dryness of the "deep or built-up litter" (page 170) is a factor in controlling embryonation— as well as the greater susceptibility of young birds, indicates the lines of preventive attack. Undrained and moist areas should be eliminated. In poultry yards and runs where many birds are confined the droppings and litter should be removed and burned frequently; the interval in this connection should not be longer than ten days. Young birds until they are at least four months of age should be reared away from the older birds. It is of especial importance that feed hoppers, and drinking troughs be kept free from droppings. This may be accomplished by elevating them, and surrounding them with wire netting platforms. (Figs. 159 and 160.)

Treatment rests on a large number of recommended remedies some of which are quite efficient though dangerous while others are less effective and less dangerous. In the former group there is included carbon tetrachloride capsules in doses of one dram for each two pounds of weight. There may be some deaths from this dosage, and egg laying is reduced for about ten days. In the less dangerous group of remedies, and when mass treatment is to be applied, tobacco dust has been used. It should contain not less than one and one-half per cent of nicotine. It may be added to the dry mash at the rate of two per cent by weight, and the feeding of the mixture continued for three to four weeks. The droppings and litter must be removed frequently to prevent reinfestation.

Phenothiazine (page 689), for the flock treatment of 1000 fowl, at the rate of one pound of the drug to 60 pounds of mash, the latter moistened to form a crumbly mass, is effective and safe.

Fowl gapeworm; Syngamous trachea.

Gapeworms of fowl lodge in the windpipe This is a small round worm producing the condition known as "gapes." The female worm from one-fourth to three-fourths inches in length is attached to the lining membrane of the windpipe, and the male one-eighth to one-fourth inch long is permanently attached to the female, so that the pair have a forked appearance. The parasite occurs in chickens and turkeys, and many wild birds so that its control is extremely difficult.

The usual life history begins with the rupture of the body of the adult female so as to liberate the contained eggs—she cannot pass them in the usual manner as the attached male permanently closes the genital opening. The eggs reach the outside and are picked up by other birds. The young worms soon migrate from the digestive tract to the windpipe. It has been demonstrated that the parasite may in some instances live for a time in the body of the earthworm, and by eating the latter fowl become infested. Apparently the role of the earthworm is to serve as a means of protection during periods that would be extremely rigorous for an unprotected gapeworm.

The symptoms produced in infested fowl depend in a measure upon the number of parasites that are in the windpipe. The gapeworm is a blood sucker, and if enough are present the total volume of blood withdrawn from the bird is sufficient to cause weakness and even death. Sneezing or gaping is always observed in the bird's attempt to dislodge the parasite.

Sanitary preventive measures consist in frequent rotation of runs with their occasional plowing under, daily change of litter—except in the built-up litter (page 170), and clean feeding and watering. The foregoing method of handling will materially reduce losses in the more or less closely confined flocks; range flocks are never seriously bothered by the parasite. In fact modern incubation and sanitary feeding methods have to a great extent eliminated this parasite.

A form of home treatment that is laborious and not very efficient is frequently applied to individual birds. It consists in stripping a feather of all its web excepting only a small tuft on the end. The latter is moistened with kerosene, introduced into the windpipe, rotated on its long axis so as to cause the parasite to become detached, after which it is coughed up.

"Barium antimonyl tartrate when inhaled by affected birds is an effective drug for the treatment of gapeworm infestations in young chickens and turkey poults. For treatment the birds are placed in a closed container or a tight box and exposed to the chemical from 15 to 20 minutes. One ounce of the finely powdered dust is sufficient for a box having a capacity of 8 cubic feet, and this will accommodate 50 chicks or 30 turkey poults. The box should be deep enough to permit the birds to stand erect, and just enough birds should be placed inside the box to fill it about two thirds full. The dust is introduced by means of a dust gun through a hole or an opening in one side of the box. At the start, one third of the total dust is blown into the box and the latter is then tilted slowly and repeated until the birds slide from one side to the other, the purpose of this being to disperse any powder that may have settled on the birds or on the floor of the box, and it causes the birds to breathe more deeply so as to cause the drug to reach the lower portion of the trachea. Five minutes after the introduction of the first third of the powder, the second third is introduced and the tilting repeated. The remaining powder is introduced ten minutes after the beginning of the treament and the box is again tilted. The birds are released five minutes after the last of the powder has been introduced, and treatment should not be continued beyond the twenty-minute period, as the birds may become overheated or suffocated. As a result of critical tests involving 1126 chicks and 236 turkey poults, the efficiency of the drug was demonstrated to be 92% for chicks and 96% for turkey poults."

A home treatment   A stock mixture consisting of garlic oil 33 parts and cottonseed oil 67 parts is used; each infested fowl is given 3 drops.

The cecal worm is important because it transmits the cause of blackhead in turkeys   *Cecal Worms; Heterakis gallinae.* This parasite is an inhabitant of those portions of the intestinal tract, known as the ceca (page 24). Chickens, and turkeys as well as other kinds of birds may be infested. The greatest importance of this parasite lies in the fact that it harbors and transmits the protozoa responsible for blackhead of turkeys (page 739). Independently of this the small parasite—it is one-third to one-half inch in length—may, in young birds particularly, be present in such large numbers as to cause severe inflammation of the ceca, which is reflected in the unthrifty condition, and even in death of young birds.

The life history of the parasite is virtually identical to that of the ascarids or roundworms of poultry (Fig. 183), and therefore its prevention is along similar methods (page 690).

Treatment of birds known to be infested may be by means of tobacco dust as described for roundworms of poultry (page 690). Another form of treatment consists in rectal injections of *one-third fluid ounce* of a mixture of one dram of oil of chenopodium (page 673) and six fluid ounces of cottonseed oil. The recommended dosage is sufficient for a bird weighing one and one-half pounds; is should be doubled for birds weighing three pounds or more. The injection is made by means of a blunt nosed hard rubber syringe. Phenothiazine (page 689) is also recommended.

The Gizzard Worm; Cheilospirura hamulosa in chickens and turkeys, and the *Amidostomum* in ducks and geese, and some other forms in other birds. Such worms are small roundworms that bury themselves under the horny membrane lining the gizzard. They are from one-fourth to three-fourths inch in length,

A worm under the gizzard lining

varying in color from white to deep red. On the outside of the gizzard the worm evidences its presence by little nodules or elevations which when opened disclose the parasite. The eggs of the parasite are passed with the droppings, eaten by grasshoppers, and go on to fowl. *Amidostomum* requires no intermediate host as ducks and geese ingest the eggs containing matured embryos.

Prevention is not too satisfactory. Having birds on ranges comparatively free from grasshoppers is a theoretical principle hard to apply. For smaller yards frequent removal of droppings is suggested. For ducks and geese the problem is still more complicated because of their aquatic habits.

The continuous feeding of tobacco dust at the rate of 1.0 per cent of the mash has been suggested. Also carbon tetrachloride and tetrachlorethylene (carbon dichloride) in doses of from 1.5 to 2.0 cc. for adult birds have been recommended.

CHAPTER XXXI

ECTOPARASITES, AND THEIR ROLE

The history of animal life indicates a continuous battle for supremacy between man and other species,

The
battle for
supremacy
between
man and
insects

in which the victory has rested usually with man because of his superior intelligence. Insects and parasites, however, have resisted to the point where eminent authorities are inclined to the belief that the outcome is still in the balance. In some parts of the world the lower forms of life as represented by insects, ticks and others still rule supreme, as witnessed by the fact that man dares not at the risk of his life trespass into some of the swamps, jungles, and lowlands. In Exodus 8:24, it is recorded, "and there came a grievous swarm of flies into the house of Pharaoh, and into his servants' houses, and into all the land of Egypt; the land was corrupted by reason of the swarm of flies," indicating that ancients as well as moderns, were subjected to insect visitations. The word "ectoparasite"—literally a parasite living on the outside of the body—is used in this paragraph in a very general and broad sense.

The House Fly. (*Musca domestica L.*) (Page 291.) The ordinary house-fly deposits its eggs mostly in

The
housefly
is a filthy
transmitter
of disease

moist barnyard manure, especially that derived from the horse and to a less extent in that of other species of animals including man. Other development places are in moist grain under feed bins, in garbage, in rejected ensilage, and in lawn grass clippings. The larvae are also found in moist earth under manure piles. Pasture and feed-lot deposited manures are favorable for growth of the larvae so long as they are not dried out. Whenever there is an abundance of houseflies in the vicinity of a dwelling, it is evidence that a fly-breeding place is probably within 300 yards, though flies have been found as far as 17,000 yards from their hatching place. The white eggs—in groups—hatch in one day to grayish maggots which feed for ten days, and then change to form the brown seed-like pupae. This is the third stage in the development of an insect, from which the adult fly emerges in three to six days.

Houseflies are non-biting. The average duration of life of the housefly is in the neighborhood of thirty days, with a maximum life span of sixty days. Flies eat animal excrement, garbage, and decomposing material, as well as the daintier foods of man. Their legs are hairy, and all manner of filth adheres to them, to be later tracked over animal feeds, as well as over the food of man. Further, they also contaminate with their excrement and vomit all substances with which they come in contact. They actually serve as bearers of the germs of typhoid fever, dysentery, tuberculosis, anthrax, and cholera, as well as carrying in their digestive tracts the eggs of certain worms, such as fowl tapeworm (page 668) and others.

The biting barnyard flies are the stablefly (Stomoxys calcitrans L.), the hornfly (Haematobia irratans L.), and the horseflies (Tabanidae).

The stablefly. (Page 291). Closely related to and resembling the housefly though somewhat larger, has a pointed beak, a grayish abdomen with four paired circular dots on the upper side. Its eggs are developed in wet straw, strawy manure and in soggy waste feed under feed racks in about the same time period as the housefly. There may be from five to ten generations a year. Areas of attack favored are the back, sides, legs and shoulders of animals. It sucks blood from animals and in this way decreases milk and meat production. It

A biting blood sucker

feeds on cattle out of doors though some **Stable fly** follow the cattle inside buildings. Probably **a blood** 80 per cent remain outdoors on the sides of **sucker** buildings, board fences, trees, etc. while the cattle are inside. In other words it stays on the cattle only long enough to get a meal of blood. The stable fly is known to be a mechanical spreader of the virus of infantile paralysis, and in the Far East of transferring a disease-producing protozoa of horses.

For the control of the stable flies the win- **Methods** ter accumulation of animal droppings **of control** should be hauled out early in the spring to be spread on cultivated ground. Spread wet or moist straw from feed racks every two weeks. All sources of wet straw are breeding places. Treatment of manure piles with D.D.T. is not satisfactory (page 169). Sanitation, and the use of residual insecticides to the premises are important. Lindane (page 303) is an approved disinfestant that has a wide use, though not on dairy cows. Pyrethrum (page 309) when activated with piperonyl butoxide, (page 310) has been recommended. Methoxychlor is a considered agent. (page 304). Malathion (page 305) has now been approved by the U. S. Food and Drug Administration to be sprayed or dusted directly on *beef* cattle, hogs, and poultry. As yet it may not be used directly on dairy cattle. Its use as a spray on or in buildings has had approval for some time. It is lethal to flies that are resistant to D.D.T. and other chlorinated hydrocarbons.

The *hornfly* (page 291) is the smallest blood sucking fly that pesters cattle during the hot days of summer. It is half as large as the housefly. **Another** It feeds on cattle with its head down, prin- **blood** cipally on their backs and shoulders. It **sucker** spends its life on the animal so its control is easier. Its eggs develop on and under fresh cow droppings so that the adult fly emerges in five days or more.

To control hornflies fresh cow droppings should

be hauled out of barn yards two or three times a week, or their drying out should be hastened by dragging a sled, brush, or rake over them. Hogs following cattle tend to reduce the breeding of the hornfly. Sanitation is the most important part of fly control. Methoxychlor sprays are effective (page 304) as well as "stable fly" agents (page 698). D.D.T. in a strength of eight pounds of the 50 per cent wettable powder in 100 gallons of water sprayed four times at monthly intervals during the summer caused the sprayed steers to make gains of 18 pounds per head over unsprayed animals. Malathion (page 305) sprayed on beef cattle is approved. Dusting with 50% methoxychlor or toxaphene at the rate of one tablespoon at three week intervals, but not within four weeks of slaughter is effective.

Horseflies, gadflies or greenheads are from two to ten times the size of houseflies. They annoy livestock
A large biting fly near streams and swampy places. Their eggs are laid in masses on plants in or near streams and persist as larvae during the cold months of the year to emerge from dry soil during the summer. There is only one generation each year.

Since the horsefly breeds in swamps and low wet places its control depends on good land drainage. If
Horse-fly control there is no need of protecting aquatic life, spread over stagnant pools a film of kerosene which destroys many female flies.

These flies also pester cattle. The pyrethrum-piperonyl butoxide spray gives some protection for a few days (page 310). Methoxychlor (page 304) will kill many of the feeding flies, as will also malathion (page 305).

The blood sucking flies torment farm animals so that they do not gain weight as readily and there is
Losses due to biting flies reduced milk flow. There is also a loss of blood that probably is not particularly serious to a vigorous well fed animal but it is harmful to the anemic, ill, under-

nourished individual. Biting flies are potential disease spreaders—anaplasmosis (page 744) is an example.

So generally are their harmful attributes understood that man keeps them out of his dwelling places by the use of screens, and traps and destroys them in various ways (page 290); their control, however, rests in the destruction of their breeding places. The proper construction of barn floors (page 125) and the sanitary handling of manures (page 163) are very important steps in fly control. If school children can be enlisted in programs of fly control, they are an important aid.

Baits do not attract blood sucking flies to any extent and therefore the flies that are caught by baiting traps with milk, diluted molasses and other such materials are houseflies and blowflies (page 702). For the blood sucking flies the so-called Hodge window trap—described in detail and illustrated in U.S.D.A. Farmers Bulletin No. 1097—gives excellent results.

Sticky flypaper can be made by heating in a double boiler one pound of rosin and eight ounces of castor oil and while hot smeared on strips of heavy paper with a paint brush. When hung on wires stretched across the inside of the barn it will catch many flies (page 290).

Electric screens and doors electrocute all insects touching the screen. They operate on low voltage, and the amount of current used by them is negligible.

Other means of protecting animals from flies are fly nets or covers, and even old trousers put on the animals' legs. At times animals will stand partly submerged in available ponds or other bodies of water for the relief afforded from the attacks of these pests.

Sprays vaporized inside a building—such as pyrethrum (page 309) have a definite value. Methoxychlor, lindane, chlordane, benzene hexachloride, etc., are of some value (pages 297 to 304).

Repellents applied to animals afford some temporary relief though not to the extent with which they are frequently credited.

The Tsetse Fly. Another member of the fly family that is a serious menace to human and animal health

The Tsetse fly not an American problem

is the Tsetse fly, whose habitat is restricted to the so-called "fly-belts" of Africa. It is both a mechanical and biological bearer of the protozoa that causes sleeping sickness in man (this disease has been estimated to be responsible for the death of one-half million humans over a period of a decade), and nagana in horses and other domesticated animals. Its control is going to be an exceedingly difficult matter, as this fly develops along river banks, but not in animal or human refuse. Bush clearance, and human settlement are helpful. Benzene hexachloride and D.D.T. are used. It is not an American problem.

Flesh flies; blowflies. The adults, and the larvae are spoken of as wool-maggots *(Lucilia cuprina),* in Australia it is the *Lucilia sericata,* and erroneously as screwworms and foot-maggots. The mature flies almost always deposit their eggs in a haphazard manner on dead animals or diseased tissues, and less frequently on decaying vegetation, and occasionally in the nose of

Blowflies usually deposit their eggs on dead animal tissue

man. The larvae usually reach full growth in three days. They are very destructive to the tissues, sometimes causing severe bleeding. When animals are infested, a veterinarian should be consulted at once to apply specific treatment. The development of the fleshflies may be largely prevented by promptly destroying all dead animals by burning or deep burial and closely watching all wounds with the destruction of the larvae as rapidly as they develop by means of benzene (not benzine) (page 317) or by the application of repellents to try to prevent the fly from depositing its eggs—oil of tar—from pine trees is used.

The true screwworm fly (Cochliomyia americana or *Callitroga hominovorax)* lays its eggs in shingle-like cemented masses on wounds of warm-blooded ani-

mals. Blowflies or fleshflies (see preceding paragraph)
eggs are placed in a haphazard fashion and are not
cemented together. True screwworms cannot get

**True
screwworms
eat deeply
into the
tissues of
the host,
and may
cause his
death**
through unbroken skin and they are not
found in cold-blooded animals such as
turtles, snakes and lizards. The front end
of the screwworm is imbedded and attached by means of two horn-like mouth
parts in the living flesh, while blow-fly
maggots are not attached and if they are
simultaneously present they will be observed crawling about on the surface of wounds. True
screwworms, uncontrolled, will eat so deeply into the
living tissues as to cause the host's death. The screwworms finally drop from a wound, burrow into the
ground and in seven to fourteen days emerge as the
adult fly, and ten days later these are ready to lay
eggs. Applying pine-tar oil to recent wounds and navels
to repel the fly, benzene (not benzine)—it is also
widely, though incorrectly, known as benzol—to infested wounds (page 317), also Formula or Smear No.
62 (page 317), or "Smear EI-335," (page 303) and the
prevention of injuries are the important control steps.

The screwworm fly is not very prevalent on open
wind-swept plains and high mountains. Sparsely settled
grazing land covered with a heavy growth of low brush
and timber favor its rapid increase. The flies cannot
survive if the average temperature is 50°F. or lower
for a continuous period of three months. Destroying
dense brush is a preventive factor. Hydrocarbon insecticides are of some help (pages 291 to 306).

On the island Curacao, in the Caribbean region, a
method of eradication practiced for sometime has been

**A unique
though
biological
method of
control**
entirely successful. The same plan has
now been instituted in the United States.
Screwworms survive during the cold season, especially in Florida. As warmer
weather sets in they migrate to other
southern states, and to an extent into

northern states. It has been definitely established, that during the mating season, *the female accepts the male only once.* *Also males are sexually sterilized by exposure, during their pupal or resting stage,* to radiation from cobalt-60, a radioactive material. Millions of these sterilized males are raised in laboratories, and released so that the sterilized males very greatly exceed or outnumber the wild nonsterilized male flies. This means that most of the females will be mated to the sterilized males, and when the females' eggs are laid they do not hatch since a potent male fertilizing element is lacking. A small percentage of the females will of course have mated with the nonsterilized wild males, but the proportion of these is so relatively small that if the program is persisted in for several years the total number of screwworms will be greatly reduced— at least that has been the experience on the island of Curacao.

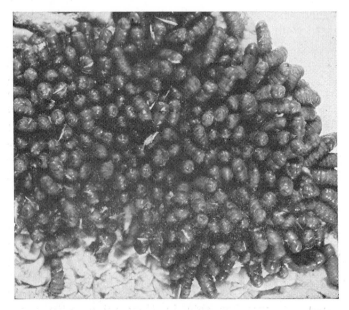

FIG. 184. Inside of a horse's stomach showing bots attached to the lining.

In areas where the above described plan is operative, the following requests are made to livestock owners:

1. Check the livestock carefully and often, and treat infested animals with one of the approved smears (pages 303 and 317).

2. Promptly report all suspected cases to the veterinarian, County Agricultural Agent, or the local screwworm inspector.

3. Cooperate in the effort by not moving screwworm infested stock.
   (The publication known as "Program Aid No. 367," U. S. Dept. of Agriculture, discusses the plan in detail.)

The horse Botfly (Gastrophilus intestinales or G. equi) is responsible for the development of stomach bots in horses. The life history, stated **The stomach** briefly, is that the eggs are deposited by **bot of horses** the mature fly on the hairs of the fore- **is responsible** legs, head and other parts of the body. **for large** Usually the horse nibbles (page 290) at **annual losses** these eggs so that as a result of friction **because it is** and moisture they hatch, thus getting into **responsible** **for loss of** the animal's mouth, and pass on to the **vigor in** stomach where they remain attached to its **the host** lining during the fall, winter and early spring months, (Fig. 184) when they loosen their hold to pass out with the intestinal contents, and then burrow into the ground from which they emerge as the mature fly after a period of from three to five weeks.

The bot is not known to be a bearer of disease to the horse, but it is frequently very injurious to its host because it may partially block the digestive tract, it draws its nourishment from the tissues of the host as well as from the contents of the stomach, and it is an irritant to the stomach. Horses badly infested are frequently at the beginning of the work season in the spring so weakened by this parasite that they are not in fit condition for labor. It is therefore important to prevent infestation by destroying the eggs on the hairs a least once every two weeks by touching them lightly with kerosene or gasoline, or by removing them with a razor blade or clippers.

For horses that are already infested, there are now many communities in the United States with veterinary-sponsored bot eradication programs.

When to medicate horses for the control of stomach bots

The best time to kill the bots is when they are in the horse's stomach and when the mature fly has been killed by frost so that no more eggs will be deposited. The time to begin handling, therefore, is about one month after the first killing frost and from that time on until about the latest killing frost. Within the limits set in the preceding sentence it is best to start treatment as early as possible in order to free the horse of a parasite that is injurious to it; however, if done too early in the season, the eggs that are on the legs and other parts of the body must at the same time be completely removed. The remedy is carbon bisulphide (page 306), but as this is a poisonous agent of a highly volatile character, and there is in its administration potential danger to the life of the horse, its application should be entrusted to no one other than the qualified graduate veterinarian.

The Warble fly; Hypoderma lineatum; the ox warble; grubs in the backs; the heel fly. (Consult "Derris Root," page 311.) This is a common pest throughout the United States, and is responsible for the warble or grub under the skin in the region of the back of cattle.

Grubs in the backs of cattle constitute a serious condition

In general appearance and size, the adult fly, like several other botflies, resembles the common honey bee. (Fig. 185). It is about one-half of an inch long, black in color, covered with yellowish-white and reddish-brown and black hairs.

In the spring, from the latter part of March to the middle of May, the flies appear about cattle, laying their eggs on the hairs of the legs, especially in the region just above the hoof. The eggs are yellowish-white, and are securely attached in rows of five or six on a single hair (Fig. 186). The animal usually licks the part of the body upon which the eggs are laid, and the saliva or moisture from the tongue softens the shell so that the larva or grub within may hatch or escape from the egg.

It has been proven that the larvae or tiny grubs enter the skin where the eggs are laid on the legs, and that they journey under the skin, usually in the subcutaneous tissue, to the esophagus or gullet, and a little later they journey from there through the flesh to their objective place beneath the skin all along the back. (Fig. 187.) This journey through the flesh takes place during the summer and fall months. In the middle west the small swellings appear along the back about the latter part of December. Very soon a small opening is made by the grub in the middle of the elevated area, through which the grub receives air. The tumor increases to the size of a small walnut, the holes become larger, and the grub becomes a thick, heavy-set, spinny maggot, brown or dark in color and about one inch in length. In the spring it works its way out through the hole, falls to the ground, burrows in the loose soil, and within a few days passes into the pupal stage. From the pupa the winged insect, or fly, emerges in from five to six weeks.

The life history of the parasite

The great economic losses caused by the ox warble must be considered from several points. The following are some of them. That produced to the hide which becomes full of holes where the grubs have emerged. (Fig. 56.) This annual loss is estimated at from

Economic loss is great

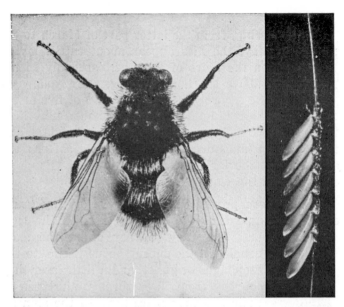

FIGS. 185 and 186. Adult female heel fly (left) enlarged about four times; (right) her eggs—enlarged ten times. The female fly dies soon after depositing the eggs on the hairs of the limbs of cattle. Eggs of the Northern species (bovis) are deposited singly. The ox warble or cattle grub is an intermediate stage.

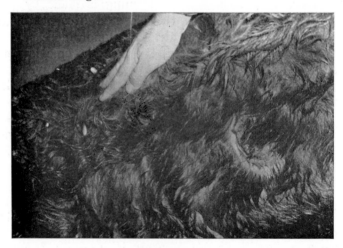

FIG. 187. Pressing ox warbles out of the subcutaneous tissue of a steer.

fifty to sixty million dollars. The heavy loss caused by
the reduction in milk secretion, which is estimated at
from 10 to 20 per cent of the normal yield. The loss of
flesh, due to the wild endeavor of the animal to escape
from the flies and the irritating larvae. The deprecia-
tion of the value of the carcass as flesh, (Fig. 188)
which becomes greenish and jelly-like in appearance at

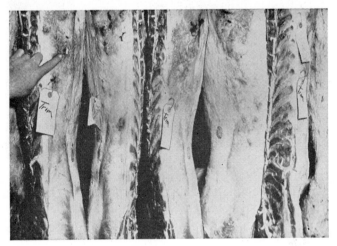

(Courtesy Oklahoma Department of Agriculture)

FIG. 188. Trimming meat because of ox warble or cattle grub
injury.

the points where the grubs are located and is really unfit for consumption.

The control of warble infestation rests very largely
in the destruction of the grubs before they drop to
the ground in the spring months. If all
Prevention   stockmen were to cooperate and practice
this method the succeeding year, the prospective crop
of flies would not make its appearance. (See pages 311-
312.)

During the latter part of January and all through
February, a better method is to remove the grubs
bodily, which can be done by squeezing them out, because the grubs are about ready to leave the tumors.
After removing them they should be destroyed. If they

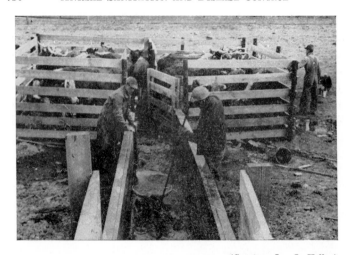

(Courtesy Ira J. Hollar)

FIG. 189. Dipping in rotenone solution to control cattle grubs.

are simply thrown to the ground or floor, they will go ahead and complete their life cycle. (For handling with derris and rotenone see page 311.)

Within the latest years—since about 1956—animal systemic insecticides have attracted much attention. At the present time, there are at least Systemic three of these, i.e., Trolene, Co-ral, and insecticides Dimethoate—the first two named have been approved for use on beef cattle, by the U. S. Dept. of Agriculture. The third named has not yet been approved since its possible toxic effects on cattle are not well understood.

Trolene (Dow-Et-57, formerly known as Viozene though this name is now obsolete; technically it is O, O-dimethyl O-2, 4, 5-trichlorophenyl phosphoratioate). The usual form of trolene is as a bolus—this is a rounded, usually elongated cylindrical mass, larger than a pill. It is administered to an animal by way of the mouth and by means of an instrument known as a "balling gun." Care must be taken not to injure the animal's throat region by careless or too vigorous use

of this instrument. In southern regions trolene should
be given during July, August, and September, and during August, September, and October in the northern
states. In the United States it is not recommended for
use after the first of November, and in Canada not
after the first of December. It is better not to treat
lactating animals with a systemic insecticide—on
these the derris scrub is best. Good subjects are beef
cattle, young heifers and the nonlactating animals.
Treated animals should not be slaughtered for sixty
days after medication. Trolene is absorbed from the
stomach, and then goes into all the juices
and tissues of the body to destroy the
grub in its pupal and larval stages as it
migrates through the body from the egg
stage—it never reaches the back to damage the hide. Trolene in powder form
mixed with the feed in daily doses of five
milligrams for each kilogram of body weight and
continued for twenty-five days gave 75 per cent control as compared with 90 per cent or even higher when
the bolus was the method of administration. Animals
primarily treated for grub control also appeared to receive a measure of control over other internal parasites
such as Haemonchus, and Ostetagia. Animals treated
showed better weight gains than those not treated.

It is ab-
sorbed into
the animal's
tissue so as
to kill
the larva

In regard to still another systemic insecticide,
"Bayer 21/199," a preliminary report late in 1957 indicated that some heavily grub-infested
yearlings were sprayed with an emulsion
of this compound—suspensions were less
effective—at the rate of one and one-half
gallons per animal under 300 pounds pressure. Results were that all sprayed cattle were—with
two minor exceptions—free of grubs. It is essential
for the success of this treatment that the emulsion,
in concentrations of either 0.25, 0.50, or 0.75 per cent,
reach the animal's skin for absorption to take place—
suspensions did not seem to penetrate the hair coat as

Spraying
with a
systemic
insecticide

well as emulsions. Preliminary estimates also show that "Bayer 21/199" sprayed on cattle at the proper time of year, and correctly applied, prevented infestation with grubs.

On sheep, spraying with "Bayer 21/199" destroyed screwworms in wounds—clipping, castration, docking and others—and in addition provided pro-

Prevent screwworms in sheep

tection against screwworm attacks for two to three weeks. Each animal was sprayed with one quart of either a suspension or an emulsion with equally good results. The suspension had been prepared from a wettable powder containing 25 per cent active ingredient so that the spray solution contained 0.25 per cent, or 0.5 per cent of insecticide. In these treatments by spraying, equally good results were obtained as by the more laborious application of a smear (EI-335, page 303) to the wounds. Treated with the spray, the screwworms in most instances did not reappear to infest wounds until ten days later, though when only the smear was used reinfestation was frequently observed two to four days following treatment.

Sheep Gadfly; Oestrus ovis. The grubs of this fly occur in the nostrils and their communicating head cavities—the sinuses—in sheep.

Grubs in the heads of sheep are a source of great annoyance

The adult fly is about the size of a large housefly. During the heat of the day in the summer months this fly deposits a very small larva or grub at the entrance of the nostrils in sheep. The larva crawls from the nose into the head cavities or sinuses, remaining there and enlarging until it is three-fourths of an inch long and one-third of an inch thick. Some of these larvae become so large that it is not possible for them to escape through the small passageway connecting the sinuses and the nostrils, so that these die in the sinuses and undergo a chalk-like change. Sometime during the spring or

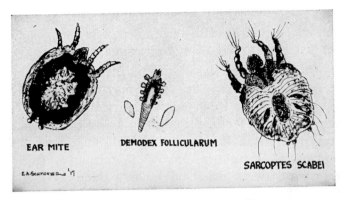

EAR MITE   DEMODEX FOLLICULARUM

SARCOPTES SCABEI

Fig. 190. Varieties of mange mites.

early summer the larvae that are not imprisoned because of their size leave the sheep to drop onto and burrow into the ground. Two or three weeks later under favorable conditions of moisture and temperature the adult fly emerges and is soon depositing its larvae on the nostrils of sheep.

Sheep infested with this parasite have a thick discharge from the nose. It creates the impression that they have a bad head cold. Sheep men refer to the condition as "snotty nose." Because of the spines on its body the grubs are a source of constant irritation to the animal—they neither rest nor sleep well—so that many of them become unthrifty. Breathing is very difficult as a sequence of the swollen air passages.

Preventive measures consist in burning or destroying all under-brush in which the mature fly can find lodging. On some farms there are so many of these flies that the owners permit the sheep to **A practical** graze only during the night time. Other **method of** sheep men plow up one or two furrows in **prevention** a pasture, and sheep soon learn to raise a dust cloud which in a measure prevents the fly from depositing its eggs. An additional preventive measure is to take a log, bore some two-inch holes in it, place salt in the bottom of the holes and smear tar around the sides. In reaching for the salt, the sheep smear the nostrils with tar, and that is obnoxious to the fly so that eggs are not deposited.

Curative treatment is not so satisfactory though it now appears that some good may result from the use of spraying a three per cent saponated cresol solution (page 263) into the nostrils under thirty-five to forty-five pounds pressure. Two fluid ounces per animal of the three per cent solution is used. During treatment the animal should be in a standing position with the nose somewhat tilted upwards. It is estimated that this treatment destroys ninety per cent of the grubs in the head.

Ticks are bearers of many diseases, such as Southern Cattle Fever, and African Cattle Fever, and in humans, Rocky Mountain Spotted Fever (page 249), and African Relapsing Fever. Less frequently, not at all in America, horses, mules, dogs, and sheep and fowl have tick-borne diseases.

Ticks are a menace to the livestock industry

In animals, Southern Cattle Fever (page 747) is undoubtedly the one of greatest importance. It is still present to a limited extent in southern United States, though approximately 500,000 square miles of territory have been freed from it, as well as in other parts of the world. The Southern Fever tick is the biological bearer of the protozoa that causes the disease; not only this, but the ticks when hatched from eggs away from cattle and then placed upon susceptible cattle will cause the fever. It has been determined that the maximum time elapsing from the period that the seed tick, which is the first of the three stages following the egg, first becomes attached to the host until the adult tick drops off is 66 days. Animals must therefore be kept on tick-free fields for this length of time in order that all may be free of ticks.

A method of eradicating Southern Fever ticks by a system of pasture rotation

Somewhat more in detail, the plan to free both cattle and pastures of ticks is to place cattle successively in a series of four pastures with drainage or slope from No. 1 to No. 4. Cattle are placed in No. 1 some time early in the spring and kept there to June 15 when they are moved to an adjoining field No. 2. Fields 1 and 2 are separated from each other by two rows of fencing 15 feet apart so that ticks cannot crawl from one to the other. On September 1, the cattle are moved to pasture No. 3, to be separated from No. 2 by 15 feet of neutral ground, and kept there until October 12 when they are moved to pasture No. 4, which is separated from No. 3 by 15 feet of space, and in which they may be kept to November 1. After this they are returned to pasture No. 1, which is by this time free from ticks, providing no animals of any kind have been permitted in this field since June 15 of the same year. In view of the fact that the colder season is now coming on, and the life of the tick is prolonged when exposed to moisture and cold, therefore field No. 2 may not be considered free of ticks until July 1 of the following year and the double line of fence may not be removed until this date. By August 1 of the second year, all the plots of pasture used in this rotation plan of eradication, as well as the cattle, are free of ticks. Cattle may also be freed of ticks by dipping them twice in an approved arsenical dip. The interval between the two dippings is from seven to ten days. After the second dipping, the animals are to be placed on a tick-free pasture, and preferably so after the first dipping. Benzene hexachloride is also highly effective (page 300). For beef cattle, use only 0.5 per cent malathion, 0.5 toxaphene, or 0.025 per cent lindane, as a dip or spray. Do not use lindane or toxaphene within four weeks of slaughter. For dairy cattle, a spray containing 12 ounces of 5 per cent rotenone powder per gallon of water may be used.

Unusual importance is attached to the discovery that the Southern Fever Tick is the biological bearer of **Importance** the protozoa causing Southern Fever as **of discovery** described in that historical Bulletin No. 1 **of the role of** of the United States Bureau of Animal In- **the Southern** dustry. This is the first time of discovery **Fever tick** indicating that diseases may be transmitted in this manner, and it formed the foundation for the latter information that such diseases as yellow fever and malaria of humans are also insect transmitted. (Page 748.) The hydrocarbon insecticides (pages 295 to 305) are of help on infested cattle.

The Spinose Ear tick: (Otobius megnini.) This parasite is so called because of the spines on the body of the young tick. It is an infestant in the **A common** ears of cattle, sheep, horses, dogs, jackrab- **infestant** bits and others. The mature ticks hide in **in the** cracks in buildings, posts, trees and other **ears of** favorable places. Here the female lays its **animals** eggs. These soon hatch into a small seed tick which attaches itself to the thin inner ear-skin of any suitable passing host to suck blood and to undergo some transformation. After several months of this location in the ears it reaches a stage where it drops to the ground, secretes itself in cracks and crevices where it becomes sexually mature, and lays its eggs.

When the ticks are small and not numerous in the ears they may escape detection. As they increase in size, and especially when they are present in large numbers, they are readily visible. Occasionally they are so numerous as to practically fill the ear. Because of their blood sucking habits, and also by their movements they are a source of great irritation to the host. This is usually manifested by shaking of the head, attempts to rub the ears, and even by rolling on the ground, or by rubbing the head against solid objects.

Prevention of the condition is difficult because, in those sections of the country that constitute its nat-

Practically impossible to control

ural place of abode, it affects so many species of animals, including some that are not domesticated, and these are practically impossible to control.

In handling this condition the first thing that should be done is to mechanically remove as many of the ticks as possible. Usually this is done with a piece of rigid wire with a loop in the end. The looped end is inserted quite deeply into the animal's ear and then by rotary and scraping movements with the loop, as many of the parasites as possible are removed, and as there sometimes are large masses of ear wax, this is at the same time broken down.

A good remedy against this tick is a mixture consisting of two parts by volume of ordinary commercial pine tar (page 316) and one part by volume of cottonseed oil. These ingredients should be thoroughly mixed so as to make a smooth preparation. In cold weather it may be necessary to heat the ingredients slightly, before they are mixed.

The best instrument to use for injecting this material into the ear is a two-ounce metal dose syringe with a blunt nozzle from 2 to 4 inches in length. A syringe of this type is not easily broken nor is it likely to cause injury to the ear.

About one-half ounce of the mixture should be injected deeply into the animal's ear, and at the same time, by means of the fingers, the outside of the ear should be manipulated so that the mixture will come in contact with all parts, especially the deeper ones, of the ear. The mixture will kill only those parasites with which it actually comes in contact.

Care should also be taken that none of the mixture gets on the outside of the face, because when exposed to the action of the sun's rays it will cause blistering. It never seems to cause any blistering on the inside of the ear.

This mixture, if thoroughly and carefully deposited, will remain in position for as long as thirty days, and during this period it will afford protection against the tick. Sometimes the protection is for even longer, but at the end of thirty days it is advisable to re-examine the animals and to give another treatment if this is needed. All animals in an infested herd should be treated immaterial whether or not there are ticks in their ears. Animals on tick infested ranges are best treated late in the fall or early in the winter.

The following in regard to the handling of the spinose ear tick is taken from Farmers Bulletin Number 980—United States Department of Agriculture, pages 5 and 6:

"The Benzene Hexachloride-Xylol-Pine Oil Remedy"

"This new remedy formulated by the Bureau of Animal Industry consists of a mixture of 1 part of benzene hexachloride (also known as hexachlorocyclohexane and gammexane), 2 parts of xylol, and 17 parts of pure pine oil, all parts by weight. The benzene hexachloride that is used in this formulation should be of a technical grade having a gamma isomer content of about 15 per cent, or more."

"To mix the ingredients, place the benzene hexachloride, and xylol in a kettle or bucket and heat to 120° F. with frequent stirring. When the mixture is largely reduced to a liquid, remove it from the source of heat and add the pine oil, with repeated stirring. Since xylol is inflammable, it should be kept away from an open flame. The mixture should be prepared in a well ventilated room, or preferably out of doors. This preparation is not unpleasant to use and will flow freely from a spring-bottom oiler, in winter as well as in summer. Furthermore, this preparation causes no irritation and does not tend to collect dirt in the ears of the animals. The mixture penetrates the masses of ear wax and ticks, and rapidly kills all larvae and nymphs. It also protects the ears against a reinfestation for about 3 weeks or longer, even where opportunity for rapid reinfestation with ear ticks is great. Livestock grazing on large pastures and ranges, or maintained under certain other circumstances where a reinfestation with ear ticks is generally more slowly accumulated, are usually given protection for more than a month."

The Pyridine-Adhesive Remedy

"A remedy developed by the Bureau of Entomology and Plant Quarantine, called Stock 1029,* is a mixture of pyridine in an adhesive containing 45 per cent rosin, 40 per cent hydrogenated methyl abietate (commercially sold as Hercolyn), and 15 per cent dibutyl phthalate."

"The adhesive base (called Adhesive A58) is made up by blending the aforementioned ingredients (except pyridine) under cautious application of heat and constant stirring until the rosin is liquefied. The operation should be carried out in a well ventilated room or in the open, and care should be taken not to overheat the mixture. After the mixture has been allowed to become almost cool, 10 per cent by weight of pyridine (practical grade) is added and the resulting product (Stock 1029) stirred into a uniform preparation. Pyridine is inflammable and must be kept away from open flame."

"Experience with Stock 1029 indicates that it destroys ear ticks effectively and provides reasonable protection from reinfestation for considerable periods of time."

For beef or dairy cattle use 0.75 lindane (page 303) in ten parts of xylene and 85 parts of pure steam-distilled pine oil. Introduce one-half ounce of this mixture into the ear with a spring-bottomed oil can with a two-inch spout that is fitted with a piece of rubber tubing.

---

*For full details of this remedy, U.S.D.A. Department Circular No. E-695, entitled "Control of the Ear Tick," should be consulted.

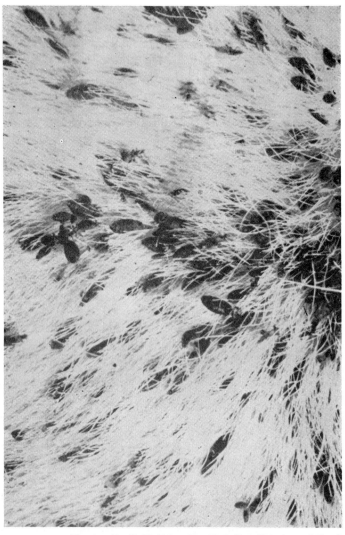

(Courtesy Dr. D. W. Baker, New York State Veterinary College)
FIG. 190-a. Sucking lice (enlarged) from small area of a leg.

Or use 20 per cent lindane, one part in nineteen parts of heavy mineral oil, and apply with a blunt nozzled bulb syringe.

Lice on domesticated animals. These parasites spend

their entire existence on the host's body. They deposit
their eggs or "nits" there, these are
Lice are hatched, and after reproduction their life
very common cycle is completed, so that they die on the
on all
domesticated host. Many of these parasites are blood
animals suckers so that they devitalize their host
in this manner, and all of them are ex-
tremely irritating so as to induce a state of restlessness
in the host. Many of them are specific for a certain
species of animal. They are always more abundant on
weakened unthrifty animals. Because of the close contact between domesticated animals, especially when
they are housed, it is practically impossible to entirely
rid herds and flocks of these pests. Whenever treatment
is instituted all members of that group must be treated
if the results are to be good. In view of the fact that
most remedial agents are not effective against or
destructive to the "nits," and as these usually hatch
in ten days or two weeks, treatment must be repeated
ten days or two weeks following the primary one. For
details regarding treatment refer to Chapter XIX.

"*Cattle Lice:* (Fig. 190-a) There are three species
of sucking lice on cattle, including the short-nosed
cattle louse, *Haematopinus eurysternus Nitzsch*, the
long-nosed cattle louse, *Linognathus vituli L.*, and the
capillate louse, *Soloneptes capillatus End.*, and one biting species, the cattle biting louse, *Bovicola bovis Nitz.*
H. eurysternus and B. bovis are the two most prevalent
species on cattle. Heavily infested animals are usually
found to be in poor condition."

"Powder and spray formulations containing D.D.T.
have proven effective against all species of cattle lice."

"The Division of Entomology, Ottawa, controlled
biting and sucking lice of cattle by applying powders
containing 3, 5, and 10 per cent D.D.T. in pyrophyllite
to different groups of infested young cattle. The
powder was dusted on the animals with a shaker can
and rubbed into the hair by hand over most of the body
except the legs, belly and brisket. Excellent control

was obtained for one month and a large measure of control for three months. The tests showed that at least four ounces of powder are required to treat a mature cow, and complete coverage of infested parts is necessary." *Do not use D.D.T. on dairy animals, and do not use within thirty days of slaughter.*

D.D.T. for lice control Lice on cattle may also be controlled by spraying (Fig. 63) the top, sides and bellies with a 0.25 per cent D.D.T. solution. Hogs have been dipped in a 0.75 per cent solution for lice control.

LICE—BEEF OR DAIRY CATTLE

The latest recommendations are as follows:

Spray

Use 0.025% pyrethrins plus 0.25% synergist (piperonyl butoxide), (page 310) or 1 to 2 pounds of 5% rotenone dust per 100 gallons water. Spray the animals thoroughly. Repeat after two to three weeks.

Dust

Use 0.5 to 1.0% rotenone. Dust animals thoroughly.

LICE—BEEF CATTLE ONLY

Dip

Use 0.5% toxaphene. Be sure to submerge the animals' heads. Dipping is preferable to either spraying or dusting. Also effective is lindane 0.05 to 0.06% or 0.5% methoxychlor, which can be repeated in two or three weeks if necessary.

Spray

Use 0.03% lindane, 0.5% methoxychlor (1.0 to 1.5% for the tail louse), 0.5% toxaphene or 0.5% malathion. Two applications may be necessary two to three weeks apart. Apply enough spray—1 to 2 gallons or more—to wet the animals thoroughly. Do not use lindane or toxaphene within 30 days of slaughter. Do not spray calves less than one month old with malathion.

Dust

Use 10% methoxychlor, or 10% D.D.T. or one per cent lindane. For the control of dog lice and fleas, sponge with a 0.5 to 1 per cent water suspension of D.D.T. immediately after bathing the animal so as to permit drying in the hair coat, or if more convenient dust the animal with a ten per cent D.D.T. powder—this to be repeated ten days later. It is best not to use D.D.T. on cats because they lick themselves. Instead, use rotenone, methoxychlor, T.D.E., lindane, chlordane, dieldrin, pyrethrum, etc.

Chicken Lice: Chickens are subject to infestation by about a dozen species of biting lice, of which three or four are serious pests causing loss of condition and reduced egg production when control measures are neglected. Painting the roosts with nicotine sulphate or dusting the birds with sodium fluoride (page 315) are widely accepted control practices. DDT appears promising as an effective and less toxic substitute for these materials (page 291).

"Dove reported that dusting hens individually with 5 per cent DDT in pyrophyllite from a can with a shaker top rid them of lice. Telford found that as little as 0.5 per cent DDT in pyrophyllite gave a complete kill of body and shaft lice (*Eomenacanthus stramineus Nitz.*, and *Menopon gallinae L.*) within 28 hours, using about one-half ounce of powder per bird." Other chlorinated hydrocarbon insecticides (pages 297 to 305) are also used.

"Telford obtained complete control of these species in two days by dipping 4 infested birds in an emulsion containing only 0.03 per cent DDT. The treated birds continued free of lice for several weeks in an infested flock, indicating residual effectiveness."

Hog Lice, (Haematophinus adventicius): This sucking louse infesting swine has the same general life history as other lice. It is irritating and causes restlessness and loss of weight, or at least poor gains, in the infested host. It has been demonstrated to be a spreader of swine pox (page 576). It may be controlled by the use of chlorinated hydrocarbons such as benzene hexachloride, lindane, chlordane, toxaphene, methoxychlor, etc., (Chapter XIX), and such agents as pyrethrum, rotenone, crude petroleum, coal-tar creosote oil, etc., (pages 316 to 323), are helpful control agents. (U.S.-D.A. "Farmers Bulletin," No. 1085 entitled "Hog Lice and Hog Mange and Control and Eradications" is recommended.)

Mosquitoes. These insects are among the most pernicious of all disease transmitters, though the male is **The life history of the mosquito** not a blood sucker and therefore not a vector. In their development, mosquitoes are first in the egg stage, the eggs being deposited on water. This is followed by the larva or "wrigglers," and it in turn by the pupa or "tumblers," and finally there is the winged insect. All stages beyond the egg are air-breathers. They are bearers of such human diseases as malaria, and yellow fever. Furthermore, in both man and animals **Mosquitoes bearers of many diseases** they may pass into the blood stream a very small worm or filaria, usually called the heart-worm. Fowlpox may be spread by them. Several other less well known diseases may be ascribed to the presence of mosquitoes. Since they are air breathers in the later stages of their development they are readily drowned by denying them access to air. This is usually accomplished by placing a film of oil over the water. A mixture of equal parts of kerosene and crude oil applied with a sprayer results in a smooth unbroken, reasonably durable film. A system of drainage to get rid of stagnant pools, as well as the removal of water from tin cans and comparable receptacles, is very helpful in controlling the development of these insects.

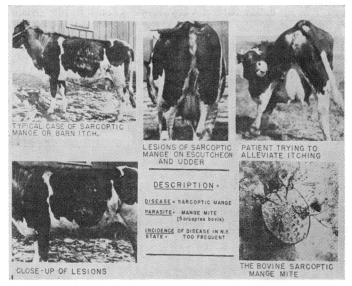

(Courtesy Dr. D. W. Baker, New York State Veterinary College)

FIG. 190-b. Sarcoptic mange (scabies or "barn itch"). Most common in housed animals where contact is close; less frequent in range animals. The causative parasite lives in burrows in the skin.

On animals, except cows in lactation, use one to two ounces of an oil solution containing three to five per cent lethane as a mist spray daily.

Fleas: (*Ctenocephalides canis.*) These insects are lodged most frequently on dogs though they may be present on other domesticated animals. They are distinguished from lice and mites in that they do not remain continuously on the host. They propagate in kennels, blankets, rugs, litter, and comparable material which necessitates either the destruction of these things, or at least their thorough disinfection, along with the animal host. Various disinfestants such as pyrethrum, kerosene, and others are destructive to these pests (pages 316 to 323).

The distinguishing feature of fleas is that they do not remain continuously on the host

Mites on domesticated animals. These parasites

(Fig. 190) constitute a very large group living in all parts of the world. They attack members of the animal and plant kingdoms. In animals, members of this group are responsible for such conditions as mange (barn itch) (scabies) (page 727) in sheep, cattle, horses, (Fig. 191) swine and others; "scaly leg" and "depluming itch" in fowls; ear mange, demodectic mange (Fig. 192) in the dog and cat; "airsac mite" disease in fowls; "red" mites of poultry; "harvest mites" or "chiggers" of man and animals and many others.

Mites are responsible for many animal ailments

Some of the mites referred to preferably spend most of their life on the host. Usually these may be destroyed by the use of "dips" (pages 288 to 325). Others, especially those of fowls, hide in cracks and crevices during the daylight hours and suck blood from them during roosting periods. Sparrows are also infested. Clean, dry, well-ventilated houses are much

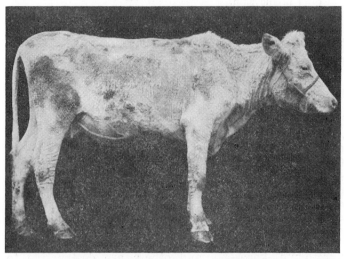

(Courtesy Dr. D. W. Baker, New York State Veterinary College)

FIG. 190-c. Sarcoptic mange (scabies). A highly contagious skin disease spread by contact, due to a small parasite. Causes intense itching, especially when animal is warmed in a barn.

less likely to be infested. Thorough cleaning of houses (page 215), the use of creosote wood preservers on woodwork, and treating fowl with kerosene emulsion, nicotine dip and others (pages 308 to 323), is advised.

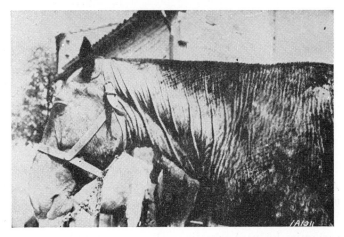

(Courtesy Dr. W. M. McLeod)

FIG. 191. Horse affected with scabies or mange.

Cattle may be infested i.e., (1) *Psoroptic*, (2) *Chorioptic*, (3) *Sarcoptic* or tunneling mite, and (4) *Demodectic* mange mite. No. 1 is in clusters all over the skin; No. 2 in clusters usually on the limbs, tail and brisket; No. 3 tunnels into the skin, and No. 4 lives in hair follicles and skin glands. Three pounds of 25 per cent lindane powder in 100 gallons of water, or seven pounds of benzene hexachloride (wettable) containing 10 per cent gamma isomer in 100 gallons used twice at a 10-day interval, saturating the hide thoroughly is effective. Also disinfect premises and manure piles.

"Hog Lice and Hog Mange, Methods of Control and Eradication," U.S.D.A., Farmers Bulletin No. 1085 is recommended.

Itchiness in Sheep: In America intense itching and loss of wool in sheep as a result of infestation with

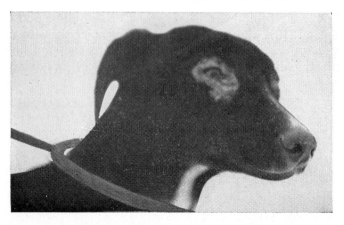

FIG. 192. Eye mange (demodectic).

A new skin mite of sheep

mange mites—*Psoroptes communis ovis* (common scab); *Sarcoptes ovis* (head scab); *Chorioptes ovis* (foot scab); *Demodex folliculorum* (rare)—have long been recognized. In Australia still another mite—*Psorergates ovis*—was held responsible for mild itching. This same parasite has now been isolated in an outbreak of mild itching and "taggy" wool in a flock of sheep in a mid-western state. Sheep harboring *Psorergates* have all the appearance and symptoms of a mild attack of scabies or mange. This comparatively new American mite is lodged very deeply in the skin of infested sheep. In order to detect it, it is necessary to take very deep skin scrapings, or even shavings or skin clippings— these to be examined microscopically for the minute mites. Handling of the condition if diagnosed is primarily by removing those having clinical manifestations from the remainder of the flock, and secondarily dipping affected ones in benzene hexachloride (page 300) or lindane solution (page 303).

No attempt has been made to offer a description of all the ailments and conditions that may be ascribed to the larger parasites—the subject is much too extensive. There are however brief statements about the

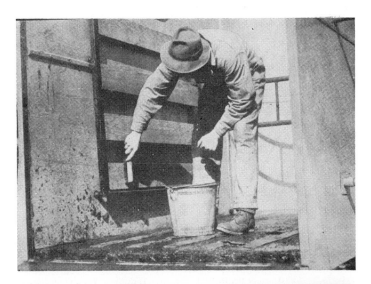

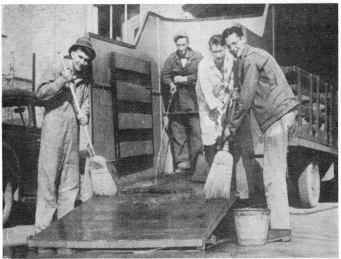

(Courtesy Dr. D. W. Baker, New York State Veterinary College)

FIG. 192-a. Since sarcoptic mange mites can be harbored in cracks and crevices of wood in barns these should have an application of lindane solution, or lime and sulphur dip. Infested animals should be similarly hand treated or dipped. (Lindane, page 303; lime and sulphur, page 321.)

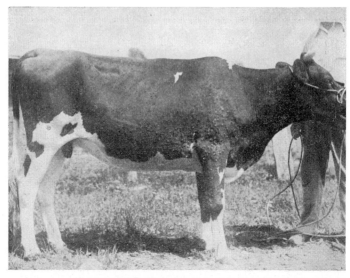

(Courtesy Dr. D. W. Baker, New York State Veterinary College)
FIG. 192-b. Demodectic mange (a form of scabies). Nodules containing the causative parasite embedded in a thick white
pus-like exudate. The mode of contamination is not well
understood though presumably by contact. (See Figs. 192,
192-c.)

parasites that are of common and frequent occurrence,
and that are also representative of several different
groups, so that the recommended, outlined preventive
and sanitary steps for the individuals described are
practically equally applicable to other members of the
same group.

(For details about the control of flies, ticks, and
others the reader is referred to Chapter XIX).

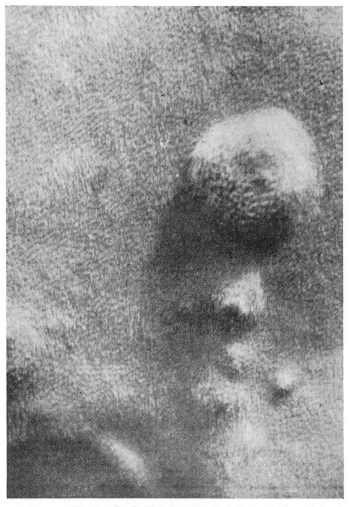

(Courtesy Dr. D. W. Baker, New York State Veterinary College)
FIG. 192-c. A demodectic mange nodule from the skin of an animal. (See Fig. 192-b.)

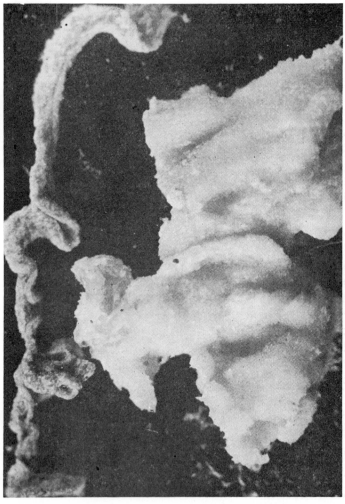

(Courtesy Dr. D. W. Baker, New York State Veterinary College)

FIG. 192-d. Contents of an opened nodule of demodectic mange. (See Fig. 192-c.)

CHAPTER XXXII

SOME SMALLER (MICROSCOPIC) PARASITES

All of the ailments described in this chapter are due to microscopic parasites grouped as protozoa. They consist of single celled animal organisms usually classed as the lowest division of the animal kingdom.

Red dysentery, or coccidiosis (page 733). This is a parasitic disease of cattle—also sheep—caused by a microscopically sized animal parasite be-

A bloody diarrhoea of cattle due to a small parasite longing to the group known as protozoa, the subdivision coccidia, and specifically as the *Eimeria zurni* in cattle. Coccidiosis occurs in all species of live stock though each of these has a coccidia peculiar to itself, and not intercommunicable. Red dysentery is not a contagious disease in the strictest interpretation of this word, but the nature of the causative parasite is such that a single infested animal is likely to contaminate a very extensive area so that other cattle of the neighborhood soon contract the same ailment. The parasite resists freezing and ordinary disinfectants, though destroyed by the sun's action and drying.

The parasite is very abundant in the intestinal evacuations of affected animals. It abounds in wet, filthy, insanitary surroundings, or in any

The parasite is readily spread area that is subjected to contamination with intestinal evacuations. It may be spread from farm to farm among cattle that drink from a common stream.

Symptoms of the disease are observed most frequently in young animals—four to twenty-four months of age. Occasionally in those one month of age or nine years old. The characteristic symptom is a more or less severe bloody diarrhoea—hence the name red dysentery. It seems that the parasite in its development destroys a superficial layer of the intestinal lining membrane thus opening the very small blood vessels or capillaries so that bleeding results. General symptoms of weakness soon appear, there may be muscular twitching, and the animal goes down. Death takes place in as high as fifty per cent of the affected ones.

Prevention consists in prompt segregation of affected animals. Portable calf pens and age-group segregation is advisable. (Fig. 23.) As their intestinal discharges teem with the highly resistant **Prevention consists largely in sanitation** parasite their destruction must be effected with the most powerful agents such as a three per cent water solution of sulphuric acid (page 278). In making this solution add the sulphuric acid slowly to the water—never the reverse as the reaction is likely to be explosive. Bear in mind that sulphuric acid is destructive to almost all substances, including human tissues, metals, paint, wood, leather, cloth, etc. Use glassware or crockery in which to store it. For the disinfestation of very small

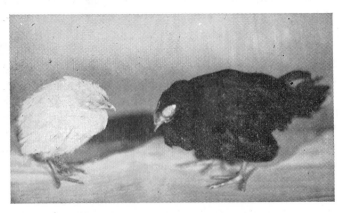

(Courtesy Dept. of Bacteriology, Kansas State University)

FIG. 193. Coccidiosis showing the general external symptoms, including eye lesions.

areas a mixture of carbon bisulphide (page 306) and two per cent of phenol (page 260) is effective. Do not permit surface drainage, or animate or inanimate forces to disseminate the parasite.

If the parasite in young calves is located in almost any section of the intestinal tract, the best success follows treatment for five days with either sulfamethazine or sulfamerazine. In older cattle the parasite is usually only in the rectum, and in these cases an enema of sulfaquinoxaline is the preferred agent.

Coccidiosis of poultry (page 144). This is one of the most prevalent diseases of poultry. It is estimated that from 12 to 20 per cent of the losses in chicks hatched in the United States are due to it. It is due to a single celled animal parasite known as coccidia—*Eimeria tenella* in the ceca (page 24) and *E. necatrix* in the other parts of the intestine. *E. acervulina*, and *E. hagani* have more recently also been isolated as causes of coccidiosis in poultry. This disease occurs in most domesticated animals (page 733) and barnyard fowl, but each species of animals is infected by a specific coccidia, or in other words there is a host specificity, which means chickens can contract the disease only from chickens, ducks from ducks, cattle from cattle and so on.

A microparasitic disease of poultry

The disease is world-wide and affects fowl of all ages, though those from three weeks to three months of age are most frequently affected. It is contracted by eating foods contaminated with intestinal discharges of sick birds. The symptoms are not at all characteristic. The affected birds appear unthrifty. (Fig. 193.) Diarrhoea, frequently with a mixture of blood in the droppings, is suggestive of the ailment. Emaciation becomes marked, and death usually results, though a varying number make an incomplete recovery. A positive diagnosis is based on the microscopic detection of the coccidia in the intestinal discharge.

There is no known entirely satisfactory method of curative treatment though the following method of feeding has been recommended. As soon as the bloody diarrhoea is first noticed all members of the flock are placed on a ration consisting of dry skim milk or buttermilk 40 pounds; wheat bran, 10 pounds; yellow cornmeal, 30 pounds; ground barley or ground whole oats, 20 pounds. In addition grain may be fed corresponding in amount to one-third to one-half of the mash consumed. This ration is continued for not longer than two weeks, by which time the outbreak is supposed to be checked, and then the fowl are gradually returned to their regular ration. This ration presumably creates an acid condition in the intestines which is unfavorable for the coccidia.

The milk-flush to control coccidiosis in fowl

The addition of two per cent of dusting sulphur to the ration has also been recommended and seems to have some merit as a preventive in chicks between four and ten weeks old, but following its use gains in weight are retarded, the rear gut shows evidence of irritation, and rickets is a common sequel even though cod liver oil was also a part of the ration. In this event, or if there is evidence of skin irritation discontinue the sulphur. The consensus is that until a method for the feeding of sulphur without unfavorable results is developed it is best not to use it.

The feeding of sulphur may be harmful

It has been found that birds that have recovered from coccidiosis are resistant to subsequent attacks. On this basis the practice is to expose chicks, between the ages of two to four weeks, to infection by placing them in pens that have previously been occupied by coccidia-infected chicks. It is known that ailing fowl start to pass immense numbers of coccidial oocysts in from two to six days

Exposure and immunity as methods of prevention

after blood is noticed in their intestinal evacuations. Thus, infected pens are created. Chicks free from disease—two to four weeks of age—are placed in these moist infected pens, and at the same time are treated with sulfonamides (pages 280-281). At the end of six days of this exposure they have acquired the infection and have recovered from it so that they are then immune to the *tenella* organism at least.

A vaccine is available—this is the Edgar or Auburn vaccine developed by Dr. Edgar of Auburn University, Auburn, Alabama, against the *Eimeria tenella* infestation as well as against *E. necatrix, E. acervulina,* and *E. hagani.* There are four other known species against which the vaccine is of no value. The vaccine consists of four separately prepared suspensions of live oocysts —this is one of the stages in the development of coccidia—of the four above mentioned species of coccidia, all tested for purity and potency before being bottled. The suspension or inoculum, that is, the vaccine, is fed to three day old chicks. The chicks, immediately after being hatched, are fed in the usual manner for the first three days of life outside the shell. On the third day after the usual feeding, the feed should be removed at about eight A.M. At noon, the vaccine is mixed with a measured amount of water, and this in turn is mixed with the feed so as to make a thick, moist mash. This is placed in hoppers or scattered on papers in the brooders or feed house so that all of the chicks will get some of the material. On the 13th day following this feeding the chicks are treated for three days with sulfaquinoxaline in the feed to protect those birds that have eaten too much of the oocyst treated mash. It is claimed that from 17 to 28 days later the birds will have developed a solid immunity.

A vaccine to protect chickens against coccidiosis

Other methods of immunization against coccidiosis in poultry are in the research stage, i.e., by Dickinson and Babcock at Oregon State College, and by Urrichio at Catholic University in Washington, D. C.

If the Auburn vaccine is used, chicks may still be susceptible to the *E. necatrix,* but this latter does not develop on dry floors; dryness and cleanliness will control it. The sulfonamides used are the comparatively insoluble sulphamerazine or sulphamethazine, and their soluble salts, sodium sulphamerazine or sodium sulphamethazine. Either of the former are put in the chick starter mash, and either of the two latter in the drinking water. The dosage is one ounce of any of these four sulfonamides (pages 280-281) daily for from 850 to 1000 chicks. If an insoluble is used mix it thoroughly by ten minutes of stirring with 40 to 60 pounds of the mash; if a soluble is used dissolve it in from six to seven gallons of water. This is to be kept up for six days, then move the chicks to a dry floor and keep under sanitary conditions so that they can contaminate neither their drinking water nor their feed with their droppings. This method of prevention will obviate sudden outbreaks and prevent extensive losses. Veterinarians should be consulted as they are fully familiar with the details of this plan.

When chicks show evidences of bloody diarrhoea they may be given one ounce of sulfamerazine in 15 pounds of mash or a corresponding amount **Handling in smaller flocks** of sulphamethazine; or one ounce of either sodium sulfamerazine or sodium sulfamethazine in three gallons of freshly prepared drinking water. Sulfaquinoxaline, one ounce to 125 pounds of feed has also been advised. Another sulfonamide known as sulfaquanidine—one-fourth pound in fifty pounds of mash—is also used as a remedy. Continue these treatments for three days, and if a further outbreak occurs in the same group four or five days later a further treatment is given for one or two days. Sulfonamides are dangerous drugs if improperly used and overdosing is to be guarded against by veterinary supervision of these treatments.

The more strictly sanitary methods of controlling the disease are very laborious but effective. The

Sanitary steps are effective

brooder houses and runs must be cleaned daily. This method of attack is based on the fact that the coccidia from the time of their passage from a diseased bird must undergo one of its developmental stages before it is capable of reproducing the disease. If all droppings and litter are removed and burned daily no infection can occur. Water troughs and feed hoppers must be placed high enough to prevent the contamination of their contents with intestinal discharges, and elevated wide-meshed wire platforms (Figs. 159 and 160) should be placed around for the fowl to stand upon. Sanitary runways (Fig. 29) are to be recommended (page 143). Frequent and thorough disinfection of all floors, drinking and feeding vessels is essential. Ordinary disinfectant solutions must be used frequently at double strength to be thoroughly effective. Scalding water alone or with lye (page 253) is helpful.

Sheep and Goats: Coccidiosis is comparatively rare. *Eimeria nina-kohlyakimovi, E. arloingi, E. faurei, E. parva* and others have been isolated. This condition should be controlled as in beef cattle, and treated with sulfas.

Swine Coccidiosis: Rare; due to *Eimeria debliecki, E. scabra* and others. Control by sanitation, and treat with sulfas.

Enterohepatitis of turkeys; blackhead of turkeys; turkey coccidiosis. This disease is probably the greatest hazard to the raising of turkeys. Chickens are occasionally affected with it.

Blackhead of turkeys was formerly the major hazard in the raising of these birds

The disease is due to a protozoa, a one celled animal parasite, known as *Histomonas meleagridis.* (Fig. 194) This protozoa is harbored (it does not need to live there for its development) in the body and eggs of the cecal worm (*Heterakis gallinae*) (page 695) of chickens, and therefore the practical impossibility of

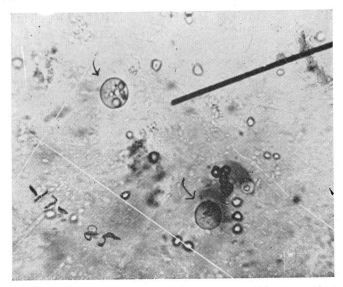

Fig. 194. A microscopic reproduction of the Histomonas maleagridis, the cause of blackhead in turkeys. Note the arrows.

permitting turkeys and chickens to occupy the same
runs because the poults are almost certain to contract
blackhead and die. The causative protozoa probably
live over on a farm from year to year unless there is a
period of zero temperatures. Also the protozoa are in
the droppings of ailing birds frequently several days
before visible illness appears.

The symptoms are most frequently observed following the fourth week of life. (Fig. 195.) Usually
one member of a flock shows listlessness by lessened
activity, and there may be some diarrhoea with orange
colored droppings especially in the older birds—in
young poults the color varies from light green to
brown. In some cases the skin of the region of the
head becomes dark in color. In young birds death takes
place in a few days, though older ones may linger for
as long as a month. In the latter event there is extreme emaciation and weakness.

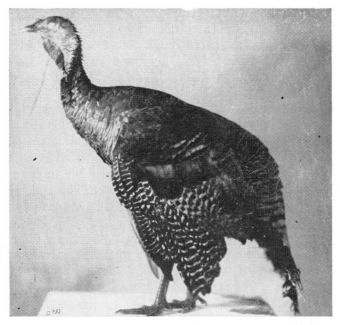

(Courtesy Department of Bacteriology, Kansas State University)

FIG. 195. Blackhead. Note the drooping wings of the sick bird.

On post-mortem examination the inside of the ceca (page 24), which are the two elongated appendix-like parts of the intestines, is found to be ulcerated, (Fig. 196) and the liver usually has dark yellow abscesses (Fig. 197).

Prevention of the condition consists in keeping both young and old turkeys away from chickens and **Keeping turkeys away from chickens is the best means of control** their droppings, and also if possible keeping the young poults away from older turkeys because these are carriers of the infection, and young turkeys contract the disease by picking food from contaminated ground. If turkeys are to be raised under natural conditions—without phenothiazine (page 689)—without the development of blackhead it must be done on land that for two years previously has had on it neither chickens nor turkeys. Artificially turkeys may be raised in dry brooder houses on contaminated land. They must be kept from contact with the soil by constructing for their use raised runways (Fig. 29) made out of boards or wire netting. Fresh green forage, and fish liver oil to the extent of three per cent in the ration are other essentials. If under the conditions described blackhead makes its appearance it is indicative of contamination, and the flock should at once be moved to clean ground.

A unique method of preventing blackhead in young turkeys consists in a surgical procedure. The abdominal cavity is opened and the ceca are per-

A unique surgical operation
manently isolated from the remainder of the digestive tract by tieing them off at their point of union with the intestines. It is not claimed to be a practical method of prevention. There are hazards in the operation and it has not been generally adopted.

In the case of valuable birds in the earlier stages of the disease curative treatment may be attempted by either the oral or rectal administration twice daily of twelve to twenty-four drops—the dose depends upon the size of the bird—of fluid extract of ipecac mixed with one-half to two ounces of water, and repeated twice daily for a week. When a cure has apparently been affected the bird should be given from fifteen to thirty drops of turpentine in order to eliminate remaining causative parasites from the ceca. There is a possibility that recovered birds may be carriers and spreaders of the infection. They are usually resistant to a second attack of the disease.

From time to time various chemicals have been recommended for both prevention and treatment. Probably the drug known as enheptin (2-amino-nitrothiazole), or in trade simply as "ANT," in a dosage of 0.05 per cent in the feed as a preventive and cure during the early stages is the best known. If the dosage is not carefully controlled it has toxic properties resulting in such conditions as reduced egg production and lowered hatchability.

Phenothiazine (page 689) used one pound in every one hundred pounds of mash fed for a three-day period every three weeks to poults after they have been turned

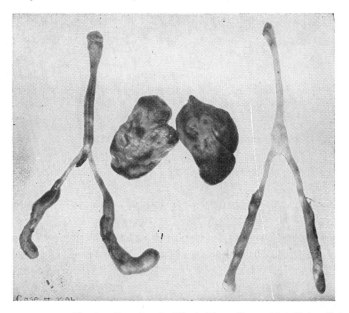

(Courtesy Department of Bacteriology, Kansas State University)

Fig. 196. Blackhead lesions showing normal ceca (right) and diseased ceca (left); (center) diseased liver. All were taken from a six-weeks-old bird.

Pheno-thiazine helpful though not a specific

out to range, is regarded as helpful in breaking the life cycle of the cecal worm (page 695). In a measure this is helpful in preventing blackhead. The 1948 Annual Report of the Chief of the United States Bureau of Industry states that the Bureau has kept its experimental flock on the same ground over a period of five years, and during the fifth year, the turkeys fed a mash containing 0.5 per cent by weight of phenothiazine (page 689) suffered a loss of eight per cent while at the same time non-

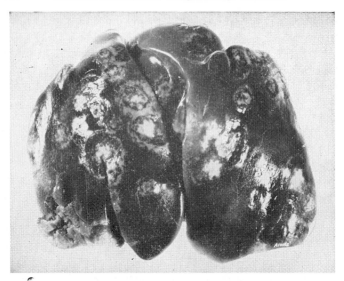

(Courtesy Department of Bacteriology, Kansas State University)
FIG. 197. Blackhead liver from a turkey poult showing typical necrotic ulcer-like areas.

medicated turkeys had a death rate of 70 per cent from blackhead. For the fiscal year 1947 the loss among the medicated was eleven per cent and the non-medicated 47 per cent. This indicates improvement of the fifth year over the fourth year.

Anaplasmosis of cattle; yellow teat disease (page 701). An ailment affecting both young and aged cattle.

It is believed due to an animal parasite—

A serious micro-parasitic disease of cattle the protozoa known as the *Anaplasma marginale* (late research is not entirely convinced of the absolute correctness of this) which in infected animals is in the red blood cells. (For the latest research information the reader is referred to page 111, Vol. 6, "Advances in Veterinary Science" by Brandly, *et al.* The book is published by Academic Press, 111 Fifth Ave., New York 3, N. Y.) The parasite, and consequently the disease, may be transmitted from animal to animal by means of biting insects, and by mechanical agencies such as bleeding needles, hypodermic needles, dehorning and other surgical instruments, sharp pronged driving contrivances, or in fact in any manner that will transfer blood. An animal that has contracted this disease permanently retains the parasite in its blood, though it may show no evidence of ill health. Such animals are "carriers," (page 210) and they are potential sources of danger to others.

The symptoms may be those of a mild, acute, or chronic condition. There is nothing characteristic about the infection in calves. They simply become "dumpy" for a few days, and then apparently recover though their blood remains the permanent abode of the parasite.

The older milk cows show more characteristic symptoms during an acute attack. The milk flow ceases, there is a marked rise in temperature, and there is almost complete collapse. If death does not take place in the course of a day or two, in light skinned animals, the hairless skin of the body such as that surrounding the eyes, mouth, genitals, udder, and teats becomes first very pale because of the destruction of the red blood cells by the parasite, and second because of jaundice they are tinged a decided yellow color— hence the cattleman's name of "yellow teat" disease. Many of the animals thus affected die while others go into a chronic stage. These latter ultimately recover in so far as clinical symptoms are concerned, and they appear to be healthy, but the parasite remains permanently, though in reduced or negligible numbers, in the blood. A small amount of blood from one of these apparently fully recovered animals when injected into a susceptible cow will produce the disease in the latter.

If these "carriers" (page 210) can be detected in a manner that is practical in its application—other than by the inoculation of a known suscep-

Detection of carriers a needed step

tible bovine—a big step will have been taken in the ultimate eradication of the disease. In this connection, the U. S. Animal Research Service, has developed a complement fixation test (page 759) that holds out some promise of success.

Animals in the acute stage of the disease, and those in the early part of the "carrier" stage, seem to have an increased amount of euglobulin—this is a blood protein—present in their blood. On the basis of the foregoing, Boynton and Woods developed the following test:—A sample of blood is collected in a test tube and this is permitted to clot so that a small amount of the clear serum may be obtained. Two drops of serum are added to two milliliters of distilled water in a tube. If the animal is not infested with the causative parasite of anaplasmosis the mixture of water and serum will remain clear. On the other hand, if the disease is present there will be immediate clouding, and about twelve or more hours later there will be a white sediment in the tube.

A simple test

Prevention is by no means entirely effective because of the difficulty of controlling the biting insects that are capable of transmitting the disease. In those regions in which the condition is known to be prevalent more than the usual precautions must be observed to prevent its spread by such mechanical means as surgical instruments, dehorners, prods, needles, and others.

Prevention only partly understood

The use of insecticide sprays—D.D.T. and others (page 291)—have only limited value in that they are not repellents, though they may be helpful in reducing the total biting insect population.

In those sections of the country where the disease results in extensive animal losses consideration should be given to the life-time protection afforded by inoculating calves shortly after birth with some virulent blood. This inoculation must not be adopted unless there is a thorough understanding of the fact that calves so inoculated become life-time carriers (page 210) of the causative protozoa, and therefore they are a source of danger for non-immune cattle. This may safely be practiced as very young calves are seldom if ever fatally affected. Others limit their cattle groups to the strictly home-bred herd; this is recommended for herds in areas where the disease is quite generally present.

Curative treatment is not at all satisfactory, though some antibiotics, terramycin and aureomycin—the former in doses of five mgs. to a pound of animal live-weight per day, intramuscularly, for two weeks, or the latter in 15 mg. doses per pound per day for two weeks will eradicate the carrier state. But, the treated animal again becomes susceptible. Good care and good nursing are the principal steps.

Southern cattle fever; tick fever; red water; cattle malaria; splenic fever (page 714) erroneously called

Southern cattle fever for many years prevented the development of the cattle industry in the southern American states

Texas Fever as it was not limited to Texas. This disease also is due to a protozoa, the *Piroplasma bigeminum.* In its usual existence it spends a portion of its life in the body of the fever tick *(Margaropus annulatus)*, which in turn passes the protozoa into the blood of cattle, in which the red blood cells are broken down so that their red coloring matter gets into the blood plasma, and thence in part is excreted with the urine—therefore, the name "red water" frequently applied to this disease. The fever tick is the only means by which the disease is naturally transmitted from animal to animal, and therefore, the destruction of these biting and blood sucking ticks will cause the disease to disappear.

The disease may be transmitted artificially by inoculating a susceptible animal with blood from a diseased one. The fever tick that has sucked blood from an infected cow has the piroplasma bigeminum in its eggs as well as in its various larval stages. The female tick lays its eggs on the ground, where they hatch. The young larvae climb onto the vegetation to await the passing of cattle to which it attaches itself and develops by biting, and sucking blood. In this process it passes the *Piroplasma bigeminum* into the blood of cattle.

Usually native cattle are but slightly affected, though in the days that the fever tick was ubiquitous in most of the territory south of the Mason and Dixon line practically all of the cattle in that territory were infected. Northern highly susceptible cattle shipped into the southern territory promptly contract an almost invariably fatal form of the disease.

The symptoms in an acute form usually consist of a high temperature, rapid pulse and breathing, pale and yellowish mucous membranes, and discolored urine varying from a light red to almost black. Sometimes these symptoms subside only to recur in a milder form at later periods. Young animals less than one year of age usually recover, older ones die in approximately fifty per cent of the cases. The blood of a recovered animal remains permanently infective.

Prevention of the disease consists in a program of tick eradication by pasture rotation (pages 220 and 715), and the dipping of tick infested cattle—crude petroleum (page 321) and the arsenical dip (page 315). The use of D.D.T. and benzene hexachloride (page 300) and other chlorinated hydrocarbons is recommended for the destruction of the fever tick.

Dipping and pasture rotation have practically stamped out the disease

It is appropriate at this time to again emphasize (page 716) the importance of the discovery by the United States Bureau of Animal Industry scientists (see bulletin number one of the United States Bureau of Animal Industry) that "Southern cattle fever" is transmissible from an infected to a susceptible bovine by means of an intermediate biological carrier—the Fever tick. No such discovery had previously been made in either human or veterinary medicine. This discovery formed the basis for many later ones indicating the method of spread of such human ailments as malaria and yellow fever—both mosquito-borne—and many others. The method of Southern cattle fever transmission opened a new era in human and animal disease control.

Trichomoniasis; bovine venereal trichomoniasis (page 801). This is a breeding disease of cattle due to the flagellate protozoa *Trichomonas foetus*—it is primarily located in the reproductive organs of cows and bulls; hence it is also named "bovine genital trichomoniasis." Its distribution is probably world wide.

A disease of the organs of reproduction of cattle
Bulls do not appear to be affected physically by the infection but transmit it to susceptible cows. In cows it may result in a genital purulent discharge, in a gathering of pus in the uterus, and abortion or premature births, as well as barrenness. If present in bulls in the preputial cavity (this is the region at the end of the penis sometimes called the foreskin) it may spread to deeper portions of the genitalia, even to the testicles.

Cows almost invariably contract the trichomonads from infected bulls through the act of coitus or service. It is therefore a true venereal disease of cattle.

The exact diagnosis of trichomoniasis presents many difficulties. However, the disease should be suspected when several heifers in a herd fail to settle after repeated services, and if they have irregular heat periods. Early abortion—between the third and sixteenth week after conception—is suggestive but certainly not conclusive as this is also observed in bovine brucellosis (page 578). Discharges appear from the vagina or uterus usually clear and colorless but frequently showing whitish flakes or even streaks of pus. During the early stages of an infection in the bull the end of the penis may be inflamed and sensitive so that he hesitates or is disinclined to serve; also at this stage small reddish elevations may be observed on the end of the penis. The clinical symptoms in the bull usually disappear in two or three weeks leaving the animal outwardly normal though infected and therefore capable of spreading the disease.

A positive diagnosis can be made only when the causative protozoa is demonstrated to be present, microscopically, in the genital discharge—obtained from the prepuce by either the pipette, the swab or douche methods—the latter is most efficacious and is the method of choice, or in the tissues or fluids of recently aborted young. Failing in this, the even more difficult laboratory technique is employed to grow the suspected protozoa on appropriate culture media, and then demonstrate it microscopically.

A final positive diagnosis depends on demonstrating the protozoa

The immunity following recovery from a primary infection with the trichomonas is rather uncertain but in general it is considered *that an infected cow taken out of the breeding line for a period of ninety days is free from the infection, and in the absence of other abnormal conditions should settle to the service of a healthy bull. Insofar as the infected bull is concerned his infection is permanent or at the best it is of indefinite duration.* Some investigators offer good evidence that an occasional bull recovers spontaneously.

The prevention of this condition—once it has appeared—depends entirely upon elimination of natural service by the bull, as he is the spreader. Even after a cow has apparently recovered there is still the danger that she may harbor some of the protozoa to infect a clean bull serving her, thus perpetuating the infection in the herd. It has been demonstrated that the good breeding performance of a previously infected cow is not clear-cut evidence that she is actually free from all infection. Rigid preventive steps therefore in large herds demand (1) the

Prevention and control

elimination of infected bulls; (2) subsequent breeding in the herd to be by artificial insemination (page 803) with semen from clean bulls; (3) clean bulls must never be used for a natural service on cows or heifers that have previously been covered by an infected bull. In smaller herds where artificial insemination cannot be adopted a fairly satisfactory plan is to use a clean bull first on all clean cows and heifers, and next on infected animals. The bull is then sent to the slaughter at the end of the breeding season, and a clean bull obtained for use during the following season. In dairy herds such a plan at least maintains the milk flow.

The following recommendations are those of Dikmans of the U. S. Animal Research Service:

"1. No mature animal should be bought as a permanent addition to the herd without a thorough investigation of the breeding record of the animal and of the herd from which it comes."

"2. No outside animals should be brought to the premises for breeding purposes without knowing the breeding history of the animals and of the herd from which they come."

"3. Cows should not be bred outside of the herd and away from the premises without taking similar precautions. If breeding troubles and difficulties occur in your herd, consult your veterinarian and try to determine the cause of these troubles. If, after examination and consultation, it is determined that the trouble is due to trichomoniasis, breeding operations should be stopped for a time and from available records it should be determined which animals are infected and which may reasonably be suspected of being infected."

"4. The use of known infected or suspected bulls should be restricted to cows that have passed through an attack of the disease and to cows that have previously been exposed to infection."

"5. A new bull should be provided for heifers coming to breeding age and for the cows that have not been exposed."

"6. In cases of early abortion due to trichomoniasis if the abortion is clean and uncomplicated the cow should be left alone and given sexual rest for about three months."

"7. If the abortion is incomplete and there are complications such as persistent discharge, and in cases of pyometra, the case should be handled by a veterinarian."

"8. In cases of temporary sterility due to trichomoniasis, breeding should be stopped until the estrual or heat periods have returned to normal for 2 or 3 periods."

There is no known cure; a three months sexual rest for infected cows, and disposal of infected bulls is the

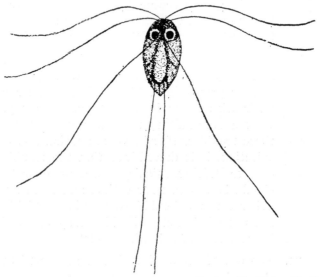

(Courtesy The Turkey World)

FIG. 198. The Hexamita maleagridis (greatly magnified).

approved procedure. In test tube tests the parasite seems to be sensitive to such antibiotics as aureomycin, and terramycin. But when these antibiotics are used on the living animals, results are discouraging. However, in clean herds some operators have adopted the routine practice of douching the bull's sheath before and after each service with a luke-warm 0.5 lactic acid; other operators have turned to various disinfectants. These are certainly highly recommended sanitary practices.

No known cure

Hexamitiasis in Turkeys; Infectious Catarrhal Enteritis. This condition is now widespread in turkey growing areas. It was formerly generally regarded as a trichomoniasis. It is due to infection with the protozoa *Hexamita meleagridis.* (Fig. 198.) In the disease there is a foamy water diarrhoea and loss in weight (Fig. 199), and finally in most instances there is a coma and death. Young poults from one to ten weeks of age are the usual victims though older birds may contract the condition. The death loss when the disease first makes its appearance in a flock may be very heavy though later the deaths taper off. Birds that do not die are unthrifty for a long time, and still more serious they

A serious disease of poults

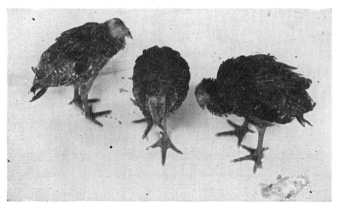

(Courtesy Department of Bacteriology, Kansas State University)
FIG. 199. Hexamitiasis in turkey poults.

are potential carriers (page 210) of the protozoa. Insect transmitters have not been found. In the field the disease appears usually in the later hatches because the "carriers" and the early poults must first build up the infection.

Prevention consists in maintaining separate units and caretakers for the breeding flock and the young poults. The use of wire platforms (pages 144 and 630-631) for water (Figs. 159 and 160) and feed (Fig. 29)—and keeping these sanitary—

Sanitation as a preventive   is important as well as cemented areas of the yard where the poults congregate. In badly diseased flocks the plan is to sell all breeding birds at least two weeks before any poults are hatched.

The success of a positive curative treatment is doubtful. Some researchers, though, attribute a measure of success following the use of enheptin (2-amino-5-nitrothiazole), aureomycin, terramycin, pennicillin G, and other antibiotics.

Dourine. This contagious disease of horses is spread by coitus (the sex act). It is due to the *Trypanosoma equiperdum*, an endoparasitic protozoa, in the blood. Indications are in the swellings observed in the disease, in the mucous material of the genitalia, and in the testicles. A characteristic symptom, in addition to swelling and discharge from the genitals (Figs. 200 and 201) is the appearance of flat, circumscribed swellings—the so-called "dollar plaques" on the skin.

A disease stamped out by sanitation   Overcoming dourine is a good example of what can be accomplished by sanitary and control measures. Formerly quite widespread in the United States, in so far as known, it has now been stamped out by hygienic breeding practices.

Balantidiosis of Swine: This condition is due to a ciliated protozoa—the *Balantidium coli* and possibly the smaller protozoa—the *Balantidium suis*. These or-

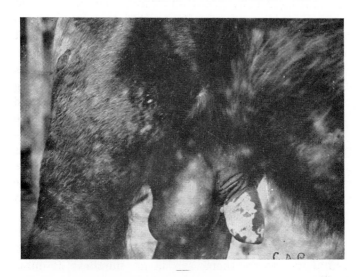

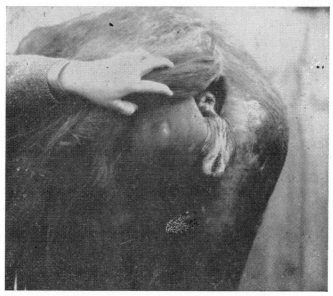

FIGS. 200 and 201. Dourine in stallion and mare.

ganisms are very generally distributed in nature—in fact placing straw, grass and other vegetation in a glass of water and permitting it to stand at room temperature for a few days will result in a swarm of this protozoa in the water. It has never been positively determined whether or not this protozoa is the cause of an ulceration, bloody diarrhoea, and general mal-
Is it a cause of disease? nutrition, or is its presence in the ulcers incidental and without particular signifi-cance. The protozoa is generally present in the lower end of the small intestine as well as in the large intestine. "It is conveyed from infested to sus-ceptible animals by microscopic bodies known as cysts. A cyst is a resistant stage in the life cycle of the para-sites. The cysts are discharged with the droppings. Pigs swallow them with contaminated feed or water." When not present in large numbers it appears to cause no harm — when there are large numbers it may take advantage of low debility of the host to cause symptoms.

At any rate pigs with bloody diarrhoea should be segregated or destroyed and the premises disinfected (page 215).

In the very early stages oil of chenopodium (page 673), phenothiazine (page 689), and a milk diet have been recommended.

Balantidiosis of swine may bear a relationship to a human dysentery. Human infestation has apparently been cured by the use of an arsenical compound, known as carbarsone ($C_7H_9AsN_2O_4$), which is classed as an antiprotozoan. One treatment was sufficient in 50 per cent of those treated, a second treatment cured the re-maining 50 per cent. The remedy has not been used in animals because of lack of a positive diagnosis, and be-cause other bloody dysenteries spread so rapidly.

PART TEN

Miscellaneous Information

⚶⚶⚶⚶

CHAPTER XXXIII

SOME SPECIAL METHODS OF DIAGNOSIS

Accurate animal disease diagnosis offers many exceedingly complex problems. The knowledge regarding the normal animal, and the animal in ill-health has during the latest decades been enormously increased. With it has come the realization that there can be no animal disease control until the exact nature of the problem is understood. Paradoxical as it may seem, increased knowledge has caused greater difficulty in arriving at precise diagnoses, though it cannot be disputed that this has resulted in a much better final solution and handling of the problems.

The diagnosis of animal diseases is a complex problem

Many of the facilities for the making of these refined diagnoses are usually available only in the larger private and public laboratories. Here also are the specialized technicians that have frequently devoted a lifetime of study to certain particular phases of animal disease. It is therefore natural that the aid of these laboratories and their staffs are sought when unusual difficulties arise. It must be said to the credit of the practitioner of veterinary medicine that he has demonstrated an almost uncanny ability based

Laboratory aids are sometimes needed

757

on broad experience and training to solve in the field by clinical methods most of the very abstruse problems presented to him. A brief statement about some of the special diagnostic methods follows.

Blood tests. (1) The agglutination test is one in which a small graduated quantity of either whole blood or blood serum derived from an animal suspected of being affected with certain disease has added to it a definite amount of a reagent known as an antigen. This reagent consists of a suspension of a homogeneous nature of the specific germ causing the disease for the diagnosis of which the test is to be conducted. A reaction consists in loss of motility, and aggregation, agglutination or clumping of the specific germs. The reaction is based on the fact that when a germ invades the animal body it produces in the blood of that animal a certain specific substance known as

During recent years blood tests are extensively employed in the diagnosis of animal diseases

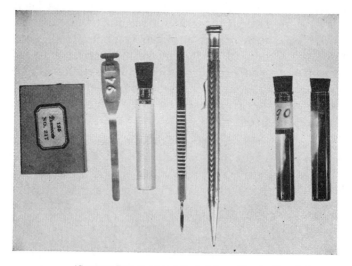

(Courtesy Department of Bacteriology, Kansas State University)

FIG. 202. Materials necessary for bleeding birds for the agglutination test: (1) Labels; (2) Leg bands; (3) Glass vial; (4) Bleeding knife; (5) Pencil; (6) Vials filled showing slant of clot and labeled vial.

an agglutinin which has the power of causing agglutination or clumping of the causative germ. Each germ stimulates the production of its own agglutinin, or this agglutinin will cause clumping only of the germ that stimulated its development in the blood. There are several modifications of the agglutination test but the basic principle is the same in all. The test is generally used in the diagnosis of Bang's disease (page 578), pullorum disease of fowl (Fig. 170) (page 651), and others. (2) The complement-fixation is also a blood test. It is much more complicated than the agglutination test, and is therefore less frequently employed. (For details consult standard textbooks on bacteriology, and serology.) In veterinary medicine it is used to a limited extent in the diagnosis of glanders. (3) The precipitation test consists in bringing together a specially prepared antigen or bacterial reagent and the suspected serum. Different types of reactions occur such as the formation of a cloudy zone at the point of contact of the two fluids; or uniform turbidity of the fluids; or the formation of a precipitate or deposit in the bottom of the test tube. The precipitation test is sometimes used in the diagnosis of anthrax (page 591), glanders (page 614), and swine erysipelas (page 620). A test for Bang's disease (page 578) applied to the milk known as the "Ring Test" (page 582) has in it the possibility of assisting considerably in the control of this disease.

The allergic tests are accurate, and much used *Allergic reactions or tests.* These are exemplified in veterinary practice by the tuberculin tests (page 598), and the mallein tests (page 614) used in the diagnosis of tuberculosis and glanders. These are highly accurate tests. A comparable test for the diagnosis of Bang's disease in cattle is seldom employed because of its lack of accuracy; abortin is the name of the diagnostic agent.

Animal inoculation tests. In these tests some diseased animal tissue is injected into a test animal such

as a guinea pig, rabbit, pigeon, white
These are usually tests of last resort mouse or rat, and occasionally into a more expensive large animal such as a dog, hog, cow, or horse. The purpose is an attempt to reproduce the suspected disease in the test animal. The diseased tissue or material is injected into the test animal either intravenously, intracranially or intracerebrally, intraperitoneally, intramuscularly, subcutaneously, intraocularly, or by other routes. It is considered to be a highly accurate method of diagnosis. Its chief disadvantage is the delay occasioned by the time it requires for the disease to develop in the test animal. It is, therefore, not in many instances a practical method. When large animals are used for testing purposes it is expensive. It is the most reliable test for the diagnosis of such diseases as swamp fever of horses (page 553), anaplasmosis of cattle (page 744), and hog cholera. It is extensively used in the diagnosis of rabies, swine erysipelas, tuberculosis, and others.

Feeding tests. It frequently happens that animals become ill and may even die, because of the consumption of suspected animal foods. In these **Feeding tests may be applied by any intelligent person** instances it is not possible in the comparatively brief time at the disposal of the person handling the investigation to conduct a detailed examination that would lead to the disclosure of the exact substance in the feed that is harmful. Under the circumstances the best that can be done is to feed the suspected material en masse to some laboratory animals, or better still to some animals of the same species as those that originally sickened. Usually the least valuable animal in a herd is selected for such a feeding test. The suspected feed should be fed under the same conditions and in the same daily amounts as that suspected of causing the trouble in the beginning. It must usually be continued for ten days or two weeks, and during this period the suspected feed must not be consumed by other valuable animals.

Occasionally harmful qualities in animal foods are more harmful to some species than others, so that the latter may be used as test animals, they giving early warnings of approaching trouble. This is exemplified in the so-called "rabbit test" (page 463) for sweet clover poisoning. Feeding tests are also employed in the testing of moldy corn poisoning in horses (page 470), forage poisoning (page 469) and others.

Biopsy. This signifies a detailed examination of tissues, normal or diseased, excised from the living body. It is a method frequently used for **An examination of abnormal tissues** diagnosis of tumors and other tissues that are easily accessible for surgical removal. In humans, less rarely in animals— though equally applicable in the latter, a biopsy may be resorted to in an attempt to determine whether or not the patient's infertility is due to a pathological condition in the testes; the test is known as "gonadal biopsy" (page 761).

Chemical tests. These are frequently resorted to for the diagnosis of a large variety of animal diseases. In cases of suspected chemical poisoning the stomach contents may be analyzed, or for that matter any tissue **Chemical tests are of great value in the diagnosis of animal ailments** in which the poison is likely to be deposited. Urine is frequently examined chemically for the presence of sugar, albumen, ketones (page 507), and other evidences of disease that are likely to manifest themselves there. Blood is frequently subjected to a chemical analysis to determine its mineral composition, especially in phosphorus and calcium. A chemical test of saliva of race horses to determine if they have been "doped" previous to racing is available (page 821). The description of the use of chemical tests in the diagnosis of disease and for other purposes may almost be extended indefinitely.

Pregnancy tests. During recent years these tests have been employed with increasing frequency though not so well established in animals as in the human female. In the latter the Friedman test which is a modification of the Zondek-Aschheim test has become almost standard. In general it consists of the injection into the blood stream of a virgin rabbit of a small amount of urine derived from the person to be tested. A positive reaction consists in certain well defined changes such as enlargement, hemorrhage, and fresh lutein cells in the ovaries of the rabbit, the latter having been anaesthetized, and her abdomen surgically opened 24 to 30 hours following the injection of the urine. If the reaction is negative there are no ovarian changes.

In animals the pregnancy tests are at this time limited in their application almost entirely to the mare. There are two types of tests, the one a chemical test of the urine—the Cuboni test—of the animal to be examined, and the second a biological test of the mare's blood serum. This latter is very similar in its details to the Friedman test in humans, differing only in that blood serum is used as a testing fluid rather than the urine. This test is applicable only between the 45th and 90th day following service. Following the 90th day a veterinarian can usually make a diagnosis about the pregnant or non-pregnant condition of a mare by a physical examination. The diagnosis previous to the 90th day is frequently of value as it may be desired to submit a barren mare to another service at the earliest possible time. From Japan there is a report that a diagnosis of pregnancy in the mare may be established fifteen days after conception by pressing a glass side against the os uteri externum (opening to the uterus.) If the mare is pregnant the slide on naked eye examination will disclose a thick tenacious, white, glossy mucus. If not

Pregnancy tests have a limited value in animals

pregnant the collection on the slide is thin, watery and almost transparent.

Autopsy; necropsy; post-mortem. This is an examination of the internal organs of a dead body for the

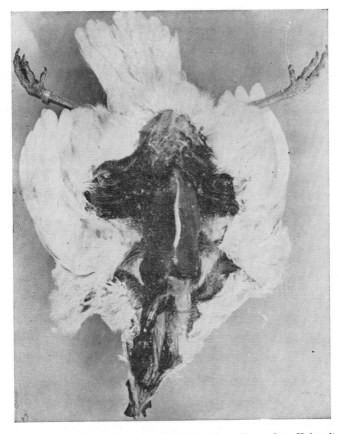

(Courtesy Department of Bacteriology, Kansas State University)

FIG. 203. Lower surface of the fowl's body in preparation for a post mortem examination. The skin has been dissected away. Also shown are the legs broken away from body.

An examination made of the organs of a dead animal is a source of valuable information

purpose of determining the cause of death, or of studying the abnormal conditions that may be present (Figs. 203 and 204). In the diagnosis of animal ailments it is very generally resorted to because the life of the individual is not of as great value as that of the flock or herd; therefore, it is not uncommon to kill a sick animal for autopsy purposes in order that the lives of the group may be safeguarded. Furthermore, there is no objection in animals to the more or less extensive mutilation necessary for a thorough examination.

It is never safe for the uninformed to open an animal carcass (Fig. 204) if the general nature of the disease is not understood (page 228). It may be a method of spreading highly contagious diseases, or the operator may expose himself to a dangerous infection.

Partial autopsy. Frequently an autopsy is performed simply to confirm or "clinch" an ante mortem diagnosis. In these instances the nature of

A limited or partial post mortem examination is frequently all that is needed to establish a diagnosis

the disease is fairly well understood so that the technician needs only a portion of the dead animal's body. A good example of this type of an autopsy is the examination conducted to determine whether death was the result of rabies (page 544). The head of the suspected animal only is needed as the changes of rabies if present are located in the brain.

Parasite identification. If a skin disease is suspected to be due to a parasite—especially mange conditions—it is a simple matter to brush away all the superficial skin debris on a small area; then apply a few drops of

Skin parasites

olive oil or mineral oil to the area, and then by means of a dull knife-edge scrape the part until a little blood is drawn. Place all these scrapings in a small bottle or box and send it to the veterinarian for a microscopic examination.

If information is desired with regard to the presence or absence of intestinal parasites place a small quantity of the animal's stool in a box.

Stool or fecal examinations Through an examination of this material —usually by the so-called flotation test— it is possible to locate parasite eggs, and

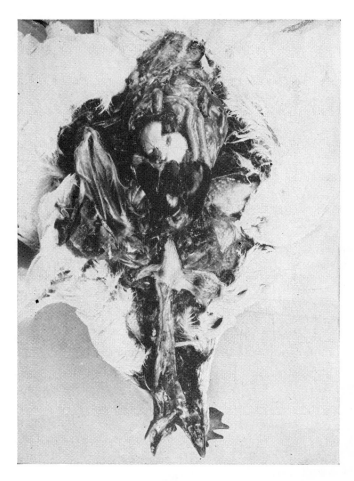

(Courtesy Department of Bacteriology, Kansas State University)

FIG. 204. A post mortem examination showing the fowl's internal organs after the skin, muscles and bone have been dissected away.

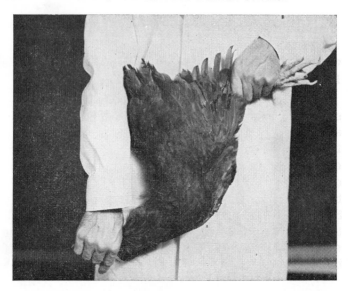

(Courtesy Department of Bacteriology, Kansas State University)

Fig. 205. Method for breaking a bird's neck preliminary to a post mortem examination.

by means of their identification determine the parasite from which they originated.

When a beast has died it may be desirable to learn whether a parasite is responsible—as in lung worms (page 678), coccidiosis (page 735), and certain other small parasites. Simply remove a piece of the involved tissue, place it in a wide-mouthed clean glass container, pour ten per cent formalin (page 266) on it, and take it or send it to the laboratory.

Rabies or dog madness   Veterinary laboratorians are frequently called upon to examine the brain of an animal that has been killed or died because of suspected rabies (pages 327 and 544). Usually these are either dog's heads or the heads of other biting animals. Occasionally the heads of larger animals—horses, cattle, swine and sheep—are also presented for a laboratory examination. If it is at all possible, and unless there is need for quick action, it is best to permit the suspected animal to die naturally rather than to kill it before brain lesions have had an opportunity to develop. The veterinarian and the physician should be consulted about this matter.

It is always undesirable to destroy the animal by shooting it through the brain as that practically destroys the evidence for laboratory purposes. The head, for rabies examination, should be packed in a double container, properly refrigerated, and sent to the laboratory by the most direct and quickest route. Laboratories are frequently closed on Saturday afternoon and Sunday so telephonic or other wire connections should be established with the laboratory to insure that there will be some one to accept the shipment and to give it the necessary attention.

In the case of diseased poultry ship or send living fowls being reasonably certain that the birds reach the laboratory in the living state. Always send **Poultry ex-** more than one bird so that there will be **aminations** plenty of material for the laboratorian. Do not send fowl tissues because of their rapid decomposition. If dead fowl are sent refrigerate them as already described in a preceding paragraph dealing **Help the** with rabies. Always help the laboratorian **laboratorian** by giving him as complete a history as possible of the outbreak; this should be done in all instances where laboratory aid is sought.

Many animal diseases, brucellosis (page 578), anthrax (page 591), anaplasmosis (page 744), leptospirosis (page 535), swamp fever (page **Blood** 553), hog cholera (page 616), and others **specimens** can be diagnosed following a laboratory examination of the animal's blood. However, the collection of blood specimens and many tissue specimens necessitating the opening of a cadaver is so fraught with danger to the operator, and from the standpoint of spreading contagious diseases, that it should be attempted by none other than the trained veterinarian.

During recent years the scope of diagnostic work has been much enlarged by two developments: (1) Photomicrography, and (2) the electron microscope.

A photograph of very small objects

Photomicrography: This is the photographing of objects so small that it requires a microscope to make them visible. Formerly a hobby, it was inevitable that photography should become an adjunct of the microscope. Photomicrography must not be confused with microphotography—this latter consists of minute photographs that can be seen in detail only under a microscope.

The electron microscope is an instrument which magnifies to an almost unbelievable degree. The virus of foot-and-mouth disease (page 605)—it is one of the smallest of all viruses in that it is in the order of ten millimicrons in diameter—a micron is one-millionth of a meter, and a millimicron is a thousandth part of a micron—indicates the power of magnification of the electron microscope. The bacteriophages (page 250) have actually been observed by means of this high magnification; the phages look like tadpoles, swimming vigorously toward bacteria, entering the latter, and destroying them in a matter of minutes.

CHAPTER XXXIV

ARTIFICIAL FEEDING OF ORPHANED ANIMALS

The feeding of newly born orphaned domesticated animals is frequently attempted, but not entirely with success because of the many and varied factors that are involved.

Newly born orphaned animals need artificial feeding

It is an established fact that in the nutrition of young animals milk derived from a member of its own species is always superior to that from others. This at once sets up a serious obstacle in the artificial feeding of all young creatures excepting the calf because cows' milk is the basis of almost all artificial feeds. A comparison for example (after Henry and Morrison) of the composition of milk of the cow, ewe, sow, and mare is as follows:

	Water Per Cent	Mineral Matter Per Cent	Protein Per Cent	Sugar Per Cent	Fat Per Cent
Cow.......	87.2	0.7	3.5	4.9	3.7
Ewe.......	80.8	0.9	6.5	4.9	6.9
Sow.......	81.0	1.0	5.9	5.4	6.7
Mare......	90.6	0.4	2.0	5.9	1.1

In addition to the above named ingredients milk also contains vitamins essential for the growth of the young.

In artificial feeding *there is danger of overfeeding.* The general rule to follow is to have the young creature still hungry when it has taken its allotted amount. There is far more danger in overfeeding than in underfeeding in the case of newly born creatures. Dur-

Danger in over-feeding

769

ing the first few days of life the feeding should be comparatively frequent—at least every two hours—and gradually reducing this to three to four times per day.

For the very young animal *it is advisable to heat the milk to body temperature,* especially during the colder seasons of the year. The attendant must exercise his judgment in this matter, based largely on his personal eating experiences.

One of the gravest errors in the artificial feeding of young animals *is a disregard for cleanliness.* The
Cleanliness is very important food, the utensils in which it is stored, those from which it is fed, and its handling *must be as scrupulously clean* as in the artificial feeding of the human infant. Otherwise diarrhoea and digestive disturbances are certain to follow.

It is generally held to be advisable, if possible, for the newly-born to receive the first milk (colostrum)
The mother's first milk is believed to protect against infections (consult page 540 for Link's "kafmalak") secreted by its mother. It is lower in water content and sugar, and higher in protein, largely because of the albumen and globulin, and fat. The belief that colostrum confers measurable immunity against infections during the highly susceptible period of early life is well substantiated because of the high concentration in colostrum of globulin, similar to blood globulin—the latter being a blood protein fraction that carries protective antibodies. For example, the blood of the newly born calf is very low in blood globulin but the amount rises quickly after a feeding of colostrum. When skim milk instead of colostrum milk is fed the globulin content of the blood remains low for some time.

In the case of foals (Gamble et al, U. S. D. A.) it has been found that if during the first 18 hours of a foal's life, instead of colostrum, the young creature is fed on "1000 cc. of horse serum incorporated in a mix-

Substitutes for colostrum
ture of dried whole cow's milk, dried skim milk, sugar and water that the foals suffer no apparent ill effects from failure to receive colostrum." On the other hand three foals fed only the dried-milk mixture as substitutes for the dam's colostrum developed joint ill (page 537) and died within two weeks after their birth.

Cow colostrum fed to lambs is a fairly good substitute for ewe's colostrum; however, lambs fed during the first 24 hours of life on sheep's serum having incorporated in the whole-milk mixture did better than those fed cow's colostrum substituted for ewe's colostrum. The evidence seems to be then that newly-born animals that do not receive colostrum or a substitute for it frequently succumb in a few days as a result of some infection. *A reliable substitute is the oral or subcutaneous administration of from one to eight ounces of blood serum* depending upon the size of the young creature, derived preferably from its mother; if not obtainable from this source it should at least be from a member of the same species.

Feeding of orphaned colts. Fresh cow's milk, preferably with a low butter fat content, is the basis of the food. Dissolve a heaping teaspoonful

Colts need their milk with sugar and lime water added
of sugar in as little warmed water as possible. To this add two tablespoonfuls of lime water. Add enough cow's milk to make the total measure one pint. Let the colt have one-fourth of this every two hours for three days. Gradually increase the amount and decrease the number of daily feedings. When the animal has reached one month of age the sugar may be left out of the ration. The whole milk may gradually be changed to skim milk at six weeks of age, and at three months of age the colt may be allowed three daily feeds of as much skim milk as it will drink. In addition to the foregoing, and as soon as it will take it, the colt should be allowed some solid food such as linseed

oil meal, oatmeal, corn or oats chops, alfalfa leaves and green grass. At six months of age the colt should be on an exclusively solid ration.

Another somewhat similar, though simpler, formula for the artificial feeding of orphan colts consists of equal parts of cow's milk, boiled water, a tablespoonful of sugar, and a tablespoonful of lime water. The method of feeding is similar to that of the formula in the preceding paragraph.

Cow's milk which is the natural food for calves is abundantly available, though it must be fed in limited amounts and in a clean manner

Feeding of orphaned calves: milk replacements and "starters" (page 51) and "kafmalak" (page 540). This also offers certain problems that are frequently disregarded or overlooked as evidenced by the very common appearance of scours and unthriftiness in artificially fed calves. Excluding infectious white scours (page 538) much of the scouring in newly born calves is the result of *overfeeding, and a lack of cleanliness in feeding.* The regimen recommended on page 540 is a satisfactory one, provided each calf has its individual thoroughly clean feeding utensil, and if, by muzzling, the closely confined animal is prevented from licking and consuming extraneous matter such as soiled bedding and intestinal discharges. When out-of-doors away from animal habitations many of these latter problems disappear.

At one month of age skim milk may gradually be substituted for whole milk. In season it is desirable to permit the calf to nibble grass, or during the winter months some succulent material such as cabbage leaves, alfalfa leaves, carrots and their tops, and comparable material may be fed. All woody and indigestible foods are to be avoided. The liquid food should be limited at all times as overfeeding is likely to prove fatal. As the calf shows a desire for it small quantities of ground grains may be allowed.

Feeding orphaned lambs (page 772). The simplest

method is to provide a foster mother. Usually there is in the flock a nursing ewe with an abundant milk supply or one with a single lamb that will by the exercise of persistence and care adopt the orphan. Smearing the orphan with the afterbirth or with some of the fluids of parturition results in its more ready acceptance by a foster mother. At other times the foster ewe must be physically restrained during nursing by the orphan.

A foster mother should be provided

Failing in the attempt to supply a foster mother, sheep's serum incorporated in a whole milk mixture (page 772) may be used, or cow's milk enriched with cream may be used. The addition of a teaspoonful of lime water to each feeding is desirable. During the first week of life not more than two tablespoonfuls should be given at a feeding, though this should be repeated once every two hours. At two or three weeks of age three daily feedings are enough. The food should be at body temperature. It may be given by means of a human nursing bottle and nipple. When about two weeks old additional solid food in the form of small amounts of mixtures of concentrates may be made available in a lamb-creep. At this age the lamb will also begin to nibble at soft forage.

Lambs need milk rich in fat

Feeding orphaned pigs (milk substitutes in the raising of pigs, page 52). The best plan is to have a nursing sow adopt the orphans. Usually she will accept them if they are placed with the foster mother when her own pigs are nursing. In the absence of a foster mother sweet whole milk from the cow, fed six to eight times daily by means of a human nursing bottle, or out of a flat pan, at body temperature, with the addition of a teaspoonful of lime water to each feeding is most satisfactory. As soon as possible they should be taught to partake of suitable concen-

Sweet whole cow's milk is satisfactory for pigs

trates in addition to the liquid diet. Yellow corn, tankage, and a salt-mineral mixture should be provided free choice. The addition of one raw egg daily to the permissible quart of cow's milk is beneficial.

Feeding orphaned puppies. Two tablespoonfuls of top milk (cream), two tablespoonfuls of sterile water, one teaspoonful of "sugar of milk," and one teaspoonful of lime-water. At one week of age add the yolk of one raw egg to the formula. Feed every two to four hours (Zepp in the June 1, 1944 number of the Bul. of the Kans. Veterinary Medical Association.)

Artificial foods for puppies should be rich in fat content

CHAPTER XXXV

METHODS OF ADMINISTERING MEDICINES TO ANIMALS

The administration of medicines or other substances is usually against the animal's will. If improperly performed the act may result in serious losses. It was rumored, for example, that during the great horse plague of 1912 on the western plains more horses died as a sequence of improper oral administration of linseed oil than from the disease itself.

Care required in administering medicine

Medicines may be administered through various channels: by way of the mouth or digestive tract; injected directly into the blood; injected under, and into the skin; introduced into the rectum; and rubbed into the skin. The first named method, by the mouth, is the one most frequently resorted to by livestock producers. It is designated as "drenching."

Channels for administering medicine

In *horses* that are accustomed to being handled the best method of administering medicines by those who have had no special training in this work is by the oral route. The medicine must be in liquid form. If the medicine is non-liquid, it must be made so by dissolving it in or mixing it with a liquid such as water, milk or one of the bland oils—raw linseed oil, mineral oil (liquid petrolatum) and others. The liquid medicine is put in a long necked bottle preferably of the collapsible rubber type, though because of ease of procurement it is most frequently of glass. In using the latter due care must be taken to avoid breaking by the horse's teeth. The horse to be medicated is placed in a single stall, and its head elevated by means of a slip-noose

Giving medicine to a horse

made of sash cord or a comparable substitute placed around the upper incisor teeth with the other end passed over an overhead rafter.

The head should be pulled up just enough so that liquids poured into the mouth will flow backward towards the stomach. Excessive head elevation causes the animal to strangle more easily. The medicine is then poured into the mouth by first passing the neck of the bottle through the side of the animal's mouth. Be certain to keep the bottle away from the incisor or molar teeth to avoid breaking of the bottle. The medicine is then slowly poured into the animal's mouth.

Coughing on the part of the animal when medicine is being given by way of the mouth is an indicator of trouble

If at any time during this step the animal coughs, its head must immediately be lowered as coughing is a symptom that the medicine is going into the lungs instead of the stomach. Any medicine finding its way into the lungs is almost certain to result in a fatal lung fever.

Some horses, because of debility or illnesses involving the brain, and throat paralysis, give no sign of the passage of medicines into the lungs. Therefore careful operators always permit the animal to depress its head frequently during the administration process and under no circumstance is an animal to be drenched during brain diseases and when affected with paralysis of the throat. Some horses swallow readily while others simply permit the medicine to stand in the mouth until this runs over.

Horses that will not swallow may safely be made to do so by pouring teaspoonful amounts of clean water into the nose. Never pour anything other than clean cold water into the animal's nose, and be cautious even about the use of water as a very small amount is sufficient to make the animal swallow. Pouring medi-

Do not rub an animal's throat

cines into an animal's nose is almost certain to be followed by an attack of fatal lung-fever. Neither is it permissible to rub an animal's throat in an endeavor to make it swallow, as this practice usually induces coughing so that some of the medicine may reach the lungs and the rest of it is expelled from the mouth.

Veterinarians prefer to administer medicine by previously passing a stomach tube and pumping it in, or for quicker results from the use of non-bulky, completely soluble drugs injected under the skin, or directly into the blood stream. If well done these methods obviate the danger of medication-lung fever.

Giving medicine to cattle

Cattle are more easily drenched as a rule than are horses because they swallow more readily. The steps in the administration of medicines to cattle by the mouth and otherwise, and the care and precautions to be followed are essentially the same as in horses with this exception in the oral administration that their heads are not elevated by means of a rope. The approved method is for the operator to stand alongside the animal's neck facing forward. The nostrils are grasped between the thumb and fingers, with the forearm resting on the front of the animal's face to function as a lever—the animal's poll is the fulcrum—so that the mouth may be pulled upward to receive the medicine.

More than usual care must be taken in administering medicine to sheep

Sheep must frequently be medicated especially in the treatment for stomach worm infestation. If precautions were necessary in the oral giving of medicines to horses and cattle, then these must be redoubled in sheep as it is not uncommon for almost immediate death to take place following drenching because of the passage of all the medicine into the lungs. The old and time proved injunction to permit sheep to remain standing on all four feet, and never to raise the animal's nose higher than the level of its eyes during the drenching process cannot be emphasized too strongly. A funnel, a piece of rubber tubing four feet long and having a piece of metal tubing from six to 12 inches long and being of a diameter to slip into the end of the rubber tubing, the funnel being fitted into the other end, is the equipment needed. The metal tube is inserted into the animal's mouth—it may chew on it if it wishes to do so, and the correct dose of the medicine is then slowly poured into the funnel. If large numbers of sheep are to be medicated a measuring device may be placed in the pathway of the medicine. In sheep, up to 2 ounces of medicine may be given with a bulb dose syringe, simply by holding the nose shut with the left hand, and injecting the medicine far back in the mouth, and releasing the nose immediately after dosing. The animal is to be on all fours.

Hogs are very difficult to medicate as individuals, and in general this should be left in the hands of the veterinarian. Many medicines, especially those that are not too pungent and bad tasting, may be given in the feed. It is best to starve the animals for 24 to 36 hours. They should be divided into lots of 12 or less, and the individual members of the lot should be approximately the same weight. The medicine is intimately mixed with a thin slop, the number of doses corresponding to the number of hogs in the lot that are to be simultaneously treated. Each member of the lot will receive about the correct dosage. Veterinarians also administer medicines to individual hogs, in capsule form, by means of a speculum to hold the mouth open and a "balling" gun to place the capsule far back in the mouth. Inexperienced laymen have attempted to do this, but instead of getting the medicine into the gullet, it is deposited in a recess just above the origin of the gullet in the wall

As individuals hogs are difficult to medicate. Medicine, in the hands of the amateur, is best given mixed with the food

of the pharynx, where it causes a severe inflammation manifested by swelling of the throat, and frequently death.

Another method of medicating hogs is to place a piece of metal tubing in the mouth through which a stomach tube is passed into the stomach, and then the medicine injected through it by means of a syringe. Even in the hands of the expert these latter methods of hog medication give rise to difficulties such as the necessary handling of very large swine, or of pregnant sows with the possibility of inducing abortion, and hogs have the ability to readily vomit material not to their liking—this being most likely to take place when nauseating drugs are placed into a starved stomach. Taken as a whole then, and unless otherwise directed by a veterinarian, the inexperienced person had best limit his attempts to medicate hogs to the method first described.

Dogs must frequently be restrained forcibly in order to administer medicines orally and therefore an assistant is needed to grasp the forelegs and at the same time allow his arms to press lightly against the animal's ribs. The medicine may be given from a spoon or from a bottle which has an extension on it consisting of a piece of rubber tubing, the latter being safe to get between the teeth. The necessary preparations having been made, one of the angles of the lips is grasped and pulled out in such a manner as to result in the formation of a distinct pocket within the cheek into which the medicine is poured in small quantities at a time. If the dog will not swallow, pinch the nostrils shut so as to shut off his breath which is usually effective, but in a very stubborn dog, it may start coughing and when this occurs the animal should be freed quickly until normal breathing is re-established after which the operation may be repeated.

In giving capsules or tablets to a dog the operator

must first grasp the upper jaw from above with the thumb and forefinger and press the cheeks against the gums just back of the corner teeth which will force the mouth open. The tablet or capsule is then placed as far back as possible on the tongue by means of the fingers or a pair of forceps and after withdrawing the hand or forceps, the mouth is tightly and rapidly closed. After it has gulped two or three times examine the mouth to ascertain if the medicine has been swallowed.

Medicines without a disagreeable taste may also be given in the food either by mixing intimately with the food or tablets may be concealed in a small ball of meat. Experts whenever possible resort to subcutaneous or intravenous medication.

Cats are even more difficult for laymen to medicate than are dogs. Their mouths are so diminutive and their cheeks so devoid of elasticity that it **Cats because of having a small mouth are difficult to medicate** is impossible to create a pocket in which to lodge the medicine. Furthermore their claws are most efficient organs of defense. In order to overcome these difficulties liquid medicine may be incorporated in the food, but it must be tasteless or nearly so, and the cat must not see the medicine or the container when the dose is prepared as it will at once arouse its suspicions. If it is offered to the animal at its regular meal time there is a greater chance of success. Such drugs as mineral oil, olive oil, and castor oil may be added to pieces of canned salmon or sardines; arsenic in the form of Fowler's solution, aspirin, bismuth salts, and calomel may be added to a little milk. By means of a medicine dropper small quantities of liquid drugs may sometimes be successfully administered by way of the very small cheek pouch, or a tablet may be placed on the back of the tongue with a pair of forceps. Liquid medicine is usually given as to dogs. If the cat does not swallow at once rub a moistened finger across pussy's lips and almost at once it will make tongue lapping motions indicating swallowing. A cat-bag, or a towel wrapped around the animal is the method of restraint. A cat resents foreign odor, therefore the operator should approach the animal for handling with thoroughly washed hands.

Fowls. Administering medicines to sick **fowls** (Fig. 206) is not encouraged as it is not likely to be

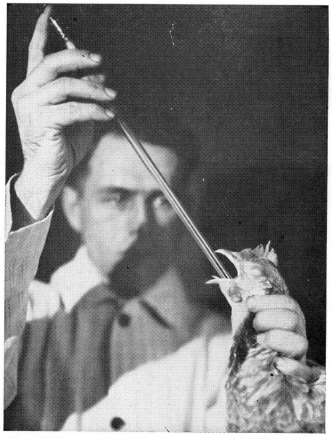

(Courtesy Dept. of Bacteriology, Kansas State University)

Fig. 206. Using a pipette in administering medicine to **a fowl.**

profitable, and it is seldom completely beneficial. In fact it may be positively harmful in maintaining a "carrier" (page 210) in the flock.

Medicating fowl is as a general rule not to be encouraged

If treatment is decided upon, solid drugs may be placed in a capsule, or in tablet form, and then pushed back into the mouth. In flock treatment a powdered drug such as some of the worm expellers may be mixed with a dry mash. Soluble solids such as epsom salts and copper sulphate may be added to the drinking water. All water is withheld the evening before the medication and until 9:00 a.m. the next day when the fowl are permitted access to the medicated water. In an hour they will have taken their fill, and fresh water is to replace the medicated. Liquid drugs in small quantities may also be given by passing a piece of rubber tubing, via the mouth, into the crop, then attaching a funnel or dose-syringe to the free exposed end and by this means introducing the medicine.

In giving medicines to animals be patient, avoid unnecessary haste, give the animal plenty of time to swallow, and above all don't get it into the windpipe and lungs as the final outcome is likely to be a dead animal.

CHAPTER XXXVI

LIVESTOCK BREEDING PROBLEMS

The value of a breeding herd is largely nullified if the semi-annual or annual crop of young is not up to a high average. It is too much to expect **A 100** each female to reproduce her kind up to **per cent crop** a maximum efficiency of 100 per cent, **of young is** though this is the breeder's ideal, and the **the breeder's** more it is departed from the less profitable **ideal** is the venture.

Sterility in either male or female is defined as un-productiveness, or inability to reproduce their kind. It is also designated infertility, and bar-**Barrenness** renness. Some animals are said to be bar-**or sterility** ren, though actually they conceive, but **is inability** expel the young when it is still so small **to produce** that the act passes unobserved. One au-**young** thority has introduced the phrase "the unseen disappearance of a fertilized ovum" as one of the conditions that may be included under the general designation of sterility. Usually the non-technical person defines sterility as a condition in which the normal mating of apparently healthy animals is not followed by conception. If a certain male fails to settle the females bred to him he is usually the one at fault, or on the other hand if a female does not settle to the service of a certain male, though other females do conceive from him then the female is the one at fault.

Sterility may be the result of any one or more of a large number of conditions including age, environment,

Barrenness may be either temporary or permanent
diet, season of the year, hybrids, disease and various other factors. Some of these factors are such as to result in permanent sterility, while others are of a more temporary character. It is an established fact that reproduction cannot take place if there exists a diseased condition of the genital organs. To continue for example, to subject a female with an abnormal discharge from the genitals to repeated services in the hope that she will settle is basing expectations on false premises. Healthy young cannot be incubated in, or produced from, sexually diseased parents.

The nature, amount and kind of food needed by a pregnant animal is a question frequently raised. The simplest answer is that the food of a pregnant animal need differ in no respect from the well balanced adequate ration of the non-pregnant—with the possible exception that as pregnancy advances more food must be offered to meet the needs of the growing young as well as of the mother. Some of the essentials of good feeding are described on pages 30 to 62 inclusive, and those constituents that are most frequently absent, such as vitamins and minerals, on pages 60 to 105. Also if the growing and developing young has improper food (Chapters IV and V) and management, it cannot develop into a healthy vigorous breeder; in other words the production of germ cells will be so delayed that the inception of vigorous breeding life is correspondingly delayed or even permanently impaired.

What food is needed by a pregnant animal?

Good management under reasonably sanitary conditions, sufficient exercise and exposure to direct sunshine must not be overlooked. Excessive fatness, especially in show animals will so lower the breeding efficiency of an animal that its value for this purpose is inhibited or lost. High "show condition" and high breeding efficiency simply do not mix.

The animal owner is frequently perplexed in his attempt to solve the question of the best breeding season. When carefully analyzed it resolves **What is the best breeding season?** itself into a conflict between nature's time, and man's desires to regulate the process for his own pecuniary benefit. In nature's plan grazing animals usually are bred rather late in the spring months when the female has had an opportunity to replenish her general condition including sexual well-being by the abundant feeding on lush vitamin-rich vegetation. In this plan parturition occurs early during the next spring months.

In a general way—without reference to the specific causes of low fertility—the practice of breeding females at the very first opportunity following **Breeding rest very important** parturition undoubtedly is an important factor in destroying high reproductive efficiency. Sexual moderation and rest are among the best preventives of genital diseases. Excesses result in loss of sexual vigor and health. For example, the cow should have a breeding rest of from sixty to ninety days following each parturition. Comparable rest periods are appropriate for other animals.

For economical reasons in the domesticated animals, cows are frequently bred so as to calve late in the fall and thus be in maximum milk production during the winter months because this is, in general, a season of milk scarcity and therefore higher prices. Ewes, if they can be made to come in heat and to ovulate by the use of gonadin (a pregnant mare serum) —the former occurs though the occurrence of the latter is doubtful,— are bred to lamb late in the summer for the production of "hot-house" lambs for the Christmas trade. In concluding this paragraph it is well to warn that parturition at unseasonable periods necessitates special care and attention to safeguard the well-being of both the dam and her offspring. The dam usually has a shorter than normal time of sexual rest which predisposes her to barrenness, and the offspring is dropped during a season of the year when inclement weather predisposes to those respiratory and germ diseases that are incidental to the unnatural conditions of housing.

The age at which animals may best be used for breeding is a question often raised. The answer is that the vigor of a certain degree **What is the best breeding age?** of maturity is essential for the best and highest degree of reproductive efficiency. Unfortunately this simple answer is in conflict with man's desire for early and late financial returns from his breeding animals. Though young animals under domestication are most frequently violated against in breeding practices it is not uncommon to attempt to prolong the breeding usefulness of aged animals almost to the point of senility and usually with very unsatisfactory results such as failure to settle or conceive, abortion, retained afterbirth and weak offspring.

The onset of puberty duration of estrus (heat) etc. is about as follows:

Animal	Onset of Puberty	Estrus Number of Days after Parturition	Length of/ or Frequency of cycle	Duration of Estrus	Time of Ovulation
Mare	1–1½ yrs. (10–24 mo.)	9 days (7–11 days)	20–22 days	3–5 days variable	1–2 days before or near end of estrus.
Cow	6–18 mo.	15–60 days	18–21 days	16–19 hrs.	After estrus 12–19 hrs.
Ewe	8–15 mo.	6–7 mo. (next breeding season) nutrition and temperature have important influence.	15–18 days	12–30 hrs.	End of estrus
Sow	4–7 mo.	3–6 days Anestrus* till pigs are weaned.	18–21 days	1–2 days	Toward end of estrus
Bitch	7–10 mo.	6 mo.	3–6 mo.	9 days	Middle of estrus

(*Anestrus—no noticeable heat.)

Male animals of a species reach puberty at the same time as female or slightly later.

The normal duration of pregnancy in the domesticated animals is a moot question. There are many factors that apparently exert an influence upon the length of time that the young shall remain in the uterus. It is well known and conceded that diseased conditions frequently cause a premature termination of pregnancy, though it is not so generally understood that sexual ill-health may also prolong the intra-uterine existence as appears to be evidenced in those instances where as a sequence of disease in the uterus the young is not properly nourished and remains unborn for some time beyond the usual duration of pregnancy. Also the offspring of some sires remain in the uterus longer than those of others. Furthermore there appears to be greater irregularity in females that give birth to their first young. The state of nutrition of the mother, the sex of the unborn—longer for males than females—and even the vagaries of the weather such as prolonged unusual cold spells may have an influence upon the length of pregnancy.

The duration of pregnancy is important information

It is generally accepted that the following are approximately the pregnancy durations:

In the mare between 340 and 350 days with a maximum of 400 days.

In the cow the average duration is 283 days or somewhat over nine months, with a minimum of 260 days and a maximum of 300 days.

Sheep and goats carry their young for an average of 149 days, about five months, with a minimum of 145 days and a maximum of 157.

The sow is pregnant for an average of 120 days or four months with 110 days as a minimum and 120 as a maximum.

The bitch has an average duration of pregnancy of

63 days or nine weeks, with a minimum and maximum of 55 and 70 days respectively.

The cat is pregnant usually for eight weeks or 56 days, with minimum and maximum of 50 to 64 days.

The duration of incubation in farmyard birds is chicken 21 days; turkey 28 days; guinea 28 days; duck 28 days, (Muscovy duck 33 to 35 days); goose 28 to 30 days.

The late Prof. W. L. Williams of Cornell University devoted a very active life to the study of *bovine* reproduction. The six rules for high reproductive efficiency enunciated by him are as follows:

1. Hold as future breeders only those animals which are the progeny of healthy parents, that have been carried in uteri for a gestation period of from 279 to 288 days, and have been born without dystocia, retained afterbirth, or metritis.

2. Handle the newborn so that its health shall be assured, in order that it may enjoy uninterrupted development.

3. Withhold the young animal from breeding until amply mature.

4. Mate only individuals of general and sexual health. Employ only vigorous, mature sires.

5. Provide ample sexual rest between pregnancies.

6. Carefully avoid overloading the male.

FEMALE BARRENNESS AND SOME OF ITS CAUSES

This is a highly technical problem. It is discussed here in order that with a better understanding abuses frequently practiced by laymen may be avoided. In no other field is the technical training of the veterinarian so necessary.

Closed womb; imperforate neck of the uterus. This condition is more imaginary than real. It is men-

It is frequently an error to "open up" a non-breeding female

tioned here because of a practice frequently indulged in by charlatans which as they express it is a manipulation of the neck of the uterus of a barren cow or mare "to open her up" under the usually mistaken notion that this organ is so closed that it will not permit the passage of the male fertilizing element. Those practicing this device fail to recognize that the male element is of microscopic size and actively motile so that it can and does traverse a passageway so small that it would be imperceptible to the touch. They base their diagnosis on the fact that they cannot feel a perceptible passageway. They fail to recognize that the male element can readily pass through a digitally imperceptible channel.

In the cow the neck of the uterus in a state of health is a rigid tortuous passageway from two to three inches in length, and closed to the touch of the operator, though actually in almost all instances there is a passageway of sufficient size to permit the male

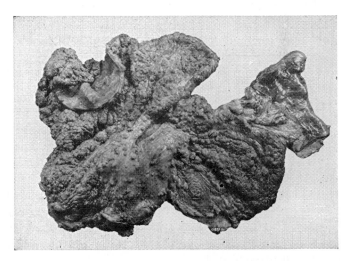

(Courtesy Dept. of Pathology, Kansas State University)

FIG. 207. Bovine uterus affected with tuberculosis; a possible cause of permanent barrenness.

element to pass through it. In the mare the neck of
the uterus is softer and more readily manipulated
than in the cow. In a filly it is usually closed to the
touch, but in older mares is quite open. This latter
leads many stallioners to the erroneous belief that all
mares, both young and old, should be equally open.

This entire unfortunate misconception of the true
state of the healthy uterine neck, has caused the breeding ruination of many females by attempts at forcible
dilation. Never permit anything of this nature to be
done excepting on the advice of the qualified graduate veterinarian.

Persistent hymen. The hymen is a fold or thin circular membrane in the genital tract located a short
distance forward from the outer opening
Surgical handling is necessary to overcome an imperforate hymen
of the vagina. It is occasionally present
in very young females and may be persistent up to the time of the first attempted breeding. The so-called persistent
hymen may be perforate or imperforate,
either of which may result in preventing
coitus. Furthermore, when imperforate, genital secretions may accumulate in the vagina so as to distend its
cavity. The persistent hymen is readily overcome by
surgical means.

Free-martin. This is a barren imperfect female
born twin to a male. The condition is most frequent
in the case of a heifer calf born twin to
A female calf born as a twin with a bull calf is almost always permanently barren
a bull. It may also occur in sheep, goats
and swine. The free-martin heifer to the
casual observer usually appears normal
and may even come in heat but seldom
does she settle to service. It is generally,
though not universally, accepted that the
barren state is due to unsexing of the female by a product of the testicles of the twin male, the
twins having a common blood supply so that testicular
hormones pass to the ovaries of the female to arrest

their development. In an examination of 74 twins—
one a male and the other a female—66 gave evidence
of a common blood supply and of these all the heifers
were barren. Eight did not have a common before birth
intra-uterine blood supply and all of the heifers later
settled to service. Free-martins are not curable, and
are usually slaughtered at an early age.

General or non-specific infections of the female
genital tract are prolific causes of barrenness. Usually
pus producing germs are the cause. It is
Infection a wise provision of nature that neither the
of the male nor female element can thrive in dis-
female eased surroundings. This important fact
organs is very frequently ignored as witnessed
of by repeated attempts to impregnate an
generation animal having genital organs so badly
is a cause diseased that there is a persistent dis-
of either charge of pus or other abnormal matter.
temporary Some animals do not present clear-cut
or evidence of these infections though their
permanent failure to conceive after several services
barrenness by a potent healthy male should arouse suspicion.
Such animals should be subjected to a careful examination by a veterinarian versed in the pathology of the genital tract. Other than a collection or
discharge of abnormal matter, which may involve any
part of the genitals from the outward opening to the
ovaries, infection or disease is evidenced by unusual
localized or general redness, and swelling of the involved area, and occasionally by partial denudation.

The point that it is desired to stress in the preceding paragraph is the futility of attempting to cause
impregnation where the "bed" or female genitals are
not qualified to receive the male element, or in case
fertilization does take place it is reasonably certain to
be followed by premature expulsion of the embryo.

At the time of the birth of their young, in all
species, a certain degree of non-specific infection of

Sexual rest is effective in minor infections in overcoming the infection naturally the uterus takes place, but if the animal is permitted to have a sexual rest period these minor infections clear up. Cattle need about three months. Occasionally the infection is more intense so that it does not clear up naturally though there is not always outward evidence of it.

In the case of cattle the first thing noticed is that after as many as three matings there still is no conception though other cows served by the same bull conceive promptly. Many of these cases conceive if a day or two following service the female is given an intra-uterine injection of a solution of an antibiotic (page 248). Veterinarians are fully familiar with the technique. If after such a treatment conception does not take place it indicates that the infection is too severe for the antibiotic to overcome. This method of handling is recommended only for apparently normal animals that fail to settle to at least three services. If it does not produce results the animal is in most cases to be sent to market for beef purposes.

Normally when a cow in heat is served, the sperm and ovum will meet and join in less than an hour after

When do sperm and ovum meet? service. This union takes place in the tube (fallopian tube) extending from each of the two ovaries to the horns of the uterus. It requires two or three days for the fertilized ovum to reach the horn of the uterus for permanent attachment and development. Therefore if the antibiotic treatment is used within a day or two following service there will be no interference with the fertilized ovum.

In the mare antibiotics and the sulfas have been helpful in treating infections of the genitalia but they do not control all of the many infections in the mare's organs of generation.

Specific diseases of the female genitals are also causes of barrenness in a manner similar to the gen-

Specific
diseased
conditions
of the
genitals
cause
barrenness

eral infections. Such diseases as tuberculosis (Fig. 207), (page 595); Hang's abortion disease (page 578); dourine (page 758) of horses; trichomoniasis (page 749), vibriosis (page 590) and others frequently localize in or involve the female organs of generation to inhibit conception. Frequently the only pronounced evidence of the presence of one of these diseases is the failure to settle to repeated services. If a correct diagnosis is established many, though not all, of these specific infectious diseases are found to be amenable to treatment so that the infected female will again become productive. Such treatment is seldom simple in character, requiring all the technical and professional resources of the trained person for its successful issue.

Diseases of the ovaries are frequent causes of barrenness in all domesticated females. The outstanding ones are retained or persistent corpora lutea or yellow bodies; cystic degeneration in the ovaries; and ovarian dysfunction.

1. *Yellow bodies* (page 102) on or in the ovaries are the physiological successors of egg laying or ovulation. If impregnation does not take place the yellow body under normal conditions gradually disappears, with the development of another yellow body at the next heat period or ovulation. On the other hand, if impregnation does occur the "yellow body" persists and serves as a physiological function in the development

There
is a
variety
of ovarian
diseases that
inhibit
conception

of the foetal membranes. If a yellow body is removed from the ovary of an animal during the earlier stages of pregnancy it is followed shortly by the expulsion of the fetus. When pregnancy is terminated normally or in some species even before this time, the "yellow body" disappears, so that the next post-partum heat period may appear. For a reason not fully understood after a heat period without impregnation, and also following a normal pregnancy, the yellow body does not disappear or shrink away with the result that no more heat periods or ovulations take place, and the affected animal as a consequence is temporarily barren.

The condition may be successfully handled by digital expression, or sometimes surgical excision, of the persistent yellow body. Such a step must not be hastily or imprudently performed as there are dangers in it. If however a non-pregnant animal goes for a prolonged time without the appearance of heat or ovulation, if there is no question about her non-pregnancy, if she is on an adequate ration, if she is free from harmful genital infections, and if she appears to be otherwise normal the operation of removing the "yellow body" may be practiced. Occasionally following this operation serious ovarian bleeding is an after-effect though the experienced technician will guard against this. Instead of this surgical handling the use of the synthetic hormone diethylstilbestrol (pages 104 and 415) is being used with a fair degree of success— as "heat" appears in less than forty-eight hours. Whether ovulation appears with "heat" has not yet been made clear.

A preparation containing a natural estrogen (heat producing)—Alpha estradiol—is frequently used for the relief of retained yellow body, pus in the uterus, and to overcome "silent heat" (anestrus).

2. *Cystic degeneration* in the ovary is the development in this organ of sacs filled with fluid. It may involve either the ovisac, or as a degenerative process of the yellow body. If the former, it usually causes sexual mania, viciousness in the mare, "bullers" in the cow, and if the latter, the opposite condition or absence of heat periods. In either event the affected animal is barren. In some cases recovery is brought about by repeatedly evacuating the cystic fluid as rapidly as it collects, though in others the mania is over-

come only by removal of the entire ovary. This latter step is serious from the standpoint of the animal's breeding value only when both ovaries must be removed.

In this connection a report in regard to a swine herd examined in one of the larger American universities revealed that out of a total of 2188 **Cystic ovaries in swine** non-pregnant females 4.1 to 6.5 per cent had cystic degeneration of the ovaries, and three per cent had distention, with a watery fluid, of the tubes leading from the ovaries to the uterus. The conclusion of the report is that "females (swine) that do not conceive after two services should not be retained for breeding purposes."

However, in cattle the treatment of this condition is somewhat more hopeful following the use of chorionic gonadotropin, than the results from surgical handling as mentioned in a preceding paragraph. This hormone stimulates a normal heat rhythm in cows having cystic ovaries prior to treatment.

3. *Ovarian dysfunction* which is a normal condition in those animals approaching senility is occasionally observed in animals of breeding age. Its exact nature is not understood though it doubtless is the result of failure of some portion of the ductless or endocrine gland system to function. Normal sexuality is not an expression from the genital organs alone, but the manifestation of an intimate relationship of several glandular and other structures. Failure of one of these to function is followed by a disturbance in the physiological reactions of the others. In such an event the ovaries become small, hard, and apparently functionless so that heat periods are in abeyance and barrenness follows. In some instances reports seem to indicate favorable response to repeated subcutaneous or intramuscular injections of ovarian extracts with the recurrence of ovulation and settling to service. In others there is no appreciable result from treatment.

The *foetal membranes* (afterbirth) are frequently *unduly retained,* or fail to become detached from the walls of the uterus. This accounts for the phrase "retained afterbirth." In the mare it is considered normal if the "afterbirth" is discharged within thirty minutes following the birth of the foal; if the cow retains hers beyond twelve hours it is considered to be abnormal. Animals normally giving birth to more than one young expel the membranes of each as they are born.

Retained membranes are doubtless associated with or the result of pathological conditions present at the time of conception. Females weak at birth, those born from dams with diseased genitalia, those bred at a time of extreme youth, those fed far beyond a maintenance ration, and those bred without permitting a period of sexual rest following a previous parturition are most prone to be affected. Several "heats" should elapse before an animal is again bred. In cattle and sheep it is frequently a sequel of specific abortion infection. It is commoner in the dairy than in the beef breeds though the latter are not free from it.

Failure of the foetal membranes —the "afterbirth" —to be expelled is the result of any one of several conditions

So frequently is the retention of the membranes observed following the conditions mentioned in the preceding paragraph that some prominent authorities regard it as a preventable condition by a careful regard for genital health in all animals intended for breeding purposes. The elimination of the sexually weak and diseased, careful feeding of an ample diet without overfeeding or underfeeding, a certain degree of maturity at the time of the first breeding, and sexual rest after a previous pregnancy are all factors conducive to normal pregnancy and parturition with a prompt discharge of the membranes.

The pathologically retained membranes result in destructive changes in the uterus, and not infrequently threaten the life of the mother. If the mother lives her future usefulness as a breeder may be impaired because of loss of a large part of the lining of the uterus, and because of chronic infection **Retained "afterbirth" may threaten the future usefulness of the mother** and inflammation. If conception follows service it is likely to terminate prematurely, or the offspring is weak at birth.

When and under what conditions a retained afterbirth is to be manually removed must be left to the judgment of the attending veterinarian. Usually he is guided by the extent of the ravages of the existing infections. In general removal is attempted where this can be done without at the same time inflicting serious damage to the uterus, that is, the uterus must in a measure have relaxed its hold on the membranes, and before the infections that are present destroy too much of the uterus. It is valueless, in fact detrimental, to remove from the uterus that part of the membranes that is practically loose and leaving that which is still firmly attached.

The introduction of cleansing and disinfecting agents following the removal of the afterbirth should be limited in quantity, and of the very mildest character. Large volumes of irritating disinfectants introduced into a uterus that has lost its tone and power of contracting are harmful. Water sterilized by boiling, with subsequent reduction to blood temperature, and with not more than one per cent of salt added to it is a safe douching agent if introduced without excessive force or volume and if carefully siphoned out. Iodoform (page 277) in mineral oil though too odorous for use in a commercial dairy, and sterilized water with the addition of one-tenth of one per cent of Lugol's solution of iodine (page 276) have also been used. During recent times there has been success immediately after the manual removal of the abnormally retained membranes by the use of antibiotics, or in other cases the antibiotic has been placed in position alongside the retained membranes and then permitting the membranes to loosen naturally.

Only a few of the commoner conditions responsible for temporary or permanent infertility have been mentioned; however enough has been presented to indicate the complexity of the problem. If there ever was a situation requiring the attention of the experienced skilled person then this is that situation.

SOME MALE REPRODUCTIVE PROBLEMS

Failure to reproduce vigorous offspring may be due to a diseased condition of the male. It is not nearly so frequently recognized in the male because **Sterility in the male is more difficult to recognize than in the female** it does not stand out so clearly. It is a comparatively easy matter to diagnose barrenness in a female simply on the basis that she does not reproduce her kind, either by failing to settle to service, or by giving birth to immature and nonviable young. The male serves many females. If all of these failed to conceive as a result of these services the male is undoubtedly at fault, but he may settle some of his females though frequently through no fault in them the offspring is born prematurely, or retained for a prolonged period, or so weak that vigorous life outside of the mother is not possible. Some of the conditions responsible for partial or complete sterility in the male are as follows:

Mechanical causes are sometimes responsible. There may be adhesions between the penis and the adjacent tissues of the sheath that prevent protrusion of this organ. In other **Adhesion and deflection may render service impossible** instances because of a previous injury the penis during erection is so bent or deflected that successful coitus is impossible. Tumors on the penis may also be included in this grouping. Some of the conditions

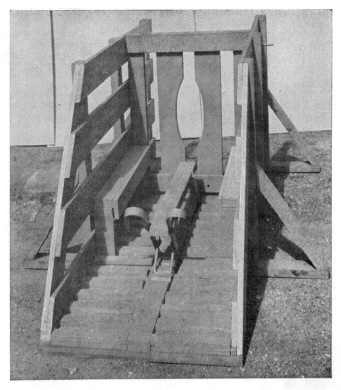

(Courtesy Dept. of Agricultural Engineering, Kansas State University)

FIG. 208. Breeding and hog ringing crate. This device may be used to confine the female when there is disparity in the size of the male and female.

mentioned in this paragraph respond quite well to surgical interference.

Low vitality in the male due to an inadequate diet especially if low in vitamins and minerals, under-feeding, overfeeding—the so-called "show" conditions—lack of exercise and compara-ble conditions are conducive to low sexual vigor. In many instances a restoration of vitality may be brought about by appropriate sane handling and feeding of the patient.

Low vitality a cause of male sterility

Impotency due to excessive exercise of the sex function may at times be observed. This is especially true when young males are used in uncontrolled pasture breeding. Even the more mature may be sexually ruined if an unusual demand is made upon **Excessive** their procreative powers. Proper manage-**sexual use** ment usually corrects this form of trouble. **a cause of** On the other hand impotency because of **impotency** advancing years cannot be overcome, though the sex strength of the aged may to an extent be conserved by moderation of the demands made upon it. During senility the sex function is in complete abeyance.

Dysfunction of the sex complex. It is **Failure of** well recognized that in neither the male or **the general** female is sex vigor dependent on the func-**sex complex** tioning of any single organ. It is a com-**to function** bination of stimuli and reflexes originat-**leads to** ing in several endocrine glands located in **sterility** different parts of the body. If the function of any one of these structures does not coordinate with the others there is a disturbance of the entire group and a dysfunction results, or there is a greater or less degree of sterility. Veterinarians are occasionally able to stimulate the lagging member of the group by the use of the appropriate endocrine principle and thus return to normal the harmonious functioning of the whole.

Inflammation and degeneration in the testicles frequently of unknown origin, or due to mechanical injury, or as a sequel of some diseases, **Testicular** or accumulations of pus in some portion **ailments** of the genitals result in the failure of **result in** secretion of living vigorous sperms and **weak sperms** infertility of the affected male.

Numerous specific disease factors may lodge in the testicles or other portions of the generative system so as to destroy the procreative power. Included in this group of diseases are tuberculosis (page 595) of the testicles, actinomycosis (page 422) of the testicles, dourine (page 754), specific venereal disease of horses;

Various specific ailments localize in the testicles to result in sterility trichomoniasis (page 749), a parasitic disease of the genitalia in cattle; Bang's abortion (page 578), infection of the testicles, and others less common. All of the conditions named in this paragraph are in the light of our present knowledge considered to be incurable, though in regard to Bang's disease and trichomoniasis the door is not entirely closed.

In many of the diseases mentioned in the preceding paragraphs the sperms in the semen, on microscopic examination of the latter, are found to be

The male element weak slow or motionless — in normal potent semen the sperms move in their fluid surroundings in swirls of motion; slow semen is entirely without potency. Some of these semen conditions improve as the male's general condition gets better, or under the influence of sunlight, exercise, and good food. A semen examination is always to be advised, sometimes supplemented by gonadal biopsy (page 761), when the male is suspected of being at fault in the breeding program. Veterinarians do work of this nature almost as a routine procedure in suspected male impotency.

Since the question is frequently raised, it is to be emphasized that on the basis of our present knowledge there is no indication that the nutritive

Feeding the bull requirements of breeding males such as bulls or other species are any different from good feeding practices, and good care and sanitary requirements in the case of any other animal. The reproductive requirements of the male are not specific. Any good well balanced ration will automatically influence the reproductive organs in the same way that other organs of the body are affected. A ration that is relatively high in carbohydrates for energy, and some-

what low in protein or about the same ration as that
which adequately nourishes the dry cow is good.

Chapter XXXVII

ARTIFICIAL INSEMINATION OR
ARTIFICIAL BREEDING

An old-time horseman's term used is "capsule breeding," though this has only the faintest relationship to modern artificial breeding. Taken as a whole artificial insemination refers to the artificial or manual introduction of the male element or sperm into the female genitals. It is thus distinguished from natural mating.

This is a practice in which a female is fecundated in an artificial manner

During a natural mating the male discharges much more semen than is needed for a fertilization. In those countries of Europe and Asia where the numbers of good sires are limited an attempt is made by artificial insemination to distribute each male seminal discharge to as many females as possible. Another reason is that the uninformed believe that "shy" breeders settle better following this practice—this is an erroneous belief because any female that does not settle to a natural mating is exceedingly unlikely to conceive by artificial methods. In America the practice is almost limited to dairy cattle. It is seldom practiced in beef cattle because there is no good standard, such as increased milk production in dairy cattle, to judge results; also beef animals are usually pasture bred, and there is a strong desire to preserve established blood lines. Several million dairy cows are now artificially inseminated annually; the greatest number is in Wisconsin followed in order by New York and Pennsylvania. Horse registration associations will not permit the official registration of an equine resulting from artificial insemination.

There are several approved methods of collecting the semen. Some of those most frequently practiced consist in:

1. Massage of the accessory genital organs in the bull.
2. Collecting excess semen from the floor of the vagina following a natural service.
3. Causing the male to discharge into an artificial vagina. In this method at the beginning of a natural service the penis is deflected into the artificial vagina in the hands of the operator, or, a phantom female with artificial genitalia is used. This is the most frequently followed practice.
4. Electrical stimulation of the spinal cord.
5. Collecting semen from the end of the penis after a natural mating.

The advantages of artificial insemination may be summarized as follows:

1. More efficient use of males over large areas of territory and maintaining community milk yields at a high level.
2. Mating animals of different sizes.
3. Mating of different species, where natural mating does not occur, to beget hybrids.
4. Some males, especially among fur bearers, are naturally monogamous (mating with one female only). Thus by artificial insemination their semen may be spread to many females.
5. To overcome female barrenness resulting from processes that inhibit natural mating.
6. To prevent the spread of certain diseases—dourine (page 754) and trichomoniasis (page 749) are examples.

Advantages and disadvantages of artificial insemination

7. Extending the usefulness of valuable males that cannot perform a natural service because of broken bones, soreness of the hind limbs and feet, excessive fat-

ness, broken and bent penis, and comparable conditions.

Some of the disadvantages of artificial insemination are:

1. If a male is genitally infected this infection may be communicated to a disproportionately large number of females, though penicillin and streptomycin control some of this (page 248).

2. Unscrupulous sire owners may substitute the sperm of less valuable animals.

3. Occasionally a pregnant female accepts a natural service with no harm to the unborn young, though artificial insemination attempted in a pregnant female frequently results in abortion.

4. Some males transmit undesirable characteristics to their offspring though outwardly such a male appears normal. By normal matings only a comparatively few undesirable offspring will result, though these will be greatly multiplied if the sire's impregnations are spread by artificial insemination.

5. Large numbers of sires which are necessary in natural matings keep blood lines open, or there is said to be genetic fluidity.

6. In America there is no scarcity of good sires, and stockmen of high intelligence desire to maintain the breeding competitive spirit in the various herds.

7. Owners of unusually valuable sires accept only a few females for submission to their males so that they may collect high service fees, and to maintain a monopoly of the progeny which they want to sell.

Research has demonstrated that semen rapidly loses its life if it is permitted to remain fully active

The male element retains its potency longest when stored at lowered temperatures

at the normal blood temperature, and when in the natural fluid of the accessory sex organs. To prolong the life of the semen after its discharge from the male and before its introduction into the female it is centrifuged with the removal of most of the actively stimulating accessory fluid, and the storage of the remaining sperms at a low temperature. The result of this method of handling is to make the sperms sluggish or at the extremely low temperature of –79° C. entirely inhibit movement thus conserving their energy and prolonging the life for many months at –79° C.

Research work in England demonstrated that semen frozen to –79° Centigrade maintained its potency for a long time. Some researchers have found that at ten months and even longer the semen so frozen was entirely viable and potent. As soon as the semen is collected it is diluted 1:25 with whole cow's milk and stored at five degrees Centigrade for 4-6 hours. It is then diluted further with an equal amount of milk buffer containing 20 per cent glycerine so as to obtain an end product of 10 per cent glycerine and 1:50 dilution. This diluted semen is placed in sealed ampules of proper dosage, about one cubic centimeter, and stored in a refrigerator surrounded by dry ice in plastic bags so as to drop in temperature at the rate of 2 degrees a minute down to 15° C. and then more rapidly to reach a temperature as low as -79° Centigrade. To prevent the glass ampules, all contained in one jar, from freezing together they are surrounded or immersed in alcohol. Before being used the contents of the ampule are thawed by holding the ampule in the protected hand or in lukewarm water for a few minutes, then the neck of the ampule is broken with a fine file and the contents used in the usual manner or following the usual technique.

Deep freezing a recent step

Normal semen usually has in it in the neighborhood of four billion sperms in the average mature bull's ejaculate of four to five ccs (roughly corresponding to a teaspoonful), and only one of these millions of sperms is needed to fertilize a female ovum. Therefore, in artificial insemination each ejaculate is diluted with a buffer or diluent solution at the rate of from one part of semen to ten to twenty-five parts of diluent. There is no exact standard; there are some indications that with improved technique the dilution in the course of time may be at the rate of one part of semen to one hundred parts of diluent. If this degree of accuracy is reached it would mean that theoretically one hundred cows could be inseminated, possibly fertilized, from a single ejaculate. Under proper kitchen refrigerator temperature and with adequate buffer the viability may be maintained for at least three to four days— much longer under deep frozen conditions. The diluent for bovine semen which may also be used for other species consists of 0.2 grams of potassium dihydrogen phosphate (KH_2PO_4) also known as monobasic potassium phosphate and 0.2 grams dibasic sodium phosphate ($Na_2HPO_4 \cdot 12H_2O$) dissolved in 100 ccs of sterile distilled water (the foregoing is the buffer solution). To the buffer solution is added the yolk of fresh eggs. The pH of the mixture must be close to 6.75; if it is lower add more of the buffer solution. This and other semen diluents are now obtainable through commercial sources.

Foreign research in regard to stallion semen followed by research work in America with bull semen has determined that boiled homogenized cow's milk is a practical, easily prepared diluter for bovine semen. The milk is heated in a covered double boiler for from 1 to 10 minutes at a temperature of 95° Centigrade (203° F.). The heated temperature of the milk is critical—not lower than 92° C., and not higher than 95° C. Main-

Another advancement

taining this temperature range is of even greater importance than the duration of heating time. It has been hypothesized that the correct temperature of heating the milk might be due to hydrolysis of lactose to glucose and galactose which provide energy, or to changes in protein. It appears that homogenized milk may replace the diluent described in the preceding paragraph.

It has been found that in many instances of bulls with low conception rates, the breeding efficiency was materially increased by the addition of 500-1000 I.U. (International Units) or micrograms (a microgram is the millionth part of a gram) of penicillin and streptomycin per milliliter of diluted semen. Crystalline sodium penicillin-G and Streptomycin sulphate were used. The addition of antibiotics to the semen of bulls having a satisfactory conception rate is without value because the added antibiotics are simply for bacterial control (page 249).

Antibiotics in semen

Most inseminators in the past have followed the practice of inseminating a cow late in the heat period because the ovum is not released from the ovary until this time or even later when the cow has overcome the "heat" period. The rule followed—the cow's visible heat period is in general of 18-24 hours duration and the ovum or egg is released 8-13 hours afterward—is if the "heat" is noticeable at milking time in the morning to inseminate the cow in late afternoon. If the "heat" appears late in the forenoon or during the afternoon inseminate the next morning. This is best for optimum conception with one service, and it gives the inseminator a definite working schedule. However, from the purely physiological aspects in both humans and animals, according to researchers, the best time for insemination is at midestrus (mid-heat) because at this time the uterus

Time of insemination

Physiological time for insemination

is most resistant to infection during this estrogenic phase, though later it is easily infected. Also in mid-estrus the secretion in the cervical canal (neck of the uterus) is at its optimum, and this fluid condition favors the migration of the sperms.

Usually the semen in artificial insemination is deposited midway in the cervical canal. If deeper deposition is attempted—especially by the **Place of** unskilled—there is danger of laceration or **insemination** otherwise injuring surrounding tissue. At any rate there is no difference in conception rate by depositing the semen in the body of the uterus or the horns of the uterus as compared with the intra-cervical method. Usually one milliliter of the diluted semen is considered an adequate amount.

The universal practice has been as indicated in the preceding paragraph. A late method occasionally re-sorted to, especially when there are ab-**A late** normalities or serious infections in the **technique** cervix is to deposit semen into the horn or horns of the uterus via the rectum. This latter organ is emptied and mechanically cleansed with an enema. Then by means of an appropriate injection apparatus a guarded hypodermic needle is passed forward into the rectum, the two horns of the uterus digitally fixed in position, and the needle passed through the wall of the rectum at two places so as to puncture each of the two uterine horns and inject the semen. From the con-ception standpoint this by-passes the frequently dan-gerous cervical canal. It is a technique devised to be used when the cervical canal is not normal.

The male fertilizing element—the semen—improp-erly or carelessly handled is easily destroyed. A few drops of water in the inseminating appara-**Some facts** tus quickly destroys it or greatly reduces **about** its potency; even, momentary exposure to **semen** direct sunlight is fatal to it. It does not remain viable very long—possibly an hour or less—

when it is subjected, under unnatural conditions, to temperatures of 100° F. or higher.

Finally it must be stressed that frequently a cow in heat does not settle to artificial insemination because for some reason or other she is mentally disturbed. This may seem strange in such a comparatively phlegmatic animal as the cow, but practice has **Don't excite** demonstrated that cows that are distracted **the cow un-** do not as a rule ovulate or release the **necessarily** necessary ovum or egg. Excitement from violent exercise, from tail twisting, from beating, or even placing the cow in a surrounding that she associates with some previous undesired experience such as vaccination and dehorning are all to be avoided. Some technicians claim better results if another cow is near at the time of insemination.

Because of a shortage of veterinarians the actual insemination is unavoidably in many regions being done by lay trained inseminators under general veterinary supervision, though better results follow the services of the veterinarian. Cattle are comparatively frequently affected with diseased conditions, either general or involving the generative apparatus alone, that interfere with or prevent conception—it is for these conditions that the veterinarian is most needed. In almost every instance the cooperative spirit existing between the lay inseminators and the local veterinarian has been most commendable. Some of the artificial insemination associations have failed because of hasty, ill-advised, underfinanced and poorly organized groups. Sometimes the hope has been held out that by resorting to artificial insemination "chronic non-breeders" could be made to conceive—it's a false hope.

Artificial Insemination of Swine: The technique of artificial insemination of swine is quite comparable to that practiced in cattle. About the same equipment is used, difference depending largely in the difference in the genitals of the two species, as that used in cattle.

The boar has a very large ejaculate as compared to that of the bull—about 125 to 400 cc. in the boar and 5 to 10 cc. in the bull. The ejaculation

Differences in swine and in cattle takes much longer in the boar—as long as twenty minutes. Boar semen is gelatinous in character and contains waxy particles derived from the urethral glands—these particles serving to seal the cervical canal. The centrifuged and thus concentrated semen has been kept viable and potent for as long as 128 hours by storing at a temperature of near 0° C.

The main advantages of artificial insemination in swine are (1) to control the spread of infectious or contagious diseases incidental to contact during a natural service; (2) the use of semen from boars, desirable in every respect, that because of size or physical conditions cannot serve naturally; (3) the wide dissemination of the semen of very highly desirable boars to many herds.

Artificial insemination of swine has not been adopted to any extent because (1) there is no means or standard to determine a boar's breeding value other than show-ring winnings, and not by high milk production as in cattle; (2) low initial cost of a boar and comparatively high resale value of the boar when his breeding days are over—usually as an emasculated animal; (3) the high cost, including the charges of the inseminator, in community artificial insemination of swine as compared with the natural services by a plentiful number of desirable boars.

If a swine breeder desires to adopt a program of artificial insemination in his herd, the entire technique is available through the services of the graduate veterinarian.

Artificial Insemination in Horses: Here also the technique is simple. The principal reason for its non-adoption—a good one by the way—is that horse registration associations refuse registration to any foal produced by any means other than natural service. If artificial insemination were permitted it would soon result in almost countless progeny from the comparatively few really desirable sires, and a corresponding drop in the value of the foals. It is therefore practiced only when a natural service might result in injury or harm to the mare or to the stallion.

Artificial Insemination in Turkeys: In turkeys fertility is an inherited trait and as a result several flocks are known as problem flocks because of the infertility of the hatching eggs.

Toms used for this purpose should be vigorous from the standpoint of ability to mate naturally; and balance since the male is largely responsible for high fertility of the eggs. The recommended age of the tom is 36 weeks. He gives little or no semen **Desirable "Toms"** during the molting time and therefore those showing signs of molt must not be used during this period.

Two operators are needed and it requires some experience, as well as habituating the tom to an ejaculation. One operator holds the tom **Collecting the semen** in a resting position on a low stool, grasping the bird's thighs so that there is a minimum of the bird's weight on its legs. At the same time the technician with the fingers of his right hand massages the soft parts of the bird's abdomen a short distance below the anus. At the same time by means of the thumb and forefinger of the left hand the cloaca (page 24) which is the common terminal organ of the digestive and sex organs is everted so as to cause the ducts of the sex organ to appear, the bird's tail is pushed forward toward its back, abdominal massage is continued, and a small glass vessel held in position the moment the sex organ appears; ejaculation ensues.

The semen is cream-like, white in color and sticky in consistency. The amount collected varies from 3 to 7 drops at a "milking." It is best to use a tom only once every other day. The semen does not survive for more than 30 minutes outside the body, it must not be exposed to direct sunlight, and it must not be chilled below 40° F.—the best temperature for survival is from 45° to 55° F.

Character of semen

During "milking" the tom must not be frightened by rough handling. The process usually requires some training on the part of the bird, as well as an experienced technician. In early attempts only feces may be voided and such contaminated semen is valueless, however, small particles of feces in the semen do not seem to be harmful.

Males should be separated from females for 3 to 4 days before semen collection is started or if early in the season hatching eggs are desired the males must have at least a 14-hour day by starting electric lights—one watt of light for each 3 to 4 square feet of floor space is enough, or this means two 50 watt lamps in a 20′ x 20′ pen.

A one cc. tuberculin glass syringe, without needle, is the injecting instrument. The female is held on a table in a manner similar to holding males. The tail is pushed forward and by pressure with the right hand the cloaca is everted completely so as to expose the oviduct on its left side. The end of the loaded syringe is inserted about one inch and 1/20 cc.—slightly less than one drop —deposited. The abdominal pressure must be relaxed before the semen is injected and the syringe removed so that the semen will not be forced out of the oviduct, and straining by the bird must also be prevented by handling her gently. One semen injection every two weeks is adequate, and hatching eggs may be saved the second day after the first insemination.

Insemination of hens

Commercial turkey hatcheries, and problem flocks almost at once show increased hatchability of eggs. However, it is said to be only an emergency measure. The real effort should be to increase the fertility of the flock by selective breeding. Finally, artificial insemination in turkeys is not a "cure-all."

CHAPTER XXXVIII

THE SOUND AND THE UNSOUND HORSE

The sale of horses and mules, in spite of mechanical motive power, is still an important commercial process. Those engaged daily in this occupation are thoroughly familiar with the rules and regulations governing their actions, though this is not the situation as applied to the occasional purchaser or seller of a horse or mule. A sound animal is free from defects of any kind.

For the benefit of the uninformed there follow some definitions and names of ailments that should be borne in mind during the legal transfer of these animals.

An unsound horse is one having some defects which interfere with the complete utilization of the animal's ability to perform a service. There are several qualifying adjectives used in connection with the word "unsoundness" that modify its meaning. Some of these are as follows:

Absolute unsoundness. This is always a cause for rejection of the animal as it renders it unfit for any kind of service. Included under this classification are such conditions as incurable lameness, blindness, deafness and various deformities. It may furthermore include those conditions that are present at the time of sale, though in such an undeveloped stage that there is no interference with the animal's usefulness, but that in the light of past experience will in the course of time develop into interfering defects. Good examples of these are the early non-painful stages of bog-spavin and thoroughpin. Neither of the conditions named for example causes any inconvenience

An unsoundness may be qualified

during their earlier stages though experience has taught that in the course of time when their fluid contents become organized they result in permanent incurable lameness.

Serviceable Soundness. In a measure this is a deceptive phrase. It means that the animal is unsound though serviceable. For example an animal may have had such a severe attack of lung fever that the proper functioning of the lungs is partially destroyed though not enough to interfere with a utilization of the animal's power at a slow pace or at light labor. It is permissible to classify as serviceably sound an animal that is not lame because of a bone spavin though from the breeding standpoint such a condition places the animal in the "breeding unsound" group.

A serviceably sound animal is unsound

Temporary Unsoundness. Under this classification there are included those conditions that interfere during their duration with the full utilization of the animal's powers. It is desirable to have this classification in order to await the outcome of what at the beginning at least appears to be a transient condition. There may, for example, be a severe lameness as a result of a sprain of some joint ligaments. Usually such a condition is overcome completely following appropriate treatment, but occasionally secondary bone disturbances, such as ringbone formation following sprain of the fetlock ligaments, follow so that it constitutes a permanent or absolute unsoundness.

Temporary unsoundness is common

Breeding Unsoundness is always a cause for rejection of animals intended for procreative purposes, though otherwise their utilization may not be impaired. This includes such conditions as malformation of the genitals and of the birth passageway, cryptorchidism (ridgling), scrotal rupture (hernia), and other comparable abnormalities.

Breeding unsoundness is serious

Hereditary Unsoundness is the most serious of all unsoundness because of the possibility of transmission from parents to offspring. Most frequently

Hereditary unsoundness is most serious

this group of unsoundnesses has as a basis an abnormal conformation of one or more parts. The sway-backed horse is unsound for load carrying purposes; the animal with narrow joints such as in the region of the hock is predisposed to bone spavin formation; in a similar manner the sickle-hocked, calf-kneed, knee-sprung, bow-legged, narrow chested animal is most likely to develop a diseased or unsound condition when the hereditary poorly formed part of the body is subjected to the strain of severe labor. In view of the fact that such conformations are hereditary therefore these animals are to be discriminated against even though no actual unsoundness exists at the time of sale.

Blemishes. A blemish on an animal is an acquired condition offensive to the sight of the examiner. It is

A blemish does not interfere with the usefulness of the animal

located in the skin or the immediately underlying tissues. It does not interfere with the animal's usefulness, though it may decrease its monetary value. The following are some of the blemishes:— scars of former wire cuts, or those following surgical operations, or the hairlessness occurring after blistering and comparable conditions. Sometimes the tissues immediately under the skin are involved such as the so-called "wind-puffs" of the region of the tendons near the fetlock. A blemish in the form of white hairs on the front of the knees is to be regarded with suspicion as it may indicate that the animal is a "stumbler."

Bad Habits. Usually these are the result of idleness. They do not prevent the utilization of the animal —they are annoying, and in some instances are destructive to the natural grace of an otherwise beautiful animal. The terms generally employed to describe these habits are so descriptive as to be self explanatory. They

are as follows:—tongue lolling, striking lower against
the upper lip, head shaking and rein jerking, wind
sucking, pawing or trotting in the stable, weaving like
a bear, and tearing off blankets. These bad habits are
causes for discrimination.

Vices. These are serious moral defects the exact
nature of which is not understood. There seems to be
some ground for the belief that bad tem-
Bad habits pers, which are responsible for some of
and vices these vices are hereditary—at least good
reduce the horsemen discriminate against the off-
animal's spring of a vicious sire or dam. At other
usefulness times disease—especially of the ovaries—
is at the bottom of the trouble. Bad training, and
interference with established habits are also of causative significance.

Some of the more serious vices are the balky horse,
the horse that backs when harnessed, the kicking and
striking horse, the animal that fights harnessing, the
biting horse, the shyer, the runaway horse, and the
horse that has aversions to special objects and things.

These vicious horses are a source of genuine danger to humans, and other animals. Sometimes they may
be cured by surgical operations upon the ovaries or
testicles, or they may in some cases be controlled by
mechanical devices. Taken as a whole however they
are not recommended for purchase as they can seldom
be made dependable or trustworthy.

For detailed information about animal conformation reference should be directed to standard text-books
about this subject.

CHAPTER XXXIX

HORSE RACE-TRACK PRACTICES

General Statement

Race track officials and associations are making a most determined effort to eliminate or prevent the entry for racing purposes of horses that are substitutes ("ringers") for others of higher or lower racing ability—and thus mislead persons that follow the races for recreational purposes. The regulations, their enforcement, and the imposed penalties for violations are severe though fully warranted for the handling of these forms of intentional fraud. Racing horses has become "big" business; figures released to the public press in January, 1949, by The Thoroughbred Racing Protective Bureau indicate that the sums **Financial investments in horse racing** involved are 175 million dollars in racing plants; 146 million dollars in breeding farms and stock in forty states; and that nearly 50 million dollars in purses were distributed in 1948. In Maryland for 1947 revenues for the state or its subsidiaries from horse racing totaled $5,095,324, this being derived from the $1000 a day licence fee and four per cent on total betting that the major tracks pay; smaller tracks in Maryland pay $50 a day license fee to the county treasurer in the county in which the race is held, one per cent on the first $500,000 bet, two per cent on the next $500,000 and four per cent on wagers over $1,000,000. The contributions on the foregoing basis to the State revenues from the various race tracks were Pimlico $1,234,402; Laurel $1,131,206; Bowie $1,054,656; Havre de Grace $1,-059,503; Bel Air $153,535; Cumberland $103,847; Hagerstown $99,571; Marlboro $124,002; and Timonium $125,815—incidental fees brought $9,173. According to Maryland law of the total Baltimore city and the counties received $2,396,094; the Fair Board $245,978; and the General Fund $2,453,251.

There are at least two methods in vogue by means of which horses may be identified for race track purposes. They are:

1. A method of tattooing developed by the U. S. Army, and advanced by The Thoroughbred Racing Protective Bureau. In this system a five digit number is applied to the underneath side of the upper lip by especially designed tattooing dies and an indelible ink. The **Identification by tattooing** work can be done in less than two minutes. The uniquely designed dies, limited in number are under the careful control of the Thoroughbred Racing Protective Bureau. Specially trained TRPB crews operate at various race tracks. Tattooing is free. The tattoo is a permanent mark, and will eliminate the underhand tactic of substituting ("ringing") a fast horse for a slow one.

2. The other identification is based on the fact that no two chestnuts—horsemen refer to them as night eyes—(the horny growths on the inner surfaces of the forearm about a handbreadth above the carpus—knee, and on the lower inner surface of the hock of the hind limbs) are exactly alike. In general **Photographing the chestnuts** the chestnuts are quite variable in form and size; on the front limbs they are usually about one and one-half inches to two and one-half inches long, oval in outline, and the upper end pointed; on the hind limbs, when well developed, they are two to two and one half inches long, broad below and a pointed upper end with a short blunt process in front. *Again no two are exactly alike.* All four are photographed—full size, and these

photographs with additional detailed descriptive material—also side and front view photographs of the animal—become permanent records maintained by the Pinkerton National Detective Agency.

Stimulating Horses for racing—usually referred to as "doping" is another highly unethical and fraudulent practice that race track authorities will not permit. Without question horses—humans also—can by the use of drugs be stimulated to unusual physical effort. In the early days of the Spaniards in Peru they were astonished to note that native Indians could apparently tirelessly maintain a rapid pace for hours at a time; it was not until it was learned that en route the Indians were chewing coca leaves—it is from these that the alkaloid cocaine is obtained—as the source of their muscular energy. When the effect wore off hours were required for recuperation, and still more serious for humans it was habit forming with complete mental and moral degeneration in the course of time.

Some of the drugs that are alleged to have been used in the stimulating of race horses are atropine, benzedrine, benadryl, brucine, caffeine, cocaine, codeine, coramine, demerol, ephedrine, met-
Some drugs used razol, morphine, novocaine, quinine, scopolamine, sodium barbital, sodium dilantin, strychnine, theophylline and several others including the so-called "Canadian elixir" which contains almost everything.

In testing for these drugs—all can be tested for—a sample of the horse's urine or saliva is collected and treated with various chemical reagents until the "dope" used crystallizes out *each in its own characteristic shape.* Occasionally a small amount of the **Tests to detect "dope"** urine or saliva of the horse being tested is injected into laboratory mice to note the physiological reaction. One of the drugs used for a long time, benzedrine—this is the proprietary name for a complex chemical compound occasionally used in weak concentration in an oil base as an inhalant for the treatment of head colds, hay fever, etc. in humans—remained undetectable until chemistry scientists by means of the spectroscope and ultraviolet light analyzed its presence. In fact a test now performed at the race track—ether extraction and acid—will disclose benzedrine by a red color, the intensity of which depends on the amount of the drug in the urine. One prominent chemist doing testing of this nature has stated that "it's usually a race between two groups of people, one inventing scientific tests and the other getting around them."

The records indicate that because of the attempts of race track officials, and the various race track associations in their efforts to detect and punish fraudulent practices and to safeguard the interests of racing devotees, and to protect the avocation of many persons by sponsoring only legitimate racing, they have succeeded in reducing "doping" of race horses. However, the National Assoc. of Racing Commissioners is now considering that horses that have been medicated for 48 hours before a race may not be entered. There is no unanimity of opinion about its value as the proposed regulation is very ambiguous. For those interested, consult Proceedings of the 5th Annual Equine Practitioners Assoc.

It is also well to know that the possession or use in an unauthorized manner of many of the agents formerly affirmed to have been used in the "doping" of race horses fall within the provisions and penalties of the federal Harrison Anti-Narcotic Act. Fines and imprisonment await offenders.

A federal offense

(For those interested in the details of the various chemistry phases of the matter reference may be had to an article entitled "The Detection of 'Doping' in Race-Horses," appearing on page 153 of the July 1951 issue of The Australian Veterinary Journal.)

CHAPTER XL

SOME DISEASES COMMON TO
MAN AND ANIMALS

All American states require physicians to report to a central state agency the contagious ailments of humans encountered by them in their general practice. In one of these states (Michigan) sixty-five human diseases are listed as reportable and of these twenty-three are either transmissible from animal to man, or from man to animal, or having an animal reservoir (page 4) and five more are milk borne. Some 80 different diseases are now recognized as transmissible from animals to man. During the last decade the actual number of diseases intercommunicable between animals and man is reported to have increased ten-fold.

Briefly some of these diseases are as follows:

Actinomycosis or *Actinobacillosis* (Lumpy-jaw, etc. of cattle) (page 422). Domesticated animals affected are cattle, swine, sheep and goats. Due to the bacteria *Actinomyces bovis* and *Actinobacillus lig.*, genera containing 64 members. It is quite doubtful that man contracts this condition from contact with animals; it is more likely that man and animals contract the infection from a common source; for man the chewing of germ contaminated straw, grain, weeds and other comparable materials may be the mode of infection.

Anthrax (page 591) affects cattle, sheep, horses and swine. Due to the *Bacillus anthracis*, humans may contract it by contact with the tissues of animals dead of the disease—hides, wool (wool-sorters disease) swine bristles as in non-disinfected shaving brushes, and blood. Malignant pustule in man is one condition observed. Precaution—do not open (page 228) animal carcasses—do not handle tissues excepting when gloves are worn, and practice disinfection, and instrument sterilization.

Botulism (page 471). Limberneck (page 650) in poultry; food poisoning in man. Cattle, horses, and chickens very susceptible; sheep and swine quite resistant. Due to *Clostridium botulinum*. Man contracts it following the ingestion of contaminated food of animal origin, and from spoiled canned food. Prevention—destroy suspected food by burial after first subjecting it to the action of lye (page 253) for at least 24 hours; do not eat questionable food or when in doubt cook thoroughly; non-acid foods (meats and vegetables) are to be processed, for canning or preserving, under steam pressure.

Brucellosis (page 578); undulant fever in man (page 588); Malta fever of man; Bang's disease of cattle. Due to *Brucella melitensis, B. abortus* and *B. suis*. Occurs in cattle, goats, swine, horses, sheep and poultry. Man contracts the infection from direct contact with infected animals, and from the consumption of dairy products. Prevention—avoid contact with infected animals, and pasteurize milk.

Bubonic plague (page 326). Caused by infection with the germ *Pasteurella pestis*. Occurs in rodents —especially rats and squirrels. Transmitted to man by rodent fleas, and the pneumonia type of the disease from man to man. Prevention—destruction of rats (page 325) and other rodents in infected areas; the use of D.D.T. (page 291) to control fleas.

Asiatic Cholera. Man is the victim as domesticated animals enjoy high resistance. The disease is due to the cholera vibrio—*Vibrio coma*. In man the disease follows the ingestion of contaminated drinking water or food—it may thus be milk borne—the latter having become contaminated by flies that carry the germ from human fecal material. The disease is endemic in India but at times has spread to Europe and Asia. Prevention—sanitation and vaccination.

Gas Gangrene. All domesticated animals are susceptible. Due to *Clostridium septicum, C. perfringens, C. novyi* and others of this group. In animals blackleg of cattle (page 551) ; enterotoxemia of sheep (page 476) ; malignant oedema (page 552) and others belong to this group of ailments. Many of these germs normally live a saprophytic (said of germs that live on decaying organic matter) existence in the intestinal canal of animals, and from this source man and animals contract wound infections. It was relatively common in man as a wartime condition. Prevention— disinfection of wounds with Carrel-Dakin chlorine-boric acid disinfectant (page 259) ; the use of antitoxin, and penicillin (page 249).

Glanders (page 614). Horses and mules are highly susceptible. Caused by the germ *Malleomyces mallei.* Man contracts the disease by contact with affected animals. Since the use of the automobile has practically placed the horse in quarantine (page 212) on the farm and therefore having no contact with diseased animals or their nasal discharges through the common hitching post and the common watering trough the disease, formerly quite common in the United States, has virtually disappeared in both man and animals. Prevention— destruction and cremation of all diseased horses and mules, and all others on the same place, unless demonstrated to be free from the disease by a non-reaction to the mallein test (page 614).

Equine encephalo-myelitis, Equine encephalitis, sleeping sickness of horses (page 555) is due to an ultramicroscopic virus that is most abundant in the blood of a horse or mule just dead of the disease. Fowl, squirrels and monkeys are also susceptible. The disease is transmitted by mosquitoes, ticks and biting intermediate hosts. The spread of this disease is relatively frequent presumably by biting insects that have fed on infected horses or on their carcasses. However, the most recent opinion (1961) is that in horses it is a "dead end disease." Prevention—infected horses to be protected against biting insects by nets and repellents (page 323) ; animals dead of the disease to be covered completely with a tarpaulin while awaiting burial or cremation (page 228).

Leptospirosis (page 535) affects rats, dogs, cats, horses, swine and foxes. Caused by the germs *Leptospira icterohemorrhagiae* and *L. canicola*. Man contracts the disease by direct contact or by the consumption of foods soiled by animals that carry the infection, and also when this soiling involves packing-house workers, those employed on wharves, fishermen that follow fishing as a vocation, veterinarians, persons working in dog-pounds, persons having contact with sewage, swimmers in polluted water and various other industrial sources. Prevention—almost purely a matter of sanitation especially in avoiding the exposure of a naked portion of the body to pollution by the materials or substances, or animals, that carry the infection, and particularly the ingestion of food that may have been contaminated.

Salmonellosis; food infection. This is a group of food infections due to almost anyone of the more than one hundred types of the *Salmonella* bacteria. In man the disease is due to the ingestion of contaminated or spoiled food of fowl or mammal origin. The outstanding symptom in man is the appearance of more or less violent involvement of the intestinal tract, not uncommonly with a fatal termination. Some of the animal tissues that may be contaminated are pork with the *S. cholerasuis* (page 531) ; poultry with *S. pullorum* (page 651) ; sheep with *S. typhi-murium* and others. Some of these infections are in the eggs of fowl, and some of the salmonella are natural pathogens of animals; some infected animals are not visibly ill, and certainly foods contaminated— in this flies have been implicated as carrying the salmonella from infected chicken droppings to human food—with salmonella frequently show no outward evidence of it. Prevention—all human food of animal origin should be thoroughly cooked—even eggs should not be eaten raw. Human food should at all times be protected against flies.

Swine erysipelas (page 620) *diamond-skin disease* (page 621). Affects swine, turkeys and sheep. Due to the germ *Erysipelothrix rhusiopathiae*. Transmitted to man through skin abrasions causing the so-called *erysipeloid* in man. Prevention — do not handle infected animals with bare hands or in case this is unavoidable disinfect the hands thoroughly and apply pure tincture of iodine (page 276) to skin abrasions.

Tetanus (page 542) lockjaw. This disease may affect all warm-blooded animals. It is due to the germ *Clostridium tetani* which is prevalent in manure, garden soil, road dust, on rusty metal and many other places. Man and animals contract the infection through lacerated or penetrating wounds—the germ remains localized at the site of invasion into the tissues where it elaborates a very powerful toxin or poison—frequently the wound heals outwardly. Prevention—all deep, lacerated and penetrating wounds must be deeply disinfected—iodine (page 276) is excellent, and as soon as possible after the injury has taken place tetanus antitoxin should be administered. Tetanus toxoid confers measurable permanent immunity.

Tuberculosis (page 595). This is a disease of cattle, swine, and fowls. It is due to the germ *Mycobacterium tuberculosis*. Man is highly susceptible (page 597) by contact, and by the ingestion of meat, and milk products of infected animals. Since the virtual stamping out of cattle tuberculosis in the United States the incidence of human bone-deforming tuberculosis, and tuberculosis of the human digestive organs of milk consumers has been lowered correspondingly. Prevention—continuation of the program of eradication of cattle tuberculosis (page 599) by frequent tuberculin testing with tuberculin; pasteurization of all dairy products unless derived from a tuberculosis clean herd; tuberculin testing and other means of diagnosis to eliminate the human tuberculous food handler, and the continuation of the system of federal meat inspection by the veterinarians of the United States Bureau of Animal Industry. Human sanitarians are also sponsoring extensive programs of tuberculosis control and eradication.

Tularemia (page 561) rabbit fever. Wild rabbits and hares are the principal infected animals by the causative germ — *Pasteurella tularense* — which is transmitted to humans by contact, and by the bite of infected fleas, flies, ticks and others. Prevention—(page 561).

Foot-and-Mouth Disease (page 605). This disease of cloven footed animals is due to a virus. Humans may contract it—usually with mild symptoms on the fingers and mouth, and malaise—by contact with infected and by the drinking of milk derived from diseased animals. Prevention—in the United States the disease has never been permitted to obtain a permanent foothold though on several occasions, when it did gain an admission it has been stamped out by the most rigorous methods. During an outbreak disinfection of hands and clothing of handlers of diseased animals, and pasteurization of milk, and dairy products are the methods of preventing human infection. The incidence of this disease in humans is so rare that it is not a problem.

Psittacosis (page 562) (parrot fever). Parrots, parakeets, finches are most frequently infected. Humans contract the etiological virus from the handling of the infected birds, and particularly by inhalation of their exhalations and effluvia. Prevention—difficult because of an inherent human affection for pets. The quarantine of birds presented for importation, and inspections of pet shops are very helpful.

Pox (page 575). Cattle-pox is the variety most frequently transmitted to humans because of milking infected cows and thus inoculating the milker with the virus of the disease. Fowl-pox (page 643) is not true variola and of little significance; swine pox (page 576) is rarely a true variola (human smallpox). Prevention—humans handling cattle affected with pox should at least thoroughly scrub the hands—certainly humans are resistant to cowpox because almost all humans now-a-days have been vaccinated against smallpox or variola.

Rabies (pages 327 and 544) dog madness, hydrophobia affects dogs, cattle, horses, sheep, squirrels and many other biting animals. It is due to a virus which is in the saliva in particular, though also in other secretions of infected animals. Man acquires the condition by being bitten, or contact with infected saliva on the abraided skin. The unprotected portions of the body—face and hands—are the most serious avenues of human contamination—the clothing of a bitten person mechanically wipes the saliva off the teeth of an infected biting animal. Prevention—compulsory annual immunization of all dogs especially in dense centers of human and dog population; quarantine of dogs, or their control on leash, for a 90-day period during an outbreak; destruction of all ownerless and stray dogs. Humans bitten or contaminated by a rabid animal should at once have the wound treated by a physician, and should be subjected to the protective vaccination.

Other diseases such as scabies (page 727), favus (page 661), ring worm (page 567), swamp-fever (page 553), listerellosis (page 535), necrobacillosis (pages 526 and 527), round worms* (pages 670 and 690), tape worms (page 665), Rocky Mountain spotted fever (pages 249 and 714), trichinosis (page 681), rat-bite fever (page 561), Q-Fever (page 563), and others are either common to man and animals, or

---

*Round-worms of swine and poultry do not develop in humans.

under varying conditions transmissible to man.* Others such as septic sore throat, diphtheria and scarlet fever —all three human—and trembles or milk sickness (page 460) are frequently milk borne or spread by contaminated milk. Only by guarding himself against these multitudinous ailments by clean food, clean water, care in the handling of animals, and endless sanitation can man hope to escape them.

---

*(For a listing of transmissible diseases, names of causative organisms, etc., animal hosts, geographical distribution, and vectors or methods of spread, consult page 205, Proceedings 51st Annual Meeting, U. S. Livestock Sanitary Association, regarding "The Importance of Animal Disease Morbidity and Mortality Statistics to Public Health.")

PART ELEVEN

Livestock Sanitary Bureaus, Boards, and Commissions, and the Veterinarian

✧✧✧✧

CHAPTER XLI

GENERAL STATEMENT

In the United States the control of animal diseases is in charge of various federal and state officials. Some of these agencies are also engaged in research work, educational campaigns, foods inspection activities, and regulatory or police duties. Some of the more important of these agencies with brief descriptive statements, are as follows:

1. The Agricultural Research Service, U. S. Dept. of Agriculture, formerly known as the United States Bureau of Animal Industry.

This is a Bureau in the federal Department of Agriculture. It came into official existence May 29, 1884, through congressional action. Doubtless the most important factor leading to the establishment of the Bureau was the presence and the spread in the United States of the highly contagious pleuro-pneumonia of cattle. This disease was introduced from Europe about 1843, but it was not until 1879 that livestock men became aroused to the seriousness of the situation.

A federal bureau that has demonstrated its usefulness

From its very beginning the Bureau has been the leader in all those programs dealing with live-stock conservation. Its standing and influence are world-wide. In America the live-stock industry could not have reached nor maintained its position of pre-eminence without the efforts and constructive work of the Bureau. There can be listed here only some of the major accomplishments in which it has been the leader:

(a) Eradication of contagious pleuro-pneumonia.

(b) The discovery of the nature of Southern cattle fever, h o w it is conveyed, and a practical method of its eradication (page 747).

(c) The discovery of the cause of hog cholera (page 616), and the development of a successful method of permanent immunization.

(d) The rapid eradication of every outbreak of foot-and-mouth disease (page 605) that has occurred in the United States.

(e) The virtual eradication of tuberculosis (page 595) of cattle. The occurrence of this disease is now less than one-half per cent of the cattle population in each state of the union.

(f) The establishment and maintenance of a national meat inspection service so that all meat food products before being permitted to enter interstate traffic must be "U. S. Inspected and Passed." (Fig. 209.)

(g) The discovery of a remedy effective against human hookworm disease of the South.

In addition to the foregoing there are endless spectacular though almost equally important contributions of this Bureau to human and animal welfare in the United States.

The U. S. Dept. of Agriculture—this is the parent organization of the former Bureau of Animal Industry —was reorganized effective Dec. 28, 1953, so that the word "Bureau" as the designation of the various subdivisions of the U.S.D.A. became obsolete. At the same time what had been in the U.S.D.A. the Agricultural Research Administration (A.R.A.) became "Agricultural Research Service" (A.R.S.). With the breaking up of what had up to this time been designated as "Bureau," the former Bureau of Animal Industry was subdivided under the "A.R.S." naming into the following:

Administrator.

Deputy Administrator, Regulatory Programs.

Assistant Administrator, Regulatory Programs.

Deputy Administrator, Production Research.

Assistant to the Administrator, Emergency Programs.

Director, Animal Disease Eradication Division.

Director, Animal Inspection and Quarantine Division.

Director, Meat Inspection Division.

Director, Animal Disease and Parasite Research Division.

Director, Animal Husbandry Research Division.

All of the foregoing are located in Washington, D.C.

The Agricultural Marketing Service, U.S.D.A.

Livestock Division, Meat Grading Branch

    Staff Veterinarian, Eastern Area, Washington, D. C.

    Staff Veterinarian, Central Area, 27 Exchange Bldg., National Stockyards, Illinois.

    Staff Veterinarian, Western Area, 403 Livestock Exchange Bldg., Denver, Colorado.

Poultry Division, Inspection Branch.

    Chief

    Assistant Chief.

    Poultry Pathologist.

    Eastern Area Veterinary Supervisor, Room 200 Customs Bldg., 2nd and Chestnut Sts., Philadelphia, Pa.

    Chicago, Ill., Area (Midwest) Veterinary Supervisor, 1014 U. S. Custom House, 610 So. Canal St., Chicago 7, Illinois.

Des Moines, Iowa, Area (Midwest) Veterinary Supervisor, Room 104, Iowa Bldg. Des Moines 9, Iowa.

Pacific Coast Area Veterinary Supervisor, Room 333 Pacific Bldg., 821 Market St., San Francisco 3, Cal.

Poultry Division, Grading Branch.

The U. S. Dept. of Health, Education and Welfare has the following:

Food and Drug Administration, Bureau of Medicine, Veterinary Medical Branch.

Veterinary Medical Director.

Associate Veterinary Medical Director.

Therapeutic Testing Section.

Staff Veterinarians—three.

It is indicated that the main purpose of the so-called "streamlining" is to strengthen and improve federal veterinary service to agriculture.

2. State Veterinarians, Sanitary Commissions, and Boards.

In most states livestock sanitary and regulatory duties center in a state veterinarian or comparable officer or officers. They are zealous in **State veter-** their efforts—a fact attested by the very **inarians** low occurrence of widespread outbreaks **render an** of animal diseases. They cannot of course **important** influence the appearance of sporadic dis- **service** eases.

In the various states the official designations and addresses are as follows:

Alabama—State Veterinarian, Montgomery

Alaska—State Veterinarian, Spenard

Arizona—State Veterinarian, Phoenix

Arkansas—State Veterinarian, Little Rock

California—Administrator, Division of Animal Industry, State Department of Agriculture, Sacramento 14

Colorado—State Veterinarian, Denver 11

Connecticut—State Veterinarian, State Office Building, Hartford

Delaware—State Veterinarian, Dover

District of Columbia—Chief, Animal Disease and Parasite Research; Health Officer, Washington D. C.

Florida—State Veterinarian, State Livestock Sanitary Board, Tallahassee

Georgia—Chief Veterinarian, State Capitol, Atlanta

Hawaii—State Veterinarian, Honolulu, Hawaii

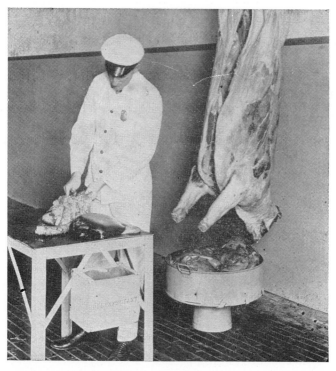

Fig. 209. A United States veterinary inspector at his work in a large meat packing establishment.

Idaho—Director, State Bureau of Animal Industry, State House, Boise

Illinois—Superintendent, Division of Livestock Industry, Springfield

Indiana—State Veterinarian, Indianapolis

Iowa—Chief, State Division of Animal Industry, State House, Des Moines

Kansas—State Livestock Sanitary Commissioner, Topeka

Kentucky—State Veterinarian, Frankfort

Louisiana—State Veterinarian, State Livestock Sanitary Board, Baton Rouge

Maine—State Veterinarian, Division of Animal Industry, State Department of Agriculture, Augusta

Maryland—State Veterinarian, Univ. of Maryland, College Park

Massachusetts—Director of Livestock Disease Control, 41 Tremont St., Boston

Michigan—State Veterinarian, Lansing

Minnesota—Secretary and Executive Officer, State Livestock Sanitary Board, 310 Globe Building, St. Paul

Mississippi—State Veterinarian, Jackson

Missouri—State Veterinarian, Jefferson City

Montana—State Veterinarian, Helena

Nebraska—Director, State-Federal Livestock Disease Eradication Program, Post Office Building, Lincoln 1

Nevada—Director, Division of Animal Industry, Reno

New Hampshire—State Veterinarian, Concord

New Jersey—Division of Animal Industry, 1 West State Street, Trenton 8

New Mexico—Veterinary Surgeon, Livestock Sanitary Board, Albuquerque

New York—Director, Animal Industry Bureau, Albany

North Carolina—State Veterinarian, Raleigh

North Dakota—State Veterinarian, Bismark

Ohio—Chief, Division of Animal Industry, Columbus

Oklahoma—State Veterinarian, Oklahoma City

Oregon—State Veterinarian, Division of Animal Industry, Oregon Department of Agriculture, Salem

Pennsylvania—Director of the Pennsylvania Bureau of Animal Industry, Harrisburg

Puerto Rico—Commissioner, Department of Agriculture and Commerce of Puerto Rico, San Juan, P. R.

Rhode Island—Chief, Division of Animal Industry, Veterans Memorial Bldg., Providence

South Carolina—Director, Federal-State Livestock Disease Eradication Program, Columbia 1

South Dakota—State Veterinarian, State Livestock Sanitary Board, Pierre

Tennessee—State Veterinarian, State Capitol, Nashville

Texas—Director, Livestock Sanitary Commission of Texas, and State Veterinarian, Fort Worth

Utah—State Veterinarian, State Capitol Building, Salt Lake City 1

Vermont—Commissioner, State Department of Agriculture, State House, Montpelier

Virginia—State Veterinarian, Richmond

Washington—Director of the State Department of Agriculture, Supervisor of Dairy and Livestock, Olympia

West Virginia—State Veterinarian, State Dept. of Agriculture, 230 Staunton Ave., South Charleston

Wisconsin—Chief Veterinarian, State-Federal Cooperative Animal Disease Eradication Programs, 6 West, State Capitol, Madison 2

Wyoming—State Veterinarian, Cheyenne

CHAPTER XLII

THE VETERINARIAN

In concluding this dissertation it would be derelict if worthy tribute were not paid to the veterinarian. He

The veterinarian is the keystone of the arch supporting livestock well-being in America

is the very keystone supporting the arch upon which rests the entire burden of all those factors concerned with the preservation of animal health.

The veterinarian of today must meet high educational and professional standards before he may practice his profession. Modern legal requirements in force in most states, adopted for the protection of the livestock industry, are that to practice veterinary medicine and surgery the applicant must be a graduate of a veterinary college of recognized standing. High School graduation and six years—two years preveterinary and four years professional curriculum—of college or university study are the requirements for the degree Doctor of Veterinary Medicine. Veterinary colleges receive their professional rating from the American Veterinary Medical Association; the Agriculture Research Service, U. S., Dept. of Agriculture; the U. S. Civil Service Commission; the U. S. Army; and from the various State Veterinary Examining Boards. At the time of this writing the Colleges of veterinary medicine are as follows:

School of Veterinary Medicine, Auburn University, Auburn, Alabama

School of Veterinary Medicine, Univ. of California, Davis

College of Veterinary Medicine, Colorado State University, Fort Collins

New York State Veterinary College at Cornell University, Ithaca

School of Veterinary Medicine, University of Georgia, Athens

College of Veterinary Medicine, University of Illinois, Urbana

College of Veterinary Medicine, Iowa State University, Ames

School of Veterinary Medicine, Kansas State University, Manhattan

College of Veterinary Medicine, Michigan State University, East Lansing

College of Veterinary Medicine, University of Minnesota, St. Paul

School of Veterinary Medicine, University of Missouri, Columbia

College of Veterinary Medicine, Ohio State University, Columbus

College of Veterinary Medicine, Oklahoma State University, Stillwater

School of Veterinary Medicine, University of Pennsylvania, Philadelphia

School of Veterinary Medicine, Purdue University, Lafayette, Indiana

School of Veterinary Medicine, Texas Agricultural and Mechanical College, College Station

Ontario Veterinary College, University of Toronto, Guelph, Canada

School of Veterinary Medicine, Tuskegee Institute, Tuskegee Institute, Alabama

College of Veterinary Medicine, Washington State University, Pullman

School of Veterinary Medicine (Affiliated with the University of Montreal), St. Hyacinthe, Quebec, Canada

This College, and University thoroughly trained person may engage in any one of several professional vocations as follows:

Veterinary vocations

1. Large animal (usual farm animals) practitioner in a rural community.

2. Small animal (pet animals, especially cats and dogs) practitioner in the larger urban centers.

3. U. S. Agr. Res. Service Inspector—engaged as veterinary (meat) inspectors (Fig. 209) in packing plants, or as field men in tuberculosis, Bang's disease, mange, tick fever and other disease eradication work, or in any other of the A.R.S. numerous activities.

4. Officer in the U. S. Army—rank from first lieutenant to colonel inclusive.

5. Foods inspectors in CCC camps under U. S. Army control.

6. State veterinarian, sanitary officers and municipal meat, milk and dairy inspectors.

7. Manufacturer of veterinary vaccines, and serums.

8. Veterinary teacher and research worker in colleges and agricultural experiment stations.

9. Commercial engagements in the sale of drugs, instruments and other supplies needed by practicing veterinarians. Also research by commercial concerns.

10. Miscellaneous occupations such as veterinarian for circuses, for exploratory organizations, foreign quarantine service, etc.

The livestock industry depends upon a well-trained veterinary personnel to safeguard the health of its charges. A good veterinarian in a community is an asset to that community not only from a professional standpoint but also as a civic leader. Many are mayors, members of boards of health, members of

The veterinarian an asset to a community

city councils and school boards, and serve in comparable positions.

The private practitioner of veterinary medicine does a thorough job, night and day, in all kinds of weather and seasons. Neither the livestock industry nor human welfare could long survive without him. Encourage him.

INDEX

A

Abomasum, 20
Abortion, contagious of cattle (see Bang's disease), 578
Abortion, nitrate, 480
Abortion, virus of sheep, 590
Acetonemia (ketosis), of cattle, 505
Acid, acetic, diluted, 279
Acid, ascorbic (vitamin C), 71
Acid, boric, 278, 468
Acid, carbolic, 260
Acid, carbolic, crude, 263
Acid fast germs, 253
Acid, folic, 69
Acid, nicotinic, 69
Acid, prussic, poisoning, 18, 437
Acids, amino, 44
Acid, sulphuric, 278
"Acorn calves," 447
Acridines, 282
Actinobacillosis ("wooden tongue"), 425
Actinomycosis ("lumpy jaw"), 422, 801, 823
Acute bloat, 361
Acute salt poisoning, 478
Administering medicines to animals, 775
Adrenals (suprarenals), 95
Afterbirth (placenta), retained, 796
Age, from horse's teeth, 9
Agglutination blood test, 580, 758
Ailments, secondary, 346
Air and ventilation for housed animals, 154
Aldrin, 304
Algae destroyed by copper sulphate, 275
Alkali disease, 449
Alkali water, 112
Allergic reactions or tests, 634, 759
Allethrin, 310
Amino acids, 44
Ammonia, quaternary, 279
Amputation of wattles or "dubbing," fowl, 404
Anal sacs in dogs and cats, 192
Analysis of water, 115
Anaplasmosis ("yellow teat disease"), 701, 744, 767
Anatomy and physiology of organs of digestion :
    cheeks, 13
    intestines, 24
    jaws, 10
    lips, 7
    oesophagus (gullet), 15
    palate, hard and soft, 14
    pharynx, 15
    rectum and anus, 24
    salivary glands, 14
    stomach, 17
    teeth, 8
    tongue, 8
Anemia in suckling pigs, 86, 494
Anestrus ("silent heat"), 794
Animal care and disease, 189
Animal housing and control, 122

Animal housing ventilators, 158
Animal inoculation test, 759
Animal surroundings and manure disposal, 163
Anoxemia, 154, 480
Anoxia, 154
Anthrax, 109, 110, 111, 591, 767, 823
Anthrax, symptomatic (blackleg), 551
Antibiotics, 248-249
Antibiotics in cattle feeds, 61
Antiseptic, definition, 235
"Antu," raticide, 339
Aphtha, epizootic (foot and mouth disease), 605
Arsenical dips, 315
Arsenic poisoning, 488
Arsenic trioxide, a rat poison, 338
Artificial breeding, sex ratio in, 186
Artificial feeding of orphans, 769
Artificial insemination, 803
Ascarids (round worms), 670
Ascarids (round worms in chickens), 690
Ascorbic acid (vitamin C), 71
Aseptic delivery of pigs, 54
Atrophic rhinitis of swine, 624
Aureomycin (chlortetracycline), 622
Autopsy (necropsy, post-mortem), 228, 763
Autopsy (partial), 764
Awns in lips, cheeks, and tongue, 352
Azoturia (Monday or holiday disease), 38, 513

B

Baby chicks, sexing of, 409
Bacillary white diarrhoea (B.W.D.) of fowl, 651
Bacitracin, an antibiotic, 249
Bacteria in ruminant's stomach, 20
Bactericide, definition of, 235
Bacteriophage, 250
Baits, rat, 334
Balano-posthitis of sheep (sheath rot), 560
Balantidiosis of swine, 754
B.A.L. (British Anti-Lewisite), 489
"Balls," hair, fur and wool, 349
"Balls," stomach, 348
Bang's disease (brucellosis), 109, 203, 205, 425, 578, 767, 801, 824
Bang's disease, "ring-test" for, 582
Bang's disease vaccination (calf vaccination), 584
"Bankrupt" worms (stomach worms) of sheep, 685
Barium carbonate, a rat poison, 337
Barn, heat or temperature in, 158
"Barn itch" (mange, lice, etc.), 722
Barn, loose housing, 130, 152, 164
Barn ventilation, 158
Barrenness, female, 788
"Bean" in horse's penis, 191
Beef cattle, starvation, 498
Benzene hexachloride (B.H.C.), 300
Benzene hexachloride-Xylol-Pine Oil for spinose ear ticks, 718

843